NUTRITION RESEARCH

CONCEPTS AND APPLICATIONS

KAREN EICH DRUMMOND, EdD, RDN, LDN, FAND
Lecturer, Gwynedd Mercy University
Gwynedd Valley, Pennsylvania
Former Principal Investigator, Eat.Right.Now Nutrition
Former Didactic Program in Dietetics Director, Drexel University
Philadelphia, Pennsylvania

ALISON MURPHY-REYES, MS, RD
Dietetic Internship Director
Sodexo Health Care Services
Allentown, Pennsylvania

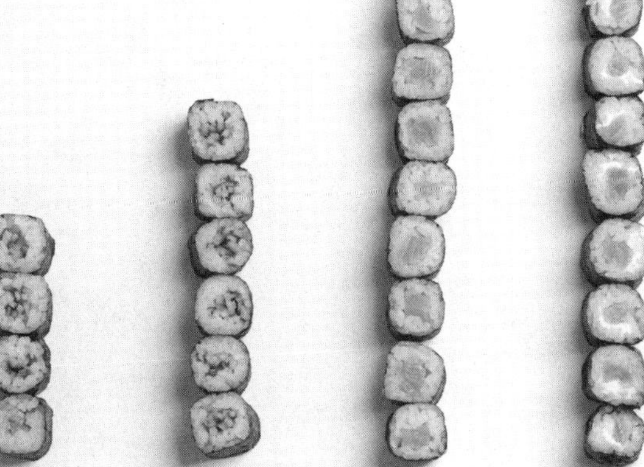

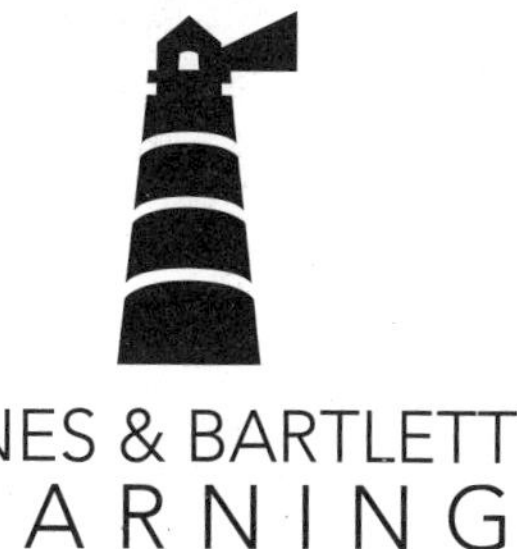

JONES & BARTLETT
LEARNING

World Headquarters
Jones & Bartlett Learning
5 Wall Street
Burlington, MA 01803
978-443-5000
info@jblearning.com
www.jblearning.com

Jones & Bartlett Learning books and products are available through most bookstores and online booksellers. To contact Jones & Bartlett Learning directly, call 800-832-0034, fax 978-443-8000, or visit our website, www.jblearning.com.

Substantial discounts on bulk quantities of Jones & Bartlett Learning publications are available to corporations, professional associations, and other qualified organizations. For details and specific discount information, contact the special sales department at Jones & Bartlett Learning via the above contact information or send an email to specialsales@jblearning.com.

12646-4

Production Credits
VP, Executive Publisher: David D. Cella
Publisher: Cathy L. Esperti
Acquisitions Editor: Sean Fabery
Associate Editor: Taylor Maurice
Director of Production: Jenny L. Corriveau
Director of Vendor Management: Amy Rose
Vendor Manager: Juna Abrams
Director of Marketing: Andrea DeFronzo
VP, Manufacturing and Inventory Control: Therese Connell
Composition: Cenveo Publisher Services
Project Management: Cenveo Publisher Services
Cover Design: Kristin E. Parker
Director of Rights & Media: Joanna Gallant
Rights & Media Specialist: Merideth Tumasz
Media Development Editor: Shannon Sheehan
Cover Image: © PhotoAlto/Ale Ventura/Shutterstock
Printing and Binding: Edwards Brothers Malloy
Cover Printing: Edwards Brothers Malloy

Library of Congress Cataloging-in-Publication Data
Names: Drummond, Karen Eich, author. | Murphy-Reyes, Alison, author.
Title: Nutrition research : concepts and applications / Karen Eich Drummond and Alison Murphy-Reyes.
Description: First edition. | Burlington, MA : Jones & Bartlett Learning, [2018] | Includes bibliographical references and index.
Identifiers: LCCN 2016050868 | ISBN 9781284101539 (pbk. : alk. paper)
Subjects: | MESH: Research Design | Nutritional Sciences | Biomedical Research--methods
Classification: LCC R850 | NLM QU 145 | DDC 610.72/4--dc23 LC record available at https://lccn.loc.gov/2016050868

6048

Printed in the United States of America
21 20 19 18 17   10 9 8 7 6 5 4 3 2 1

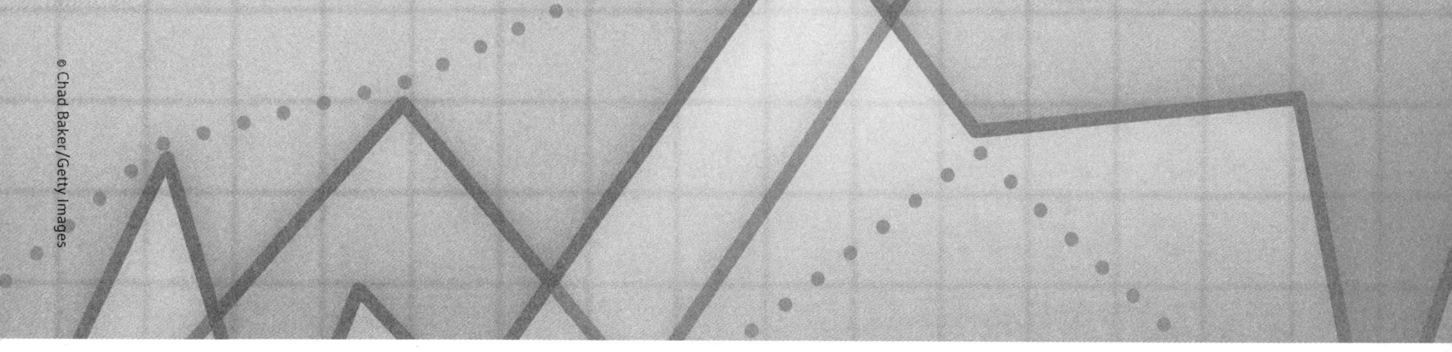

For Caitlin.
K.E.D.

To my late mother. Thank you for being my very first English teacher and giving me the best writing advice. Thanks, Dad, for being a great role model and teaching me to work hard in all that I do. To my loving husband Robert, who devotes his life to our family and medical research.
A.R.

CONTENTS

	Preface	xiii
	The Pedagogy	xvii
	Contributors	xxi
	Reviewers	xxii
Part 1	**Foundations**	**1**
Chapter 1	**Introduction to Research**	**3**
	Introduction	3
	What Is Research?	4
	Purposes of Nutrition Research	7
	Ways to Classify Research	9
	Major Types of Nutrition Research Studies	15
	Practice-Based Research Networks	21
	Researcher Interview: Translational Research	22
	Summary	24
	Review Questions	25
	Critical Thinking Questions	26
	Suggested Readings and Activities	27
	References	28
Chapter 2	**How to Find Appropriate Research Articles**	**31**
	Introduction	31
	Everything You Need to Know About Journals	33
	Scientific Literature Not Found in Journals	36
	How to Use Databases to Find Articles	37

	Checklist for Selecting Articles	44
	Principles of Scientific Writing	45
	Researcher Interview: Bioactive Compounds in Fruits and Vegetables	46
	Summary	47
	Review Questions	48
	Critical Thinking Questions	49
	Suggested Readings and Activities	50
	References	50
Chapter 3	**Ethics in Nutrition Research**	**53**
	Introduction	53
	History of Research Ethics	54
	Responsible Conduct of Research	56
	Ethics and Human Subjects Research	60
	Institutional Review Boards	66
	Researcher Interview: Management Research	70
	Summary	71
	Review Questions	72
	Critical Thinking Questions	73
	Suggested Readings and Activities	74
	References	74
Part 2	**How to Read, Interpret, and Evaluate Quantitative Nutrition Research**	**75**
Chapter 4	**Key Concepts in Quantitative Research**	**77**
	Introduction	78
	Foundations	78
	Reliability and Validity	86
	Error and Bias	90
	Sampling	92
	Instruments and Measurement	98
	Anatomy of a Research Article	101
	Researcher Interview: Outcomes Research	107
	Summary	108

Review Questions 109

Critical Thinking Questions 110

Suggested Readings and Activities 112

References 113

Chapter 5 What Do the Quantitative Data Mean? 115

Rosalind M. Peters, Nola A. Schmidt, Moira Fearncombe, and Karen Eich Drummond

Introduction 116

Levels of Measurement 116

Using Frequencies to Describe Samples 118

Measures of Central Tendency 120

Measures of Variability 124

Distribution Patterns 127

Inferential Statistics: Can the Findings Be Applied to the Population? 130

Reducing Error When Deciding About Hypotheses 132

Using Statistical Tests to Make Inferences About Populations 136

Effect Size 144

Risk Statistics: Risk Ratio, Odds Ratio, and Hazard Ratio 145

What Does All This Mean for Evidence-Based Practice? 147

Summary 149

Review Questions 150

Critical Thinking Questions 151

Suggested Readings and Activities 152

References 153

Chapter 6 Quantitative Research Designs: Experimental, Quasi-Experimental, and Descriptive 155

Introduction 155

Experimental Study Designs 157

Quasi-Experimental Designs 168

Descriptive Quantitative Designs 171

Additional Types of Designs 177

Researcher Interview: Intervention Research 178

Summary 179

	Review Questions	180
	Critical Thinking Questions	181
	Suggested Readings and Activities	182
	References	182
Chapter 7	**Epidemiologic Research Designs and Predictive Correlational Designs**	**185**
	Introduction	185
	Epidemiologic Research Designs	186
	Causality in Epidemiological Designs	196
	Predictive Correlational Designs	197
	Researcher Interview: Epidemiology	211
	Summary	212
	Review Questions	213
	Critical Thinking Questions	215
	Suggested Readings and Activities	216
	References	216
Chapter 8	**Putting It All Together: Understanding and Evaluating Quantitative Research Studies**	**219**
	Introduction	219
	Research Title and Authors	220
	Introduction of Article	222
	Methods	224
	Results	228
	Discussion and Conclusion	230
	Additional Evaluation Tools	232
	Researcher Interview: Food Science/Sensory Evaluation	233
	Summary	236
	Review Questions	239
	Critical Thinking Questions	239
	Suggested Readings and Activities	240
	References	240

Part 3 **How to Read, Interpret, and Evaluate Qualitative Nutrition Research** **241**

Chapter 9 **The Basics of Qualitative Research** **243**

L. Suzanne Goodell, Natalie K. Cooke, and Virginia C. Stage

Introduction 244

The Problem Statement 245

Literature Review 246

Methods 247

Data Analysis 262

Results 273

Discussion and Conclusions 278

Summary 278

Review Questions 280

Critical Thinking Questions 281

Suggested Readings/Activities 282

References 282

Chapter 10 **Qualitative Research Study Designs** **285**

Virginia C. Stage, Natalie K. Cooke, and L. Suzanne Goodell

Introduction 285

Thematic Analysis 286

Phenomenology 288

Grounded Theory 289

Case Studies 292

Conclusion 293

Researcher Interview: Qualitative Research 294

Summary 296

Review Questions 297

Critical Thinking Questions 297

Suggested Readings and Activities 298

References 298

Chapter 11 **How to Evaluate Qualitative Research** **301**

Natalie Cooke, L. Suzanne Goodell, and Virginia C. Stage

Introduction 301

Statement of the Problem 302

Literature Review 306

Research Design 307

Subject Selection 308

Data Collection 309

Data Analysis 310

Results 311

Discussion 311

Conclusions 312

Trustworthiness 313

Summary 313

Review Questions 314

Critical Thinking Questions 314

Suggested Readings and Activities 315

References 315

Part 4 Using Research in Practice and Reporting Research 317

Chapter 12 Understanding and Using Sources of Evidence: Systematic Reviews and Evidence-Based Nutrition Practice Guidelines 319

Introduction 319

Systematic Reviews 320

Systematic Review Process for the Evidence Analysis Library 332

Using the Evidence Analysis Library of the Academy of Nutrition and Dietetics 338

Additional Systematic Reviews and Guidelines 342

Summary 345

Review Questions 346

Critical Thinking Questions 347

Suggested Readings and Activities 348

References 348

Chapter 13 How to Develop and Use Surveys in Research 351

Karen Eich Drummond and Natalie K. Cooke

Introduction 351

Survey Basics 353
Pick a Sample 357
Construct and Refine the Cover Letter and Questionnaire 365
Test the Reliability and Validity of a Survey 372
Collect and Analyze Survey Data 377
Summary 381
Review Questions 382
Critical Thinking Questions 384
Suggested Readings and Activities 384
References 385

Chapter 14 Writing and Disseminating a Research Proposal and Paper 387

Introduction 387
Identify a Topic and Research Question/Objective 388
Search the Literature and Write the Literature Review 391
Write the Introduction 395
Write the Methods 396
Use a Style Manual to Format Your Paper 398
Write the Results, Discussion, and Conclusion 402
Write a Title and Abstract 406
The 3 P's of Dissemination: Posters, Presentations, and Publications 408
Summary 411
Review Questions 413
Critical Thinking Questions 414
Suggested Readings and Activities 414
References 415

Chapter 15 Securing Grants for Nutrition Research 417

Introduction 417
Government Funding 418
Nongovernment Funding 422
Plan Your Application 425
Develop and Write Your Grant Proposal 426
Summary 433

Review Questions 434

Critical Thinking Questions 434

Suggested Readings and Activities 435

References 435

Appendix A Full Length Quasi-Experimental Research Article: Garden-Based Nutrition Education Affects Fruit and Vegetable Consumption in Sixth-Grade Adolescents 437

Abstract 437

Methods 438

Results and Discussion 439

Conclusions 441

References 441

Appendix B Full Length Experimental Research Article—Clear Liquid Diet vs Soft Diet as the Initial Meal in Patients With Mild Acute Pancreatitis: A Randomized Interventional Trial 443

Abstract 443

Keywords 444

Methods 444

Results 446

Discussion 448

Conclusion 451

Acknowledgment 451

References 451

Appendix C CONSORT 2010 Checklist of Information to Include When Reporting a Randomized Trial 453

Appendix D STROBE Statement—Checklist of Items That Should Be Included in Reports of Observational Studies 457

Appendix E PRISMA 2009 Checklist 461

Glossary 463

Index 485

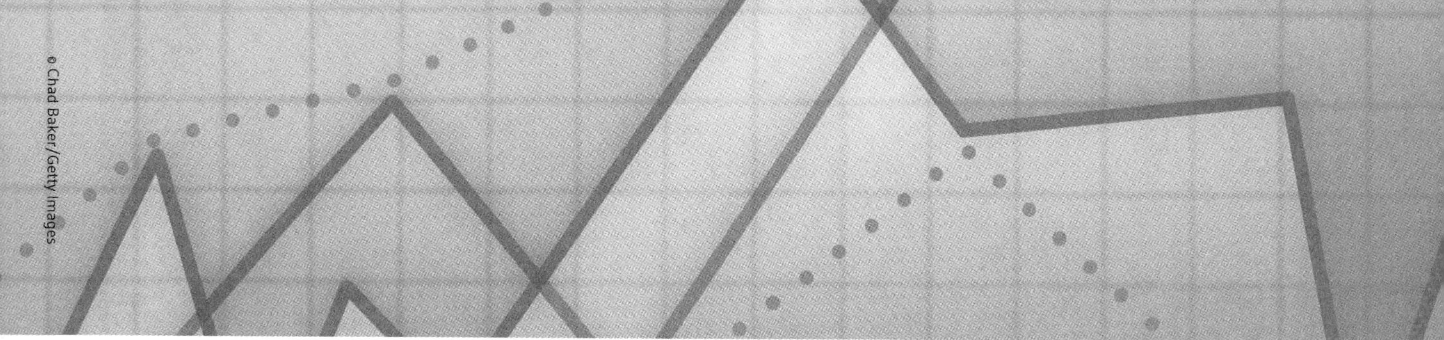

PREFACE

Reading and evaluating research articles is a vital skill for nutrition students and practitioners, and it is critical for our profession. From teaching in didactic nutrition programs and dietetic internships, we saw a need for a nutrition research methods book to get students interested and proficient in reading and appraising research. Research can be exciting for students (after all, research can be like a good mystery), as long as students understand what they are reading. Using a step-by-step approach that combines discussion of research concepts with applications using research articles, *Nutrition Research: Concepts and Applications* helps students experience each stage in the research process.

Changes in the field of nutrition research present challenges to students. The amount of nutrition research published has grown tremendously over the years, mirroring the growth in medical and nursing research. The annual number of MEDLINE articles increased 46% between 1978 to 1985 and 1994 to 2001, and the proportion of reported randomized controlled trials jumped from 1.9% to 6.2% over these same time periods (Druss & Marcus, 2005). With so much published research, it can be difficult for students to locate the most appropriate articles on a specific topic. In addition, many open-access journals featuring free online articles have entered the market over the past 20 years. Although Björk and Solomon (2012, p. 9) found that many open-access journals are of "high quality and widely cited," students must be able to evaluate and appraise each journal article they read, whether from open-access or subscription journals.

In addition to the explosion of published research, a knowledge of statistical tests beyond correlation, t-tests, and ANOVA is very important to understand research today. Nutrition students need to grasp what is meant by effect size, how to translate results from linear or logistic regression models, and how to interpret relative risk and hazard ratios—concepts not often included in a basic statistics class.

Nutrition Research: Concepts and Applications is appropriate for undergraduate students as well as graduate students who have minimal skills for reading research. This text will help students develop the skills necessary to:

- become knowledgeable consumers of research,
- conduct and document research projects, including a master's thesis, and
- use research findings in the classroom and supervised practice.

Our aim is to make research articles approachable and understandable to students so they feel confident reading and interpreting not just primary research but also narrative and systematic reviews. Because systematic reviews serve as the foundation for evidence-based practice guidelines, this text also helps students understand and access practice guidelines to enable their participation in evidence-based nutrition and dietetics practice.

APPROACH

Learning research methods should not be dull or overwhelming. The approach taken in this text is based on giving the student:

- *step-by-step* mastery of concepts; and
- lots of *examples* of concepts in each chapter; and
- ample *practice* using actual studies to answer simple questions, such as identifying the independent variable, as well as questions involving more critical thinking, such as explaining a study's results or writing an abstract.

For example, in the chapter on systematic reviews, a table explains each of the 10 steps in the process alongside a description of how this actually occurred in a study. The Critical Thinking Questions (at the end of each chapter) then ask students to practice identifying and explaining these steps after reading a systematic review article (answers are in the Instructor's Manual). Throughout the book, an incremental approach is used so that students first learn to identify original research, then decide if it is quantitative or qualitative, then identify types of variables, next determine whether an intervention took place, and so on. Two full-length studies are provided in the appendices to help students make connections to concepts discussed in the text.

This is the first nutrition research text that starts with the basics and is very comprehensive in approach. For example, two entire chapters help students find appropriate research studies for class assignments, use databases, write like scientists, organize and write research proposals and complete studies, and make and present a poster. Because surveys frequently are used in student research, another chapter is devoted to survey development and testing. Students also learn the nuts and bolts of using the Academy of Nutrition and Dietetics Evidence Analysis Library (EAL) and searching for grants.

ORGANIZATION

Nutrition Research: Concepts and Applications is organized into four parts.

- Part 1 includes three foundational chapters: an introduction to research, how to find appropriate research articles, and research ethics. The first chapter describes the research process, ways to classify research, and major types of research such as intervention and translational research. In the second chapter, much help is given to students on using databases to find *appropriate* journal articles for assignments, as well as guidance on writing scientific papers. The last chapter in Part 1 discusses the history of research ethics, responsible conduct of research, informed consent, privacy, and institutional review boards.
- Part 2 includes five chapters on quantitative research. The first chapter introduces foundations such as reliability, validity, bias, sampling, instruments, statistical significance, as well as a walk-through of a research study with many examples. Next in Part 2 are chapters on statistics and research designs, ending with a chapter that explains and demonstrates how to critique a study.
- Part 3 on qualitative research includes three chapters on foundational concepts, research designs, and how to critique a study.
- Part 4 includes four chapters on understanding systematic reviews and evidence-based practice guidelines, developing surveys, writing research proposals and papers, and finding grants. The first chapter explains and demonstrates how a systematic review is conducted, including how to read and interpret the results of a meta-analysis. Students also go through the systematic review process used by the EAL to see how conclusions from evidence analysis questions are used to

develop recommendations and guidelines. An entire chapter is devoted to helping students develop and use surveys. Part 4 also includes a complete guide to writing a research proposal and paper, and tips on disseminating study results. A sample research proposal is available on the Navigate Companion Website.

Several appendices appear at the end of this text, including study checklists and two full-length studies (one randomized controlled trial and one quasi-experimental study) that are used as examples in a number of chapters.

Features and Benefits

Nutrition Research: Concepts and Applications uses a variety of strategies to enhance student learning.

- *Outline*: The Outline at the beginning of each chapter helps students organize what they are going to learn as well as anticipate what will be covered.
- *Learning Outcomes*: Each chapter's Learning Outcomes can be used by students to help guide and focus study.
- *Tips*: Each chapter contains several Tips, a special feature that is used to make a concept easier to understand or to pull several ideas together.
- *Applications*: Each chapter also contains Applications—another special feature—that pose one or more questions to students to help them apply the information in the text. Answers to questions posed in the Application feature are in the Instructor's Manual.
- *Key Terms*: All bolded terms are defined in the Glossary, which is found at the back of the book.
- *Tables and Figures*: The text uses many tables and illustrations to further explain concepts and make it easy for students to find and review information.
- *Researcher Interview*: Eight chapters contain interviews with researchers in different areas in which they discuss their research, what they enjoy about research, and tips for anyone who wants to get involved in research.
- *Summary*: Designed to help students focus on the important concepts within the chapter, a numbered summary is provided at the end of each chapter.
- *Review Questions*: These questions, from multiple-choice to short essays, check the comprehension of factual material in the chapter. Answers for these questions and the Critical Thinking Questions are in the Instructor's Manual.
- *Critical Thinking Questions*: These exercises ask students to apply the chapter's concepts to a variety of studies, so students gain a deeper understanding. From determining which variable is independent and which is dependent in one study, students begin to understand these concepts. But they need to repeat this by looking at more studies and different types of studies to really make it second nature to them. Critical Thinking Questions are provided for a number of articles to allow for practice. The studies chosen are from the *Journal of the Academy of Nutrition and Dietetics*, open-access journals, or another journal to which students typically have access.
- *Suggested Readings and Activities*: At the end of each chapter are citations for readings that are particularly useful as well as Websites with helpful exercises, videos, and so on.

In addition, a Navigate Companion Website offers students additional learning opportunities to understand and apply concepts, such as watching videos and completing an interactive chapter summary.

INSTRUCTOR RESOURCES

Qualified instructors can receive access to the full suite of Instructor Resources, including the following:

- *Slides in PowerPoint format*, featuring more than 400 slides.
- *Test Bank*, containing more than 700 questions.
- *Instructor's Manual*, providing Outlines, Slide Guide, Classroom Activities and Worksheets, and Answer Keys to the in-text Application Questions, Review Questions, and Critical Thinking Questions.

STUDENT RESOURCES

By accessing the Navigate Companion Website—access to which accompanies every new print copy of this text—students will have these useful resources at their fingertips:

- *Video Lectures* for each chapter help explain specific chapter topics. The purpose of these videos is to help students understand some of the more difficult concepts. Many of the videos demonstrate how to read and understand a part of a study, such as statistical results. Some chapters may have more than one video.
- An *Interactive Summary* of each chapter contains blanks that students fill in using a drop-down menu. This tool helps with comprehension and retention of factual material.
- An *Interactive Glossary* and *Flashcards* help students learn definitions.
- *Web Links* take students to Websites that can enhance learning through videos and other methods.
- A *Sample Research Proposal* helps students get an idea of what the finished product should look like.
- *Practice Quizzes* allow students to test their knowledge of important concepts by answering Multiple Choice and True/False questions.

REFERENCES

Björk, B., & Solomon, D. (2012). Open access versus subscription journals: A comparison of scientific impact. *BMC Medicine, 10*(73), 1–10.

Druss, B. G., & Marcus, S. C. (2005). Growth and decentralization of the medical literature: Implications for evidence-based medicine. *Journal of the Medical Library Association, 93*, 499–501.

THE PEDAGOGY

Nutrition Research: Concepts and Applications uses a variety of techniques, many interactive, to address different learning styles, increase interest and participation, as well as enhance mastery of key concepts.

The **Outline** at the beginning of each chapter helps students see the big picture and organize what they are going to learn. The **Learning Outcomes** provide instructors and students with a snapshot of the key information and skills they will encounter, which students can use as a checklist to help focus their study.

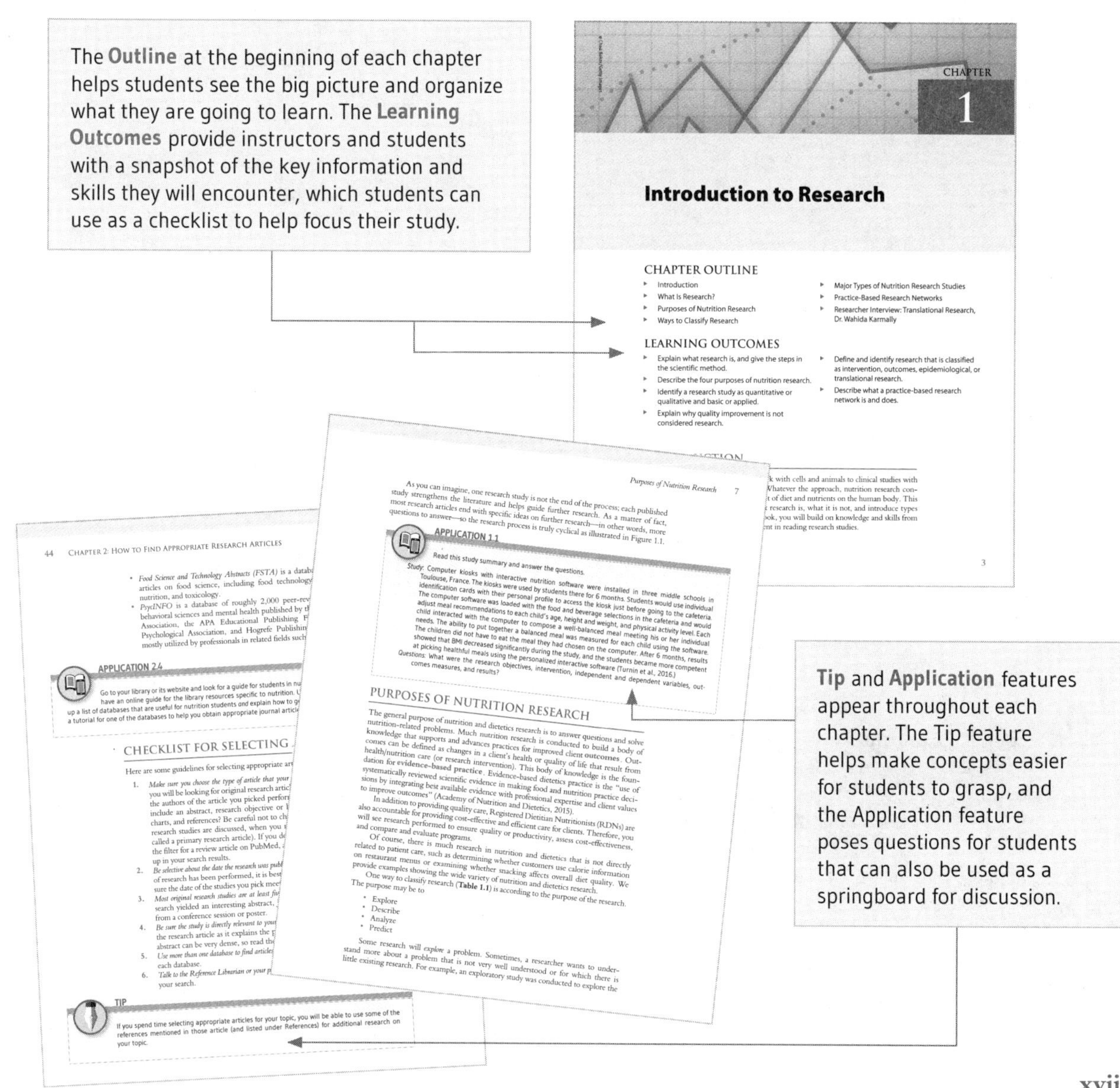

Tip and **Application** features appear throughout each chapter. The Tip feature helps make concepts easier for students to grasp, and the Application feature poses questions for students that can also be used as a springboard for discussion.

142 CHAPTER 5: WHAT DO THE QUANTITATIVE DATA MEAN?

Other Tests of Significance

Table 5.13 shows that a number of other inferential statistics can be used to determine whether there are statistically significant differences between groups. These include the Kolmogorov-Smirnov test, sign test, Wilcoxin matched pairs test, signed rank test, median test, and Mann-Whitney U test (Hayes, 1994; Plichta & Kelvin, 2013). These tests are used when ordinal level data are involved; thus, they are categorized as nonparametric tests. Tests are selected based on considerations such as the number of groups being compared, the distribution pattern of the data (normal or skewed), and other nuances that can be found in the data.

TESTING FOR RELATIONSHIPS AMONG VARIABLES

To find whether there are relationships among variables, a variety of statistical tests is used to examine the relationships (see Table 5.13). Decisions about which statistical tests to use are based on the number of variables and their level of measurement. Understanding how decisions are made allows you to ascertain the quality of the findings.

Correlation and Pearson's r

Bivariate analyses are performed to calculate **correlation coefficients**, which are used to describe the relationship between two variables. Correlation coefficients provide information regarding the degree to which variables are related. **Correlations** are evaluated in terms of magnitude, direction, and sometimes significance. Scatterplots of data can provide hints about direction and magnitude of the correlation (**Figure 5.13**).

Direction refers to the way the two variables covary. A positive correlation occurs when an increase in one variable is associated with an increase in another, or when a decrease in one variable is associated with a decrease in the other. For example, if a researcher found that as weight increased so did systolic blood pressure, or if weight decreased so did systolic blood pressure, a "positive" relationship between weight and blood pressure exists. A negative correlation occurs when two variables covary inversely; that is, when one decreases, the other increases. For example, as exercise increases, body weight decreases.

Magnitude refers to the strength of the relationship found to exist between two variables. A correlation can range from a perfect positive correlation of 1.00 to a perfect

Large Magnitude, Positive Correlation

Large Magnitude, Negative Correlation

No Correlation

FIGURE 5.13 Scatterplots of Correlational Relationships

Key Terms are bolded in the text, with definitions provided in the end-of-text Glossary.

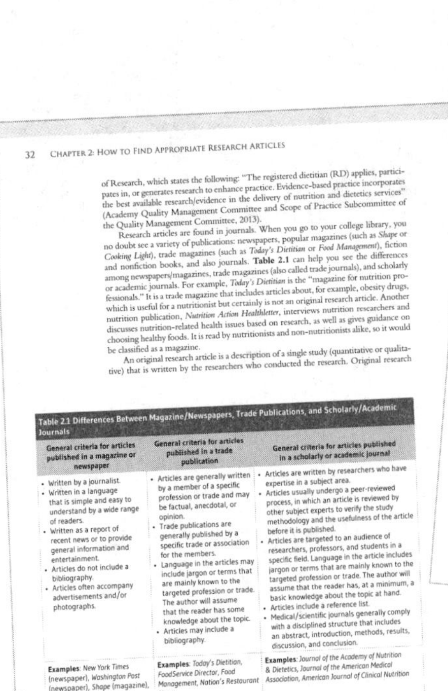

32 CHAPTER 2: HOW TO FIND APPROPRIATE RESEARCH ARTICLES

of Research, which states the following: "The registered dietitian (RD) applies, participates in, or generates research to enhance practice. Evidence-based practice incorporates the best available research/evidence in the delivery of nutrition and dietetics services" (Academy Quality Management Committee and Scope of Practice Subcommittee of the Quality Management Committee, 2013).

Research articles are found in journals. When you go to your college library, you no doubt see a variety of publications: newspapers, popular magazines (such as *Shape* or *Cooking Light*), trade magazines (such as *Today's Dietitian* or *Food Management*), fiction and nonfiction books, and also journals. **Table 2.1** can help you see the differences among newspapers/magazines, trade magazines (also called trade journals), and scholarly or academic journals. For example, *Today's Dietitian* is the "magazine for nutrition professionals." It is a trade magazine that includes articles about, for example, obesity drugs, which is useful for a nutritionist but certainly is not an original research article. Another nutrition publication, *Nutrition Action Healthletter*, interviews nutrition researchers and discusses nutrition-related health issues based on research, as well as gives guidance on choosing healthy foods. It is read by nutritionists and non-nutritionists alike, so it would be classified as a magazine.

An original research article is a description of a single study (quantitative or qualitative) that is written by the researchers who conducted the research. Original research

Table 2.1 Differences Between Magazine/Newspapers, Trade Publications, and Scholarly/Academic Journals

General criteria for articles published in a magazine or newspaper	General criteria for articles published in a trade publication	General criteria for articles published in a scholarly or academic journal
• Written by a journalist. • Written in a language that is simple and easy to understand by a wide range of readers. • Written as a report of recent news or to provide general information and entertainment. • Articles do not include a bibliography. • Articles often accompany advertisements and/or photographs.	• Articles are generally written by a member of a specific profession or trade and may be factual, anecdotal, or opinion. • Trade publications are generally published by a specific trade or association for the members. • Language in the articles may include jargon or terms that are mainly known to the targeted profession or trade. The author will assume that the reader has some knowledge about the topic. • Articles may include a bibliography.	• Articles are written by researchers who have expertise in a subject area. • Articles usually undergo a peer-reviewed process, in which an article is reviewed by other subject experts to verify the study methodology and the usefulness of the article before it is published. • Articles are targeted to an audience of researchers, professors, and students in a specific field. Language in the article includes jargon or terms that are mainly known to the targeted profession or trade. The author will assume that the reader has, at a minimum, a basic knowledge about the topic at hand. • Articles include a reference list. • Medical/scientific journals generally comply with a disciplined structure that includes an abstract, introduction, methods, results, discussion, and conclusion.
Examples: *New York Times* (newspaper), *Washington Post* (newspaper), *Shape* (magazine), *Nutrition Action Healthletter* (magazine)	**Examples**: *Today's Dietitian, FoodService Director, Food Management, Nation's Restaurant News*	**Examples**: *Journal of the Academy of Nutrition & Dietetics, Journal of the American Medical Association, American Journal of Clinical Nutrition*

Tables and **figures** are used to explain and summarize key concepts.

22 CHAPTER 1: INTRODUCTION TO RESEARCH

RESEARCHER INTERVIEW Translational Research

Wahida Karmally, Dr.PH, RDN, CDE, CLS, FNLA
Associate Research Scientist and Director of Bionutrition Research Core for the Irving Center for Clinical and Translational Research, Columbia University Medical Center, New York, NY

1. **Briefly describe the areas in which you do research.**

The mission of Columbia University Medical Center's Clinical and Translational Science Award (CTSA) is to transform the culture of research to hasten the discovery and implementation of new treatments and prevention strategies. In October 2006, the Irving Center for Clinical Research joined a national consortium created by the National Center for Research Resources (NCRR) branch of the NIH to energize the discipline of clinical and translational research, ultimately enabling researchers to provide new treatments more efficiently and quickly to patients.

My interest in research began when I was a graduate student in India conducting experiments on hundreds of albino rats to study bioavailability of iron from green leafy vegetables that grow on the roadside and are accessible to anyone who desires to pick them. This research was of public health significance because iron is a shortfall micronutrient in many populations. The results showed that the greens provide nutritional benefits that were cost-effective.

My interest in research continued during my postgraduate studies in London, UK. As an intern, I helped with clinical research at the Middlesex Hospital in London. I started working in research studies at the Mount Sinai Medical Center in New York with Dr. Virgil Brown in the early 1980s in the Diabetes Demonstration Project and on studies examining the effectiveness of statins.

I moved to Columbia University in 1987 as the director of nutrition in the General Clinical Research Center, and in 2006 the center became the Irving Institute for Clinical and Translational Research. In my current position as director of the Bionutrition Research Core, I had the opportunity to run the diet component of a multicenter landmark study: DELTA (Dietary Effects on Lipoproteins and Thrombogenic Activity). This study in essence determined that one standard macronutrient distribution in the diet does not "fit" all sections of the population. In individuals with insulin resistance, the results suggested that the replacement of dietary saturated fatty acids with monounsaturated fatty acids rather than carbohydrate is preferred because of associated smaller reductions in high-density lipoprotein cholesterol (HDL-C) and a trend toward reduction in fasting triglycerides (TG). Diets lower in saturated fat and higher in monounsaturated fat may benefit individuals with normal HDL-C levels or with high TGs. DELTA's results added to the body of evidence for the Therapeutic Lifestyle Changes (National Cholesterol Education Program), which stated that rather than relying on a single dietary recommendation for all, individualized nutrition counseling ("personalized nutrition") should be provided based on risk factors for the treatment and prevention of coronary artery disease.

I have been an investigator on several diet-related studies, including examining the effects of different intakes of dietary cholesterol in young men and women, beta-glucan from a ready-to-eat cereal on LDL-C in Hispanic Americans, the effects of diacylglycerol on TGs, very low calorie diets on insulin sensitivity and beta cell function in patients with type 2 diabetes, and studies on lipoprotein metabolism. The bionutrition core has supported protocols on energy homeostasis and osteoporosis as well as several pharmacokinetic studies, to name a few.

A collaboration with the National Heart, Lung, and Blood Institute (NHLBI) on the Latino and African American Initiatives resulted in the development of materials with culturally appropriate heart-healthy recipes for Latino and African Americans based on evidence-based recommendations for the prevention and treatment of cardiovascular risk factors. This was a "translational" strategy to improve the health of minority communities.

Found in eight chapters, **Researcher Interviews** provide students with a unique opportunity to learn from researchers about how they do research in their specialty areas and what they enjoy about it. The researchers also provide tips for students on how to get involved in research.

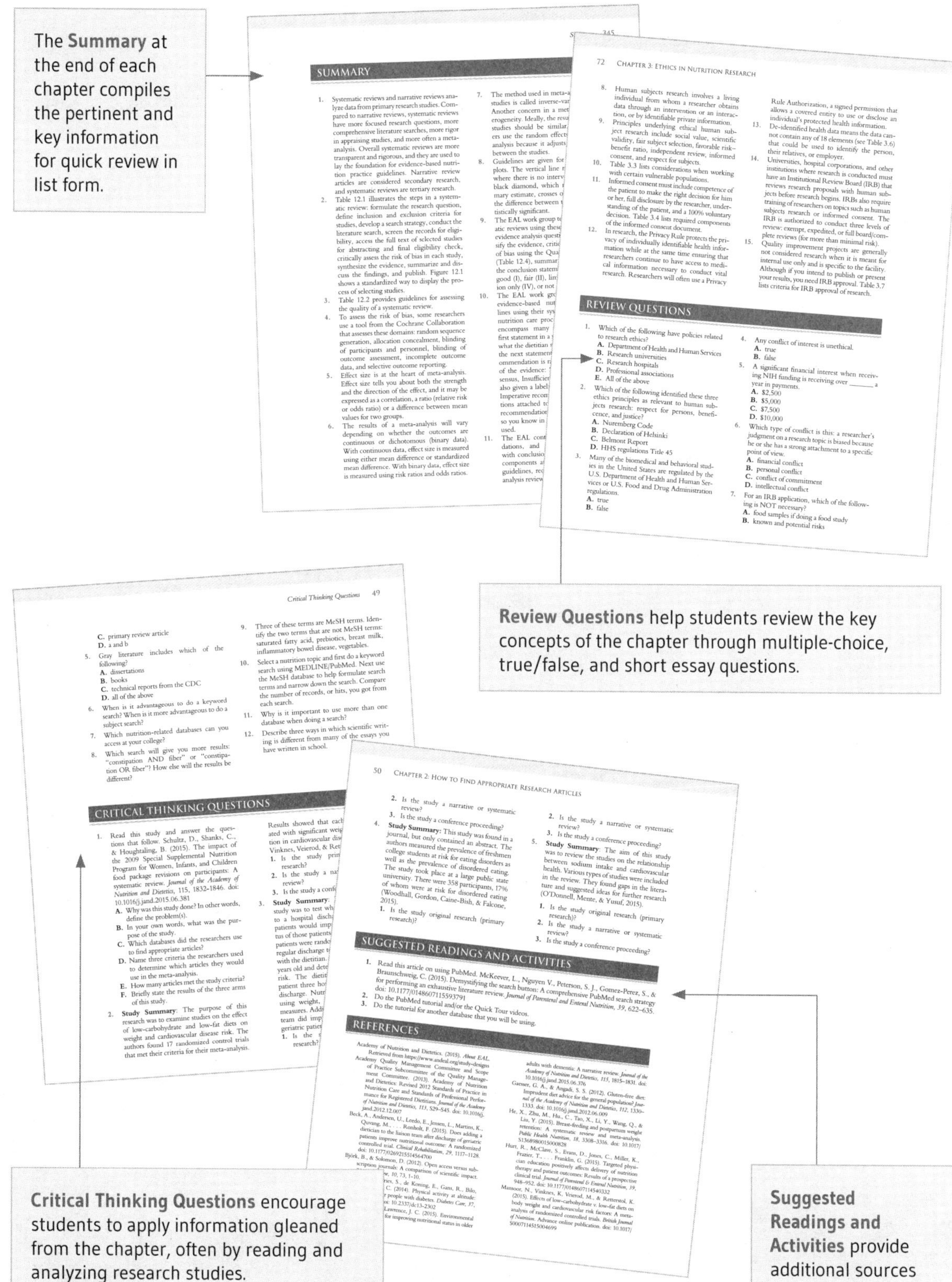

The **Summary** at the end of each chapter compiles the pertinent and key information for quick review in list form.

Review Questions help students review the key concepts of the chapter through multiple-choice, true/false, and short essay questions.

Critical Thinking Questions encourage students to apply information gleaned from the chapter, often by reading and analyzing research studies.

Suggested Readings and Activities provide additional sources of information or activities.

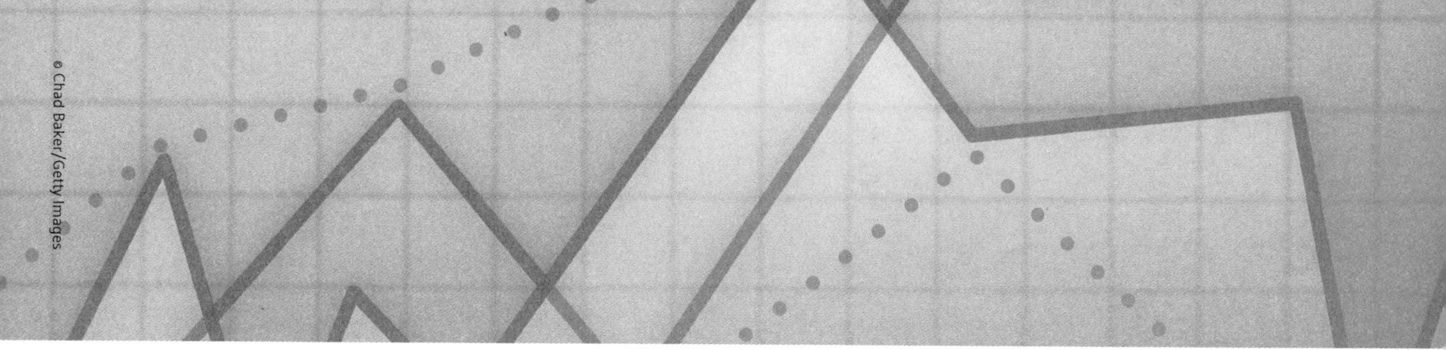

CONTRIBUTORS

Natalie K. Cooke, PhD
Teaching Assistant Professor
Coordinator, Undergraduate Nutrition Program
Department of Food, Bioprocessing, and Nutrition Sciences
North Carolina State University
Raleigh, North Carolina

Moira Fearncombe
Associate Professor
The Illinois Institute of Art
Schaumburg, Illinois

L. Suzanne Goodell, PhD, RD
Associate Professor of Nutrition
Department of Food, Bioprocessing, and Nutrition Sciences
North Carolina State University
Raleigh, North Carolina

Rosalind M. Peters, PhD, RN, FAAN
Associate Professor
College of Nursing
Wayne State University
Detroit, Michigan

Nola A. Schmidt, PhD, RN, CNE
Professor
College of Nursing and Health Professions
Valparaiso University
Valparaiso, Indiana

Virginia C. Stage, PhD, RDN, LDN
Assistant Professor of Nutrition Science
College of Allied Health Sciences
East Carolina University
Greenville, North Carolina

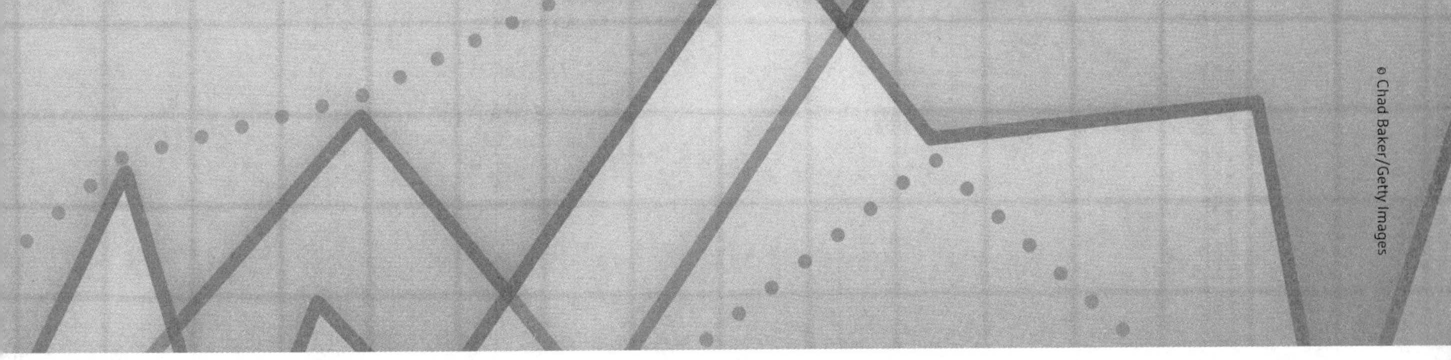

REVIEWERS

John J. B. Anderson, PhD
Professor Emeritus
Department of Nutrition
University of North Carolina
Chapel Hill, North Carolina

Jameela Banu, PhD
Assistant Professor
Department of Biology
University of Texas–Pan American
Edinburg, Texas

Detri Brech, PhD
Professor
Department of Dietetics
Ouachita Baptist University
Arkadelphia, Arkansas

Nina Crowley, PhD, RD, LD
Metabolic and Bariatric Surgery Program Coordinator
Medical University of South Carolina
Charleston, South Carolina
Adjunct Faculty
Stony Brook University
Stony Brook, New York

Diane M. DellaValle, PhD, RDN, LDN
Associate Professor
Research Dietitian
Department of Nutrition and Dietetics
Marywood University
Scranton, Pennsylvania

Kathryn Hillstrom, EdD, RD, CDE
Assistant Professor
School of Kinesiology and Nutritional Science
California State University, Los Angeles
Los Angeles, California

Michelle Lee, PhD, RDN, LDN
Assistant Professor
Graduate Coordinator for MS in Clinical Nutrition
East Tennessee State University
Johnson City, Tennessee

Diane Longstreet, PhD, MPH, RDN, LDN
Instructor
Keiser University
Lakeland, Florida

Gretchen Lynn George, PhD, RD
Assistant Professor
Consumer & Family Studies/Dietetics Department
San Francisco State University
San Francisco, California

Sara Plaspohl, DrPH, CHES
Assistant Professor
Master of Public Health Program Coordinator
Department of Health Sciences
Armstrong State University
Savannah, Georgia

Kimberly Powell, PhD, RD
Assistant Professor
Department of Human Sciences
North Carolina Central University
Durham, North Carolina

Hollie Raynor, PhD, RD
Associate Professor
Department of Nutrition
University of Tennessee
Knoxville, Tennessee

Jesse Stabile Morrell, PhD
Undergraduate Program Coordinator
Principal
Lecturer
Department of Molecular, Cellular, and Biomedical Science
University of New Hampshire
Durham, New Hampshire

Diane K. Tidwell, PhD, RD
Professor and Dietetic Internship Director
Department of Food Science, Nutrition, and Health Promotion
Mississippi State University
Mississippi State, Mississippi

Grenith J. Zimmerman, PhD
Professor
School of Allied Health Professions
Loma Linda University
Loma Linda, California

PART

1

Foundations

CHAPTER 1

Introduction to Research

CHAPTER OUTLINE

- Introduction
- What Is Research?
- Purposes of Nutrition Research
- Ways to Classify Research
- Major Types of Nutrition Research Studies
- Practice-Based Research Networks
- Researcher Interview: Translational Research, Dr. Wahida Karmally

LEARNING OUTCOMES

- Explain what research is, and give the steps in the scientific method.
- Describe the four purposes of nutrition research.
- Identify a research study as quantitative or qualitative and basic or applied.
- Explain why quality improvement is not considered research.
- Define and identify research that is classified as intervention, outcomes, epidemiological, or translational research.
- Describe what a practice-based research network is and does.

INTRODUCTION

Nutrition research is varied—from work with cells and animals to clinical studies with humans to population-based studies. Whatever the approach, nutrition research contributes to our knowledge of the impact of diet and nutrients on the human body. This chapter will help you understand what research is, what it is not, and introduce types of nutrition research. Using this textbook, you will build on knowledge and skills from one chapter to the next to become fluent in reading research studies.

Quality research is the foundation for nutrition practice. Without it, we would not be able to counsel a client on how to lose weight or help a client with diabetes improve his hemoglobin A1c results. Although the concept of research may seem intimidating, you have no doubt already done some personal research. For example, if you need to buy a new laptop, you will consider what features you want and use a variety of sources to compare features and prices of new ones. You will probably read reviews and examine how many customers were satisfied overall with different computers, as well as ask others for advice. In the end, you will make a decision based on the data you collected. Personal research is similar to scientific research, but there are some important differences.

WHAT IS RESEARCH?

Before defining what research is, let's look at what it is *not*.

- *Research is not when you look really hard for information on a topic.* You may spend hours looking for some reliable information on a narrow topic in sports nutrition, for example. That is not really researching; it is more like finding information.
- *Research is not when you read a number of journal articles on a nutrition topic*, such as the effect of vitamin D on muscles. Yes, you certainly know more about this topic now, but what you did is not true formal research; that was done by the authors of the articles you read.
- Let's say you went further than just reading articles. You wrote what is commonly called a "research paper." After reading and highlighting lots of articles (we hope you were picky about which articles you selected), you organized your paper and proceeded to write it up, including supporting and referencing your statements using the articles you read. *Research is not when you simply transfer and summarize facts from what you read.* This is definitely closer to real research than simply reading journal articles. By interpreting and drawing conclusions from the facts, you are starting to get more involved in the research process.

Now that we know what research is not, we can look at how research is defined.

Research is a systematic process of collecting, analyzing, and interpreting information/data to answer questions to *extend knowledge*. A systematic process means that research is completed using a system, and that system is usually the **scientific method** (**Figure 1.1**). The scientific method is a step-by-step process used for investigating questions, interpreting data, and expanding our understanding. Researchers use the scientific method to guide their research studies. (This should be a review for most readers. If so, be sure you know all the boldface key terms.)

1. *First, the researcher considers and develops a specific* **research question** *designed to shed light on a current or potential problem, such as obesity. A research question poses a relationship between two or more variables. A* **statement of the problem** *explains the problem and provides the context for why this research is needed.* For example, the treatment of obesity is an area of concern because obesity affects health in many negative ways and treatment is difficult, but even a small amount of weight loss can improve health. An obesity researcher may then develop a research question such as: "Do obese adults who weigh themselves every day lose more weight and keep it off than obese adults who weigh themselves less than 7 days a week?" Research questions can be developed on the basis of problems, for example, in clinical nutrition, community nutrition, business/management, or food science. Consider a community nutrition research question such as this: "What is the impact of teaching children to eat more fruits and vegetables on plate waste in child feeding programs?"

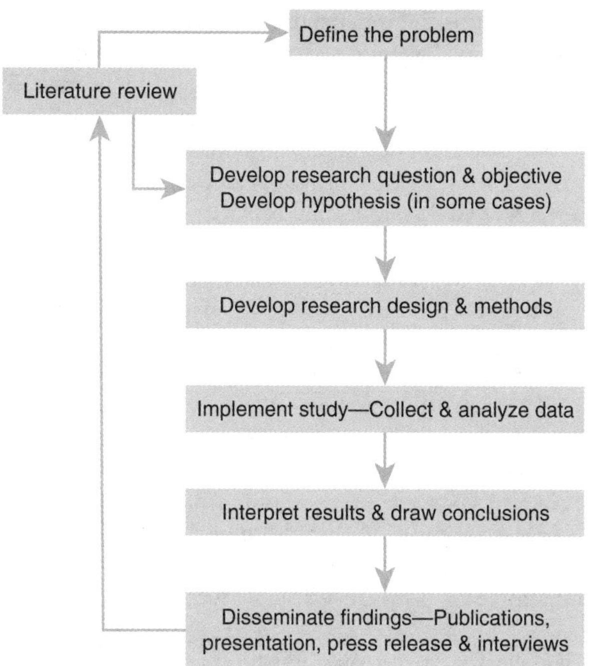

FIGURE 1.1 Scientific Method

2. *The statement of the problem is based on a review of research already completed—commonly called a* **literature review**. Prior research provides the foundation of what is known on the topic.
3. *Based on the literature review and the research question, the researcher clearly states the* **objective** *(or purpose) of the study*. For example, the objective for the obesity study could be stated this way: "To examine whether weighing every day produces greater weight loss compared with weighing less than daily for obese adults." The objective needs to be clear, objective, and identify the key variables in the study.

   Study **variables** are any characteristic that can take on different values, such as BMI or social support, and are measured, controlled, or manipulated in research. Variables are **categorical** when they take on values that are names or labels, such as sex, or **continuous** when they can be counted and have an infinite number of possible values. In the obesity study, the variables are weight and the frequency of weighing (using a scale). If you look at the abstracts of the original research papers in the *Journal of the Academy of Nutrition and Dietetics*, each study has an objective with variables.
4. *Many, but not all, studies state a* **hypothesis**. A hypothesis is a statement of what the researchers predict the relationship will be between two (or more) variables, and it must be able to be tested. Quantitative research designs are used to look at causal relationships as well as associations or relationships between variables. For example, in the obesity study, the hypothesis is that daily weighing will lead to greater weight loss at 6 months when compared with less frequent weighing. The hypothesis shows a relationship between two variables: an **independent variable** (what the researcher manipulates in certain studies) and a **dependent variable** (sometimes also called the **outcome measure**). In the obesity study, the researchers manipulate how often the study participants weigh

themselves—so that is the independent variable. Then the researchers measure the study participants' weight—the dependent variable. Research examines whether the independent variable affects the dependent variable. Many research studies that are more descriptive in nature, such as examining trends in global obesity, do not have a hypothesis and only have a research objective.

5. *Once the researcher has a problem statement, research question(s), and possibly a hypothesis, the researcher works on a detailed research plan that states precisely what data are required, where the data will come from, which methods will be used to collect the data, and how the data will be analyzed.* This series of decisions is called **research design**, and it focuses on the end product: getting the evidence required to adequately and accurately answer the research question(s).

   A research design, such as a randomized controlled trial, is like a blueprint for a house. The blueprint can be used for a number of homes, but most blueprints will be changed to meet the specific needs of each homeowner. A good research design ensures that the evidence obtained answers the research question as accurately as possible (keep in mind that some research questions cannot be tested). Also keep in mind that although many research studies *generate new data*, some *analyze existing data*, such as from the National Health and Nutrition Examination Survey, to answer new questions (known as **secondary data analysis**).

   If data is collected at just one point in time, this is referred to as a **cross-sectional study**. In a **longitudinal study**, participants are observed and multiple measurements taken over a long period of time. Longitudinal studies either go forward in time (**prospective**) or backward in time (**retrospective**).

6. *When you read a study, the "Methods" section addresses the research design, including how variables will be measured, the setting, how participants will be chosen (if used), and the statistical analysis.* **Research methods** refer to the many kinds of tools, techniques, and processes used in research to obtain data, such as questionnaires, case studies, and interviews. Measurement devices are also often referred to as **instruments**. In the obesity study, study participants are enrolled and randomly put into the **intervention group** or the **control group**. The intervention group (receives the treatment or intervention) is instructed to weigh daily using a smart scale (a scale that sends data directly from the scale to a website). Members of the control group also get smart scales and are instructed to use the scales less than daily. Participant weights at 3 months and 6 months are used to determine statistically whether the daily weighers lose significantly more weight compared with those weighing less than daily.

7. *Once the data are collected and statistical tests have been run, researchers interpret the meaning of the results as related to the problem and the research question.* Researchers also have to take into account possible **extraneous variables** (factors other than the variables being studied that might influence the outcome of a study) that can cause incorrect conclusions. Results are compared to other similar studies, and conclusions are drawn. Good research builds on previous studies and contributes to a broader knowledge of the topic. In the obesity study, it was found that weighing every day led to significantly more weight loss compared with the control group, leading the researchers to conclude that daily weighing is an effective weight loss tool.

8. *The last step is to report or disseminate the results.* This could take the form of an article published in a journal or another publication; presentation or a poster at a professional conference, meeting, or workshop; a press release to the media; or interviews.

As you can imagine, one research study is not the end of the process; each published study strengthens the literature and helps guide further research. As a matter of fact, most research articles end with specific ideas on further research—in other words, more questions to answer—so the research process is truly cyclical as illustrated in Figure 1.1.

APPLICATION 1.1

Read this study summary and answer the questions.

Study: Computer kiosks with interactive nutrition software were installed in three middle schools in Toulouse, France. The kiosks were used by students there for 6 months. Students would use individual identification cards with their personal profile to access the kiosk just before going to the cafeteria. The computer software was loaded with the food and beverage selections in the cafeteria and would adjust meal recommendations to each child's age, height and weight, and physical activity level. Each child interacted with the computer to compose a well-balanced meal meeting his or her individual needs. The ability to put together a balanced meal was measured for each child using the software. The children did not have to eat the meal they had chosen on the computer. After 6 months, results showed that BMI decreased significantly during the study, and the students became more competent at picking healthful meals using the personalized interactive software (Turnin et al., 2016.)

Questions: What were the research objectives, intervention, independent and dependent variables, outcomes measures, and results?

PURPOSES OF NUTRITION RESEARCH

The general purpose of nutrition and dietetics research is to answer questions and solve nutrition-related problems. Much nutrition research is conducted to build a body of knowledge that supports and advances practices for improved client **outcomes**. Outcomes can be defined as changes in a client's health or quality of life that result from health/nutrition care (or research intervention). This body of knowledge is the foundation for **evidence-based practice**. Evidence-based dietetics practice is the "use of systematically reviewed scientific evidence in making food and nutrition practice decisions by integrating best available evidence with professional expertise and client values to improve outcomes" (Academy of Nutrition and Dietetics, 2015).

In addition to providing quality care, Registered Dietitian Nutritionists (RDNs) are also accountable for providing cost-effective and efficient care for clients. Therefore, you will see research performed to ensure quality or productivity, assess cost-effectiveness, and compare and evaluate programs.

Of course, there is much research in nutrition and dietetics that is not directly related to patient care, such as determining whether customers use calorie information on restaurant menus or examining whether snacking affects overall diet quality. We provide examples showing the wide variety of nutrition and dietetics research.

One way to classify research (**Table 1.1**) is according to the purpose of the research. The purpose may be to

- Explore
- Describe
- Analyze
- Predict

Some research will *explore* a problem. Sometimes, a researcher wants to understand more about a problem that is not very well understood or for which there is little existing research. For example, an exploratory study was conducted to explore the

Table 1.1 Research Purposes and Examples

Research purpose	Study example	Possible research designs
Exploratory	Explore the barriers to eating healthy foods for Hispanic women in an urban community.	Qualitative study.
Descriptive	Examine the availability and price of low-fat and higher-fat milk in stores across the United States.	Descriptive cross-sectional study. Descriptive correlational design.
Analytic	Test the effect of a high-fiber diet on blood glucose control in people with type 2 diabetes.	Randomized controlled trial. Cohort study.
Predictive	Predict the rate of weight loss based on patient characteristics and intervention strategies.	Predictive correlational design.

barriers to eating healthy foods for Hispanic women in an urban community (Suplee, Jerome-D'Emilia, & Burrell, 2015). Exploratory studies are often based on qualitative research, and most exploratory studies are also descriptive studies.

Descriptive research attempts to *describe* a wide variety of phenomena often at a specific point in time—such as the nutrition knowledge, attitudes, and behaviors of youth athletes or the dietary quality of preschooler sack lunches. Descriptive research may measure, classify, and compare phenomena. For example, Rimkus et al. (2015) undertook a study that looked at the availability and price of low-fat and high-fat milk in stores across the United States. One of their findings was that the odds of finding low-fat milk were 32 to 44% lower in low-income communities when compared to high-income communities. Also, pricing of low-fat and nonfat milk was higher on average in grocery stores in majority black compared to majority white communities.

Descriptive studies often aim to provide information about relevant variables, but they do not test hypotheses or examine possible cause and effect. Good descriptive studies provoke the "why" questions of analytic research.

Analytic research goes beyond describing and looks at cause and effect. An analytic study tries to quantify the relationship between either an intervention *on* an outcome or an exposure *on* an outcome.

First, let's look at a study with an intervention. A researcher may test a hypothesis such as this: "Eating a high-fiber diet improves glycemic control in people with type 2 diabetes." To test this hypothesis, an **experimental design** is used. Requirements of true experimental research include a controlled manipulation of the independent variable, administration of the treatment to the experimental group, and random assignment of participants to the experimental or control groups.

Using the high-fiber diet hypothesis, the independent variable is the high-fiber diet, and the dependent variable is glycemic control. To figure out which is the independent or dependent variable, fill in the sentence: "The study is looking at the effect of variable A on variable B." In this case, the study is looking at the effect of a high-fiber diet (A is the independent variable) on glycemic control (B is always the dependent variable).

Now, let's look at the relationship between an exposure on an outcome. Sometimes researchers perform analytic studies, such as **prospective cohort studies**, to look for causes of a disease when it would not be safe or ethical to expose participants to a factor suspected to be harmful. In a cohort study, researchers form a hypothesis about the potential causes of a disease and then they *observe* a group of nondiseased people (the cohort) over a (usually) long period of time to detect any changes in health (outcomes such as the presence of coronary artery disease) in relation to *exposure* to certain *risk factors* (such as obesity).

For example, The Nurses' Health Studies is a prospective cohort study started in 1976 that continually collects information from more than 100,000 nurses. The researchers obtain accurate information about exposures before disease develops in any of the participants. The data are then used to answer a variety of research questions about how risk factors affect disease outcomes, such as grouping participants based on their body mass index and then comparing their risk of developing heart disease (or cancer). Cohort studies such as the Nurses' Health Studies have provided important information about the link between lifestyle factors and disease. Prospective cohort studies are a good example of analytic studies that are observational, *not* experimental.

Another purpose of research may be to predict something, such as a questionnaire that can predict young adults at risk for eating disorders or a formula to predict resting metabolic rate in college adults. Being able to predict something does not mean that we can always explain why the phenomenon occurs or control the outcome. But predictive studies are good at isolating an independent variable that may enhance successful outcomes. For example, researchers have examined factors such as initial body weight and frequency of diet counseling to help predict the rate of weight loss (Finkler, Heymsfield, & St-Onge, 2012).

APPLICATION 1.2

Read this study summary and answer the questions.

Study: In the Swedish mammography cohort, the researchers used food frequency questionnaires from 33,747 female participants to calculate each participant's Dietary Inflammatory Index. During 15 years of follow-up, the researchers identified deaths due to cancer, digestive-tract cancer, and cardiovascular disease. Statistical tests were performed to examine the association between the Dietary Inflammatory Index and mortality (all causes, cancer, digestive cancer, and cardiovascular disease). Higher Dietary Inflammatory Index scores were associated with all-cause and digestive-tract cancer mortality (Shivappa, Harris, Wolk, & Hebert, 2015).

Questions: What was the purpose of this research: to explore, describe, analyze, or predict? Was this an experimental or a cohort study? Why is it an experimental or cohort study? What is meant by "higher Dietary Inflammatory Index scores were associated with all-cause and digestive-tract cancer mortality"?

WAYS TO CLASSIFY RESEARCH

When discussing research in this section, we will only be talking about original research studies. An **original research study** is a narrative of a single study designed and conducted by the researchers themselves. Original research articles are also called **primary research**. Other types of research articles that you may read are narrative reviews or systematic reviews. **Secondary research** includes **narrative reviews** in which authors organize, interpret, and summarize evidence from a number of primary studies in a particular research area. **Systematic reviews**, which are more rigorous than narrative reviews, belong in the category of **tertiary research** because they collect and distill information from both primary and secondary sources. Narrative and systematic reviews are both examples of synthesizing research (**evidence analysis**) and are discussed in Chapter 12.

You can classify research studies in many ways. For example, you can classify research by purpose (just discussed) or by research design (such as a randomized controlled trial or cohort study). In this section, we look at two additional ways to classify research: Is the study quantitative or qualitative? Is the study basic or applied research? When you first read a research study, you should try to answer these questions.

QUANTITATIVE AND QUALITATIVE RESEARCH

You have probably read a number of quantitative studies. **Quantitative studies** use a formal, objective, and systematic process of collecting, analyzing, and interpreting information/data—in other words, the scientific method. Quantitative data is expressed numerically and can be analyzed in a variety of ways. The goal of quantitative research is generally to describe and examine relationships among variables (descriptive studies) and examine cause-and-effect relationships (analytic studies). One thing to keep in mind is that no matter how powerful the findings of a quantitative study are, nothing is ever proven. The most that can be claimed is that the hypothesis is either supported or unsupported.

The concept of **control** is very important in a quantitative study, and it is even more important in an experimental study than in a descriptive study. Control is used to prevent *outside* factors from influencing the study outcome. Common areas in which researchers exert control include how participants are selected and how much they know about the study, selection of the research setting, and measurement of variables.

Qualitative research is quite different from quantitative studies. **Qualitative research** does not manipulate variables or put a group through an intervention. The qualitative researcher gets into the shoes of the study participants to capture information not conveyed in quantitative data, such as values, beliefs, or motivations behind behaviors. For example, Schindler, Kiszko, Abrams, Islam, and Elbel (2013) used **focus groups** to ask 105 New York City residents about factors that affected whether they used, or did not use, the calories posted on fast-food menus. Most participants knew the calorie information was there, but few used that information due to reasons such as a lack of understanding about calories or giving priority to what has been ordered in the past (habit). Qualitative research has been used for many years in social and behavioral sciences such as anthropology or sociology, and it is also used in nutrition research.

Like quantitative research, qualitative research is a systematic process, involves **rigor** in implementation, and generates knowledge. But the two types of research seem to have more differences than similarities (**Table 1.2**). The quantitative approach is objective, which means that it tries to be unbiased toward the participants. The qualitative approach is just the opposite: the researcher wants to understand the participant's experience. Whereas the qualitative researcher may conduct an open-ended interview with a participant, the quantitative researcher often counts and measures behavior with instruments such as food frequency questionnaires. Typical qualitative methods used in nutrition research are focus groups, observations, and document analysis.

The differences between quantitative and qualitative research spring from the researcher's paradigm on how the world works. Much nutrition (and medical) research is based on a **positivist paradigm** in which reality is ordered and events can be studied empirically and explained with logical analysis. Using a positivist paradigm, a researcher uses objectivity and control to study a world driven by natural causes. In contrast, qualitative researchers operate from a **constructivist paradigm** in which reality is mentally constructed by individuals. Therefore, they value the uniqueness of each individual and focus on the subjective. Data in qualitative research takes the form of words, sounds, and pictures, which are captured in field notes, transcripts, or photographs. Qualitative

Table 1.2 Comparing Quantitative and Qualitative Research

	Quantitative	Qualitative
Researcher's focus	• To describe and test relationships among variables. • Examine cause and effect by testing hypotheses. • Make predictions.	• To provide details about human behavior, emotion, personality, and interactions; describe a problem or condition from the point of view of those experiencing it. • To formulate theory or hypothesis after data is collected.
Reasoning	• Deductive: the researcher tests the hypothesis with the data.	• Inductive: the researcher formulates a hypothesis after data is collected.
Objectivity/subjectivity	• Objectivity is critical.	• Subjectivity is expected.
Setting	• Controlled environment: try to control all factors that could affect the results.	• Natural social settings without controls.
Sampling	• Sample population of interest, preferably random sample. • Larger numbers of participants.	• Nonrandom purposeful sampling. • Smaller numbers of participants give more in-depth information.
Methodology	• Experimental or quasi-experimental designs to test for group differences, relationships, etc. • Fixed design.	• Methods that explore and describe, such as case study, focus group, observation, or semi-structured interviews. • Flexible design.
Data	• Number based: precise, objective, measurable data.	• Mostly narrative: text based, images, objects.
Analysis	• Statistical analysis.	• Interpretive analysis. • Interviews and other data are often categorized or coded to identify themes and subthemes.
Reporting results	• Statistics, tables, graphs.	• Organized by research question and presented as themes.
Study validation	• Can be valid and reliable; largely depends on research design and measurement instruments.	• Can be valid and reliable, although validity and reliability are seen a little differently (Leung, 2015). • Largely depends on skill and diligence of the researcher.
Generalize the findings to a larger population	• More generalizable.	• Less generalizable.
Strengths	• Allows for greater objectivity, control, and accuracy. • Can examine possible causes under controlled circumstances. • Tests theories or hypotheses. • Can be replicated.	• Provide a holistic view and understanding of complex situations through rich detail of participants' personal experiences, etc. • Gain initial insights into a new area of research. • Describes phenomena and possibly generate a theory. • Can respond to changes that occur during the study.

(*continues*)

Table 1.2 Comparing Quantitative and Qualitative Research (continued)

	Quantitative	Qualitative
Weaknesses	• Does not work as well with phenomenon that are hard to measure accurately (such as stress) or complex phenomenon. • Does not provide information on the context of the situation. • Does not capture the full breadth of human experiences.	• Time consuming to collect and analyze data. • Smaller number of participants. • Not usually generalizable. • Results more easily influenced by researcher's personal biases. • Difficult to compare to other studies.

researchers tend to gather data and analyze it to generate a theory or hypothesis (inductive reasoning), whereas quantitative studies often test a theory or hypothesis (deductive reasoning).

Although researchers often have a preference for one or the other, quantitative and qualitative research complement each other because they generate different kinds of knowledge. Qualitative research provides insight into problems, may identify variables important for future quantitative research projects, and can help researchers explore and develop a theory. Table 1.2 explains some of the major differences between the two types of research.

Mixed methods research "mixes" quantitative and qualitative research within a single investigation to provide a more complete data picture. Mixed methods research originated in the social sciences and has expanded into the health and medical sciences, including nursing and nutrition. It developed in part due to increased acceptance of qualitative research in the United States, increasing complexity of issues being researched, and a recognition that both quantitative and qualitative research have strengths that can be combined. Mixed methods research may also be referred to as multi-method or triangulated design.

Mixed methods research has several important characteristics (Creswell, Klassen, Plano Clark, & Clegg Smith, 2011).

1. The collection of both quantitative (close ended) and qualitative (open ended) data to answer research questions.
2. The analysis of both qualitative and quantitative data.
3. Integration of the two data sources in the results. The numbers provide the precision and the narratives supply the background texture.

By joining quantitative with qualitative methods, biases associated with one design alone are reduced, insight into the complexity of the problem is provided, and rigor in the study design is maintained (Creswell et al., 2011).

A study of parents of young children with type 1 diabetes mellitus is an example of how the use of mixed methods can uncover perceptions that might otherwise be missed (Patton, Clements, George, & Goggin, 2015). Because research shows that many young children with type 1 diabetes do not have healthy diets, the researchers wanted to learn more about what the parents know about healthful eating for their child, how they choose foods for their child, and any possible barriers to a healthful diet.

In this study, qualitative data was derived using semistructured interviews with parents, and the data was coded to identify themes and subthemes. Quantitative data came from an analysis (using the Healthy Eating Index-2010) of 3-day weighed food records of each child's intake, the Behavioral Pediatric Feeding Assessment Scale filled out by a parent, and the most recent HbA1c values. Results showed that "although parents may believe they know what constitutes a healthful diet (for T1DM), they do not always feed their child a healthful diet" (Patton et al., 2015, p. 279). This conclusion was possible to report because the quantitative data showed the quality of the children's diets, and the qualitative data showed that parents perceived their child's diet as healthful. Another interesting qualitative finding was that many parents didn't want their children to feel "different" or be seen as "different" by their peers because of their diet needs and restrictions (Patton et al., 2015).

TIP

To tell if a study is quantitative or qualitative, carefully read the title of the study and the research methods and instruments used to collect the data. If the methods involve focus groups, in-depth interviewing, observations, or a case study, then it is clearly qualitative. If you see a lot of numerical data and statistics, it is likely to be quantitative.

APPLICATION 1.3

You are in charge of a nutrition education program that includes cooking classes taught at farmers' markets to SNAP recipients in an urban setting. The purpose of your program is to improve eating habits by helping participants plan, buy, and prepare healthy meals using produce from the farmers' market. Describe one way to evaluate the program using quantitative methods and two ways to evaluate it using qualitative methods. Also, describe two ways that the quantitative and qualitative data will be different from each other.

Basic and Applied Research

Another way to classify research is whether it is basic or applied. As is often the case, there is no clear-cut line between them. Consider a research study using mice in which leptin (a hormone made by the adipose cells that inhibits hunger) is found to suppress the response of taste cells to sweet compounds. This type of study is referred to as **basic research**—research performed without a specific application in mind and completed for the sake of knowledge alone. Much basic research, also called bench research, is conducted in laboratory settings, often using animals. Experimental conditions are strictly controlled. However, basic research is also done with humans. Whether using animals or humans, the intent is to build a knowledge base—usually by testing theories.

The complexity of diseases, such as obesity or cancer, provides the impetus for using animal models in much basic research. Many research questions cannot be answered using humans due to safety and ethical concerns, so animal models are quite useful. A model is not the real world, but simply a representation to help explain and predict observed phenomena. Mice, for example, are comparative living systems that enable researchers to explore areas such as cancer and answer questions about the underlying basis of how and why cancers arise. The most commonly used animal models for cancer research are mice and rats.

Whereas basic research is completed for the sake of gaining knowledge alone, **applied research** is done to solve real-world problems and to directly influence or improve nutrition practice. Applied research may be used to identify factors associated with weight loss or to determine whether a nutrition education program changes eating habits. Applied research can inform decisions in many nutrition areas.

The distinction between basic and applied research lies mostly with its application. Although it may seem that applied research is more useful, basic research questions often inform applied research.

When you address problems in *your own work setting* with the goal of solving an ongoing problem, this is known as **quality improvement**. Quality improvement (QI) consists of identifying problems and testing solutions to improve a process, a system, or an outcome. Ultimately, we want to improve delivery of care (services) within a department or an institution. For example, if a clinical nutrition manager in a hospital is concerned about how long it takes to get patient screenings done, he or she may start the QI process to improve timeliness. **Figure 1.2** shows the steps involved.

Although QI uses many components of the research process, it is not considered research using the definition provided by the Department of Health and Human Services (DHHS). DHHS defines research as "a systematic investigation, including research development, testing, and evaluation, designed to develop or contribute to *generalizable* knowledge" (U.S. DHHS, 2009, Code of Federal Regulations, Title 45, Part 46.112). The knowledge gained from QI is for a single institution and is not generalizable outside of that institution, so QI really cannot be considered research. Also, whereas a protocol in a research study is fixed, the steps taken in a QI project are flexible because the goal is improvement. The Academy of Nutrition and Dietetics provides an excellent resource on QI: "Using Academy Standards of Excellence in Nutrition and Dietetics for Organization Self-Assessment and Quality Improvement" (Price, Kent, Cox, McCauley, Parekh, & Klein, 2014).

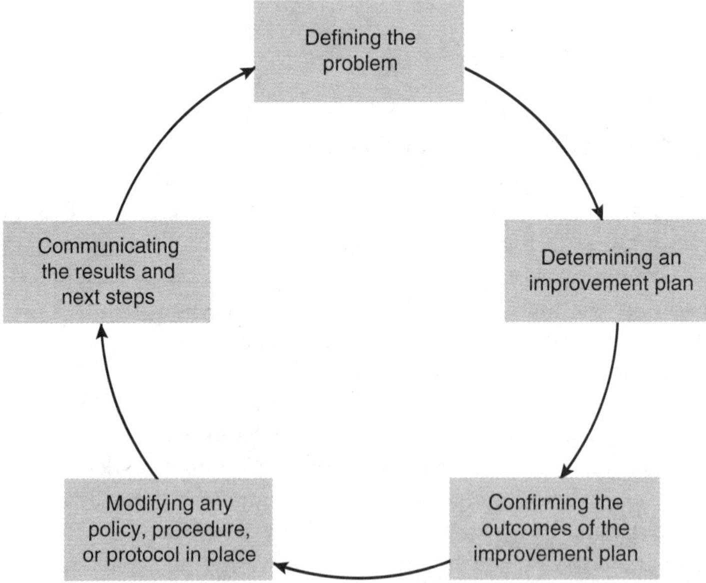

FIGURE 1.2 Steps in Quality Improvement

MAJOR TYPES OF NUTRITION RESEARCH STUDIES

When looking at nutrition research studies, it is helpful to know that there are some specific types of research being done, such as the following.

- Intervention research
- Outcomes research
- Epidemiological research
- Translational research

This does not mean that all the studies you read will fall into one of these categories; that is not the case. Also, you may read a study considered to be intervention or outcomes research that is also translational research. Therefore, some studies will fall into two categories. Each type of research is special in its own way, and knowing and understanding them will help you navigate the huge volume of nutrition studies. Following is an introduction to intervention, outcomes, epidemiological, and translational research.

Intervention Research

Intervention research is a specialized type of research in the medical, nursing, and nutrition fields. It is distinguished by an intervention that can be quite varied: from treatment of patients with parenteral nutrition to a new behavioral intervention in a health care program. Interventions are techniques, treatments, or actions that are taken in a study to produce outcomes, such as successful management of a disease. Intervention studies also may be referred to as **clinical studies** because clinical studies use human participants to help researchers understand a certain condition or disease as well as how best to treat patients.

Intervention studies often use a research design known as a **clinical trial**, which is considered experimental research. In a clinical trial, researchers test new treatments, drugs, or medical devices to add to medical knowledge related to the treatment, diagnosis, and prevention of diseases and conditions. The Food and Drug Administration (FDA) requires (and regulates) clinical trials before a new drug, medical product such as vaccines, or medical device is sold in the United States. Clinical trials are often done in stages or phases.

Many clinical trials randomly assign participants to a group to test a specific treatment or to a control group; these are called **randomized controlled trials (RCT)**. RCTs are the gold standard because randomizing helps to reduce the risk that the effects of the intervention were due to the groups being different. The experimental group receives the treatment, and the comparison (control) group receives a dummy treatment or no treatment at all, with outcomes measured at certain points. Some RCTs are blinded, which means the participants do not know if they are getting the treatment or a placebo. In double-blind studies, the researchers also do not know which participants are receiving the treatment or a placebo. In triple-blind studies, anyone involved in data management is also blinded.

Compher (2010) states that "randomized clinical trials of drugs or procedures are most often **efficacy** studies that are designed to show whether the drug or procedure produces the desired clinical outcome under optimal conditions" (p. 598). Demonstration of efficacy (ability of a treatment to provide a beneficial effect) in an RCT does not guarantee that the treatment will work in actual practice settings because RCTs are very controlled and don't normally represent the wide range of patients and settings encountered in everyday practice. To see if a treatment will work in practice settings, researchers do effectiveness studies (or outcomes research).

Intervention research is not as simple as saying "let's try a diet low in _____ to decrease the risk of __________ in patients with __________." Planning an intervention study is a lengthy specialized process, starting with an in-depth understanding of the problem and working with a team to develop a theory to guide the research. Only then can the team conceptualize a research design and go through many steps, such as talking with patients who may benefit from the research and doing pilot studies, before implementing the intervention study.

OUTCOMES RESEARCH

Before talking about outcomes research, let's take a look at what outcomes are. Outcomes can be defined as changes in a client's health or quality of life that result from health/nutrition care. Outcomes look at how a patient does after treatment; in other words, what the consequences (outcomes) are. According to Splett (2008), outcomes can be grouped into these categories.

1. *Direct Nutrition Care Outcomes.* These outcomes are due directly to a nutrient intervention such as medical nutrition therapy or counseling. For example, a client who is counseled on eating changes to reduce LDL levels may improve her nutrient intake and reduce her LDL levels (two outcomes).
2. *Clinical Outcomes.* These outcomes look at changes in the progression or severity of a disease or condition, such as a reduced risk of heart attack after implementing appropriate lifestyle changes. Clinical outcomes may also look at whether a complication was avoided.
3. *Patient Outcomes.* Patient outcomes look at what is important to the patient. Were symptoms relieved? Has the quality of life improved or gotten worse? Is the patient more confident about treatment or the future? Is the patient better able to complete the activities of daily living?
4. *Cost Outcomes.* As health care costs climb, cost outcomes have become more and more important. You can think of health care costs as coming from two places: the actual cost of the intervention (such as the cost of enteral nutrition) and the costs associated with the health effects (outcomes) of the intervention. If the intervention decreases the length of a patient's stay, that is an outcome that saves money. However, keep in mind that sometimes an intervention has outcomes that do not save money.

Table 1.3 gives an example of how researchers might look at an intervention (a weight management program) and the chain of possible outcomes. Note that Splett (2008) groups clinical, cost, and patient outcomes together as health care outcomes. Depending on the exact nature of the study, only certain outcomes are chosen to be measured.

Whereas intervention research looks at whether the intervention works under controlled conditions, **outcomes research** is undertaken to test the **effectiveness** of an intervention; that is, whether it works under *usual* circumstances. Just because an intervention worked in a hospital-based RCT does not mean that it will work equally well in a community setting such as a physician's office. Outcomes research is the crucial building block for evidence-based nutrition practice.

Outcomes research is also used to test the **cost-effectiveness** of a new treatment with the standard treatment, and whether it is a good value. Cost-effectiveness analysis tells us how much an intervention will cost to extend life by a given amount, enabling

Table 1.3 Chain of Outcomes Resulting from Weight Management Program (12-Month Period)

	Direct Nutrition Care Outcomes			Health Care Outcomes		
	Nutrition-related behavior and environment outcomes →	Food and nutrient intake outcomes →	Nutrition-related physical sign and symptom outcomes →	Clinical outcomes →	Cost outcomes →	Patient outcomes →
12-week group weight management program leads to	• Knowledge of food choices • Awareness of eating cues and responses • Self-efficacy • Increased physical activity	• Reduced energy intake • Healthful eating pattern consistent with Dietary Guidelines	• 12-week weight loss • 12-month weight loss • Reduced weight circumference • Decreased serum cholesterol	• Improved blood pressure	• Reduced hypertension medication	• Increased quality of life • Improved self-confidence

us to compare the costs and outcomes of two interventions. Along with other methods such as cost-benefit analysis, cost-effectiveness analysis is useful evidence of a treatment's value for reimbursement by insurance companies and others.

The **Academy of Nutrition and Dietetics Health Informatics Infrastructure (ANDHII)** collects data, such as outcomes data, from practitioners using easy-to-use formats and standardized terminology so that the data can be selectively analyzed in research projects and the results added to the nutrition evidence base. One component of ANDHII is a **Dietetics Outcomes Registry (DOR)**. The DOR makes anonymous data available for outcomes research and QI projects. The database includes data related to nutrition assessment, diagnosis, interventions, monitoring, evaluation, and outcomes.

TIP

Intervention studies test the *efficacy* of an intervention (whether it can work under very controlled conditions, often a RCT). Outcomes research tests the *effectiveness* (whether it achieves the desired treatment goal in a real-world setting) or the *cost-effectiveness* of an intervention. Intervention studies and outcomes studies both use quantitative research designs. Most outcome studies do not randomly assign patients to treatment or control groups, as is done in RCTs.

Epidemiological Research

Epidemiology is a discipline within public health that looks at the rates of health-related states (such as disease) in different groups of people and why they occur. Originally, epidemiology looked at communicable diseases, but now it includes noncommunicable diseases, chronic diseases, injuries, birth defects, environmental health, and other areas. Epidemiologists, sometimes called disease detectives, try to connect the dots between risk factors (sometimes called exposures) and health or disease outcomes. The studies have provided the crucial link between, for example, cholesterol and heart attacks.

Nutrition epidemiology is a subdiscipline of epidemiology. Epidemiology includes descriptive and analytic areas of study.

1. **Descriptive epidemiology** provides information about who has a disease in a population and the frequency of the disease in that population. In addition, it can tell us about the pattern of the disease, describing the time, place, and personal characteristics of those with the disease (such as age, race, socioeconomic status, or behaviors). Descriptive epidemiology is vital to assess the health of a population or a community, and it provides clues about possible contributing factors and causes of diseases and other health-related states.
2. **Analytic epidemiology** digs deeper to determine the strength of the association between a risk factor and the health-related state. For example, let's look at soda drinking by obese children. As a child drinks more soda, studies have found that the odds (or risk) of becoming obese increase. Finding an association, in this case between soda drinking and obesity, does not necessarily make it a causal relationship. Intervention studies may also be used to prove or disprove causality. Criteria for causality for epidemiological studies are discussed in Chapter 7.

Some epidemiologists work in the field of **applied epidemiology**. They address public health issues regarding control and prevention of disease in the community using data from descriptive and analytic epidemiological research.

TRANSLATIONAL RESEARCH

Translational research generally can be described as a systematic process of transforming findings from basic science or clinical studies into practical applications and evidence-based practice that improves the health of individuals and populations. That's quite a mouthful, so some people refer to it as research that *goes from the researcher's bench to the patient bedside and then to the community*.

Translational research got its start in the medical field because of impatience with the length of time it took for discoveries in the lab to translate into changes in health practices or treatments. The National Institutes of Health (NIH) funds a number of centers and institutes for translational research. Social scientists also are now getting involved in this type of research.

A model of the stages of translational research for RDNs is summarized in **Table 1.4**. and described below. Each stage builds on and informs the others. Translational research involves aspects of basic research, preclinical research, clinical research, effectiveness studies, evidence-based practice guidelines, and population health.

1. Basic research helps researchers learn about the pathophysiology of a disease or the potential for intervention. Animal models of human disease or other experimental methods may be used. Preclinical research starts to connect basic science with human medicine. Research at this point is usually not ready to be done in humans, but scientists use basic research findings to increase their understanding of a disease and ways to treat it. A hypothesis may be tested using animal models, computational models, or samples of human tissues.

Table 1.4 Translational Research Phases, Definitions, and Examples for Registered Dietitian Nutritionists

Research phase	Definition	Type of research	Research question
T1	Identification of disease mechanisms and health problem	Basic research, animal research, preclinical, and preintervention studies	What is the mechanistic action of dietary fiber sources on serum lipids?
T2	Discovery of application to human health and clinical settings	Human clinical studies, efficacy studies, and controlled observational studies	Among patients with cardiovascular disease, what is the effect on serum lipids from dietary fiber from whole foods as compared to dietary supplements?
T3	Health applications to evidence-based practice guidelines, practice guidelines to health practices, and practice to population health impact	Effectiveness research, dissemination research, implementation research, scale-up and spread research	What is the degree to which registered dietitian nutritionists in community health clinics can adopt, implement, and maintain an evidence-based nutrition program to improve cardiovascular risk factors?

Reproduced from "What Is Translational Research? Concepts and Applications in Nutrition and Dietetics," by J. Zoellner, L. Van Horn, P. M. Gleason, and C. J. Boushey, 2015, *Journal of The Academy of Nutrition and Dietetics, 115*, p. 1065. Copyright 2015 by the Academy of Nutrition and Dietetics. Reprinted with permission.

2. Both basic and preclinical studies then inform and shape the next steps, which will now involve clinical studies, perhaps starting small with case studies and then moving to larger clinical trials (early phase clinical trials are smaller). Clinical trials will test clinical efficacy and safety, as well as identify knowledge gaps. Controlled observational studies are also used.
3. Next, the results from the efficacy studies are tested and refined using effectiveness research, which tests how an intervention works under usual circumstances. Effectiveness research findings are used to develop evidence-based practice guidelines, which can be used in hospital and other settings, and with small and large populations. Scientists continue to do research to determine whether the evidence-based interventions engage the participants for optimal impact (dissemination research), are well integrated within a specific setting (implementation research), and can be successfully disseminated and implemented with large populations (scale-up and spread research) (Zoellner, Van Horn, Gleason, & Boushey, 2015).

Table 1.4 shows the three research phases designated in translational research: T1, T2, and T3.

A number of models are used for translational research within the medical field, and they may include from two to five research phases. Many researchers use two-phase models, in which case T1 refers to applying basic lab research findings to preclinical and clinical trials (T1 and T2 in Table 1.4), and T2 refers to applying clinical research findings in practice settings and communities (T3 in Table 1.4). In **Figure 1.3**, T1 is

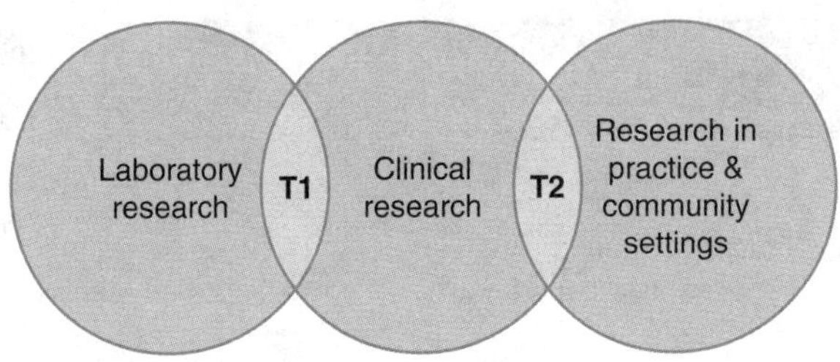

FIGURE 1.3 Research Continuum from Laboratory to Practice Settings and Communities

the shaded area between Laboratory research and Clinical research, and T2 is the shaded area between Clinical research and Research in practice & community settings.

Table 1.5 summarizes the types of research just discussed. Keep in mind that a research study may very well fit into more than one of the categories. Also, although these types of research are often clinical, you will see research on nonclinical topics such as management and economic research, sensory evaluation research, and consumer research.

Doing research requires you to maintain certain ethical standards and to protect the rights of others. Institutions engaged in research involving human participants must

Table 1.5 Types of Research in Nutrition

Type of research	Definition	Example
Intervention Research	Research involving development and testing of an intervention. Often uses clinical trials. Tests efficacy of an intervention.	A randomized clinical trial evaluates whether eating less fat (target 15% from fat) influences breast cancer recurrence in early stage breast cancer patients receiving standard cancer care.
Outcomes Research	Research designed to document nutrition-related, clinical, and patient outcomes (end results). Undertaken to test the effectiveness of an intervention under normal circumstances and its cost-effectiveness.	An experimental study evaluates whether psyllium fiber improves glycemic control in clinic patients with type 2 diabetes.
Epidemiological Research	Research that focuses on the frequency and pattern of disease in a population and on identifying possible risk factors.	An epidemiological study evaluates whether increased body weight/central obesity is related to asthma in children.
Translational Research	A systematic process of transforming findings of basic science or clinical studies into practical applications and evidence-based practice that improves the health of individuals and populations. Research that goes "from bench to bedside to community."	Preclinical animal studies are performed to determine the optimal dose of tea polyphenols needed for maximum osteoprotective effects, which will then be tested in postmenopausal osteopenic women. Results will be used to inform randomized controlled trials, which will inform effectiveness research.

APPLICATION 1.4

Using the title of these research studies, identify whether each study is an example of intervention, outcomes, epidemiological, or translational research.

A. "Association between inflammatory potential of diet and mortality among women in the Swedish mammography cohort" (Shivappa et al., 2015).
B. "Effect of nutrition intervention on food choices of French students in middle school cafeterias, using an interactive educational software program (Nutri-Advice)" (Turnin et al., 2015).
C. "Persistent effects of early infant diet and associated microbiota on the juvenile immune system" (Narayan, Mendez-Lagares, Ardeshir, Lu, Van Rompay, & Hartigan-O'Connor, 2015).
D. "In-hospital hyperglycemia: Effects of treatment protocol on glycemic control and clinical outcome" (Clinical Trials.gov NCT00302874).

satisfy an **Institutional Review Board (IRB)**, a group of people who review and monitor biomedical research. They have the authority to approve, require modifications, or disapprove research. The purpose of IRB review is to ensure that appropriate steps are taken to protect the rights and welfare of human participants. IRBs and research ethics are discussed in Chapter 3.

PRACTICE-BASED RESEARCH NETWORKS

Practice-based research networks (PBRNs) are "groups of primary care clinicians and practices working together to answer community-based healthcare questions and translate research findings into practice" (Agency for Healthcare Research and Quality, 2016). PBRNs link practicing clinicians with each other to create and run studies, which is useful because each clinician will likely only have a small sample. PBRNs also link clinicians with researchers experienced in clinical research. Primary care practitioners are well positioned to do effectiveness (outcomes) research and comparative effectiveness research (comparing the effectiveness of one treatment with another) with the assistance offered by PBRNs.

The Academy of Nutrition and Dietetics created the Dietetics Practice-Based Research Network (DPBRN) in 2003. Membership is open (and free) to all academy members, and DPBRN members include researchers, practitioners, and students. As a DPBRN member, you can be involved with any of these functions:

- Participate in research in varying capacities, such as collecting data, analyzing data, or being the investigator.
- Propose research questions.
- Serve on an advisory group to select studies to pursue.
- Take part in disseminating results (poster, research publication).
- Get help to design or carry out a study.

The DPBRN has been involved in a number of research projects, such as outpatient care, evidence-based guidelines for diabetes care, and the *Guide for Effective Nutrition Interventions and Education* (Stein, 2016).

RESEARCHER INTERVIEW Translational Research

Wahida Karmally, Dr.PH, RDN, CDE, CLS, FNLA
Associate Research Scientist and Director of Bionutrition Research Core for the Irving Center for Clinical and Translational Research, Columbia University Medical Center, New York, NY

1. **Briefly describe the areas in which you do research.**
The mission of Columbia University Medical Center's Clinical and Translational Science Award (CTSA) is to transform the culture of research to hasten the discovery and implementation of new treatments and prevention strategies. In October 2006, the Irving Center for Clinical Research joined a national consortium created by the National Center for Research Resources (NCRR) branch of the NIH to energize the discipline of clinical and translational research, ultimately enabling researchers to provide new treatments more efficiently and quickly to patients.

My interest in research began when I was a graduate student in India conducting experiments on hundreds of albino rats to study bioavailability of iron from green leafy vegetables that grow on the roadside and are accessible to anyone who desires to pick them. This research was of public health significance because iron is a shortfall micronutrient in many populations. The results showed that the greens provide nutritional benefits that were cost-effective.

My interest in research continued during my postgraduate studies in London, UK. As an intern, I helped with clinical research at the Middlesex Hospital in London. I started working in research studies at the Mount Sinai Medical Center in New York with Dr. Virgil Brown in the early 1980s in the Diabetes Demonstration Project and on studies examining the effectiveness of statins.

I moved to Columbia University in 1987 as the director of nutrition in the General Clinical Research Center, and in 2006 the center became the Irving Institute for Clinical and Translational Research. In my current position as director of the Bionutrition Research Core, I had the opportunity to run the diet component of a multicenter landmark study: DELTA (Dietary Effects on Lipoproteins and Thrombogenic Activity). This study in essence determined that one standard macronutrient distribution in the diet does not "fit" all sections of the population. In individuals with insulin resistance, the results suggested that the replacement of dietary saturated fatty acids with monounsaturated fatty acids rather than carbohydrate is preferred because of associated smaller reductions in high-density lipoprotein cholesterol (HDL-C) and a trend toward reduction in fasting triglycerides (TG). Diets lower in saturated fat and higher in monounsaturated fat may benefit individuals with normal HDL-C levels or with high TGs. DELTA's results added to the body of evidence for the Therapeutic Lifestyle Changes (National Cholesterol Education Program), which stated that rather than relying on a single dietary recommendation for all, individualized nutrition counseling ("personalized nutrition") should be provided based on risk factors for the treatment and prevention of coronary artery disease.

I have been an investigator on several diet-related studies, including examining the effects of different intakes of dietary cholesterol in young men and women, beta-glucan from a ready-to-eat cereal on LDL-C in Hispanic Americans, the effects of diacylglycerol on TGs, very low calorie diets on insulin sensitivity and beta cell function in patients with type 2 diabetes, and studies on lipoprotein metabolism. The bionutrition core has supported protocols on energy homeostasis and osteoporosis as well as several pharmacokinetic studies, to name a few.

A collaboration with the National Heart, Lung, and Blood Institute (NHLBI) on the Latino and African American Initiatives resulted in the development of materials with culturally appropriate heart-healthy recipes for Latino and African Americans based on evidence-based recommendations for the prevention and treatment of cardiovascular risk factors. This was a "translational" strategy to improve the health of minority communities.

I am very interested in obesity and diabetes prevention. I initiated the anti-overweight campaign "Be Fit to Be'ne'Fit" at the New York Presbyterian/Columbia University Medical Center campus to increase awareness of obesity-associated diseases and provide tools and motivational messages for behavior modification.

The Community Engagement Resource (CER) at the Irving Institute provides another opportunity to engage the community with managing dietary risk factors, incorporating healthy eating patterns, and preventing disease. I have given lectures to the community on management of obesity, lipid disorders, and diabetes.

2. **With your experience in translational research, what should students/practitioners know about this area of research?**

Translational research is a multidirectional and multidisciplinary integration of basic research, patient-oriented research (bedside research), and population-based research, with the goal of improving the health of the public in a cost-effective manner.

The NIH has traditionally supported the training of basic and clinical scientists in a variety of disciplines. More recently, it has supported the training of scientists in translational research through the K30 and Clinical and Translational Science Award (CTSA) programs.

NIH defines translational research to include "two areas of translation. One is the process of applying discoveries generated during research in the laboratory, and in preclinical studies, to the development of trials and studies in humans. The second area of translation concerns research aimed at enhancing the adoption of best practices in the community. Cost-effectiveness of prevention and treatment strategies is also an important part of translational science (NIH, 2007)."

According to this definition, translational research is part of a unidirectional continuum in which research findings are moved from the researcher's bench to the patient's bedside and community. In the continuum, the first stage of translational research (T1) transfers knowledge from basic research to clinical research, and the second stage (T2) transfers findings from clinical studies or clinical trials to practice settings and communities, where the findings improve health.

Several nutrition studies have been "translational." Understanding the role of nutrition to health began as early as 400 BCE when Hippocrates stated: "Food is medicine, medicine is food." We began to learn about micronutrient deficiencies that led to fortification of foods to improve health. The policy for the removal of transfatty acids from foods was fast tracked to lower risk for cardiovascular disease: this was translational. Both DELTA and DASH (Dietary Approaches to Stop Hypertension) are examples of translational research studies.

3. **What do you enjoy most about the research process?**

Each day comes with an opportunity to learn and contribute to research in different areas of medicine. My work includes helping with research design, implementation, data collection, and analysis for a variety of studies. The work is never routine. I also introduce dietetic interns to nutrition research methodology during their rotations, and I teach in the medical and dental schools at Columbia University.

I have been inspired by a number of nutritionists in research such as Audrey Cross, Penny Kris-Etherton, Judith Wylie-Rosett, Theresa Nicklas, Linda Delahanty, Cynthia Thomson, Linda VanHorn, Linda G. Snetselaar, and my fantastic colleagues in the National Association of Bio-nutritionists. I had the opportunity to work with outstanding RDNs on the Academy of Nutrition and Dietetics Evidence Analysis Library (EAL) projects on Disorders of Lipid Metabolism and chaired the expert committee. My research interests gave me opportunities to serve on the Research Committee and Evidence-Based Practice Committee. As a national spokesperson for the Academy of Nutrition and Dietetics for 11 years, I had an extraordinary opportunity to translate research findings to the American public through television, print, and radio.

4. **What tips do you have for practitioners who want to do practice-based research?**

The advice I would give to a young researcher looking to develop a successful line of research is that the research process begins with ideas generated through a review of literature in the area of interest. These ideas lead to the development of research questions and hypotheses. Also, young researchers need to find mentors in their areas of interest.

Research is the backbone of our profession. Research gives credibility to the profession. RDNs have the responsibility to make evidence-based diet and lifestyle recommendations to their patients, clients, and fellow Americans. Nutrition research provides the tools for practice and provides an understanding of the role of diet in the prevention of disease and promotion of health. In the past two decades, nutrition research has clearly demonstrated that diet is the cornerstone in the prevention and lowering of risk for several chronic diseases.

RDNs interested in getting involved in research can learn about the Dietetics Practice Based Research Network (DPBRN). This network is a membership benefit and gives practicing RDNs access to researchers who can mentor them to use practice settings to conduct research. Prior research experience is not necessary to participate in the DPBRN. You can start with this web page: http://www.eatrightpro.org/resources/research/projects-tools-and-initiatives/dpbrn/

SUMMARY

1. Research is a systematic process of collecting, analyzing, and interpreting information/data to answer questions to extend knowledge. A systematic process means that research is completed using a system; that system is usually the scientific method.
2. The scientific method (see Figure 1.1) is a step-by-step process involving defining the problem, reviewing the literature, developing a research question (or hypothesis) and objective, developing the research design and methods to be used, collecting and analyzing data, interpreting results, drawing conclusions, and disseminating findings.
3. Study variables are any characteristic that can take on different values (such as BMI or social support) and are measured, controlled, or manipulated in research. Variables can be categorical or continuous. In an experimental study, the hypothesis shows a relationship between an independent variable (what the researcher manipulates, such as diet) and a dependent variable (what the researcher measures, the outcome measure).
4. Quantitative research designs are used to look at causal relationships as well associations or relationships between variables.
5. One way to classify research is according to its purpose: studies may explore, describe, analyze, or predict. Exploratory studies are often qualitative research. Descriptive research describes a wide variety of phenomena. Analytic research tries to quantify the relationship between an intervention on an outcome (an experimental study) or an exposure on an outcome (such as in a prospective cohort study).
6. Quantitative research uses the scientific method to describe and examine relationships among variables (descriptive studies) and examine cause-and-effect relationships (analytic studies). Control is used to prevent outside factors from influencing the results.
7. Qualitative research does not manipulate variables or put a group through an intervention. The qualitative researcher gets into the shoes of the study participants to capture information not conveyed in quantitative data, such as values, beliefs, or motivations behind behaviors. Qualitative research uses a systematic process.
8. The differences between quantitative and qualitative research spring from the researcher's paradigm on how the world works—either a positivist paradigm or a constructivist paradigm. Both types of research have advantages and uses (see Table 1.2).
9. Intervention studies test the efficacy of an intervention (whether it can work under controlled conditions, often using randomized controlled trials). Outcomes research tests the effectiveness (whether it achieves the desired treatment goal in a real-world setting) and cost-effectiveness of an intervention. Intervention studies and outcomes studies both use quantitative research designs. Outcomes may include direct nutrition care outcomes, clinical outcomes, patient outcomes, and cost outcomes.

10. Epidemiology is a discipline within public health that looks at the rates of health-related states (such as disease) in different groups of people (descriptive) and why they occur (analytic). Nutrition epidemiology is a subdiscipline.
11. Translational research is a systematic process of transforming findings of basic science or clinical studies into practical applications and evidence-based practice that improves the health of individuals and populations. In brief, it is research that goes "from bench to bedside to community."
12. The Dietetics Practice-Based Research Network (DPBRN) links practitioners with each other and with researchers to do effectiveness (outcomes) research and additional types of research and projects.

REVIEW QUESTIONS

1. A statement of the problem:
   A. is the same as a research question
   B. includes a hypothesis
   C. explains the context for why the research is needed
   D. includes the research design
2. Most research:
   A. uses the scientific method
   B. involves finding answers to a question
   C. includes variables
   D. all of the above
3. An experimental study is an example of what type of research?
   A. qualitative
   B. analytic
   C. descriptive
   D. associative
4. A randomized controlled trial is an example of a research:
   A. design
   B. question
   C. problem
   D. control
5. In an experimental study looking at the effects of a weight loss drug on weight loss, which is the independent variable?
   A. weight loss
   B. drug
   C. physical activity
   D. all of the above
6. A study examined two variables: the density of fast-food restaurants in communities and the BMI of the residents. What type of relationship are the researchers looking at?
   A. association
   B. relative risk
   C. causation
   D. confounding
7. Qualitative research is most likely to have what type of research purpose?
   A. explore
   B. describe
   C. analyze
   D. predict
8. A prospective cohort study, such as the Nurses' Health Studies is a(n):
   A. experimental study
   B. quantitative study
   C. qualitative study
   D. exploratory study
9. A study that uses focus groups and in-depth interviews with participants is likely to be a(n):
   A. experimental study
   B. quantitative study
   C. qualitative study
   D. analytic study
10. Which type of study is more likely to use animals?
    A. qualitative
    B. applied
    C. basic
    D. action
11. List and briefly describe the steps in the scientific method.
12. List five differences between quantitative and qualitative research. Name an advantage and a disadvantage for each type of research.
13. What is mixed methods research?

14. Compare and contrast a prospective cohort study with an experimental study. Are they both analytic studies?
15. The National Health and Nutrition Examination Survey (NHANES) assesses the health and nutritional status of about 5,000 adults and children each year in different locations. Find an example of a study using NHANES data and explain its research objective.
16. Describe a research question for which a qualitative study would be most useful. Also describe a research question for which a quantitative study would be most useful.
17. Compare and contrast intervention research with outcomes research.
18. List five examples of outcomes that you might find in a study.

CRITICAL THINKING QUESTIONS

1. Read this study and answer the following questions. (Open-Access Article) Fildes, van Jaarsveld, Wardle, & Cookie. (2014). Parent-administered exposure to increase children's vegetable acceptance: A randomized controlled trial. *Journal of the Academy of Nutrition and Dietetics, 114,* 881–888. doi: 10.1016/j.jand.2013.07.040
   - **A.** Why was this study done? In other words, define the problem(s).
   - **B.** In your own words, what was the purpose of the study.
   - **C.** What was the hypothesis?
   - **D.** The research design was a randomized controlled trial. What elements of the study methods indicated that it was a RCT? Describe them briefly.
   - **E.** What were the independent and dependent variables?
   - **F.** Explain the tasting game that the intervention group played.
   - **G.** What does Figure 1.2 tell us about the intake and liking of vegetables in the intervention versus the control group from T2 to T3?
   - **H.** Summarize the study findings in two sentences or less.
2. **Study Summary**: The objective of the study was to interview current vegetarians and former vegetarians to explore their perceptions of the vegetarian diet and whether their perceptions had changed over time. The instruments used were semistructured interviews and focus groups. The study was a cross-sectional study, meaning that the study took place at the same point in time in the given population (Barr & Chapman, 2002).
   - **A.** Is the study quantitative or qualitative?
   - **B.** Is the study basic or applied?
   - **C.** Is the primary purpose of the study to explore, describe, analyze, or predict?
   - **D.** Is the study experimental? If so, name the independent and the dependent variables.
   - **E.** Is the study a randomized controlled trial? Could it be an intervention or outcomes study?
   - **F.** Is the study epidemiological or translational in nature?
3. **Study Summary**: The objective of the study was to test whether adding a dietitian to a hospital discharge team for geriatric patients would improve the nutritional status of those patients over 6 months. Geriatric patients were randomly assigned to either the regular discharge team or the discharge team with the dietitian. All patients were at least 70 years old and determined to be at nutritional risk. The dietitian gave each discharged patient three home visits within 8 weeks of discharge. Nutritional status was measured using weight, muscle strength, and other measures. Adding a dietitian to the discharge team did improve the nutritional status of geriatric patients (Beck et al., 2015).
   - **A.** Is the study quantitative or qualitative?
   - **B.** Is the study basic or applied?
   - **C.** Is the primary purpose of the study to explore, describe, analyze, or predict?
   - **D.** Is the study experimental? If so, name the independent and the dependent variables.

E. Is the study a randomized controlled trial?
F. Describe the intervention.
G. Is the study epidemiological or translational in nature?

4. **Study Summary**: The researchers examined the association between consumption of coffee with the risk of mortality in the Nurses' Health Study over a 25-year period. Results showed that higher consumption of coffee was associated with a lower risk of total mortality (Ding et al., 2015).
   A. Is the study quantitative or qualitative?
   B. Is the study basic or applied?
   C. Is the primary purpose of the study to explore, describe, analyze, or predict?
   D. Is the study experimental? name the independent and the dependent variables.
   E. Is the study epidemiological or translational in nature?

5. **Study Summary**: This study aimed to determine whether vitamin D supplementation can reduce the risk of developing type 2 diabetes in adults (30 or older) with prediabetes. Participants were randomly assigned to receive either a vitamin D pill or a placebo. The study was double-blinded and ran long enough to determine whether vitamin D made a difference (Pittas et al., 2014).
   A. Is the study quantitative or qualitative?
   B. Is the study basic or applied?
   C. Is the primary purpose of the study to explore, describe, analyze, or predict?
   D. Name the independent and dependent variables.
   E. Is the study a randomized controlled trial?
   F. Describe the intervention.

6. **Study Summary**: The aim of the study was to feed fruit flies (in the very young larval stage) a control diet or a high-sugar diet to see whether they became insulin resistant and obese, risk factors strongly associated with type 2 diabetes. Results showed that larvae on the high-sugar diet became insulin resistant, hyperglycemic, and fat (Palanker Musselman et al., 2011).
   A. Is the study quantitative or qualitative?
   B. Is the study basic or applied?
   C. Is the primary purpose of the study to explore, describe, analyze, or predict?
   D. Is the study experimental? name the independent and the dependent variables.

7. **Study Summary**: The aim of the study was to see if there is a link between children being overweight or obese and developing asthma. Using results from 48 previously published studies, the researchers found a significant, but weak, association between high body weight and asthma (Papoutsakis et al., 2013).
   A. Is the study quantitative or qualitative?
   B. Is the study basic or applied?
   C. Is the primary purpose of the study to explore, describe, analyze, or predict?
   D. Is the study experimental? If so, name the independent and the dependent variables.
   E. Is the study epidemiological in nature?

SUGGESTED READINGS AND ACTIVITIES

1. Zoellner, J., Van Horn, L., Gleason, P. M., & Boushey, C. J. (2015). What is translational research? Concepts and applications in nutrition and dietetics. *Journal of the Academy of Nutrition and Dietetics, 115*, 1057–1071. doi: 10.1016/j.jand.2015.03.010
2. To learn more about descriptive and analytic epidemiology, visit the Centers for Disease Control and Prevention (CDC) website for Self-Study Course SS1978, "An Introduction to Applied Epidemiology and Biostatistics." Sections 6 and 7 in Lesson One cover descriptive and analytic epidemiology.
3. To learn more about evidence-based practice, go to the Evidence Analysis Library (www.andeal.org). Read "Methodology" and "Why Use Evidence-Based Practice" under the Methodology tab.
4. To learn more about the Dietetics Practice-Based Research Network, go to the DPBRN page at eatrightpro.org and listen to the recorded presentation.

REFERENCES

Academy of Nutrition and Dietetics. (2015). *About EAL*. Retrieved from http://www.andeal.org/content.cfm?content_code=about:EAL

Agency for Healthcare Research and Quality. (2016). *Practice-based research networks*. Retrieved from https://pbrn.ahrq.gov

Barr, S., & Chapman, G. (2002). Perceptions and practices of self-defined current vegetarian, former vegetarian, and nonvegetarian women. *Journal of the American Dietetic Association, 102*, 354–360. doi: 10.1016/S0002-8223(02)90083-0

Beck, A., Andersen, U., Leedo, E., Jensen, L., Martins, K., Quvang, M., … Ronholt, F. (2015). Does adding a dietician to the liaison team after discharge of geriatric patients improve nutritional outcome: A randomized controlled trial. *Clinical Rehabilitation, 29*, 1117–1128. doi: 10.1177/0269215514564700

Compher, C. (2010). Efficacy vs effectiveness. *Journal of Parenteral and Enteral Nutrition, 34*, 598–599. doi: 10.1177/0148607110381906

Creswell, J. W., Klassen, A. C., Plano Clark, V. L., & Clegg Smith, C. (2011). *Best practices for mixed methods in the health sciences*. Retrieved from https://obssr.od.nih.gov/training/mixed-methods-research/

Ding, M., Satija, A., Bhupathiraju, S., Hu, Y., Sun, Q., Han, J., … Hu, F. (2015). Association of coffee consumption with total and cause-specific mortality in three large prospective cohorts. *Circulation,* 132. doi: 10.1161/CIRCULATIONAHA.115.017341

Fildes, A., van Jaarsveld, C. H. M., Wardle, J., & Cookie, L. (2014). Parent-administered exposure to increase children's vegetable acceptance: A randomized controlled trial. *Journal of the Academy of Nutrition and Dietetics, 114*, 881–888. doi: 10.1016/j.jand.2013.07.040

Finkler, E., Heymsfield, S. B., & St-Onge, M. (2012). Rate of weight loss can be predicted by patient characteristics and intervention strategies. *Journal of the Academy of Nutrition and Dietetics, 112,* 75–80. doi: 10.1016/j.jada.2011.08.034

Hand, R. K. (2014). Research in nutrition and dietetics—What can the Academy do for you? *Journal of the Academy of Nutrition and Dietetics, 114*, 131–135. doi: 10.1016/j.jand.2013.11.007

Leung, L. (2015). Validity, reliability, and generalizability in qualitative research. *Journal of Family Medicine and Primary Care, 4*, 324–327. doi: 10.4103/2249-4863.161306

Lindbloom, E., Ewigman, B. G., & Hickner, J. M. (2004). Practice-based research networks: The laboratories of primary care research. *Medical Care, 42*, 45-49.

Narayan, N., Mendez-Lagares, G., Ardeshir, A., Lu, D., Van Rompay, K., & Hartigan-O'Connor, D. (2015). Persistent effects of early infant diet and associated microbiota on the juvenile immune system. *Gut Microbes, 6*, 284–289. doi: 10.1080/19490976.2015.1067743

National Institutes of Health. (2007, March). Definitions under Subsection 1 (Research Objectives), Section I (Funding Opportunity Description), Part II (Full Text of Announcement), of RFA-RM-07-007: Institutional Clinical and Translational Science Award (U54). Retrieved from http://grants.nih.gov/grants/guide/rfa-files/RFA-RM-07-007.html

Palanker Musselman, L., Fink, J., Narzinski, K., Ramachandran, P., Hathiramani, S., Cagan, R., & Baranski, T. (2011). A high-sugar diet produces obesity and insulin resistance in wild-type Drosophia. *Disease Models & Mechanisms, 4*, 842–849. doi: 10.1242/dmm.007948

Papoutsakis, C., Priftis, K., Drakouli, M., Prifti, S., Konstantaki, E., Chondronikola, M., … Matzious, V. (2013). Childhood overweight/obesity and asthma: Is there a link? A systematic review of recent epidemiologic evidence. *Journal of the Academy of Nutrition and Dietetics, 113*, 77–105. doi: 10.1016/j.jand.2012.08.025

Patton, S. R., Clements, M. A., George, K., & Goggin, K. (2015). "I don't want them to feel different": A mixed methods study of parents' beliefs and dietary management strategies for their young children with type 1 diabetes mellitus. *Journal of the Academy of Nutrition and Dietetics, 116*, 272–282. doi: 10.1016/j.jand.2015.06.377

Pittas, A., Dawson-Hughes, B., Sheehan, P., Rosen, C., Ware, J., Knowler, W., … D2d Research Group. (2014). Rationale and design of the vitamin D and type 2 diabetes (D2d) study: A diabetes prevention trial. *Diabetes Care, 37*, 3227–3234. doi: 10.2337/dc14-1005

Price, J. A., Kent, S., Cox, S. A., McCauley, S. M., Parekh, J., & Klein, C. J. (2014). Using Academy Standards of Excellence in Nutrition and Dietetics for organization self-assessment and quality improvement. *Journal of the Academy of Nutrition and Dietetics, 114,* 1277–1292. doi: 10.1016/j.jand.2014.04.011

Rimkus, L., Isgor, Z., Ohri-Vachaspati, P., Zenk. S., Powell, L., Barker, D., & Chaloupka, F. (2015). Disparities in the availability and price of low-fat and higher-fat milk in US food stores by community characteristics. *Journal of the Academy of Nutrition and Dietetics, 115*, 1975–1985. doi: 10.1016/j.jand.2015.04.002

Schindler, J., Kiszko, K., Abrams, C., Islam, N., & Elbel, B. (2013). Environmental and individual factors affecting menu labeling utilization: A qualitative research study. *Journal of the Academy of Nutrition and Dietetics, 113*, 667–672. doi: 10.1016/j.jand.2012.11.011

Shivappa, N., Harris, H., Wolk, A., & Hebert, J. (2015). Association between inflammatory potential of diet and mortality among women in the Swedish mammography cohort. *European Journal of Nutrition.* Advance online publication. doi: 10.1007/s00394-015-1005-z

Splett, P. L. (2008). Outcomes research and economic analysis. In E. R. Monsen & L. Van Horn (Eds.), *Research:*

Successful approaches (pp. 281–299). Chicago, IL: American Dietetic Association.

Stein, K. (2016). Propelling the profession with outcomes and evidence: Building a robust research agenda at the academy. *Journal of the Academy of Nutrition and Dietetics, 116,* 1014–1030. doi: 10.1016/j.jand.2016.02.018

Suplee, D, Jerome-D'Emilia, B., & Burrell, S. (2015). Exploring the challenges of healthy eating in an urban community of Hispanic women. *Hispanic Health Care International, 13,* 161–170. doi: 10.1891/1540-4153.13.3.161

Turnin, M., Buisson, J., Ahluwalia, N., Cazals, L., Bolzonella-Pene, C., Fouquet-Martineau, C., … Hanaire, H. (2016). Effect of nutritional intervention on food choices of French students in middle school cafeterias, using an interactive educational software program (Nutri-Advice). *Journal of Nutrition Education and Behavior, 48,* 131–137. doi: 10.1016/j.jneb.2015.09.011

U.S. Department of Health and Human Services. (2009). *Protection of human subjects* (Code of Federal Regulations, Title 45, Part 46). Retrieved from http://www.hhs.gov/ohrp/regulations-and-policy/regulations/45-cfr-46/index.html

Zoellner, J., Van Horn, L., Gleason, P. M., & Boushey, C. J. (2015). What is translational research? Concepts and applications in nutrition and dietetics. *Journal of the Academy of Nutrition and Dietetics, 115*, 1057–1071. doi: 10.1016/j.jand.2015.03.010

CHAPTER 2

How to Find Appropriate Research Articles

CHAPTER OUTLINE

- Introduction
- Everything You Need to Know About Journals
- Scientific Literature Not Found in Journals
- How to Use Databases to Find Articles
- Checklist for Selecting Articles
- Principles of Scientific Writing
- Researcher Interview: Bioactive Compounds in Fruits and Vegetables, Dr. Joan G. Fischer

LEARNING OUTCOMES

- Identify scientific journals and the different types of articles they contain.
- Describe and give examples of gray literature.
- Use a variety of databases (such as MEDLINE/PubMed) to find relevant research articles.
- Use a checklist to select appropriate journal articles.
- Apply basic principles of scientific writing.

INTRODUCTION

Throughout your career as a Registered Dietitian Nutritionist (RDN), it will be necessary to read, interpret, and evaluate research studies, as well as keep abreast of evidence-based practice in your practice area. Nutrition advice and recommendations communicated by RDNs must be based on scientific studies and is one of our professional obligations. The Academy of Nutrition and Dietetics' Standards of Professional Performance defines six standards that dietetics professionals are obligated to comply with regardless of setting, project, case, or situation. Knowledge of research and using research in practice is acknowledged throughout the six standards, and particularly in Standard 4: Application of Research, which states the following: "The registered dietitian (RD) applies, participates in, or generates research to enhance practice. Evidence-based practice incorporates the best available research/evidence in the delivery of nutrition and dietetics services" (Academy Quality Management Committee and Scope of Practice Subcommittee of the Quality Management Committee, 2013).

Research articles are found in journals. When you go to your college library, you no doubt see a variety of publications: newspapers, popular magazines (such as *Shape* or *Cooking Light*), trade magazines (such as *Today's Dietitian* or *Food Management*), fiction and nonfiction books, and also journals. **Table 2.1** can help you see the differences among newspapers/magazines, trade magazines (also called trade journals), and scholarly or academic journals. For example, *Today's Dietitian* is the "magazine for nutrition professionals." It is a trade magazine that includes articles about, for example, obesity drugs, which is useful for a nutritionist but certainly is not an original research article. Another nutrition publication, *Nutrition Action Healthletter*, interviews nutrition researchers and discusses nutrition-related health issues based on research, as well as gives guidance on choosing healthy foods. It is read by nutritionists and non-nutritionists alike, so it would be classified as a magazine.

An original research article is a description of a single study (quantitative or qualitative) that is written by the researchers who conducted the research. Original research

Table 2.1 Differences Between Magazine/Newspapers, Trade Publications, and Scholarly/Academic Journals

General criteria for articles published in a magazine or newspaper	General criteria for articles published in a trade publication	General criteria for articles published in a scholarly or academic journal
• Written by a journalist. • Written in a language that is simple and easy to understand by a wide range of readers. • Written as a report of recent news or to provide general information and entertainment. • Articles do not include a bibliography. • Articles often accompany advertisements and/or photographs.	• Articles are generally written by a member of a specific profession or trade and may be factual, anecdotal, or opinion. • Trade publications are generally published by a specific trade or association for the members. • Language in the articles may include jargon or terms that are mainly known to the targeted profession or trade. The author will assume that the reader has some knowledge about the topic. • Articles may include a bibliography.	• Articles are written by researchers who have expertise in a subject area. • Articles usually undergo a peer-reviewed process, in which an article is reviewed by other subject experts to verify the study methodology and the usefulness of the article before it is published. • Articles are targeted to an audience of researchers, professors, and students in a specific field. Language in the article includes jargon or terms that are mainly known to the targeted profession or trade. The author will assume that the reader has, at a minimum, a basic knowledge about the topic at hand. • Articles include a reference list. • Medical/scientific journals generally comply with a disciplined structure that includes an abstract, introduction, methods, results, discussion, and conclusion.
Examples: *New York Times* (newspaper), *Washington Post* (newspaper), *Shape* (magazine), *Nutrition Action Healthletter* (magazine)	**Examples**: *Today's Dietitian, FoodService Director, Food Management, Nation's Restaurant News*	**Examples**: *Journal of the Academy of Nutrition & Dietetics, Journal of the American Medical Association, American Journal of Clinical Nutrition*

articles are also called primary research articles or simply research articles. Scientists have to submit manuscripts to journals for publication. Journals have the right to decide whether they will publish the manuscript, and they can ask the author(s) for revisions. Thousands of scientific journals publish research articles, and each journal specializes in a certain area(s).

Having some knowledge about how to find appropriate research articles is a great place to start. As a student and as you advance in your nutrition-related career, many of you will also have the opportunity to participate in nutrition research and medical writing. Without proper training, research articles can be difficult to read and interpret and even more challenging to write. This chapter helps you to understand various types of articles found in journals, use databases and other information to find appropriate research journal articles, and follow guidelines to ensure quality writing in a scientific manner.

EVERYTHING YOU NEED TO KNOW ABOUT JOURNALS

Scientific journals present research studies to further the progress of science. Most are specialized for a certain discipline or subdiscipline. Many, but not all, journals use a process called **peer review** to ensure that articles they publish are accurate, meet their standards, and advance the knowledge base. A peer-reviewed journal also may be called a referred journal. You can usually tell if a journal uses the peer-review process by consulting its "Instructions for Authors." In the peer-review process, manuscripts are evaluated and critiqued by others not employed by the journal. Their job is to evaluate the quality of each part of the research, judge whether the article meets certain criteria, and determine the article's relevance and interest to the readers of that journal. Often reviewers recommend changes to the manuscript that must be completed and reviewed before publication.

To see how one journal is set up, let's take a look at an issue of the *Journal of the Academy of Nutrition and Dietetics (JAND)*. Each issue is split up into three sections: "Practice Applications," "Research," and "From the Academy." The "Practice Applications" section normally has a message from the president, letters to the editor, and a few articles about new or emerging topics of interest to RDNs, such as informatics, a new scientific advancement, or even a nutrition-related case study.

"From the Academy" includes news from the professional association as well as Academy Position or Practice Papers. A Position Paper, such as "Use of Nutritive and Nonnutritive Sweeteners," uses an analysis of the research literature to present the Academy's stance on an issue. A Practice Paper also analyzes research but in an effort to guide and improve nutrition and dietetics practice. Two examples of Practice Papers are "Critical Thinking Skills in Nutrition Assessment" and "Principles of Productivity in Food and Nutrition Services."

TYPES OF RESEARCH ARTICLES

The "Research" section of *JAND* contains the following types of articles.

- Original research *includes quantitative and qualitative studies that are generally limited to about 5,000 words. JAND* also publishes shorter versions of original research that are labeled as "Research Brief." In either case, original research includes an abstract, introduction, methods and materials, results, discussion, conclusions, references, and tables/figures.

- *Occasionally an original research article may be accompanied by a* **research editorial**, *which is not simply an expression of someone's opinion.* Editorials are written by subject matter experts who often discuss the topic within a broader context, and they are usually very interesting to read. Because they provide evidence, they contain references at the end.
- *Although original research is the heart of a journal, additional types of articles are important for readers as well.* For example, *JAND* publishes three types of **review articles**: narrative reviews, systematic reviews, and evidence analysis library reviews.
  - **Narrative reviews** are sometimes confused with original research, but they are easy to keep separate because authors of narrative reviews do not conduct a research study. Instead, they evaluate and summarize the evidence (from many studies) in a particular research area. Review authors also report inconsistencies in the literature and research gaps, as well as give ideas for future research. For example, "Environmental Considerations for Improving Nutritional Status in Older Adults with Dementia: A Narrative Review" is a narrative review published in *JAND* (Douglas & Lawrence, 2015). After searching multiple databases for research articles and determining which studies to include using eligibility criteria, the authors selected 30 research articles to explore how feeding assistance, meal service delivery styles, and the dining room environment might be used to improve nutritional status in this population. They concluded that a variety of interventions, such as changing lighting and adding music in the dining area, may improve client eating.
  - **Systematic reviews** are more rigorous than narrative reviews. Systematic reviews are a "summary of the scientific literature on a specific topic or question that uses explicit methods to conduct a comprehensive literature search and identify relevant studies, critically appraise the quality of each study, and summarize the body of literature or evidence to answer the question" (Academy of Nutrition and Dietetics, 2015). The objective is to present a balanced and unbiased summary of the existing research. Here is an example of a systematic review article from *JAND*: "The Impact of the 2009 Special Supplemental Nutrition Program for Women, Infants, and Children Food Package Revisions on Participants: A Systematic Review" (Schultz, Shanks, & Houghtaling, 2015). This study found that the revised food package did improve dietary intake of the participants. *Often systematic reviews use a statistical technique* called a **meta-analysis** to combine the results of a number of independent studies into a single result. The studies pooled together must be similar in type, such as all randomized controlled trials, and may include published and unpublished results. A meta-analysis, when done correctly, has greater statistical power than a single study.
  - **Evidence Analysis Library Reviews** are also systematic reviews. They follow the Evidence Analysis Process of the Academy of Nutrition and Dietetics. The Evidence Analysis Process is the basis for evidence-based practice guidelines so practitioners make appropriate nutrition care decisions for patients.

JAND also occasionally publishes a commentary article on controversial or emerging nutrition issues. It is expected to be a scholarly article that is thoroughly referenced and does not show bias. A good example of a commentary article is "Gluten-Free Diet: Imprudent Dietary Advice for the General Population?" (Gaesser & Angadi, 2012).

Every journal is a little different in how it is set up. For example, the *American Journal of Clinical Nutrition* separates the research articles into specialties, such as "Obesity and Eating Disorders," and also includes Editorials and Letters to the Editor. In addition to original research, *JAMA* contains Reviews, Viewpoints, Editorials, Comments

& Response, Clinical Trails Updates, Health Agencies Updates, JAMA Patient Page (excellent patient education materials that are always free online), and more.

TIP

Make sure you can identify whether an article is an example of primary, secondary, or tertiary research. Original research articles are primary research. Secondary research includes narrative reviews in which authors organize, interpret, and summarize evidence from numerous primary studies in a particular research area into one article. Systematic reviews belong in the category of tertiary research because they collect and distill information from both primary and secondary sources. Overall, a systematic review is a much more rigorous and comprehensive summary of research than a narrative review.

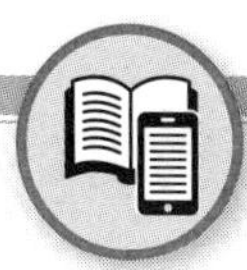

APPLICATION 2.1

Using the title of these research studies, identify each study as an example of original research, research editorial, narrative review, or systematic review.

A. "Breast-feeding and postpartum weight retention: A meta-analysis" (He et al., 2015).
B. "Are dietary guidelines sensible to consumers?" (Pérez-Rodrigo & Tseng, 2013).
C. "Targeted physician education positively affects delivery of nutrition therapy and patient outcomes: Results of a prospective clinical trial" (Hurt et al., 2015).
D. "Physical activity at altitude: Challenges for people with diabetes" (de Mol et al., 2014).

Nutrition-Related Journals

Table 2.2 lists some of the journals commonly read by RDNs.

APPLICATION 2.2

Many of the journals in Table 2.2 are published by professional associations. Identify the professional associations that publish five of the journals in the table.

Digital Object Identifiers, Impact Factors, and Open-Access Journals

When an article is published, the publisher assigns it a **digital object identifier (DOI)**. A DOI is a unique string of letters and numbers that can be used to identify the article and keep it accessible over its lifetime even if a journal changes its domain name. You will see the DOI on the first page of the article, and it always starts with a 10. DOIs are assigned and maintained by registration agencies.

Another concept to understand about journals is their **Impact Factor**. A journal's Impact Factor is related to how often articles from that journal are cited in other articles. You can find information about how often an article is cited using Web of Science or

Table 2.2 Nutrition-Related Journals	
American Journal of Clinical Nutrition	*Journal of Parenteral and Enteral Nutrition*
American Journal of Epidemiology	*Journal of the Academy of Nutrition and Dietetics*
American Journal of Preventive Medicine	*Journal of the American College of Nutrition*
Annual Review of Nutrition	*Journal of the American Medical Association*
Critical Reviews in Food Science and Nutrition	*Lancet*
Diabetes Care	*Nutrition and Metabolism*
Diabetes Educator	*Nutrition Reviews*
European Journal of Clinical Nutrition	*Nutrition Journal*
International Journal of Obesity	*Nutrition Research*
Journal of Nutrition	*Public Health Nutrition*
Journal of Nutrition Education and Behavior	

Google Scholar. (Both databases will be discussed.) A journal's Impact Factor is the frequency with which an article in a journal has been cited within a specific time frame (usually 2 to 5 years). It can be found using Journal Citation Reports (which is integrated in the Web of Science) or Google Scholar. For example, if a journal has an Impact Factor of 1 on Journal Citation Reports, it means that articles published over the past 2 years have been cited one time on average. Google Scholar publishes an index called the h5-median, which covers a 5-year period and represents the median number of citations for a journal article over 5 years. Impact Factors are interesting but have been criticized for being manipulated, among other concerns.

In contrast to subscription journals, which you will be reading most frequently, the mission of **open-access journals** is to provide unrestricted access (and reuse) of journal articles, many of which are peer reviewed and all of which are published free online only. As a university student, you can access many subscription journals online for free, and the university is paying handsomely for the licenses to provide you with that content. You can get a subscription to many popular magazines for under $20 a year, but one year of *JAND* costs an individual $370 in 2016. A number of open-access journals require payment of a publication fee in order for a research article to be published. Although there has been controversy about the quality of open-access journals, Björk and Solomon (2012, p. 9) found that many open-access journals are "high quality and widely cited."

SCIENTIFIC LITERATURE NOT FOUND IN JOURNALS

When you are looking for research articles, at some point you will come across what is called "gray literature," documents published outside of the traditional journal and academic book publishers. They can be useful sources of information and often include the following:

- *Dissertations and theses*. Sometimes when you use a database, one of your citations will be a dissertation completed by a doctoral student or a thesis completed by a Master's student. It is common practice that completed dissertations and theses are bound into a book format and placed in the university library.

- *Conference proceedings*. At scientific conferences, researchers present their findings in front of an audience, or they may simply present a poster. An abstract of either presentation may be published in a volume referred to as the "Proceedings of the Such-and-Such Conference." When you find an abstract like this in a database, that is all there is; there is normally no research paper. Every September, *JAND* publishes a supplement of abstracts from the poster sessions of its Food and Nutrition Conference and Expo, normally held in October.
- *Books*. Books report on many people's research, so they can't be considered primary research. Also, by the time a book is published, the content may be out of date.
- *Technical reports*. Government agencies and nongovernmental organizations (such as the Union of Concerned Scientists) often do scientific work that contributes to scientific knowledge. For example, the Centers for Disease Control and Prevention published a report on "Reducing Alcohol-Exposed Pregnancies: A Report of the National Task Force on Fetal Alcohol Syndrome and Fetal Alcohol Effect."
- *Commentaries and opinion pieces*. These can help give you an overview of what is going on in a specific research area, including authors' opinions.

Before using any of these sources in a research project, you may want to check with your professor.

APPLICATION 2.3

The database PubMed includes literature not found in journals. Go to the PubMed home page, enter a search term such as "hypertension/diet therapy," and click the "search" button. To the left, click on "Article Types." A number of types of gray literature are listed here such as books and clinical conferences. Name four other types of gray literatures found in the list.

HOW TO USE DATABASES TO FIND ARTICLES

Some of the important science databases for nutrition include the following.

- MEDLINE/PubMed
- Web of Science
- Scopus
- Science Direct

TIP

Although anyone can use a database such as PubMed or Google Scholar, *be sure you know which databases are available through your college library*. Libraries spend a lot of money to have databases and journals available (mostly online) for your use, and *the databases are more targeted to find the types of journal articles needed for your classes and offer more content and search features*. Talk to the Reference Librarian if you have any questions. In a matter of minutes, the Reference Librarian can improve the quality of your search results.

TIP

Journals generally allow you to search for articles on their websites using keywords. For example, if you go to the *Journal of the Academy of Nutrition and Dietetics*, you can use keywords that search entire articles or just the abstract, title, or author. Most subscription journals will give you access to any abstract, and a few articles may be available in full text. If the abstract sounds like it would be a good article, the college library may subscribe to that journal and you can get the full article online.

Each of these databases selectively chooses which journals and publications will be listed. Google Scholar is not technically a database; it is really an Internet search engine as it is created by a computer that searches scholarly literature and academic resources. MEDLINE/PubMed, Web of Science, Scopus, and Science Direct are all curated by people.

The first step in conducting a literature search is to familiarize yourself with the software that enables you to conduct the search. Software applications generally have options to expand or narrow your search, combine searches, and save searches.

SEARCHING DATABASES USING KEYWORDS OR SUBJECT HEADINGS

Software programs require the user to enter **keywords** into a database to secure matches for relevant studies. If you look at a research article or abstract, you will usually find the keywords for that article listed by the abstract. For example, in a study that evaluated the dietary quality of preschoolers' sack lunches using the Healthy Eating Index, the keywords were *early care and education, sack lunch, preschool children, Healthy Eating Index*, and *parents*.

When choosing keywords for searching, think of keywords that describe your population, intervention, control/comparison, outcome, or study design (referred to as PICOS). For example, if you are looking for research studies on the prevalence of red meat allergies following a Lone Star Tick bite in Texas, you might identify the keywords in **Table 2.3** for your search.

Keyword searching brings up all articles that contain the word(s) you have typed in, whether the word(s) appeared in the abstract, discussion, references, or anywhere else. This has advantages and disadvantages. A disadvantage is that it brings up a lot more results than a subject heading search, and many of those results will not be useful. But it can be worthwhile when you are looking for a topic with little information, brand

Table 2.3 Using PICOS to Identify Keywords

PICOS	Keywords
Population: Texas	Texas, Population
Intervention: Lone Star Tick Bite	Lone Star Tick
Control/Comparison: No Red Meat Allergy	Not Included in Literature Search
Outcome: Red Meat Allergy	Red Meat Allergy
Study Design: Randomized Controlled Trial	Randomized Controlled Trial

names, personal names, or terms that are not included in the database's list of subject headings.

Some databases also have a feature called "mapping," which translates or maps your keywords into similar terms or concepts to yield more results. Once the database locates citations of articles on your topic, the titles and abstracts can help you decide whether the articles will be helpful in your research.

Many databases, such as MEDLINE/PubMed, allow searching by subject headings. The database sets what the subject headings are, which can normally be found in the database's *thesaurus*. Using the thesaurus will help you select the most effective subject term. Because a subject search only looks in one field of each record (the subject field), your search is more specific than a keyword search.

For example, in MEDLINE, subject headings are referred to as **MeSH Headings (Medical Subject Headings)**. Other databases may call them "descriptors." Creating your own subject headings may result in not getting the correct or complete results in your search. Review the approved subject headings that the database uses to get the most appropriate results.

Table 2.4 describes some of the differences, including advantages and disadvantages, of keyword and subject searching. They both have good points. You might want to start your search with keyword searching. Once you find some good articles, look for appropriate subject headings in them, and then turn to subject headings for more searching.

Using MEDLINE/PubMed

Evidenced-based practice in the field of dietetics begins with a thorough review of existing literature. MEDLINE was started in the 1960s as the National Library of Medicine (NLM) database and contains more than 22 million life sciences journal articles that date back to 1946. The NLM also houses more than 7 million books, technical reports, manuscripts, microfilms, photographs, and images. NLM is part of the National Institutes of Health, which is an agency within the United States Department of Health and Human Services.

The MEDLINE database encompasses citations from more than 5,600 journals published globally in 39 languages. Research journal articles must undergo approval from MEDLINE before being included in the database. Journal articles are submitted to the National Institute for Health (NIH) chartered advisory committee. The advisory committee appoints a Literature Selection Technical Review Committee (LSTRC), which reviews and approves journals for MEDLINE. The LSTRC is a quality review

Table 2.4 Comparing Searching by Keywords to Subject Headings

Searching by keywords	Searching by subject heading
You choose the keywords.	You need to use specific subject headings set by the database (usually in a thesaurus).
Database searches all fields for your keywords.	Database searches the subject field.
The results are less focused and include many irrelevant records.	The results are more focused and include more relevant records.
Most helpful when you are not sure where to start, or when you need to search with a keyword that is not a valid subject in the database.	Most useful once you have determined appropriate subject headings. When your get too many results, use subheadings to narrow your focus.

board that examines scientific content, originality, and relative importance to the scientific community. Only about 25% of the journal articles submitted to MEDLINE are chosen, and the selection process is based on the following criteria: quality, scope, content, and target audience.

MEDLINE is available free on the Internet through PubMed (www.ncbi.nlm.nih.gov/pubmed/) or through several vendors, such as Web of Knowledge.

PubMed is a global database that is monitored by the National Center for Biotechnology, a subset of the NLM. PubMed includes all of the articles you would get in MEDLINE, but you also get access to PubMed Central papers, which contain some open-access articles and also articles that have not yet been indexed by MeSH headings. In other words, publishers submitted these articles "ahead of print." MEDLINE searches are comprehensive and capture approximately 89% of the total available PubMed citations. The remaining 11% of the citations include the most current research, and for this reason a comprehensive search should include both MEDLINE and PubMed or another database.

MeSH (Medical Subject Headings) is an online thesaurus created and maintained by the NLM for indexing and filtering medical journals using a controlled vocabulary. MeSH provides a consistent way to retrieve information for similar concepts. When an article is submitted to the NLM, subject analysts review each article and assign specific MeSH headings; typically 10 to 12 per citation. PubMed can then be searched using the specific MeSH headings. MeSH will also yield a "Scope Note," which defines the MeSH heading.

If you do a keyword search, PubMed takes your keywords and "maps" them to MeSH vocabulary to yield results. For example, if you enter the search term "low blood sugar," it will not only show results with these three words but will also include any articles that contain "hypoglycemia." In the "Search Details" box on the right, you will see all the terms it is using to search. The search for "low blood sugar" yields over 35,000 records—way too many! Be sure to use the "Filters" on the left to narrow down the types of studies you get.

The most effective way to get good search results with PubMed or MEDLINE is to use the MeSH database (a link is on the home page) to narrow down your search terms. Let's say you want to do a search related to heart attacks and diet. If you enter "cardiovascular" into the MeSH database, you will get some suggested MeSH terms to use such as "cardiovascular drugs" or "cardiovascular diseases." By selecting "cardiovascular diseases," which is a MeSH term, we get the following information:

1. A definition of cardiovascular diseases.
2. The subheadings for cardiovascular diseases (almost 70, from abnormalities to diet therapy to virology). At this point, if you want articles just on one or more of the subheadings, you can click boxes and do your search, or simply enter heading/subheading into the PubMed search box (such as Cardiovascular disease/Diet therapy). In any case, seeing the subheadings will help you narrow down your search. Diet therapy is often a subheading under a disease.
3. It also tells you the "Entry Terms" for cardiovascular diseases, such as "diseases, cardiovascular." If you enter "diseases, cardiovascular" into the PubMed search box, it will also search for the MeSH term "cardiovascular diseases."
4. MeSH headings are organized in a hierarchical structure, much like a tree with 16 main branches. Two of the branches are "Anatomy" and "Diseases." Of course cardiovascular diseases are classified under "Diseases" as shown in **Figure 2.1**. (Note that some MeSH terms are found in more than one branch of the tree).

Diseases
- Cardiovascular Diseases
  - Cardiovascular Abnormalities
    - Heart Defects, Congenital*
    - Vascular Malformations*
  - Cardiovascular Infections
    - Endocarditis, Bacterial*
    - Syphilis, Cardiovascular
    - Tuberculosis, Cardiovascular*
  - Heart Diseases
    - Heart arrest*
    - Heart failure*
    - Myocardial ischemia*
    - Plus over 20 more diseases
  - Pregnancy Complications, Cardiovascular
    - Embolism, Amniotic Fluid
  - Vascular Diseases
    - Aneurysm*
    - Hypertension*
    - Varicose veins*
    - Plus over 40 more diseases

An entry with an asterisk (*) means that there is a further hierarchy below that term. So, for example, if you click on "Hypertension," six categories are listed: malignant, pregnancy-induced, white coat, and three more.

FIGURE 2.1 MeSH Hierarchy for "Cardiovascular Diseases"

Modified from MeSH Database by U.S. National Library of Medicine, 2016. Retrieved from http://www.ncbi.nlm.nih.gov/mesh/?term=cardiovascular+diseases

With the MeSH database, you can use the subheadings and also the hierarchical structure to help you narrow down your search. The higher up the hierarchy your MeSH term is, the more results will show up in your searches (way too many results!) because your searches will include all the terms BELOW it in the hierarchy (unless you click the box that says "Do not include MeSH terms found below this term in the MeSH hierarchy." So if you are really looking for heart attack, use "heart arrest." A subheading under "heart arrest" is "diet therapy," so enter "heart arrest/diet therapy" in the search box.

To narrow down your search, also use the "Filters" on the left side of the "Search Results" page. You can filter by the types of articles, text availability, publication dates, and species (human or other animals). The filters are *very* helpful.

Here are some tips to get the most out of your PubMed search if you are using keywords.

1. *Enter phrases using double quotation marks only if you want to yield an exact match. For example, "Cerebrovascular Accident."*
   This will ensure your results yield an exact match for the phrase entered. If you choose not to use quotation marks, the search will be broadened and will yield results for comparable terminology such as a stroke.
2. *Avoid truncation.*

Truncation is the act of shortening a word and searching for all terms that begin with a specific string of text. For example, one might search for "cardio," which would yield numerous matches including cardiovascular, cardiogenic, and cardiomyopathy. Truncation is generally not recommended when using PubMed because the search will bypass automatic term mapping and yield far too many results. PubMed uses the asterisk symbol (*) for truncation, and it is sometimes referred as the "wildcard." For example, if one were to enter, Cardi*, PubMed would yield multiple results including cardiology, cardiovascular, cardiomyopathy, cardiopulmonary, and cardiogenic.

3. *Utilize and capitalize all Boolean operators.*
   The Boolean operators are simple words including AND, OR, NOT. They help to make a search more precise and, more important, save you time. Using AND, will help to narrow your search by telling the database that all keywords must be found. Using OR will broaden your search by telling the database that it only needs to match with one of the words in your search. Using NOT will narrow your search for combinations that you do not want to yield results. Let's take a look at an example for a search on food allergy to milk.

Food **AND** Milk **AND** Allergies	Food **OR** Milk **OR** Allergies	Food **AND** Milk **AND** Allergies **NOT** Intolerances

   When OR was used, the number of results exploded.
4. *Do not use acronyms or abbreviations.*
   Although PubMed can recognize some medical abbreviations, many will not be identified in your search. For this reason, it is best to avoid all abbreviations and spell out the words. For example, use "Hypertension" as opposed to "HTN."
5. *Identify important concepts in your research to help you identify search words.*
   Before starting your search, it is important to state your research question. For example, if your research was "To identify the prevalence of milk protein allergies in children 18 years and under," you could use the following keywords or phrases to help narrow your search: "Allergy AND Milk AND Children AND Prevalence."
6. *Avoid multiple search terms to avoid minimal results.*
   Generally speaking, PubMed searches will be narrowed based on the number of search terms entered. For this reason, avoid using too many search terms as you run the risk of yielding little to no matches. For example, if you were researching the prevalence of milk protein allergies in children 18 years and under, you would not want to use all of these search terms: Food AND Allergy AND Milk AND Protein AND Children AND Prevalence AND Pediatrics.
7. *Avoid using search terms that are not precise.*
   Common words that might not be used consistently in research should be avoided to yield more matches. Some examples of words to avoid include *increased, decreased, better, worse, less*, and *greater*. Using the milk protein allergy example, just by adding the search term "Increased" in front of "Prevalence" would greatly narrow your results.
8. *If searching for research outside the United States, use geographic MeSH tags.*
   When searching for research outside the United States, use geographic MeSH tags if you are searching for a specific region, such as Europe, Africa, or Asia.
9. *Avoid using prepositions in your search.*
   Prepositions are parts of speech not recognized by PubMed that will limit your search. Examples include *during, excluding, until, versus*, and *besides*.

10. *Use the filters.*
    Use the "Filters" on the left side of the "Search Results" page. You can filter by the types of articles, text availability, publication dates, and species (human or other animals).

Using Google Scholar

When using Google Scholar, keep in mind that it is a multidisciplinary search engine. It brings up a lot of sources that are *not* journal articles, such as conference proceedings, books, technical reports, and so on. Google Scholar searches complete articles (unlike PubMed), so your search results are usually quite large. This can come in handy if you are searching for a detail that would not surface in a PubMed search. Search results are normally given by relevance, but you can get them by date. For comparison, PubMed also can search by relevance or date.

If you use Google Scholar, keep the following two things in mind:

1. Click on the down arrow in the search box to refine your search.
2. Use another database in addition to Google Scholar because you are likely to miss some key articles using just Google Scholar. For instance, PubMed has many features to get good search results and tends to be more precise.

Using Other Databases

Some other databases can be helpful, depending on your topic. AGRICOLA, the Cochrane Database of Systematic Reviews and ERIC are available online to anyone. The others are available through college libraries.

- *AGRICOLA (Agricultural Online Access)* is a comprehensive online database established in 1970 and maintained by the U.S. Department of Agriculture (USDA). This database catalogs research from the National Agriculture Library (NAL) encompassing animal and veterinary sciences, entomology, plant sciences, forestry, aquaculture and fisheries, farming and farming systems, agricultural economics, extension and education, food and human nutrition, and earth and environmental sciences. Using the NAL catalog (AGRICOLA), start your search by entering keywords into the "Articles" box. Advanced search options are available.
- *CINAHL (Cumulative Index of Nursing and Allied Health)* is an online database for nurses and allied health professionals. The database offers complete indexing for nursing journals printed in the English language. The database includes journals related to nursing, biomedicine, health sciences librarianship, alternative/complementary medicine, consumer health, and 17 other allied health disciplines. You can use keywords or subject headings. Their subject headings sometimes overlap with MeSH headings. When entering your search terms, click on "Suggest Subject Terms" to get subject headings.
- *Cochrane Database of Systematic Reviews (CDSR)* is a quarterly publication of the Cochrane Library and was formed by the Cochrane Collaboration in 1993 and named after a British epidemiologist, Archie Cochrane. The Cochrane Collaboration is a nonprofit organization committed to providing accurate global health information to the public. The Cochrane database contains a collection of systematic reviews of health care (you can browse by topic) and clinical trials (you can search by keywords or MeSH terms).
- *ERIC* contains articles in education and related topics from more than 750 professional journals.

- *Food Science and Technology Abstracts (FSTA)* is a database updated weekly with articles on food science, including food technology, biotechnology, human nutrition, and toxicology.
- *PsycINFO* is a database of roughly 2,000 peer-reviewed journals related to behavioral sciences and mental health published by the American Psychological Association, the APA Educational Publishing Foundation, the Canadian Psychological Association, and Hogrefe Publishing Group. The database is mostly utilized by professionals in related fields such as psychiatric professionals.

APPLICATION 2.4

Go to your library or its website and look for a guide for students in nutrition. Most college libraries have an online guide for the library resources specific to nutrition. Use library resources to write up a list of databases that are useful for nutrition students *and* explain how to get full-text journal articles. Do a tutorial for one of the databases to help you obtain appropriate journal articles.

CHECKLIST FOR SELECTING ARTICLES

Here are some guidelines for selecting appropriate articles.

1. *Make sure you choose the type of article that your professor has requested.* In most cases, you will be looking for original research articles from scientific journals. If so, did the authors of the article you picked perform a research study? Does the article include an abstract, research objective or hypothesis, methods, results, tables/charts, and references? Be careful not to choose a review article, in which many research studies are discussed, when you need an original research article (also called a primary research article). If you do want a review article, you can check the filter for a review article on PubMed, and only review articles will then show up in your search results.
2. *Be selective about the date the research was published.* In research areas where quite a bit of research has been performed, it is best to select the most recent studies. Make sure the date of the studies you pick meet the requirements your professor has set.
3. *Most original research studies are at least five pages long and include an abstract.* If your search yielded an interesting abstract, just make sure the abstract is not simply from a conference session or poster.
4. *Be sure the study is directly relevant to your topic.* To do this, read the introduction to the research article as it explains the problem and the purpose of the study. The abstract can be very dense, so read the introduction for the bigger picture first.
5. *Use more than one database to find articles*, and use the advanced search guidelines for each database.
6. *Talk to the Reference Librarian or your professor* if you need help to broaden or narrow your search.

TIP

If you spend time selecting appropriate articles for your topic, you will be able to use some of the references mentioned in those article (and listed under References) for additional research on your topic.

APPLICATION 2.5

You are looking for articles about the relationship between hypertension and sodium. The amount of research in this area is huge, so you first want to select some review articles. Here are some search results. Which article will be most useful and why? What makes each of the other articles undesirable?

Pharmacological effect of functional foods with a hypotensive action. Hieda K, Sunagawa Y, Katanasaka Y, Hasegawa K, Morimoto T. *Nihon Yakurigaku Zasshi.* 2015 Jul;146(1):33–39. doi: 10.1254/fpj.146.33. Review. No abstract available.

Absence of an effect of high nitrate intake from beetroot juice on blood pressure in treated hypertensive individuals: a randomized controlled trial. Bondonno CP, Liu AH, Croft KD, Ward NC, Shinde S, Moodley Y, Lundberg JO, Puddey IB, Woodman RJ, Hodgson JM. *Am J Clin Nutr.* 2015 Aug;102(2):368–375. doi: 10.3945/ajcn.114.101188. Epub 2015 Jul 1.

Dietary Approaches to stop hypertension diet retains effectiveness to reduce blood pressure when lean pork is substituted for chicken and fish as the predominant source of protein. Sayer RD, Wright AJ, Chen N, Campbell WW. *Am J Clin Nutr.* 2015 Aug;102(2):302–308. doi: 10.3945/ajcn.115.111757. Epub 2015 Jun 10.

Start of the salt reduction campaign. Hubert M. *MMW Fortschr Med.* 2015 Apr 16;157(7):74. doi: 10.1007/s15006-015-2985-6. German. No abstract available.

Sodium intake and cardiovascular health: A review. O'Donnell M, Mente A, Yusuf S. *Circ Res.* 2015 Mar 13;116(6):1046–1057. doi: 10.1161/CIRCRESAHA.116.303771.

PRINCIPLES OF SCIENTIFIC WRITING

Scientific writing is a vehicle to communicate scientific knowledge with members of the medical community and academia. Interpreting research and writing effective articles is difficult and time-consuming, that challenges even the most highly accomplished person. Learning to read, interpret, and write effective articles poses a significant challenge for many students.

Here are some guidelines for writing a research paper or simply writing about scientific studies you have read.

1. *Scientific writing is very business-like; it is organized, professional, unemotional, and practical.* This is not the time to use your creative writing techniques or to talk about yourself. Until you are well versed in reading and critiquing studies, you will not be giving many opinions. Write in an *objective* manner; in other words, avoid using "I."
2. *Even though scientific writing may seem wordy and complex, keep it simple with short sentences and keep the subject and verb together.* Avoid starting sentences with long clauses and phrases.
3. *Limit one thought to each paragraph, and tie your paragraphs together so they flow.* Use transitional sentences between paragraphs so readers can follow your train of thought.
4. *Use the active voice most often, and pick good action verbs to convey meaning.* Although the passive voice sounds scientific, use the active voice more often because it is easier to read.
5. *Write concisely and omit needless words.*
6. *Before you start on your rough draft, carefully read everything and write some notes or an outline to help you through the rough draft.* Some students (and authors) want to write

perfect copy when they start typing on the computer, but no one can do that, not even the best. Some people think they can read and write at the same time. but you should have done a lot of reading and thinking before you even start the rough draft (otherwise you will get frustrated quickly!). Also, be prepared to write a really rough and tumble draft the first time.

7. *Then revise and edit*, because relying 100% on your spell and grammar checkers is no guarantee of a good grade. Ask a close friend to read your draft and give you feedback.
8. *Finally, but possibly most important, is to use your own words.* If you want to use something you read in your writing as is, that's fine; be sure to put it in quotation marks and write up the appropriate reference. Be careful, though, that you don't use too much quoted material. What the professor wants to read is what *you* have to say about a topic.

TIP

Don't assume that you can cut and paste material that you find online into your writing without using quotation marks and a footnote/reference. *Assume* that online materials are copyrighted and that anything you use in your paper that is not original will be picked up by a plagiarism checker such as Turnitin.

RESEARCHER INTERVIEW Bioactive Compounds in Fruits and Vegetables

Joan G. Fischer, PhD, RDN
Professor, Department of Foods and Nutrition, University of Georgia, Athens, GA

1. **Briefly describe the areas in which you do research.**
   Many bioactive compounds found in fruits and vegetables may contribute to lower risk for a number of chronic diseases. My research has examined the mechanisms through which polyphenols may reduce disease processes, with the primary area of focus being the effect of these compounds on oxidative stress and inflammation. We have studied both isolated polyphenolic compounds and whole foods.

   A second component of our work bridges the laboratory and the consumer. Being able to communicate the health benefits of fruit and vegetable intake to the community is essential. Thus, we have participated in studies that assess knowledge of recommendations for fruit and vegetable intake among older adults and have assisted with development and evaluation of interventions to increase healthy eating behaviors.
2. **With your experience researching bioactive plant compounds, what would students find compelling about this area of research?**
   Although epidemiological and clinical studies suggest that higher intakes of fruits and vegetables are associated with lower risk for some chronic diseases, there is still much work to be done to determine which compounds in plant foods provide health benefits. Further, developing an understanding of how the bioactive components in fruits and vegetables protect against disease development has opened up a whole field of new research opportunities. Our most recent work focuses on the role of anthocyanins and high anthocyanin foods on health. Anthocyanins are the blue and red pigments found in plant foods such as berries. Similar to work by others, we have shown that anthocyanins have antioxidant effects and may not only act directly as antioxidants, but may also act indirectly by affecting antioxidant enzyme activities.

Even though many polyphenols such as anthocyanins are thought of primarily as antioxidants, they have many other roles that may affect chronic disease development. For example, some of these compounds can influence cell proliferation and cellular apoptosis, which suggests a possible role in cancer prevention. We have found that blueberry polyphenolic extracts and isolated anthocyanins can alter cell proliferation and apoptosis of colon cancer cells in culture. Anthocyanins and anthocyanin-containing foods also have anti-inflammatory effects. Thus, we are currently studying the effect of blueberry supplementation on biomarkers of intestinal, systemic, and adipose tissue inflammation and oxidative stress in a rodent model of obesity. Further, because new research suggests that changes in intestinal microbiota may affect not only gastrointestinal health but also may be related to obesity-related inflammation and insulin resistance, we are examining the impact of blueberry supplementation on intestinal microbiota to determine whether this is associated with changes in intestinal health, systemic inflammation, and glucose tolerance.

In addition to studying possible mechanisms through which anthocyanins and other polyphenolic compounds can affect health, there are other interesting areas of research that are key to understanding a food's potential impact. Identifying the possible bioactive components in a food is a necessary first step for this type of research. Bioactive composition of many plant foods is dependent on cultivar and growing conditions. One of our first studies with blueberries was in collaboration with food scientists to assess the anthocyanin composition of several blueberry cultivars and determine whether this could result in different effects on cell proliferation.

Determining whether it is specific bioactives or the whole food that is necessary for disease prevention is also a key question for researchers in this area. Similar to others, we have found that the effects of isolated phytochemicals, such as isolated anthocyanins, can differ from that of a whole food or extract containing multiple components.

3. **Is some of your research considered basic research?**
Yes, much of my research is considered basic research. Our laboratory group examines the impact of anthocyanins or anthocyanin-containing foods on body composition, tissue morphology, biomarkers of oxidative stress, enzyme activity, and gene expression in rodent models. Some of our work has focused on the impact of anthocyanins on cell proliferation and apoptosis of cancer cells in culture. This type of research is important to the understanding of how these compounds function in cells and why they may affect disease risk. Although we have predominantly conducted research in animal and cell culture models, many of the assays we conduct are also used in human clinical studies.

4. **What do you enjoy most about the research process?**
I enjoy research because there is always something new to learn, whether it is from studies conducted by others or from work in our own laboratory. Research never becomes routine, and gaining an understanding of how foods influence health is fascinating. I also enjoy working with teams of colleagues and students to solve research problems. Everyone brings different perspectives and expertise to the discussion, which often generates new areas of research. Finally, helping graduate students identify a research question and carry out that research is very rewarding.

SUMMARY

1. Scientific journals present research studies to further the progress of science. Most are specialized for a certain discipline or subdiscipline. Many, but not all, journals use peer review to ensure that what they publish is accurate, meets their standards, and advances the knowledge base. Trade magazines or publications are not journals. They include informational articles but not original research articles that describe a single study (quantitative or qualitative) written by the researchers who conducted the research.

2. In a peer-reviewed journal, research articles must be accepted and pass review before being published.
3. Each issue of *JAND* is split into three sections: "Practice Applications," "Research," and "From the Academy." The "Practice Applications" section normally has a message from the president, Letters to the Editor, and a few articles about new or emerging topics of interest to RDNs, such as informatics, a new scientific advancement, or even a nutrition-related case study. "From the Academy" includes news from the professional association as well as Academy Position or Practice Papers.
4. In *JAND*, the research section includes original research (also called primary research), research editorials, and three types of review articles: narrative reviews (an evaluation and summary of evidence from many studies in a research area), systematic reviews (a more rigorous review that usually uses a statistical technique called meta-analysis, which combines the results of a number of independent studies into a single result), and Evidence Analysis Library Reviews (also systematic reviews, but they may not use meta-analysis). Review articles are categorized as secondary research.
5. Gray literature (not found in journals) include dissertations and theses, conference proceedings, books, technical reports, and commentaries/opinion pieces.
6. You can use a number of different databases to search for journal articles. Google Scholar is not technically a database; it is a search engine of the Internet as it is created by a computer. MEDLINE/PubMed, Web of Science, Scopus, and Science Direct are all curated by people.
7. Table 2.4 compares searching by keywords or subject headings. Some databases have their own dictionary of subject terms you can use for your search. Start your search with keyword searching. Once you find some good articles, look for appropriate subject headings in them, and then use the subject headings in a new search.
8. For best results using PubMed/MEDLINE, use the MeSH database to identify appropriate search terms that are not too broad in scope. Also use the filters. Tips are given to get the most out of a PubMed search.
9. Other databases include AGRICOLA (public), Cochrane Database of Systematic Reviews (public), CINAHL (private index for nursing and allied health), ERIC (public index for education), Food Science and Technology Abstracts (private database for food science), and PsycINFO (private database for psychology).
10. When selecting articles, make sure you choose the type your professor has requested and be sure the article is relevant. Be selective about the research date, and make sure any abstract has a research study to go with it. Use more than one database to find articles, and talk to the Reference Librarian when you need help.
11. Use the eight guidelines for scientific writing.

REVIEW QUESTIONS

1. Which of the following is a source of original research?
   A. *Today's Dietitian*
   B. *FoodService Director*
   C. *International Journal of Obesity*
   D. *Washington Post*
   E. a and c
2. Which of the following is an example of secondary research?
   A. original research
   B. editorial
   C. commentary
   D. review articles
3. Which type of review article is more rigorous?
   A. narrative review
   B. systematic review
   C. primary review article
   D. a and b
4. Which type of review article uses a statistical technique called a meta-analysis?
   A. narrative review
   B. systematic review

C. primary review article
D. a and b

5. Gray literature includes which of the following?
A. dissertations
B. books
C. technical reports from the CDC
D. all of the above

6. When is it advantageous to do a keyword search? When is it more advantageous to do a subject search?

7. Which nutrition-related databases can you access at your college?

8. Which search will give you more results: "constipation AND fiber" or "constipation OR fiber"? How else will the results be different?

9. Three of these terms are MeSH terms. Identify the two terms that are not MeSH terms: saturated fatty acid, prebiotics, breast milk, inflammatory bowel disease, vegetables.

10. Select a nutrition topic and first do a keyword search using MEDLINE/PubMed. Next use the MeSH database to help formulate search terms and narrow down the search. Compare the number of records, or hits, you got from each search.

11. Why is it important to use more than one database when doing a search?

12. Describe three ways in which scientific writing is different from many of the essays you have written in school.

CRITICAL THINKING QUESTIONS

1. Read this study and answer the questions that follow. Schultz, D., Shanks, C., & Houghtaling, B. (2015). The impact of the 2009 Special Supplemental Nutrition Program for Women, Infants, and Children food package revisions on participants: A systematic review. *Journal of the Academy of Nutrition and Dietetics,* 115, 1832-1846. doi: 10.1016/j.jand.2015.06.381
   A. Why was this study done? In other words, define the problem(s).
   B. In your own words, what was the purpose of the study.
   C. Which databases did the researchers use to find appropriate articles?
   D. Name three criteria the researchers used to determine which articles they would use in the meta-analysis.
   E. How many articles met the study criteria?
   F. Briefly state the results of the three arms of this study.

2. **Study Summary**: The purpose of this research was to examine studies on the effect of low-carbohydrate and low-fat diets on weight and cardiovascular disease risk. The authors found 17 randomized control trials that met their criteria for their meta-analysis. Results showed that each diet was associated with significant weight loss and reduction in cardiovascular disease risk (Mansoor, Vinknes, Veierod, & Retterstol, 2015).
   1. Is the study primary or secondary research?
   2. Is the study a narrative or systematic review?
   3. Is the study a conference proceeding?

3. **Study Summary**: The objective of the study was to test whether adding a dietitian to a hospital discharge team for geriatric patients would improve the nutritional status of those patients over 6 months. Geriatric patients were randomly assigned to either the regular discharge team or the discharge team with the dietitian. All patients were at least 70 years old and determined to be at nutritional risk. The dietitian gave each discharged patient three home visits within 8 weeks of discharge. Nutritional status was measured using weight, muscle strength, and other measures. Adding a dietitian to the discharge team did improve the nutritional status of geriatric patients (Beck et al., 2015).
   1. Is the study primary or secondary research?

2. Is the study a narrative or systematic review?
3. Is the study a conference proceeding?

4. **Study Summary:** This study was found in a journal, but only contained an abstract. The authors measured the prevalence of freshmen college students at risk for eating disorders as well as the prevalence of disordered eating. The study took place at a large public state university. There were 358 participants, 17% of whom were at risk for disordered eating (Woodhall, Gordon, Caine-Bish, & Falcone, 2015).
   1. Is the study original research (primary research)?
   2. Is the study a narrative or systematic review?
   3. Is the study a conference proceeding?

5. **Study Summary**: The aim of this study was to review the studies on the relationship between sodium intake and cardiovascular health. Various types of studies were included in the review. They found gaps in the literature and suggested ideas for further research (O'Donnell, Mente, & Yusuf, 2015).
   1. Is the study original research (primary research)?
   2. Is the study a narrative or systematic review?
   3. Is the study a conference proceeding?

SUGGESTED READINGS AND ACTIVITIES

1. Read this article on using PubMed. McKeever, L., Nguyen V., Peterson, S. J., Gomez-Perez, S., & Braunschweig, C. (2015). Demystifying the search button: A comprehensive PubMed search strategy for performing an exhaustive literature review. *Journal of Parenteral and Enteral Nutrition, 39*, 622–635. doi: 10.1177/0148607115593791
2. Do the PubMed tutorial and/or the Quick Tour videos.
3. Do the tutorial for another database that you will be using.

REFERENCES

Academy of Nutrition and Dietetics. (2015). *About EAL.* Retrieved from https://www.andeal.org/study-designs

Academy Quality Management Committee and Scope of Practice Subcommittee of the Quality Management Committee. (2013). Academy of Nutrition and Dietetics: Revised 2012 Standards of Practice in Nutrition Care and Standards of Professional Performance for Registered Dietitians. *Journal of the Academy of Nutrition and Dietetics, 113*, S29–S45. doi: 10.1016/j.jand.2012.12.007

Beck, A., Andersen, U., Leedo, E., Jensen, L., Martins, K., Quvang, M., . . . Ronholt, F. (2015). Does adding a dietician to the liaison team after discharge of geriatric patients improve nutritional outcome: A randomized controlled trial. *Clinical Rehabilitation, 29*, 1117–1128. doi: 10.1177/0269215514564700

Björk, B., & Solomon, D. (2012). Open access versus subscription journals: A comparison of scientific impact. *BMC Medicine, 10*, 73, 1-10.

de Mol, P., de Vries, S., de Koning, E., Gans, R., Bilo, H., & Tack, C. (2014). Physical activity at altitude: Challenges for people with diabetes. *Diabetes Care, 37*, 2404–2413. doi: 10.2337/dc13-2302

Douglas, J. W., & Lawrence, J. C. (2015). Environmental considerations for improving nutritional status in older adults with dementia: A narrative review. *Journal of the Academy of Nutrition and Dietetics, 115*, 1815–1831. doi: 10.1016/j.jand.2015.06.376

Gaesser, G. A., & Angadi, S. S. (2012). Gluten-free diet: Imprudent diet advice for the general population? *Journal of the Academy of Nutrition and Dietetics, 112*, 1330–1333. doi: 10.1016/j.jand.2012.06.009

He, X., Zhu, M., Hu., C., Tao, X., Li, Y., Wang, Q., & Liu, Y. (2015). Breast-feeding and postpartum weight retention: A systematic review and meta-analysis. *Public Health Nutrition, 18*, 3308–3316. doi: 10.1017/S1368980015000828

Hurt, R., McClave, S., Evans, D., Jones, C., Miller, K., Frazier, T., . . . Franklin, G. (2015). Targeted physician education positively affects delivery of nutrition therapy and patient outcomes: Results of a prospective clinical trial. *Journal of Parenteral & Enteral Nutrition, 39*, 948–952. doi: 10.1177/0148607114540332

Mansoor, N., Vinknes, K, Veierod, M., & Retterstol, K. (2015). Effects of low-carbohydrate v. low-fat diets on body weight and cardiovascular risk factors: A meta-analysis of randomized controlled trials. *British Journal of Nutrition*. Advance online publication. doi: 10.1017/S0007114515004699

McKeever, L., Nguyen V., Peterson, S. J., Gomez-Perez, S., & Braunschweig, C. (2015). Demystifying the search button: A comprehensive PubMed search strategy for performing an exhaustive literature review. *Journal of Parenteral & Enteral Nutrition, 39*, 622–635. doi: 10.1177/0148607115593791

O'Donnell, M., Mente, A., & Yusuf, S. (2015). Sodium intake and cardiovascular health. *Circulation Research, 116*, 1046–1057. doi: 10.1161/CIRCRESAHA.116.303771

Pérez-Rodrigo, C., & Tseng, M. (2013). Are dietary guidelines sensible to consumers? *Public Health Nutrition, 16*, 761–762. doi:10.1017/S136898001300089X

Schultz, D., Shanks, C., & Houghtaling, B. (2015). The impact of the 2009 Special Supplemental Nutrition Program for Women, Infants, and Children food package revisions on participants: A systematic review. *Journal of the Academy of Nutrition and Dietetics, 115*, 1832–1846. doi: 10.1016/j.jand.2015.06.381

Woodhall., A. Gordon, K., Caine-Bish, N., & Falcone, T. (2015). The risk and prevalence of disordered eating behaviors in freshmen college students. *Journal of the Academy of Nutrition and Dietetics, 115*, A32.

CHAPTER 3

Ethics in Nutrition Research

CHAPTER OUTLINE

- Introduction
- History of Research Ethics
- Responsible Conduct of Research
- Ethics and Human Subjects Research
- Institutional Review Boards
- Researcher Interview: Management Research, Dr. Carol W. Shanklin

LEARNING OUTCOMES

- Discuss the important events leading to current ethical principles and guidelines in research and why ethical standards in research are important.
- Give examples of responsible conduct of research and research misconduct.
- Describe three ways in which conflict of interest can get in the way of ethical research.
- Describe seven principles underlying ethical human subjects research and identify principles in the ADA/CDR Code of Ethics that relate to these principles.
- Explain the process of informed consent and the impact of the Privacy Rule on researchers.
- Explain the purposes of Institutional Review Boards, where they are found, who are members of IRBs, and what they do.
- Distinguish between exempt, expedited, and full board/complete reviews.

INTRODUCTION

Ethics is often defined as norms for conduct that describe acceptable and unacceptable behavior. Many disciplines and professions (such as the Academy of Nutrition and Dietetics [AND]) have their own code of ethics to guide their members and establish the public's trust. Ethical conduct in research, or research ethics, is a specialized discipline. According to Resnik (2015), having norms for conduct in research is very important.

1. *Ethics standards in research promote knowledge and avoid errors in the pursuit of knowledge.* Falsification and fabrication of data are considered research misconduct.
2. *Ethics standards in research promote collaborative work among researchers who are often from different disciplines and institutions.* Collaborative work requires values such as trust, fairness, and accountability. Ethics standards, such as guidelines on authorship for research articles and data sharing, are designed to promote collaboration while safeguarding intellectual property interests.
3. *Ethics norms in research, such as policies on conflicts of interest, help keep researchers accountable to the public*, and also encourage public funding of research.
4. *Ethics norms promote values such as human rights and compliance with regulations to help prevent ethical lapses in research*, which could harm human and animal participants.

As you can imagine, government agencies, hospitals, universities, and professional associations have adopted rules and policies related to research ethics.

The ethics guidelines in place today for research were primarily a response to past abuses, the most notorious of which in the United States was an experiment in Tuskegee, Alabama. In this infamous experiment, treatment was withheld from 400 African American men with syphilis in the mid 1900s so scientists could study the course of the disease. Various ethics guidelines were developed in response to such studies. Today, participants in research are protected in three ways (NIH, 2015):

1. *Ethics guidelines.* The purpose of ethics guidelines is both to protect patient volunteers and to preserve the integrity of the science.
2. *Informed consent.* Informed consent is a process of information exchange, not just a form, and the process continues after the participant agrees to take part in a study.
3. *IRB review.* Most, but not all, clinical trials in the United States are approved and monitored by an Institutional Review Board (IRB) to ensure that the risks are minimal and are worth any potential benefits. An IRB is an independent committee that consists of physicians, statisticians, and members of the community (such as a university or hospital) who ensure that clinical trials are ethical and that the rights of participants are protected.

These topics are discussed in some depth in this chapter because they are key pieces in research with human subjects.

This chapter begins with some history on research ethics and then discusses the responsible conduct of research, institutional review boards, and ethics in research involving human participants, including informed consent and privacy.

HISTORY OF RESEARCH ETHICS

Prior to World War II, there was no international guidance on conducting human subjects research. Around World War II, the amount of biomedical research grew in the United States. Human subjects were often institutionalized individuals who were not told all the facts about the study. Some people didn't even know they were in a study. At that time, one way to study infectious disease was to intentionally infect subjects with the pathogen. Understanding infectious diseases, such as syphilis (studied in Tuskegee), was important to the U.S. government because these diseases were taking a toll on the armed forces.

Unethical experiments were also performed by the Nazis before and during World War II. These abuses led to the **Nuremberg Code** (1949), which outlined ten principles for ethical biomedical research, including the following:

- Subjects' must voluntarily consent to be in the study.
- Subjects have the right to stop participating in a study.
- Subjects should be protected from unnecessary physical and mental suffering and injury, disability, and death.
- The benefits of the study will justify the costs.

The Nuremberg Code was the basis for the **Declaration of Helsinki** in 1964 by the World Medical Association. The Declaration of Helsinki describes ethics principles for medical research with human subjects and is a guide for physicians directing research. It has been amended seven times since 1964, and the current version (2013) is used by physicians and institutions conducting clinical research around the world. Here are some of its principles (World Medical Association [WMA] General Assembly, 2013):

- Medical research should, first and foremost, protect the health, well-being, and rights of human subjects.
- Physicians involved in a human subjects study must be sure that the risks have been adequately anticipated and can be managed in a satisfactory manner. The importance of the research objective must outweigh the risks.
- Medical research with a vulnerable group should only be done if it would benefit the health needs of this group and the research cannot be carried out in other groups that are not vulnerable.
- At the end of a study, efforts should be made to provide access to interventions (such as medicines) that have been proven effective in the study.

In the United States, the Public Health Service issued a policy requiring informed consent in research in 1966. In response to the mistreatment of human subjects in the Tuskegee study, Congress passed the National Research Act in 1974. The National Research Act created the National Commission for the Protection of Human Subjects of Biomedical and Behavioral Research, which was asked to draft ethics principles and guidelines for human subjects research.

The commission drafted the **Belmont Report** in 1979, which defined ethics principles for research including respect for persons, beneficence, and justice:

- *Respect for persons.* Individuals have the right to self-determination and to choose whether or not to participate in a research study.
- *Beneficence.* Individuals in a study should not be harmed, and researchers should minimize harms and maximize potential benefits.
- *Justice.* Individuals in a study should be treated fairly, and the benefits and risks should be distributed fairly.

In 1981, based on the Belmont Report, the Department of Health and Human Services (HHS) and the Food and Drug Administration (FDA) issued these regulations (U.S. DHHS, 2009; U.S. FDA, 2010a, 2010b), which guide almost all research in the United States.

- The HHS issued the *Code of Federal Regulations* Title 45, Part 46 (Protection of Human Subjects).
- The FDA issued the *Code of Federal Regulations* Title 21, Parts 50 (Protection of Human Subjects) and 56 (Institutional Review Board).

Part of the HHS regulations (Title 45, Part 46, Subpart A) just noted became what is known as the **Common Rule**, or the "Federal Policy for the Protection of Human Subjects," in 1991. The Common Rule has established core procedures to protect human research subjects, including the following:

1. Guidelines to ensure compliance by research institutions.
2. Guidelines for securing and documenting informed consent.
3. Guidelines for IRB operation.
4. Protections for vulnerable research participants such as pregnant women, children, and prisoners.

The Common Rule has been adopted and codified into regulations by 15 federal departments and agencies.

Many of the biomedical and behavioral studies in the United States are regulated by the HHS regulations (Title 45, Part 46, Protection of Human Subjects) or the FDA regulations (Title 21, Part 50, Protection of Human Subjects, and Part 56, Institutional Review Board). The FDA regulations cover, for example, clinical trials of new drugs. The HHS and FDA regulations are mostly similar.

APPLICATION 3.1

Go to this website (http://www.hhs.gov/ohrp/regulations-and-policy/regulations/45-cfr-46/index.html) to look at the HHS regulations: Title 45, Part 46, Protection of Human Subjects. You will see that part A, part of the Common Rule, is titled "Basic HHS Policy for Protection of Human Research Subjects." What are the titles for subparts B, C, D, and E?

RESPONSIBLE CONDUCT OF RESEARCH

All research, whether it involves human participants or not, is governed by certain ethics principles. In the United States, we call this the **Responsible Conduct of Research (RCR)**. According to the National Institutes of Health (NIH, 2009), RCR is "the practice of scientific investigation with integrity. It involves the awareness and application of established professional norms and ethics principles in the performance of all activities related to scientific research." The NIH, the National Science Foundation, and the U.S. Department of Agriculture require certain categories of researchers (including students) to receive RCR training.

Responsible Conduct of Research includes policies related to many facets of research:

- Policies regarding human subjects, live vertebrate animal subjects in research, and safe laboratory practices.
- Mentor and mentee responsibilities and relationships.
- Conflict of interest—personal, professional, and financial.
- Collaborative research including collaborations with industry.
- Peer review.
- Data acquisition and management.
- Research misconduct and policies for handling misconduct.
- Responsible authorship and publication.

Congress has enacted laws establishing the Office of Research Integrity (ORI) to promote integrity in biomedical and behavioral research supported by the U.S. Public

Health Service. The *ORI Introduction to the Responsible Conduct of Research* is an excellent online resource for the basics of responsible conduct, including the following key shared values:

1. "*Honesty*—conveying information truthfully and honoring commitments.
2. *Accuracy*—reporting findings precisely and taking care to avoid errors.
3. *Efficiency*—using resources wisely and avoiding waste.
4. *Objectivity*—letting the facts speak for themselves and avoiding improper bias." (Steneck, 2007, p. 3)

Integrity of research is not limited to these values.

Responsible Conduct of Research materials and courses are just one source of rules for the researcher. Other rules can be found in government regulations (federal and state), professional codes (such as the *AND Code of Ethics*), and institutional policies (such as those of universities or hospitals).

This section discusses conflict of interest and research misconduct. In addition, you should be aware that responsible authorship means that each author in a study should have made significant contributions to the paper and taken responsibility for certain section(s). More information on defining the role of authors and contributors can be found at the website of the International Committee of Medical Journal Editors.

APPLICATION 3.2

The Collaborative Institutional Training Initiative (CITI) at the University of Miami provides online ethics courses for researchers. Go to their website (www.citiprogram.org) and list three courses related to Responsible Conduct of Research.

Conflict of Interest

A conflict of interest is "a conflict between the private interests and the official or professional responsibilities of a person in a position of trust" (Merriam Webster, 2016). Unfortunately, a conflict of interest has the potential to compromise professional objectivity and judgment when conducting or reporting research. Every researcher has responsibilities to his or her employer as well as to the agencies that fund the research and publishers that publish the research. Dietetics practitioners also have responsibilities (as described in the Academy of Nutrition and Dietetics' *Code of Ethics*) to the public and the profession to provide accurate complete information, as well as responsibilities to clients, colleagues and other professionals.

Having a conflict of interest is not automatically bad or wrong. With all the competing responsibilities and demands on researchers, conflicts of interest are *not* unusual. However, researchers do need to make sure that conflicts in the following areas do not interfere with responsible, ethical research or harm the public in any way (Steneck, 2007).

1. *Financial conflicts*. Financial conflicts can occur in a number of ways. When you read a journal article, you may see a disclosure from one or more of the authors that they received funding from a corporation, such as a drug company or food manufacturer, to do the study. This does not make the article biased. You will need to read and critique the article like any other. Of course, if a researcher is not honest or accurate with a study's design, conduct, or reporting in order to receive (or continue to receive) such research funding, that is unethical conduct.

Anyone who wants to publish should first check to be sure he or she is compliant with a publication's conflict of interest policies, which may require disclosure of real or potential financial conflicts.

According to Steneck (2007), "While financial interests should not and in most instances do not compromise intellectual honest, they certainly can, especially if the financial interests are *significant*" (p. 69). Federal funding agencies such as the NIH and National Science Foundations have conflict of interest policies that spell out exactly what a **significant financial interest** is, as well as procedures for reporting and managing significant conflicts of interest. **Figure 3.1** defines a significant financial interest for institutions receiving NIH funding: basically whenever a researcher gets more than $5,000 a year in payment, including salary; payments for consulting, honoraria, and paid authorship; and/or equity (stock, etc.).

Researchers with significant financial interests must disclose them to the institution. A *financial conflict of interest* exists if the research institution feels that a researcher's significant financial interest can affect the design, conduct, or reporting of the NIH-funded research. If this happens, the institution will usually decide on an appropriate management plan to reduce, manage, or eliminate the conflict.

As of 1980, federal law allowed universities to let researchers benefit financially from work such as patents, as well as university-owned businesses based on researchers' ideas. Many universities have thrived with these changes, but sometimes they have created financial conflicts of interest.

2. *Conflict of commitment.* Researchers have many commitments that can create competing demands on their time. Most universities have policies on faculty responsibilities to students, teaching, advising, departmental and college activities,

The 2011 regulation defines a "Significant Financial Interest" as follows:

(1) A financial interest consisting of one or more of the following interests of the Investigator (and those of the Investigator's spouse and dependent children) that reasonably appears to be related to the Investigator's institutional responsibilities:

(i) With regard to any publicly traded entity, a significant financial interest exists if the value of any remuneration received from the entity in the twelve months preceding the disclosure and the value of any equity interest in the entity as of the date of disclosure, when aggregated, exceeds $5,000. For purposes of this definition, remuneration includes salary and any payment for services not otherwise identified as salary (e.g., consulting fees, honoraria, paid authorship); equity interest includes any stock, stock option, or other ownership interest, as determined through reference to public prices or other reasonable measures of fair market value;

(ii) With regard to any non-publicly traded entity, a significant financial interest exists if the value of any remuneration received from the entity in the twelve months preceding the disclosure, when aggregated, exceeds $5,000, or when the Investigator (or the Investigator's spouse or dependent children) holds any equity interest (e.g., stock, stock option, or other ownership interest); or

(iii) Intellectual property rights and interests (e.g., patents, copyrights), upon receipt of income related to such rights and interests."

FIGURE 3.1 2011 Financial Conflict of Interest (FCOI) Regulation for Institutions Receiving or Applying for National Institutes of Health (NIH) Funding

Reproduced from: "Financial Conflict of Interest" by the National Institutes of Health, 2014, Retrieved from http://grants.nih.gov/grants/policy/coi/index.htm.

mentoring and supervising research, and consulting for industry. For example, if a researcher wants to do some consulting, one university may not allow him or her to use university time or facilities, and may ask that the work not overlap with the researcher's university job. Another university may simply limit the number of days per year that the researcher can do consulting.

To avoid conflicts of commitment, researchers need to honor time commitments to each of their activities. Since grants typically pay a percentage of a researcher's salary, researchers need to put in the appropriate time, and be careful that they do not charge two sources of funding for the same time. Rules for consulting need to be adhered to, and researchers should seek appropriate guidance when uncertain about spending time on a certain activity.

Likewise, a healthcare-based nutritionist doing research in addition to another set of duties needs to review and abide by pertinent policies and secure permission from appropriate personnel as required.

3. *Personal and intellectual conflicts*. Personal conflicts are, for example, when you review articles for a scientific journal and you are asked to review an article that a good friend of yours coauthored. This conflict of interest can easily be resolved (ask the editor to get another reviewer for that article). Most journals and granting agencies require reviewers to disclose conflict of interest to avoid this situation.

   Intellectual conflicts are not as obvious. An intellectual conflict of interest occurs when an individual's judgment on a research topic is biased because he or she has a strong attachment to a specific point of view. This can be a real problem when researchers do research or act as advisors or expert witnesses.

Funding agencies, publishers, hospitals and other healthcare institutions, and research institutions have conflict of interest policies. At places of work, conflict of interest must be reported, and then managed as appropriate by, for example, requiring full disclosure, monitoring the research, removing the researcher from certain steps in the research process, or eliminating the conflict (Steneck, 2007).

Several principles in the "Code of Ethics for the Profession of Dietetics" (American Dietetic Association/Commission on Dietetic Registration [ADA/CDR], 2009) are pertinent to this discussion on conflict of interest for researchers (**Table 3.1**). Principle 15 speaks directly about conflict of interests, but the other principles noted are also relevant.

Table 3.1 Principles Pertinent to Conflict of Interest from the "Code of Ethics for the Profession of Dietetics"
Principle 1 The dietetics practitioner conducts himself/herself with honesty, integrity, and fairness.
Principle 6 The dietetics practitioner does not engage in false or misleading practices or communications.
Principle 13 The dietetics practitioner presents reliable and substantiated information and interprets controversial information without personal bias, recognizing that legitimate differences of opinion exist.
Principle 15 The dietetics practitioner is alert to the occurrence of a real or potential conflict of interest and takes appropriate action whenever a conflict arises. a. The dietetics practitioner makes full disclosure of any real or perceived conflict of interest. b. When a conflict of interest cannot be resolved by disclosure, the dietetics practitioner takes such other action as may be necessary to eliminate the conflict, including recusal from an office, position, or practice situation.
Principle 18 The dietetics practitioner does not invite, accept, or offer gifts, monetary incentives, or other considerations that affect or reasonably give an appearance of affecting his/her professional judgment.

RESEARCH MISCONDUCT

Research misconduct is "fabrication, falsification, or plagiarism in proposing, performing, or reviewing research, or in reporting research results, and it does not include honest error or differences of opinion" (ORI, 2011). Here are definitions for these terms:

- **Fabrication** is making up data or results and recording or reporting them.
- **Falsification** is manipulating research materials, equipment, or processes, or changing or omitting data or results such that the research is not accurately represented in the research record.
- **Plagiarism** is the appropriation of another person's ideas, processes, results, or words without giving appropriate credit. (Steneck, 2007, p. 21)

Many research institutions have adopted these federal policies on misconduct to cover all research being done at the facilities, and in some cases, they have included additional misconduct guidelines.

In their policies, research institutions must provide a method for individuals to report possible misconduct, procedures to investigate allegations, and the actions that could be taken. To find someone guilty of research misconduct in accordance with federal regulations, what the researcher did must be a "significant departure from accepted practices, the misconduct be committed intentionally, knowingly, or reckless; and the allegation be proven by a preponderance of the evidence" (NIH, 2010). In some cases, such as when public health or safety is at risk, findings of research misconduct are reported to federal agencies such as the Office of Research Integrity and the funding agency.

ETHICS AND HUMAN SUBJECTS RESEARCH

Human subjects research, according to federal regulations, is a research involving a living individual about whom a researcher conducting research obtains data

1. through an intervention,
2. through an interaction with the individual, or
3. by identifiable private information.

Human subjects research forms the evidence base used to develop the practice guidelines practitioners use when making nutrition care decisions for patients/clients. Practice guidelines also have a direct impact on third party payer reimbursement for medical nutrition therapy and public policy in dietetics practice.

If research involving humans exploits people or in some other way is unethical, then researchers will have a hard time finding subjects to take part in studies, and this can slow down the development of new treatments. Emanuel, Wendler, and Grady (2000) proposed seven requirements for evaluating whether a human subjects research study is ethical.

1. *Social value.* The study should help researchers determine how to improve people's health or well-being. Research can do this directly by providing results that lead to better tests and treatments for disease. Research can also help indirectly, by generating information that increases understanding and guides future research. If the research does not help in either of these ways, it wastes money and resources. Most important, it is unethical to put people at risk of harm or even discomfort when neither they nor society can benefit.
2. *Scientific validity.* It is only fair to ask people to donate their time and take risks for research that is scientifically valid. This means a research study must be carefully planned to answer a specific question. There should be a hypothesis to be tested, a

control, and controlled variables when appropriate. No experiment is 100% valid, but researchers should design their experiments to be as good as possible.

3. *Fair subject selection.* Researchers should use fair subject selection; that is, they should be fair in both recruiting and deciding which people can be in the study. The goal of this practice is to be fair both to the people who might be subjects and to those who might benefit from the treatment or method being studied. All different kinds of people are needed to participate in research. It is not fair to only use people who are easy to talk into participating, such as past cases when researchers used prisoners because they were easy to recruit. Given all of these considerations, researchers must carefully consider the research question and which people best can help answer it when deciding whom to recruit and whom to select for participation in their studies.
4. *Favorable risk-benefit ratio.* For research to be ethical, any risks must be balanced by the benefits to subjects, and the important new knowledge society will gain. This comparison is known as the risk–benefit ratio. The riskier the research study, the more benefit it must offer to be considered ethical. As a part of this, the risks and burdens should be as low as possible. A research burden can be the time it takes people to participate or the inconvenience or discomfort it causes them. Researchers must show that they cannot answer their question in a less risky or burdensome way.
5. *Independent review.* Not only does independent review (by an Institutional Review Board) help make sure research studies fulfill all of the ethics principles, but it is also important for building society's trust in research. If people know that research has been reviewed and approved by an independent group, they will be more confident that it is ethical and that the people who participate will be treated fairly.
6. *Informed consent.* There are four components of informed consent. First, the subject must be competent. This means that he or she is mentally capable of understanding the facts about the research and making a decision on them. Second, the researcher must give a full disclosure about the details of the study. Third, subjects must understand what the researcher tells them. A full disclosure is useless if the subject does not understand. Fourth, the subject's decision to participate must be voluntary, rather than the result of pressures such as undue inducement or coercion.
7. *Respect for subjects.* To show respect to human subjects, researchers must continue to check the well-being of each subject as the study proceeds, keep any information about the subjects confidential, allow subjects to quit the study any time they want, tell subjects about any new information they may need to know (such as new risk the researchers learn about after the study starts), and share the results of the study with the subjects (Emanuel, Abdoler, & Stunkel, 2014, pp. 4–7).

Table 3.2 lists principles from the ADA/CDR Code of Ethics that correspond to the requirements just discussed.

When some or all of the participants in a study are likely to be vulnerable to coercion or undue influence, additional safeguards must be included in the study to protect the rights and welfare of these participants. Vulnerable populations could include children, prisoners, pregnant women, people with a mental disability, or people who are economically

APPLICATION 3.3

Explain how each of the principles from the Code of Ethics in Table 3.2 relates to each of the seven principles for ethical research. Look at the full Code of Ethics to see if any additional principles may apply to the research setting.

Table 3.2 How Principles from the ADA/CDR Code of Ethics Correspond to the Seven Principles for Ethical Research

Seven principles for ethical research (Emanuel, Abdoler, & Stunkel, 2014)	Corresponding principles from ADA/CDR Code of Ethics
Social Value (Studies should improve people's health or well-being.)	Principle 3: The dietetics practitioner considers the health, safety, and welfare of the public at all times.
Scientific Validity (Only ask people to take risks for research that is scientifically valid.)	Principle 12: The dietetics practitioner practices dietetics based on evidence-based principles and current information.
Fair Subject Selection (Be fair in both recruiting and deciding which people can be in the study.)	Principle 1: The dietetics practitioner conducts himself or herself with honesty, integrity, and fairness. Principle 5: The dietetics practitioner provides professional services with objectivity and with respect for the unique needs and values of individuals.
Favorable Risk–Benefit Ratio (Any risks must be balanced by the benefits to subjects, and/or the important new knowledge society will gain.)	Principle 3: The dietetics practitioner considers the health, safety, and welfare of the public at all times.
Independent Review (Research should be reviewed and approved by an independent group.)	Principle 8: The dietetics practitioner recognizes and exercises professional judgment within the limits of his or her qualifications and collaborates with others, seeks counsel, or makes references as appropriate.
Informed Consent (Informed consent, involving voluntary participation and full disclosure about the study that the subject understands, is needed.)	Principle 3: The dietetics practitioner considers the health, safety, and welfare of the public at all times. Principle 5: The dietetics practitioner provides professional services with objectivity and with respect for the unique needs and values of individuals.
Respect for Subjects (Through a variety of ways, the researcher must show respect to subjects by, for instance, checking on their well-being and allowing them to quit the study.)	Principle 9: The dietetics practitioner treats clients and patients with respect and consideration. Principle 10: The dietetics practitioner protects confidential information and makes full disclosure about any limitations on his or her ability to guarantee full confidentiality.

Reproduced from *Research Ethics: How to Treat People Who Participate in Research*. pp. 4–7, by E. Emanuel, E. Abdoler, & L. Stunkel, 2014, Washington DC: National Institutes of Health, Clinical Center Department of Bioethics; and reproduced from: "Code of Ethics for the Profession of Dietetics and Process for Consideration of Ethics Issues," by the American Dietetic Association/Commission for Dietetic Registration, 2009, *Journal of the American Dietetic Association*, 109, pp. 1461–1462. Copyright 2009 by the American Dietetic Association. Reprinted with permission of Elsevier.

or educationally disadvantaged. **Table 3.3** lists some considerations when working with some of these groups. The *Code of Federal Regulations* Title 45, Part 46 (Protection of Human Subjects) from HHS includes regulations (Subparts B, C, and D) on protections for pregnant women, human fetuses, neonates, children, and prisoners involved in research.

APPLICATION 3.4

After reviewing Table 3.3, what considerations would you use for these vulnerable populations: people with a mental disability, or people who are economically or educationally disadvantaged?

Table 3.3 Considerations When Working with Certain Vulnerable Populations

Vulnerable population	Considerations
Pregnant women, fetuses, and neonates	Research with pregnant woman should potentially benefit the woman and/or the fetus. If the research may benefit only the fetus, then informed consent is necessary from the mother and father. Avoid unnecessary risk to the fetus. Research with neonates is to develop important biomedical knowledge that cannot be obtained by other means, and there will be no added risk to the neonate.
Children (under 18 years of age)	A child must actively show his or her willingness to take part in research. "Assent" refers to a child's agreement to be in a research study (may be verbal or written, depending on the study). To take part in the assent process, children must be mature enough to understand the trial and what they are expected to do. This usually starts when a child is about 7 years old. The IRB considers the nature of the proposed research study and the ages, maturity, and psychological state of the children involved when reviewing the proposed assent procedures and how the trial will be explained to the child. To obtain informed consent, assent of the child and permission of parent(s)/guardian(s) is required.
Prisoners	Research must be relevant to prison life and prisoners, such as incarceration, criminal behavior, conditions affecting prisoners as a class, practices to improve well-being of prisoners. Prisoners can receive compensation, but only comparable to what he or she receives in terms of earnings, amenities, food, and so on at prison. The risks must be similar to risks that would be accepted by nonprisoners.

Modified from "Code of Federal Regulations, Title 45, Part 46, Protection of Human Subjects." U.S. Department of Health and Human Services, 2009. Retrieved from: http://www.hhs.gov/ohrp/regulations-and-policy/regulations/45-cfr-46/index.html

Now, we discuss two additional facets of human subject research: informed consent and privacy.

Informed Consent

Informed consent is a process, not just a form. Most research studies require informed consent, which has four elements:

1. *Competence.* The individual must be capable of understanding everything in the informed consent to be able to make a decision.
2. *Full disclosure.* The researcher must fully explain what will be involved as a participant in this study, from the study purpose to its risks and discomforts and how long it will last.
3. *Understanding.* The researcher has to confirm whether the individual really understands everything that is discussed. Any written materials must be at an appropriate reading level and in "layman's terms." Materials will be available in various languages as needed.
4. *Voluntary.* The decision must be 100% voluntary, so you have to ensure that there is no undue pressure on potential participants.

During the informed consent process, the researcher must make sure these fundamental elements are carried out.

The Common Rule outlines the basic requirements for informed consent documents, which are listed in **Table 3.4**, along with other elements that may be needed as appropriate to the study. Many IRBs or research institutions have templates that can be used. Any topic on an informed consent form must be discussed with potential participants.

The process of informed consent begins from the moment a researcher discusses a study with a potential participant or hands out a recruitment brochure. Whether recruiting or screening participants, the researcher is also explaining the goals and structure of the study, along with each of the required elements shown in Table 3.4. The idea is to give the potential participants all the information so that they can make an informed decision.

During the discussions with the potential participants, it is important to ask for questions and assess whether the individual is understanding what you are saying. To promote understanding, information should be given at an appropriate level and be available in a written format for the participant to take home. Researchers need to give time for each person to assess the risk and benefits, and ultimately decide whether to voluntarily enter the study or not. If the individual does decide to enter into the study, in most cases, you will need his or her signature.

Table 3.4 Required Components of Informed Consent Document

Required Components

1. *Purpose*: A statement that the study involves research and the purpose of this research study.
2. *Study Length*: The expected length of time the participant will participate in the study.
3. *Required Procedures*: A description of the required procedures to be followed (including frequency) and identification of any that are experimental.
4. *Risks and Discomforts*: A description of any reasonably foreseeable risks or discomforts to the participant.
5. *Benefits*: A description of any reasonably foreseeable benefits (payment is not a benefit) to the participant or others.
6. *Alternates*: Disclosure of any alternative options that could be beneficial to the participant (including not taking part in the research study).
7. *Compensation and Medical Treatment in Event of Injury*: A statement as to whether there will be any compensation or reimbursement for expenses such as travel, as well as medical treatment available in case of injury.
8. *Contact Person for Questions*: Who the participant can contact with any questions about the research and their rights, and who the participant should contact in the event of a research-related injury.
9. *Confidentiality*: A statement about confidentiality of the participant's records.
10. *Noncoercive Disclaimer and Right to Withdraw*: A statement that the participation is voluntary, the participant may discontinue being in the study at any time without penalty.

Additional Components If Needed

11. *Unforeseeable Risks*: A statement that there are unforeseeable or unknown risks to the participant.
12. *Involuntary Termination*: A statement that participation may be terminated under certain circumstances.
13. *Costs*: Any costs to the participant.
14. *Consequences of Withdrawal*: A statement explaining the consequences if the participant withdraws and procedures to follow in the event of withdrawal.
15. *Notification*: A statement that the participant will be notified about new findings from the study that could affect their willingness to continue participation.
16. *Size of Study*: The number of participants in the study.

Reproduced from "Code of Federal Regulations, Title 45, Part 46.116 Protection of Human Subjects." U.S. Department of Health and Human Services, 2009. Retrieved from: http://www.hhs.gov/ohrp/regulations-and-policy/regulations/45-cfr-46/index.html#46.116

PRIVACY

The Health Insurance Portability and Accountability Act (HIPAA) of 1996 required the Department of Health and Human Services (HHS) to implement a rule to protect and keep health information private for all individuals, living or deceased. In 2000, HHS issued the *Standards for Privacy of Individually Identifiable Health Information* (Privacy Rule). The standards in the Privacy Rule address the use and disclosure of an individual's health information—called **protected health information (PHI)** by organizations subject to the rule. The Privacy Rule applies to **covered entities**, and **Table 3.5** gives some specific examples. A major goal of the Privacy Rule is to protect health information while at the same time allowing the flow of health information needed to provide high-quality health care and public well-being.

The Privacy Rule protects all **individually identifiable health information (IIHI)**. IIHI can include an individual's demographic data, information about provision of health care, payments for health care, and anything about the individual's past, present, or future physical or mental health. If an individual's health information is de-identified (meaning removing your name and so forth so no one could identify you), then there are no restrictions on the use or disclosure of the health information; it is not covered by the Privacy Rule. **De-identified health data** means the data cannot contain any of 18 elements (see **Table 3.6**) that could be used to identify the person, their relatives, or employer.

In research, the Privacy Rule protects the privacy of IIHI while at the same time ensuring that researchers continue to have access to medical information necessary to conduct vital research. Researchers often use a **Privacy Rule Authorization**, a signed permission that allows a covered entity to use or disclose an individual's PHI. When an authorization is signed by a participant in a research study, it is only valid for that study. An authorization may be combined with an informed consent document, but whether it is part of the informed consent or separate, the authorization must contain certain required elements and statements.

The Privacy Rule protects the rights of research participants by requiring covered entities to inform them of uses and disclosures of their medical information for research

Table 3.5 A Covered Entity

A healthcare provider	A health plan	A healthcare clearinghouse
This includes providers such as: • Doctors • Clinics • Psychologists • Dentists • Chiropractors • Nursing Homes • Pharmacies but only if they transmit any information in an electronic form in connection with a transaction for which HHS has adopted a standard.	This includes: • Health insurance companies • HMOs • Company health plans • Government programs that pay for health care, such as Medicare, Medicaid, and the military and veterans healthcare programs	This includes entities that process nonstandard health information they receive from another entity into a standard format (i.e., standard electronic format or data content), or vice versa.

Reproduced from: "Covered Entities and Business Associates." U.S. Department of Health & Human Services, 2016. Retrieved from http://www.hhs.gov/hipaa/for-professionals/covered-entities/

Table 3.6 Elements That Need to Be Removed in De-identification of Protected Health Information

1. Names
2. All geographical subdivisions smaller than a state, including street address, city, county, precinct, zip code, and their equivalent geocodes, except for the initial three digits of a zip code, if according to the current publicly available data from the Bureau of the Census: (1) The geographic unit formed by combining all zip codes with the same three initial digits contains more than 20,000 people, and (2) The initial three digits of a zip code for all such geographic units containing 20,000 or fewer people is changed to 000.
3. All elements of dates (except year) for dates directly related to an individual, including birth date, admission date, discharge date, date of death; and all ages over 89 and all elements of dates (including year) indicative of such age, except that such ages and elements may be aggregated into a single category of age 90 or older.
4. Phone numbers
5. Fax numbers
6. Electronic mail addresses
7. Social security numbers
8. Medical record numbers
9. Health plan beneficiary numbers
10. Account numbers
11. Certificate/license numbers
12. Vehicle identifiers and serial numbers, including license plate numbers
13. Device identifiers and serial numbers
14. Web Universal Resource Locators (URLs)
15. Internet Protocol (IP) address numbers
16. Biometric identifiers, including finger and voice prints
17. Full face photographs and any comparable images
18. Any other unique identifying number, unless allowed for re-identification codes

Modified from: "Guidance Regarding Methods for De-identification of Protected Health Information in Accordance with the Health Insurance Portability and Accountability Act (HIPAA) Privacy Rule." U.S. Department of Health and Human Services, 2016. Retrieved from http://www.hhs.gov/hipaa/for-professionals/privacy/special-topics/de-identification/index.html#standard

purposes. Generally speaking, the Privacy Rule allows research participants free access to their medical records as long as they are maintained by the covered entity. In some cases, such as a double-blind research study, the participants may not have access to their medical information while the study is in progress; however, they will have free access once the study is completed. In this case, the covered entity must inform the research participants in writing that they will temporarily be denied access to their medical information during the course of a clinical trial.

INSTITUTIONAL REVIEW BOARDS

Universities, hospital corporations, and other institutions where research is conducted must have a formal committee that reviews research proposals with human subjects *before research begins*. This committee is known as an Institutional Review Board and functions as an independent committee of at least five members. The main purpose of IRBs is to protect human subjects, especially vulnerable groups such as children, prisoners, pregnant women, people with mental disabilities, or people who are economically or educationally disadvantaged. The IRB determines whether your research is ethical and safe to carry out, and monitors your research via annual reviews and sometimes random study audits.

IRB members may be physicians, statisticians, or other members of the healthcare or research institution community, as long as they are knowledgeable and competent with research proposal review, federal and institutional guidelines and regulations, and professional practice. The IRB must represent diverse backgrounds, and it also has to include at least one person whose work is primarily in nonscientific areas and one person not affiliated with the institution. Each IRB must register with the Department of Health and Human Services and comply with HHS regulations that largely revolve around protecting human subjects.

Before starting any research activities, a researcher (including student researchers) must

- complete and file an IRB application for the study and wait for approval, and
- complete mandated training.

Required training typically includes information on human subjects research, health information privacy and security, and possibly other topics such as conflict of interest, good clinical practice, good laboratory practice, or animal care and use, as appropriate.

APPLICATION 3.5

Review the study in Appendix B on clear liquids versus soft diets. Was this study reviewed and approved by an IRB, or similar group, in India where the study took place? Do the researchers mention that they obtained consent from participants?

The IRB application requires the following information, as appropriate:

1. *A detailed description of your planned research* (also called the **protocol**). This includes objectives, hypotheses, background and rationale, participants and how they will be chosen, detailed study procedures including measurement, and data analysis.
2. *Length of study*.
3. *Risks-benefits*. This includes known risks, such as risks from a procedure, emotional or psychologist risks, or breach of confidentiality, along with potential risks.
4. *Any surveys or questionnaires* you will use (participants must have the option to skip sensitive topics to avoid the risk of emotional distress).
5. *Any consent forms or* **assent forms** (a child's affirmative agreement to participate in research) you will use.
6. *Privacy and confidentiality for participants*. Participants must give permission for research uses of their identifiable health information, and they have the right to know who sees the information. Authorization forms must be submitted.
7. *Any recruitment materials* you will use to find participants.
8. *Any compensation or benefits* the participants will receive.
9. *How you will store your data and keep it safe*.
10. *Budget information*.
11. *A detailed description of any secondary data you may use*, including where it came from, what it contains, and permissions to use the data.

Also, anyone who will be involved in the research has to be listed on the application. The **principal investigator** is the lead researcher responsible to direct the research.

The IRB members continually review submissions and meet once a month to discuss applications and make decisions. The IRB is authorized to conduct three levels of review: exempt reviews, expedited reviews, or full board/complete reviews.

An **exempt review** is for proposed research studies that involve no risk or minimal risk. Minimal risk is defined as the risk someone would encounter in their daily life, or in routine medical, dental, or psychological examinations (for a healthy person). Examples of exempt categories include the following (U.S. DHHS, 2009):

- Research in established or accepted educational settings.
- Research involving the use of surveys, interviews, or observation of public behavior if subjects cannot be identified.
- Analysis of previous collected data with no identifiable information; in other words, the participants cannot be identified. If these data are publically available, you may not need IRB approval.
- Consumer acceptance, taste, and food quality studies.
- Research to study or evaluate public benefit or service programs.

At least one member of the IRB must review each exempt application. The IRB does not actually approve an exempt study but instead makes a determination that the project meets at least one of the exempt categories criteria. An exempt study does not mean the study is exempt from IRB review: it will still be reviewed and recommendations given.

An **expedited review** procedure is for proposed research studies that do not present more than minimal risk and fit into one of the expedited categories. Here are some examples of the expedited categories (U.S. DHHS, 2009):

- Collection of blood samples by finger stick, heel stock, ear stick, or venipuncture in certain groups and within certain time frequency and amounts.
- Collection of data through noninvasive procedures, such as moderate exercise, muscular strength testing, body composition assessment, and flexibility testing where appropriate given the age, weight, and health of the individual.
- Prospective collection of biological specimens by noninvasive means.
- Research employing survey, interview, oral history, focus group, program evaluation, human factors evaluation, or quality assurance methodologies.

At least one member of the IRB must review and approve each expedited application. An expedited or exempt review can only be disapproved after a complete review by the entire IRB.

If your research proposal does not qualify for exempt or expedited review, in other words it involves more than minimal risk, it will require a **full board review** at the IRB meeting and the attending IRB members will vote. (If an IRB member has a conflict of interest related to an application, that member is excused from the review process.) To obtain IRB approval, the application must meet the criteria or requirements listed in **Table 3.7**.

For any type of application, the IRB members may ask for clarifications and additional information, along with revisions, additions, or deletions, on the application before it will be approved. Every application that is approved is given a number, and you will need that number for future interactions with the IRB. If you modify or amend the study's protocol after approval, the changes *must be submitted again to the IRB before*

APPLICATION 3.6

Find the website for the IRB for your college/university. What training is required? How often does the IRB meet? What is the deadline for getting in applications?

Table 3.7 Criteria for IRB Approval of Research

(1) Risks to subjects are minimized: (i) By using procedures which are consistent with sound research design and which do not unnecessarily expose subjects to risk, and (ii) whenever appropriate, by using procedures already being performed on the subjects for diagnostic or treatment purposes.
(2) Risks to subjects are reasonable in relation to anticipated benefits, if any, to subjects, and the importance of the knowledge that may reasonably be expected to result. In evaluating risks and benefits, the IRB should consider only those risks and benefits that may result from the research (as distinguished from risks and benefits of therapies subjects would receive even if not participating in the research). The IRB should not consider possible long-range effects of applying knowledge gained in the research (e.g., the possible effects of the research on public policy) as among those research risks that fall within the purview of its responsibility.
(3) Selection of subjects is equitable. In making this assessment the IRB should take into account the purposes of the research and the setting in which the research will be conducted and should be particularly cognizant of the special problems of research involving vulnerable populations, such as children, prisoners, pregnant women, mentally disabled persons, or economically or educationally disadvantaged persons.
(4) Informed consent will be sought from each prospective subject or the subject's legally authorized representative, in accordance with, and to the extent required by the Code of Federal Regulations Title 45, Part 46.116.
(5) Informed consent will be appropriately documented, in accordance with, and to the extent required by the Code of Federal Regulations, Title 45, Part 46.117.
(6) When appropriate, the research plan makes adequate provision for monitoring the data collected to ensure the safety of subjects.
(7) When appropriate, there are adequate provisions to protect the privacy of subjects and to maintain the confidentiality of data.

When some or all of the subjects are likely to be vulnerable to coercion or undue influence, such as children, prisoners, pregnant women, mentally disabled persons, or economically or educationally disadvantaged persons, additional safeguards have been included in the study to protect the rights and welfare of these subjects.

Reproduced from: "Code of Federal Regulations, Title 45, Part 46.111 Protection of Human Subjects." U.S. Department of Health and Human Services, 2009. Retrieved from: http://www.hhs.gov/ohrp/regulations-and-policy/regulations/45-cfr-46/index.html#46.111

implementation. If the research is completed within 12 months, the termination of the study is reported to the IRB. Otherwise, the researcher must report progress to the IRB every 12 months until completion of the study.

If a RDN working in a hospital, for example, wants to do any type of research using patient information, it is essential to consult the IRB. You cannot go into patient's charts to get information without prior IRB approval. If you want to work with already de-identified patient information, you still need IRB approval, although it will likely be an exempt review.

When a RDN is involved in a quality improvement project at work (often focused on policies and procedures such as checking whether patients are screened in a timely manner), the project is generally not considered "research" when it is meant for internal

APPLICATION 3.7

A RDN is working in a large, urban hospital while completing a graduate degree in the evenings. She has to complete a written research project for her graduate degree and has obtained permission to use some de-identified patient information at the hospital. Once the project is completed and written up, she has to present it at the university. Does she need to submit an application to the IRB? Why or why not?

use only and is very specific to the facility. The most common test of whether a project is research is whether the results will be published or presented. If you intend to publish or present something (even if it is a poster at a local professional meeting), you need to get IRB approval before you start. Also, if you use a rigid protocol or randomize participants, that would need IRB approval.

RESEARCHER INTERVIEW Management Research

Carol W. Shanklin, PhD, RDN
Dean of Graduate School & Professor in Department of Food, Nutrition, Dietetics and Health, Kansas State University, Manhattan, KS

1. **Briefly describe the area in which you do research.**
   I currently and recently have been engaged in research in the following areas:
   - Food Safety in Child Nutrition Programs including using the theory of planned behavior to identity factors influencing employees to engage in proper food safety practices, including behavioral intentions, and to assess the effectiveness of using storytelling in training employees on selected food safety practices including hand washing, the proper use of thermometers, and proper cleaning and sanitizing of work surfaces.
   - Environmental issues and sustainability in food service operations including the characterization of food and packaging waste and exploration of strategies to decrease wasted food and decrease the use of related resources such as energy, water, and labor. My current research focuses on the identification and characterization of preconsumer wasted food in child nutrition programs.
   - Clinical nutrition management in healthcare systems. This research focused on the identification and validation of roles and management responsibilities of clinical nutrition managers and educational needs and preparation for the role.
   - Customer satisfaction in continuing and long-term care facilities.
2. **With your experience in management research, what should students/practitioners know about this area of research?**
   Students and researchers should recognize that problems to be explored through research are limitless, and only a few researchers are engaged in conducting operational research in management practice in dietetics—both food service operations and clinical management practice. Management research should be conducted not only in food service operations but in all areas of dietetics practice as effective and efficient management is essential for success. It is important to recognize that generalizations of findings are often limited due to differences in operational practices and the scope of the problem being explored. The benefits of conducting operational research in management practice is that the results can be used immediately to advance practice.
3. **What do you enjoy most about the research process?**
   The aspect of the research process that I enjoy the most is designing studies that result in data that can address operational problems and challenges, and analyzing the data to identify strategies that management practitioners can use to improve their operations. I also enjoy collecting data in operations because I can interact with dietetics professionals and identify other research needs. The most rewarding aspect of conducting research as an educator with students and practitioners is experiencing how much team members grow professionally.
4. **What tip(s) do you have for practitioners and academic researchers who want to do practice-based research?**
   Here are some tips I have for practitioners who want to do practice-based research:
   - Establish a research team that is multidisciplinary in thought and use the expertise of each team member in the design, implementation, and dissemination of the results?

- Explore the feasibility of working collaboratively with educators in your area or state?
- Select a problem that can be clearly defined and narrow in scope so that you can identify specific research questions. Determine the intended outcome of the research so you can best determine the scope of the study. For example, are the results being used to make operational decisions at one or multiple locations, or are the outcomes to be generalizable to the larger population of the target audience?
- Control as many variables as possible when conducting operational research, but acknowledge those variables that cannot be controlled and should be considered when analyzing the data?
- Schedule data collection at times that least interfere with normal operations to the best of your ability?

Here are some additional tips for academic researchers who want to do practice-based research:

- Create partnerships with management practitioners through engagement in your state dietetic association or the Academy of Nutrition and Dietetics?
- Network with your partners to identify problems in most urgent need of being resolved and data needed for making strategic decisions?
- Engage your partners in your research and acknowledge their contributions in publications and presentations?

SUMMARY

1. Research ethics is important to promote knowledge and avoid errors in the pursuit of knowledge, promote collaborative work, keep researchers accountable to the public, and promote values such as human rights to prevent ethical lapses.
2. After unethical experiments performed by the Nazis before and during World War II, the Nuremberg Code outlined 10 principles for ethical biomedical research including voluntary consent and balancing the benefits and costs. The Nuremberg Code was the basis for the Declaration of Helsinki (1964) by the World Medical Association, a set of ethics principles that provides guidance to physicians and other researchers in medical research involving human subjects.
3. In the United States, the Belmont Report (1979) defined ethics principles for research (respect for persons, beneficence, justice). Based on the Belmont Report, the Department of Health and Human Services issued a *Code of Federal Regulations* Title 45, Part 46 (Protection of Human Subjects). The Food and Drug Administration also issued federal regulations.
4. Part of the HHS regulations (Title 45, Part 46, Subpart A) became what is known as the Common Rule, or "Federal Policy for the Protection of Human Subjects" in 1991. The Common Rule includes guidelines for IRB operation, documenting informed consent, and protections for vulnerable populations.
5. Responsible Conduct of Research means applying ethics principles in all facets of research work, such as collaborating with others, dealing with conflicts of interest, and being a responsible author.
6. With all the competing responsibilities and demands on researchers, conflicts of interest are not unusual. However, researchers do need to make sure that conflicts in the following areas do not interfere with responsible, ethical research or are harmful to the public in any way: financial conflicts, conflict of commitment, and personal or intellectual conflicts. Federal funding agencies have conflict of interest policies that spell out exactly what a significant financial interest is, as well as procedures for reporting and managing significant conflicts of interest. See Figure 3.1 for NIH rules. Table 3.1 lists several ADA/CDR ethics principles related to conflict of interest.
7. Research misconduct includes fabrication, falsification, or plagiarism.

8. Human subjects research involves a living individual from whom a researcher obtains data through an intervention or an interaction, or by identifiable private information.
9. Principles underlying ethical human subject research include social value, scientific validity, fair subject selection, favorable risk–benefit ratio, independent review, informed consent, and respect for subjects.
10. Table 3.3 lists considerations when working with certain vulnerable populations.
11. Informed consent must include competence of the patient to make the right decision for him or her, full disclosure by the researcher, understanding of the patient, and a 100% voluntary decision. Table 3.4 lists required components of the informed consent document.
12. In research, the Privacy Rule protects the privacy of individually identifiable health information while at the same time ensuring that researchers continue to have access to medical information necessary to conduct vital research. Researchers will often use a Privacy Rule Authorization, a signed permission that allows a covered entity to use or disclose an individual's protected health information.
13. De-identified health data means the data cannot contain any of 18 elements (see Table 3.6) that could be used to identify the person, their relatives, or employer.
14. Universities, hospital corporations, and other institutions where research is conducted must have an Institutional Review Board (IRB) that reviews research proposals with human subjects before research begins. IRBs also require training of researchers on topics such as human subjects research or informed consent. The IRB is authorized to conduct three levels of review: exempt, expedited, or full board/complete reviews (for more than minimal risk).
15. Quality improvement projects are generally not considered research when it is meant for internal use only and is specific to the facility. Although if you intend to publish or present your results, you need IRB approval. Table 3.7 lists criteria for IRB approval of research.

REVIEW QUESTIONS

1. Which of the following have policies related to research ethics?
   A. Department of Health and Human Services
   B. Research universities
   C. Research hospitals
   D. Professional associations
   E. All of the above
2. Which of the following identified these three ethics principles as relevant to human subjects research: respect for persons, beneficence, and justice?
   A. Nuremberg Code
   B. Declaration of Helsinki
   C. Belmont Report
   D. HHS regulations Title 45
3. Many of the biomedical and behavioral studies in the United States are regulated by the U.S. Department of Health and Human Services or U.S. Food and Drug Administration regulations.
   A. true
   B. false
4. Any conflict of interest is unethical.
   A. true
   B. false
5. A significant financial interest when receiving NIH funding is receiving over _______ a year in payments.
   A. $2,500
   B. $5,000
   C. $7,500
   D. $10,000
6. Which type of conflict is this: a researcher's judgment on a research topic is biased because he or she has a strong attachment to a specific point of view.
   A. financial conflict
   B. personal conflict
   C. conflict of commitment
   D. intellectual conflict
7. For an IRB application, which of the following is NOT necessary?
   A. food samples if doing a food study
   B. known and potential risks

C. recruitment and consent materials
D. budget

8. If your research involves a survey, it is likely to fit into which IRB category?
   A. expedited
   B. exempt
   C. full board review
   D. none of the above
9. If a RDN is involved in a quality improvement project at work, the project is generally not considered research when it is meant for internal use only and is specific to the facility.
   A. true
   B. false
10. At about what age is a child able to take part in the assent process?
    A. 5 years old
    B. 7 years old
    C. 9 years old
    D. 11 years old
11. Give three reasons research ethics is important.
12. Explain what Responsible Conduct of Research is, and list five areas in which a researcher should demonstrate responsible conduct.
13. If a researcher receives money from a food company to do a research study, does that mean the study is biased? Explain why or why not.
14. Describe the three forms of research misconduct.
15. What is the major purpose of an IRB? Describe the members of an IRB.
16. What is the difference between a consent form and an assent form?
17. Distinguish between exempt, expedited, and full board review IRB applications.
18. Briefly describe seven requirements for evaluating whether a human subjects research study is ethical.
19. Explain the informed consent process.
20. Explain the Privacy Rule.
21. What is de-identified health data?

CRITICAL THINKING QUESTIONS

1. Complete the required IRB training for your institution.
2. Read the 19 Principles in the ADA/CDR Code of Ethics and explain how 5 of them are related to research ethics.
3. Go to this website: http://ori.hhs.gov/the-research-clinic. View the video "The Research Clinic," an interactive training video on selection of research subjects and research misconduct and make choices for each character in the video.
4. Go to this website: http://ori.hhs.gov/thelab. View the video "The Lab," an interactive training video that addresses Responsible Conduct of Research topics and allows you to make decisions for each character.
5. View "The Elements of a Successful Informed Consent Video" by the National Institute of Mental Health: https://www.youtube.com/watch?v=l26hdCD9g2I. In this video, they discuss important aspects of the informed consent discussion and you view an actual meeting for informed consent between a physician and a patient with depression. Critique how the physician handled this discussion.
6. Of these following activities, which are considered research? If it is research, does it involve human subjects?
   A. Analysis of NHANES data, which is de-identified and publically available, to be used to publish a research article.
   B. Analysis at ABC Hospital for Children to determine how many minutes it takes for trays to reach patient rooms, to be used by the Food Service Director to speed up tray service.
   C. Comparison of two nutrition education programs for children in elementary schools, including dietary recalls, to be used to present a poster at a professional meeting.

D. Comparison of bread made with and without flax seeds to determine acceptability, to be done to complete a college required project including paper and presentation.

E. Testing the effects of a quercetin glycoside on endothelial function and blood pressure in 15 volunteers. This study requires blood samples and will be published.

7. Which of the studies listed in question 6 require IRB approval? Which level of approval would be appropriate?

SUGGESTED READINGS AND ACTIVITIES

1. Steneck, N. H. (2007). *ORI introduction to the responsible conduct of research.* Washington, DC: U.S. Department of Health and Human Services.
2. Academy of Nutrition and Dietetics. *Online Self-Study Modules: Research Ethics for the Registered Dietitian/Nutritionist.* Retrieved from http://www.eatrightpro.org/resource/research/projects-tools-and-initiatives/dpbrn/steps-to-developing-a-research-project-resources-to-help

REFERENCES

American Dietetic Association/Commission on Dietetic Registration. (2009). Code of ethics for the profession of dietetics and process for consideration of ethics issues. *Journal of the American Dietetic Association, 109*, 1461–1467. doi: 10.1016/j.jada.2009.06.002

Busey, J. C. (2006). Recognizing and addressing conflicts of interest. *Journal of the American Dietetic Association, 106*, 351–355. doi: 10.1016/j.jada.2006.01.024

Emanuel, E., Abdoler, E., & Stunkel. L. (2014). *Research ethics: How to treat people who participate in research.* Washington, DC: National Institutes of Health, Clinical Center Department of Bioethics. Retrieved from http://bioethics.nih.gov/education/FNIH_BioethicsBrochure_WEB.PDF

Emanuel, E. J., Wendler, D., & Grady, C. (2000). What makes clinical research ethical? *JAMA, 283*, 2701–2711.

Merriam Webster Law Dictionary. (2016). *Conflict of interest.* Retrieved from http://www.merriam-webster.com/dictionary/conflict%20of%20interest

National Institutes of Health. (2009). *Update on the requirement for instruction in the responsible conduct of research* (Notice Number: NOT-OD-10-019). Retrieved from https://grants.nih.gov/grants/guide/notice-files/NOT-OD-10-019.html

National Institutes of Health. (2010). *Research integrity.* Retrieved from https://grants.nih.gov/grants/research_integrity/research_misconduct.htm

National Institutes of Health. (2015). *Learn about clinical studies.* Retrieved from https://clinicaltrials.gov/ct2/about-studies/learn#Questions

Office of Research Integrity. (2011). *Definition of research misconduct.* Retrieved from http://ori.hhs.gov/definition-misconduct

Pech, C., Cob, N., & Cejka, J. T. (2007). Understanding institutional review boards: Practical guidance to the IRB review process. *Nutrition in Clinical Practice, 22*, 618–628. doi: 10.1177/0115426507022006618

Resnik, D. B. (2015). *What is ethics in research & why is it important?* (National Institute of Environmental Health Sciences). Retrieved from http://www.niehs.nih.gov/research/resources/bioethics/whatis/index.cfm

Stang, J. (2015). Ethics in action: Conducting ethical research involving human subjects: A primer. *Journal of the Academy of Nutrition and Dietetics, 115*, 2019–2020. doi: 10.1016/j.jand.2015.10.006

Steneck, N. H. (2007). *ORI introduction to the responsible conduct of research.* Washington, DC: U.S. Department of Health and Human Services.

U.S. Food and Drug Administration. (2010b). Institutional review boards. *Code of Federal Regulations*, Title 21, Part 56. Retrieved from http://www.accessdata.fda.gov/scripts/cdrh/cfdocs/cfcfr/CFRSearch.cfm

U.S. Food and Drug Administration. (2010a). Protection of human subjects. *Code of Federal Regulations*, Title 21, Part 50. Retrieved from http://www.accessdata.fda.gov/scripts/cdrh/cfdocs/cfcfr/CFRSearch.cfm

U.S. Department of Health and Human Services. (2009). Protection of human subjects. *Code of Federal Regulations*, Title 45, Part 46. Retrieved from http://www.hhs.gov/ohrp/regulations-and-policy/regulations/45-cfr-46/index.html

World Medical Association General Assembly. (2013). *WMA declaration of Helsinki— Ethical principles for medical research involving human subjects.* Retrieved from http://www.wma.net/en/30publications/10policies/b3/index.html

Woteki, C. E. (2006). Ethics opinion: Conflicts of interest in presentations and publications and dietetics research. *Journal of the American Dietetic Association, 106*, 27–31. doi: 10.1016/j.jada.2005.11.011

PART

2

How to Read, Interpret, and Evaluate Quantitative Nutrition Research

CHAPTER 4

Key Concepts in Quantitative Research

CHAPTER OUTLINE

- Introduction
- Foundations
- Reliability and Validity
- Error and Bias
- Sampling
- Instruments and Measurement
- Anatomy of a Research Article
- Researcher Interview: Outcomes Research, Dr. Geoffrey Greene

LEARNING OUTCOMES

- Use research terminology, such as Type II error, correctly, and identify different variables (independent, dependent, extraneous) and explain their roles in a study.
- Given a hypothesis, identify it as the research or null hypothesis, causal or associative, directional or nondirectional, and simple or complex.
- Explain how to test a hypothesis, and compare statistical significance with effect size.
- Compare and contrast reliability and validity.
- Describe threats to interval validity, external validity, statistical conclusion validity, and construct validity, and strategies to reduce these threats.
- Distinguish between random and systematic errors or bias.
- Identify types of bias in research studies and strategies to reduce bias.
- Differentiate between probability and nonprobability sampling and give examples of each.
- Explain how sampling size may be determined and identify factors related to sampling that must be considered when evaluating the quality of a study.
- Describe ways to test the reliability and validity of instruments, and distinguish between sensitivity and specificity of an instrument.
- Identify what is accomplished in each section of a research article.
- Identify a research design as experimental, quasi-experimental, or observational.

INTRODUCTION

From constructs to reliability and validity, this chapter begins with many crucial concepts in quantitative research. Procedures, such as sampling and measuring, are also discussed. This chapter ends by explaining each section of a quantitative research article, including hints on where to find certain key elements, such as the research objective or a quick summary of the results. We start with key foundation concepts.

FOUNDATIONS

CONCEPTS, CONSTRUCTS, AND VARIABLES

Before we can talk about theories, we need to look at concepts and constructs because they are the building blocks of theories.

1. **Concepts** abstractly describe a general phenomenon, idea, or object and give it a name. Examples of concepts include *moderation* or *weight*.
2. A **construct** is also abstract but is usually more complex than a concept. Often a construct is purposely invented or mentally constructed such as *IQ* or *diet quality*. Some researchers use the terms concepts and constructs interchangeably.

A concept or construct, such as weight or diet quality, is usually called a **variable** in a quantitative study (once it has been operationally defined). A variable is simply any quality of a person, group, thing, or situation that varies or changes, such as age. Many, but not all, variables are quantitative. For example, gender is a variable: male or female. Many variables are human characteristics: age, weight, LDL level, and presence or absence of disease. Some variables, such as LDL level, can vary a lot, whereas other variables, such as whether someone has diabetes or not, is considered **dichotomous**. A dichotomous variable has only two possibilities or levels.

A construct, such as diet quality, has a **theoretical definition**, such as "how well an individual's diet conforms to healthy eating patterns." Numerous instruments have been developed and tested to measure different aspects of diet quality, with varying levels of sophistication. To measure diet quality in a study, researchers have to decide on the *specific* way in which the variable will be measured, which is called the **operational definition**, *Variables are really the operational definitions of constructs.* For example, one way to operationalize "diet quality" and make it a variable in a study would be to use the Healthy Eating Index. The Healthy Eating Index assesses overall diet and categorizes individuals according to the extent to which their eating behaviors conform to the Dietary Guidelines for Americans.

Diet quality is not that hard to operationalize. Think of how you might operationalize a more complex construct such as cognitive decline, mindful eating, or family connectedness. They are much harder but could also be operationalized in a number of different ways.

Keep in mind in this discussion that not *all* study variables need to be measured; the independent variable is simply **manipulated**. **For example, in a weight control study, a special weight control program is the independent variable.** The suspected cause or influence is the **independent variable**, and the effect or outcome (such as weight loss) is the **dependent variable**. In quantitative research, researchers are generally trying to answer one of these types of questions to better understand something:

1. *Is there a difference among the groups?* This type of study involves a treatment or intervention (independent variable) manipulated by the researcher and looks at

whether it creates an effect (dependent variable) on the experimental group when compared to the control group. For example, the study may look at the use of chromium supplements (independent variable) in people with diabetes to see how it affects their glycemic control (dependent variable) compared to a group of people with diabetes who do not take the supplement.

2. *Is there an association or relationship among the variables?* In quantitative studies that do not manipulate an independent variable (meaning there is no intervention), researchers usually have an idea of a possible relationship. For example, researchers may observe a large group of individuals over time to see whether exposure to certain factors (such as a diet high in fruits and vegetables—independent variable) affects their risk of disease (such as heart disease—dependent variable). Other researchers may examine the relationship between the diet quality of a parent and his or her child to see if a parent's diet (independent variable) has a substantial impact on a child's diet (dependent variable). In an **associative relationship**, two variables are statistically related; as one variable increases or decreases, so does the other, or there may be an inverse relationship. But one variable *does not cause* the other.

Some studies have more than one independent variable or dependent variable.

Of course, there are other variables besides the independent and dependent variables in a study. **Extraneous variables** may affect research outcomes as they may or may not be recognized or controlled. Extraneous variables can affect measurement of the dependent variable and the relationships among the study's variables. As shown in **Figure 4.1**, an extraneous variable, such as smoking, could affect the results in a study of coffee drinkers and heart disease because coffee drinkers are more likely to smoke. As the extraneous variable, smoking may compete with the independent variable in explaining the outcome of the study. Researchers try to find and control as many extraneous variables as possible.

To control extraneous variables, researchers must first identify them. Common extraneous variables in nutrition studies are age, gender, education, socioeconomic status, level of health, severity of disease, and nutrition knowledge and attitudes. When the study is designed, researchers implement a number of strategies to control for extraneous variables (**Table 4.1**). Through good research design and statistical procedures, researchers can control the effects of many extraneous variables.

You may have heard the term "confounding variables." Many researchers consider extraneous and confounding variables to be basically the same. For some researchers, a **confounding variable** is a type of extraneous variable that either cannot be controlled or is not recognized until after the study begins (Grove, Burns, & Gray, 2013, p. 152). We use the terms extraneous variable and confounding variable interchangeably in this book.

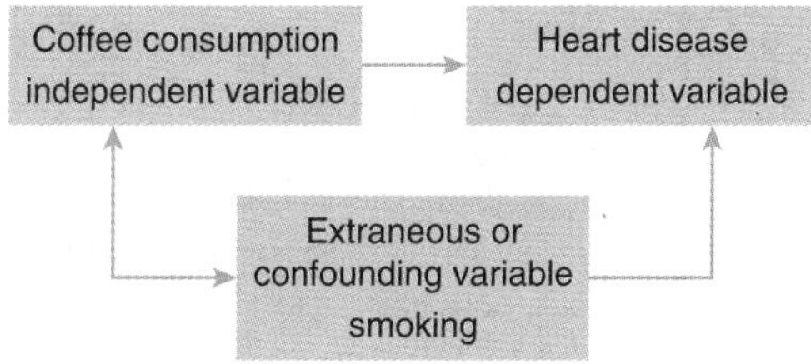

FIGURE 4.1 Relationship Among the Independent Variable, Dependent Variable, and the Extraneous or Confounding Variable

Table 4.1 Design Strategies to Control for Extraneous Variables
Design Strategies to Control for Extraneous Variables
1. Use **random sampling** to pick your participants.
2. Randomly assign participants to groups (called **randomization**) so the presence of extraneous variables is equivalent among the groups.
3. Use blocking. In a randomized block design, the participants are first split into homogeneous groups or blocks (based on age or gender for instance) before being randomly assigned to either the treatment or control group within the block.
4. Match a participant randomly selected to the experimental group with someone who is very similar (in terms of the important extraneous variables) in the control group. (This creates dependent groups, which are important for statistical purposes.)
5. If randomization is not possible, choose groups in which only people who are similar with respect to the confounding variable(s) are included (such as all women or all people more than 60 years old).
6. Depending on the statistical procedures used, you may be able to control for extraneous variables such as age, gender, and so forth. (When using regression models, for example, you can control for extraneous variables.)
7. Monitor **treatment fidelity**, implementing the intervention as planned and making sure it is delivered in a comparable manner to all study participants.

Covariates, also known as *covariables*, are another term you will see in research, but usually just in studies using regression techniques. A covariate is a variable that affects the dependent variable but is not the independent variable of interest to the researcher. *Often covariates are extraneous variables*. Using statistics such as regression, you can control for covariates such as age or gender, meaning they do not influence the study's results.

TIP

A variable may be referred to as continuous or categorical. A **continuous variable** can be counted and has an infinite number of possible values. Continuous data are measured at an interval or ratio level (see **Table 4.2**). Examples include height, blood urea nitrogen, or the total sugar in an apple. **Categorical variables** represent types of data that can be divided into groups with an inherent order (ordinal) or no defined order (categorical). Examples of categorical variables are race, sex, age group, and educational level. See Table 4.2 for the four levels of measurement. It is important to understand the levels of measurement because the level often determines which statistical test you can use.

THEORIES, MODELS AND FRAMEWORKS

A **theory** describes a set of relationships among constructs that, when taken together, attempt to explain or predict related phenomena, such as behavior change. Theories explain why things are the way they are. For example, social cognitive theory explains how personal factors, behavioral factors, and environmental factors continuously interact to determine a person's motivation and behavior. It provides guidance to nutrition educators on how to translate client motivation into action through activities such as self-monitoring, goal setting, and self-regulation. **Table 4.3** includes examples of other health behavior theories used in research that looks at changing nutrition and health behaviors. Theories from many fields of study, such as psychology, education, and biology, are used in nutrition research.

Table 4.2 Levels of Measurement

Level of measurement	Definition	Examples
Ratio	A continuum of numeric values with equal intervals between them and a meaningful zero point.	Weight, height, number of credits completed
Interval	A continuum of numeric values with equal intervals, but the zero point is not meaningful.	Celsius scale, standardized IQ, grade point average (GPA)
Ordinal	Using numbers to rank order an attribute. The intervals are not equal.	Student's level of standing (freshman, sophomore, junior, senior); a Likert scale such as "1-Strongly Agree, 2-Agree, 3-Neither Agree Nor Disagree, 4-Disagree, 5-Strongly Disagree"
Nominal	Using numbers to categorize or label attributes into groups or categories.	Gender: male is coded as "1" and female as "2"

Models also describe relationships between constructs, particularly focusing on how the constructs relate. Models may draw on a number of theories to help explain a particular problem in a certain context. Often a model is represented graphically, such as the Transtheoretical Model (or Stages of Change) shown in **Figure 4.2**.

Table 4.3 Selected Health Behavior Theories (Individual Level)

Theory	Focus	Key concepts
Health Belief Model	Individuals' perceptions of the threat posed by a health problem, the benefits of avoiding the threat, and factors influencing the decision to act.	Perceived susceptibility Perceived severity Perceived benefits Perceived barriers Cues to action Self-efficacy
Stages of Change Model (Transtheoretical Model)	Individuals' motivation and readiness to change a problem behavior.	Precontemplation Contemplation Decision Action Maintenance
Theory of Planned Behavior	Individuals' attitudes toward a behavior, perceptions of norms, and beliefs about the ease or difficulty of changing.	Behavioral intention Attitude Subjective norm Perceived behavioral control
Precaution Adoption Process Model	Individuals' journey from lack of awareness to action and maintenance.	Unaware of issue Unengaged by issue Deciding about acting Deciding not to act Deciding to act Acting Maintenance

Modified from *A Guide for Health Promotion Practice* (2nd ed.), p. 45, by K. Glantz & B.K. Rimer, 2005, Washington, DC: National Cancer Institute. National Institutes of Health Publication No. 05-3896.

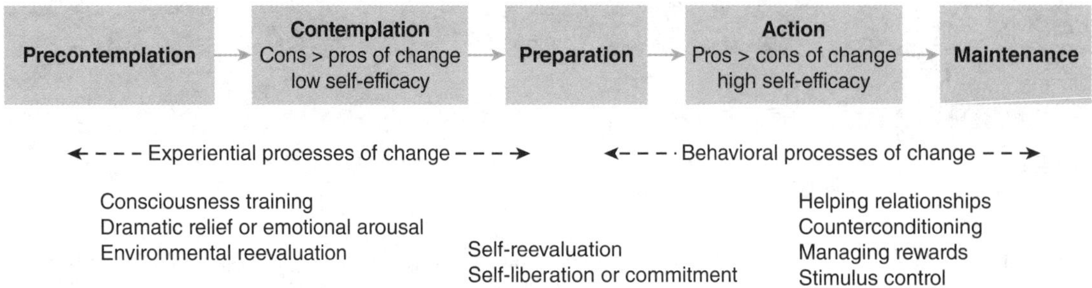

FIGURE 4.2 Transtheoretical Model

A **research framework**, which is usually less formal than a theory or model, illustrates the relationships between variables and the theoretical structure to be used or tested in a study. Theoretical frameworks are not highly developed and have not been rigorously tested.

In practice, theories, models, and research frameworks are often used interchangeably because they overlap a lot and the definitions are not standardized (Contento, 2016). Basically models and research frameworks can be considered as "theories" when we define theory in a general way.

RELATIONSHIP OF THEORY, RESEARCH, AND PRACTICE

The relationships among theory, research, and practice are dynamic as illustrated in **Figure 4.3**. Theories are tested in research, and in turn, research generates new theories. Theory provides a road map for approaching and studying problems, developing appropriate studies, and evaluating their successes. Nutritionists use and adapt theories from research in practice and develop new theories in practice when something does not work. In other words, practice informs and is informed by theory development and research.

Research also forms the basis for evidence-based practice guidelines so practitioners make appropriate nutrition care decisions for patients. These guidelines serve as a foundation for RDNs and nutrition professionals when communicating nutrition recommendations. Research also provides documentation of the impact of nutrition care on

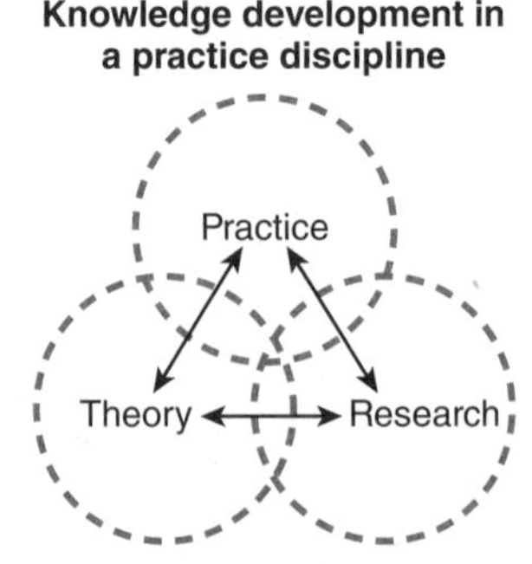

FIGURE 4.3 The Relationships of Theory, Research, and Practice

health outcomes, which increases third-party payer reimbursement for medical nutrition therapy.

HYPOTHESES

A **hypothesis** is a prediction about relationships among variables in a study. In brief, it is an educated guess. Not every research article will state a hypothesis, although sometimes you can infer what it is. Most experimental or quasi-experimental studies include a hypothesis. Studies may also have a secondary hypothesis, which can answer additional questions. In the gardening study found in Appendix A, the hypothesis is stated as follows: "The primary study hypothesis was to determine whether adolescents who participated in a garden-based nutrition intervention would increase their fruit and vegetable consumption more than those participating in a nutrition education intervention without any garden activities" (McAleese & Rankin, 2007, p. 662). This hypothesis is also called a **research hypothesis**.

A hypothesis can show either a causal or an associative relationship among variables (**Figure 4.4**). In an **associative hypothesis**, two variables are statistically related. As one variable increases or decreases, so does the other variable, or there may be an inverse relationship. *But one variable does not cause the other.* When one variable increases (or decreases) along with another variable, the variables are said to be positively correlated. An example of a positively correlated relationship is added sugar intake and education. Men and women who eat higher levels of added sugars tend to have lower education levels.

A **causal hypothesis** identifies a possible cause-and-effect relationship between two or more variables, as shown in Figure 4.4. The letter "X" represents the independent variable, and the letter "Y" represents the dependent variable. An example of a causal relationship can be seen in the lack of folate (independent variable) causing some cases of neural tube defects (dependent variable).

A hypothesis can also be directional or nondirectional. A **directional hypothesis** states the direction of the relationship between two (or more) variables. A **nondirectional hypothesis** states simply that there is a relationship between the variables, but does not give any direction. In the gardening study, the intervention is hypothesized to *increase* fruit and vegetable consumption, so it is directional.

A hypothesis can also be simple or complex. A **simple hypothesis** predicts a causal or associative relationship between just two variables. A **complex hypothesis** does

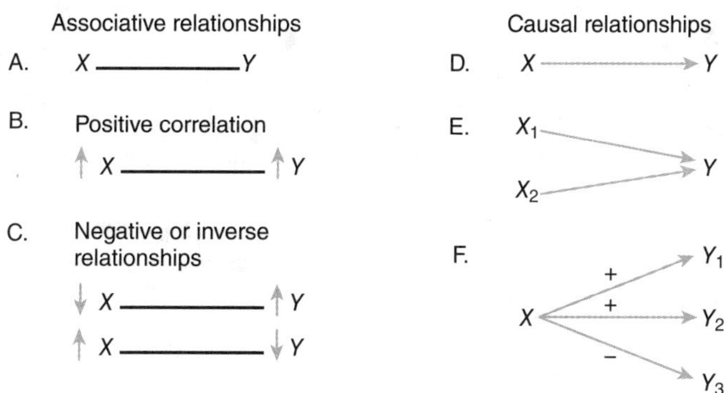

FIGURE 4.4 Associative and Causal Relationships

the same for three or more variables. Therefore, a complex hypothesis has more than one independent variable or more than one dependent variable. In the gardening study, there is one independent variable (the garden-based intervention) and two dependent variables (fruit and vegetable intakes were measured separately), so this is an example of a complex hypothesis.

The hypothesis stated by McAleese & Rankin (2007) for their gardening study is a research hypothesis. and is indicated by the symbol H_1. Every study with a research hypothesis also has a null hypothesis. The **null hypothesis** (indicated by the symbol H_0) states that if there is a difference in the dependent variable at the end of the study, *it is due to chance and is not due to the independent variable*. So the null hypothesis and research hypothesis are in some ways like opposites. The research hypothesis is also called the **alternative hypothesis** because it is the alternative hypothesis to the null.

APPLICATION 4.1

Answer the following questions about this hypothesis: "We hypothesized that a healthy dietary pattern would be associated with a decreased risk for cognitive decline" (Haring et al., 2016, p. 922).

1. Is this a causal or an associative hypothesis?
2. Is the hypothesis directional or nondirectional?
3. Is the hypothesis simple or complex?
4. What would be the null hypothesis for this study?

When we pose a hypothesis, we want to know whether the outcome is due to the independent variable or to chance. *Inferential statistics cannot test the research hypothesis directly; instead the null hypothesis is tested.* This is the reason the null hypothesis is also referred to as a **statistical hypothesis**. When testing the null hypothesis, we hope to reject it because then there is support for the research hypothesis (H_1). *Hypothesis testing is not just for causal hypotheses, it also applies to hypotheses involving associations and predictions.* To test a hypothesis, a researcher must do the following.

1. State the research hypothesis and null hypothesis.
2. Specify the **level of significance**. The level of significance refers to the probability of rejecting the null hypothesis when it is true. Often it is set at 0.05 or lower, meaning that the chance of rejecting the null hypothesis when it is true is 1 in 20 or lower.
3. Run the statistical test on your sample data. The results will include what is called the ***P*-value (probability value)** of the test. The *P*-value of any statistical test represents the probability that the results were due to chance alone, and it is sometimes called the *probability of chance*. The smaller the *P*-value computed from sample data, the more likely it is that the null hypothesis is not supported.
4. *If the P-value of the test is less than or equal to the level of significance (0.05) you set, then you reject the null hypothesis and accept the research hypothesis.* On the other hand, if the *P*-value is greater than the level of significance, then you *accept* the null hypothesis that the independent variable did not truly affect the dependent variable.
5. When the *P*-value is less than or equal to the level of significance, we say that the results are **statistically significant**. Significance means that at the level chosen (such as 0.05), the *evidence from the data rejects the null hypothesis*.

In summary, hypothesis testing tells us if one variable is really influencing another variable, or if it is due to chance. Keep in mind that no matter how powerful the findings of a quantitative study are, nothing is ever totally proven. The most that can be claimed is that the research hypothesis is either supported or unsupported.

For example, a research study tested the effects of a childhood obesity prevention program in elementary schools. The study also included a control group. The main outcome measure for each group was weight change. The research hypothesis was that the program would lead to greater weight loss in the experimental group than in a control group. The null hypothesis was that there would be no difference in average weight loss between the groups at the end of the study. The researchers set a level of significance of 0.05 and used a *t*-test (statistical test) to determine whether the means of the groups were significantly different from one another at the end of the study. The *P*-value of the *t*-test was less than 0.05, so the researchers rejected the null hypothesis and supported the research hypothesis that the program led to significantly greater weight loss in the experimental group. Because the average weight loss was statistically significant, the difference between the groups is unlikely to have occurred by chance.

The level of significance is set to avoid what is called a type I error (**Table 4.4**). A **type I error (also called α error)** is when you reject the null hypothesis when the null hypothesis is true. So a type I error is when you think the independent variable caused the difference between the groups when the groups were truly no different from each other. A **type II error (also called β error)** is when you accept the null hypothesis when it is false. So a type II error is when you think the independent variable did not have any effect, but it really did and the groups are truly different from each other.

In the gardening study, a type I error would occur if the researchers concluded the children who went through the program did eat more fruits and vegetables, when in reality both groups were the same. If the researchers found no differences between the groups, when the children who received the program were truly eating more fruits and vegetables, that would be a type II error.

TIP

To help you remember type I and type II error, use this acronym RAAR (Gillis & Jackson, 2002). RAAR stands for **R**eject the null hypothesis when you should **A**ccept it (type I) and **A**ccept the null hypothesis when you should **R**eject it (type II). You can also think of the type I error as a false positive, and the type II error as a false negative.

RAAR

Table 4.4 Type I and Type II Errors

	The null hypothesis is true in the real world	The null hypothesis is false in the real world
Researcher accepts the null hypothesis	No error	Type II error
Researcher rejects the null hypothesis	Type I error	No error

STATISTICAL SIGNIFICANCE AND EFFECT SIZE

Hypothesis testing and statistical significance can tell you whether the findings are due to chance or not, but they do not tell you if:

- the findings are necessarily *clinically important*, or
- anything about the *size* of the difference between the groups on an outcome variable, or the strength of the relationship between two variables.

Effect size is the magnitude of an effect. It could be the size of the difference in an outcome measure between the experimental and control groups in an experimental or quasi-experimental study. It could also be the strength of the relationship between two variables, as seen, for example, in a correlation.

When you want to examine the size of the difference in means between two groups in a study, all you have to do is subtract the means. For example, if the intervention group in a weight loss study lost 8 pounds (−8) while the control group lost 2 pounds (−2), the difference (or *effect size*) is −6 pounds. The effect size tells you about how powerful the effect of the independent variable is on an outcome variable, as well as the direction of the relationship. *Keep this in mind: along with statistical significance, effect size can help you evaluate the clinical importance of a study.*

Another reason you do not want to completely rely on statistical significance is that even a small difference between two variables will become statistically significant if you have a large enough sample. Effect size is not related to sample size, so effect size does not have that issue.

TIP

Statistical significance answers the question "Does it work?" whereas effect size answers the question "How well does it work?" You can also say that a *P*-value tells you whether the results are real, and the effect size tells you how important the results are. Use *both P*-values and effect sizes to evaluate the results of a study.

RELIABILITY AND VALIDITY

Reliability focuses on the repeatability of a particular set of research findings. If a study is replicated, researchers hope to get similar results, which confirms their earlier findings. Because reliability looks at the consistency of data, it is very important that any instruments used for measuring in a study are reliable. Later you will learn about how to test the reliability of instruments such as tests and questionnaires. For now, you need to know that for any observed measurement or score, such as a Healthy Eating Index score of 70, there are two components: the true score and the error score (See **Figure 4.5**). If reliability is high, the observed score will be very close to the true score. When reliability is low, the observed score contains more error.

Validity refers to the degree to which the conclusions drawn from the study are accurate and well founded. Validity also looks at whether instruments and measurements are accurate; in other words, are they truly measuring what they are intended to measure? Without accuracy (validity) and reliability in measuring variables, research results will not be useful.

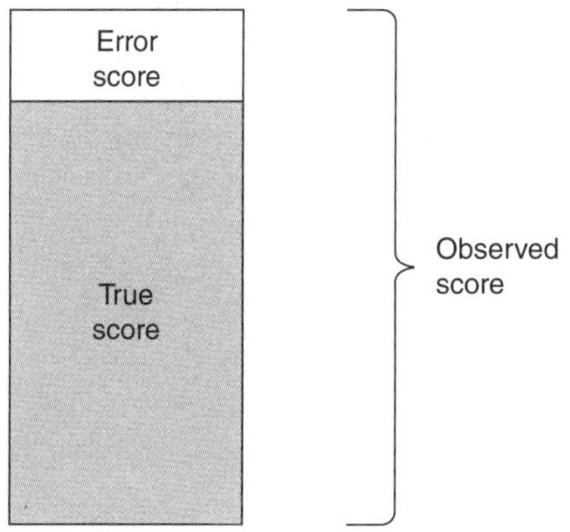

FIGURE 4.5 Relationship Between the Observed Score, the True Score, and Error Score

Shadish, Cook, and Campbell (2002) describe four types of validity:

1. **Internal validity** is the extent to which the independent variable, rather than some extraneous variable(s), actually caused the outcome of the study. Although it is most important in studies looking at causality, internal validity is a concern for all studies. At the end of a study, researchers like to see that their hypothesis appears correct, but they need to ask themselves if there is *another* reasonable explanation for the findings (in other words, a rival hypothesis).
2. **External validity** is the extent to which a study's findings can be generalized "externally," meaning beyond the study's subjects, setting, and time. In other words, are the study's results applicable to other people in different settings at a different time? For example, if adolescents exposed to growing vegetables in a program in Minneapolis ate significantly more servings of vegetables at the end of the study, will the same thing happen with adolescents exposed to the same program in rural Texas? External validity depends quite a bit on how the sampling was done.
3. **Statistical conclusion validity** is the extent to which inferences about relationships among variables *from the statistical analysis of the data are accurate*. It does not involve looking at whether there really is a causal or other relationship between certain variables; that is what internal validity looks at. Instead, statistical conclusion validity looks at whether the results of the statistical procedures accurately reflect the real world. With the proper use of statistics and statistical tests, there will be less chance of type I or type II errors.
4. **Construct validity** is the extent to which the researchers are actually measuring the theoretical concepts or constructs in the study. It is the highest standard of validity, and not easy to prove. A concept or construct such as "self-care" has a theoretical definition, which provides the basis for the development of an operational definition. However, is the researcher's operational definition of "self-care" able to accurately measure all relevant aspects of the theoretical construct? Construct validity looks at how well the dependent variable, as well as the intervention, represent the underlying constructs in an experiment.

Now we take a more in-depth look at each type of validity.

INTERNAL VALIDITY

In a randomized controlled trial (RCT), participants are randomly assigned to the intervention or control group, and then followed forward in time to compare the outcomes. Randomization, when done properly, creates equivalent groups so that differences between the groups can be attributed to the independent variable. Randomization helps rule out many threats to internal validity, but not all of them. In quasi-experimental or correlational studies, there are even more threats to internal validity—more competing explanations for why a study turned out the way it did.

Shadish, Cook, and Campbell (2002) explained a number of threats to internal validity:

- **History**: Did some current event occur during the study (and unrelated to the study) that affected the dependent variable?
- **Maturation**: Did the normal maturation of the participant (getting older, more experienced, and so forth) affect the dependent variable?
- Selection: Did any factor that was involved in creating the groups produce differences between the kinds of people in one group as opposed to another group?
- Mortality/**Attrition**: Did participants who dropped out of the study affect the dependent variable?
- Testing: Did familiarity with the pretest affect the scores on the posttest (assuming use of the same test)?
- Instrumentation: Did any change in measurement over the course of the study affect the scores on the dependent variable?
- **Regression to the mean**: If participants had very high or very low pretest scores, did their scores move closer to the mean on the posttest (due to natural variability) and affect the dependent variable?

Another threat to internal validity is an inability to determine whether the independent or dependent variable occurred first. To establish causality, it must be clear that the independent variable occurred first.

EXTERNAL VALIDITY

External validity looks at whether the results of your study can be generalized to another place, with different people and conditions, and at a later time. In other words, if a study showed that variable A heavily influenced variable B, would that still be the case in another location with different participants at a different time and under another set of conditions? Major threats to external validity are people, place, and time. A study would be much more generalizable, for example, if the researchers drew a random sample, the dropout rate was low, and the study took place in a number of locations. If the sample was not random, it would be important for the study to use a sampling plan that minimized bias, such as using eligibility criteria or choosing groups in which only people who are similar with respect to the confounding variable(s) are included.

Multisite studies provide large, diverse samples in different locations (with differing conditions), and are certainly more generalizable than a study that took place in four schools in one town in California, for instance. If a study has been replicated (meaning a new setting, people, and time) with similar results, that certainly increases its generalizability.

Systematic reviews are studies in which the researchers put together results from many primary research studies on the same topic, such as if dietary potassium affects blood pressure in hypertensive patients. Systematic reviews normally include quantitative studies with similar research designs, such as randomized controlled trials, but the studies took place at different times in different places and with different people. They are helpful in looking at external validity because they look at results across people, place, and time.

Statistical Conclusion Validity

To have statistical conclusion validity, the study must first have enough power. **Power** refers to the ability of a study to detect statistically significant differences or relationships in the groups when they really do exist. In other words, the power of a hypothesis test is the probability of rejecting the null hypothesis when you should reject it. The ability to detect significant differences is dependent on the sample size. If sample size is low, you run more of a chance of accepting the null hypothesis when it is false (type II error).

Some additional threats to statistical conclusion validity include the following (Shadish et al., 2002):

1. *Violation of assumptions of statistical tests.* Every statistical test works best when certain assumptions are met. Statistics books lay out the assumptions for statistical tests, such as that one-way ANOVA requires the distribution of the dependent variable be normally distributed, the grouping variable has at least three categories, and so on. Before running a statistical test, you should check to be sure your data meet the assumptions.
2. *Fishing.* Because research that fails to reject the null hypothesis is less likely to be published, researchers may do hundreds of tests on different variables (known as **fishing**) looking for significant differences or relationships, and then choose to write up the results from the tests that were significant. When you conduct multiple statistical tests of the same data, it increases the chance of finding a relationship that does not really exist.
3. *Reliability of measures.* When unreliable measures, such as a questionnaire or a scale, are used in a study involving two variables, they can reduce the size of any effect caused by the independent variable. When there are three or more variables, unreliable measures may increase or decrease the size of any effect.
4. *Reliability of treatment implementation.* This refers to treatment fidelity, which was mentioned earlier. When treatment differs from one participant to another, it may decrease or (less commonly) increase the chance of seeing true differences in the groups.

Table 4.5 explains consequences of these threats to statistical conclusion validity.

Table 4.5 Consequences of Threats to Statistical Conclusion Validity

Threat	Can result in
Low statistical power	Increasing risk of type II error.
Fishing	Increasing risk of type I error.
Violated assumptions of statistical tests	Overestimating or underestimating the size and significance of an effect.
Unreliability of measures	Weakening the relationship between two variables.
Unreliability of treatment implementation	Underestimating or, in some cases, overestimating effect of the treatment.

CONSTRUCT VALIDITY

Threats to construct validity can make it hard for you to conclude that a study was an accurate operationalization of the constructs. Here are some examples of threats to construct validity (Shadish et al., 2002):

1. If the theoretical construct or its operational definition are not well developed, this can lead to low construct validity.
2. When only one method is used to measure a construct, such as only using a clinical exam to assess nutrition status, fewer dimensions of the construct are measured. Using more than one instrument to measure a construct improves construct validity, especially if the two instruments vary in how data are gathered (such as written, oral, and observation).
3. Another threat is expectation bias on the part of the researcher. **Expectation bias** is when researchers' expectations of what they believe the study results should be get in the way of accurately taking measurements and reporting results.

To avoid construct validity issues, it is important for researchers to have accurate operational definitions and to use multiple validated measures. Using blinding in the study also reduces problems with expectation bias.

To summarize, here are definitions for the four types of validity.

1. Internal validity is the extent to which the independent variable actually caused the outcome of the study.
2. External validity is the extent to which a study's findings can be generalized externally, meaning beyond this study's participants, setting, and time.
3. Statistical conclusion validity is the extent to which inferences about relationships among variables from the statistical analysis of the data are accurate.
4. Construct validity is the extent to which the researchers are actually measuring the theoretical concepts or constructs in the study.

APPLICATION 4.2

An experiment was done to test a nutrition education intervention to increase calcium and vitamin D consumption among older women. A small convenience sample was found at two senior centers: one center was the experimental group and the other center was the control group. Eligibility criteria were not used. Name one threat in this experiment to each of the following: internal validity, external validity, and statistical conclusion validity.

ERROR AND BIAS

In a research study, error is defined as the difference between the *true* value of a measurement and the actual recorded measurement. All errors fit into one of two categories: random or systematic. A **random error**, also known as random variation or imprecision, is due to chance or simply the normal variability in people. **Precision** is when you get a similar result every time you measure something, so random errors decrease your precision. The impact of random error can be minimized with a large enough sample.

Systematic errors, also called **bias**, are not due to chance, meaning that multiple replications of the same study, on average, would still reach the wrong answer. Biases can operate in either direction. Some will lead to underestimation of the intervention's effect; others will lead to overestimation. Some biases have small effects, others have much larger effects. In any case, systematic errors affect **accuracy** (the degree to which a measurement approximates the true value). Increasing sample size will not help, so designing and implementing studies properly should focus on removing known biases.

An example of a random error would be the variation in response when you perform a 24-hour diet recall with a client on three separate occasions. An example of a systematic error might occur if a question on supplement use in a survey was not clear, and respondents checked off "Not Applicable" due to confusion.

Table 4.6 lists some examples of potential biases in research. There can be biases in any part of a research study, such as the research design, sampling, measurement, or reporting results. For example, participants are prone to change their behavior or responses to questions because they are being studied. This is known as the **Hawthorne effect** and is a type of measurement bias. When using surveys, **nonresponse bias** occurs when the percentage of people who do not respond to the survey varies among the different groups in the survey sample. Other disciplines sometimes use different names to refer to the same bias, so you may see other terms used.

Researchers can certainly bring their own biases to the research process.

- **Confirmation bias** is when a researcher selectively interprets information to confirm his or her own beliefs and opinions.
- **Publication bias** refers to the tendency for researchers to seek publication only of studies with statistically significant findings; studies that do not support a hypothesis often are not submitted.
- **Allegiance bias** occurs when a researcher's results risk being biased, or a study not published, because of allegiances to a funder or an employer, for example.

Because of these concerns, it is important to critique a study and focus on the quality of each study you read.

Table 4.6 Examples of Bias in Research

Type of bias	Description
Selection bias	Systematic differences between baseline characteristics of the groups that are compared.
Performance bias	Systematic differences between groups in the care that is provided, or in exposure to factors other than the interventions of interest.
Detection bias	Systematic differences between groups in how outcomes are determined.
Attrition bias	Systematic differences between groups in withdrawals from a study.
Noncompliance bias/ nonresponse bias	Systematic differences between groups in compliance with protocol.
Reporting bias	Systematic differences between reported and unreported findings.
Measurement bias	Systematic differences between true and recorded measurements. Errors in measurement may be due to the study participant (responder bias), the instruments being used to make the measurement, such as weighing scales (instrument bias), or the observer (observer bias).
Confounding bias	Systematic differences due to extraneous/confounding variables that are not controlled.

Modified from "A Common Classification Scheme for Bias" in the *Cochrane Handbook for Systematic Reviews of Interventions* (Version 5.1.0, Table 8.4a) by J. Higgins and S. Green (Eds.), Copyright © 2011, Wiley. Reproduced with permission of John Wiley & Sons Ltd.

According to Lipman (2013), "bias can be reduced only by proper study design and execution. Bias is a direct reflection of the methodological **rigor** or quality in a study—the higher or better or more rigorous the methodological quality, the lower the risk of bias" (p. 161). Some ways to reduce bias are the same things done to improve validity. They include randomization into groups, blinded studies in which the researchers/outcomes assessors and participants are blinded to group assignment, and intervention fidelity.

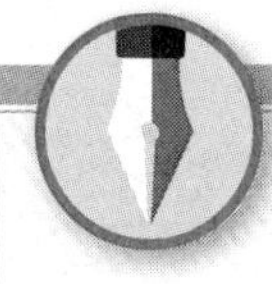

TIP

Do not confuse validity and bias. They are different but related concepts. High bias in a study means low validity, and a study with excellent validity will have little bias.

APPLICATION 4.3

When you take college courses, you usually have to complete a survey about the course/instructor at the end of the term. Describe at least two ways in which the survey results could be biased.

SAMPLING

Most researchers aim for a sample that is representative of the population of interest in order to get data that accurately reflects the population. Depending on the population of interest, researchers may use selection criteria (such as inclusion or exclusion criteria) to make sure they get representative participants. To do sampling, you need to distinguish between the following terms:

- The **target population** refers to the people the study is focused on. For example, a population might be postmenopausal women with breast cancer. The target population is the group *to whom you want to apply your results*.
- The **accessible** or **source population** is a subset of the target population to whom you can get access. It is crucial that the accessible population accurately reflects the target population. For a researcher studying postmenopausal breast cancer, a specific accessible population may be members of several cancer registries. A list of names of women with postmenopausal breast cancer from these registries are then called a **sampling frame**. A sampling frame is a list of members of the accessible population from which the sample is drawn.
- The **sample** includes the people from the accessible population who you have asked to participate. Keep in mind that some members of the sample may be eliminated if they do not completely meet the eligibility criteria for the study/survey.

Figure 4.6 displays these concepts.

Once the accessible population is identified, you can identify potential respondents in one of two ways: probability sampling or nonprobability sampling. In probability sampling, each person in the population has an equal probability, or chance, of being selected because the method for choosing respondents is random. Using probability sampling allows you to use probability-based statistics, such as hypothesis tests, with your data.

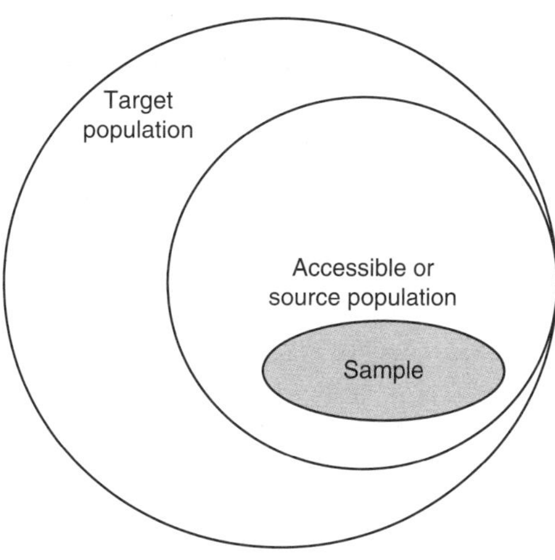

FIGURE 4.6 Target Population, Accessible Population, and the Sample

PROBABILITY SAMPLING

A variety of random probability methods can be used to pick a sample:

- **Simple random sampling** involves randomly selecting individuals on a numbered list using either a table of random numbers or an online random sample generator. Using a table of random numbers can be cumbersome when you are seeking a larger sample.
- **Systematic random sampling** involves selecting every *n*th individual from a list after a random start point, such as choosing every 35th person after starting with the 23rd person. The interval (every *n*th person) is determined by dividing the number in the sampling frame by the desired sample size.
- **Stratified random sampling** involves dividing the accessible population into groups (based on age or gender, for example) and then using simple or systematic random sampling for each group (also called strata). The random sampling is usually, but not always, done proportionally so that more respondents are drawn from the larger strata.
- **Cluster random sampling** involves dividing the population into clusters (such as geographic clusters), randomly picking some of the clusters, and then randomly sampling within each of those clusters.

Stratified sampling is used when you split up the accessible population into groups (or strata) based on a factor that could influence the variable being measured (such as age, gender, or urban/rural location), and then you use simple random sampling within each group. It is only possible when you know what proportion of the population belongs to each group. Researchers use stratified sampling to make sure that the sample accurately represents the different groups in the population.

In cluster sampling, the population is separated into groups called clusters, such as schools or nursing homes. Clusters are more or less alike, each resembling the overall population. Cluster sampling is useful when the population is widely distributed geographically and occurs in natural clusters. To use cluster sampling, the researcher randomly picks some clusters, and then randomly obtains the sample from just those clusters. Cluster sampling is used to make sampling more practical or affordable.

Many large national studies use **multistage sampling**. Multistage sampling refers to sampling plans where the sampling is carried out in stages using smaller and

TIP

Keep in mind that cluster sampling differs from stratified sampling in that cluster sampling only draws a sample from the randomly chosen clusters. With stratification, researchers draw a sample from *all* of the groups. See **Figure 4.7** for a graphic displaying this.

smaller sampling units at each stage. In reality, cluster sampling is an example of multistage sampling because it involves at least two stages. In **multistage (or multilevel) cluster sampling**, a large area, such as the United States, is first divided into smaller units, such as states, and some of these smaller units are randomly selected. In the second stage, the selected states are split into smaller units (such as counties), and a random selection is made of counties within each state. In the third stage, a random selection is made of yet smaller areas (such as census tracts) of the counties. Often this will yield an area that can be randomly sampled without being too large. **Table 4.7** gives examples of each probability sampling method.

NONPROBABILITY SAMPLING

Nonprobability sampling is based on respondents being selected by convenience or judgment. These methods are much less likely than probability samples to produce representative samples. Here are common nonprobability sampling methods:

- **Convenience sampling** is when members of the population are chosen simply because they are easy to reach and the researcher often has a comfort level asking them to participate. It is the weakest form of sampling but is frequently used in research.

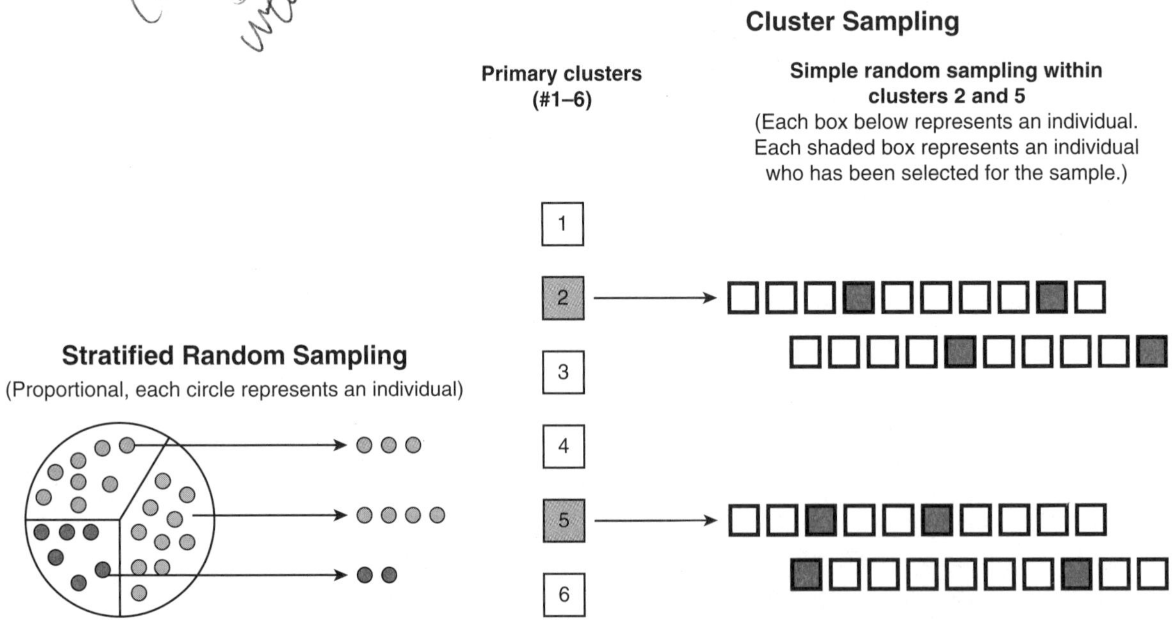

Stratified Random Sampling
(Proportional, each circle represents an individual)

Cluster Sampling
Primary clusters (#1–6)
Simple random sampling within clusters 2 and 5
(Each box below represents an individual. Each shaded box represents an individual who has been selected for the sample.)
1
2
3
4
5
6

FIGURE 4.7 Stratified Random Sampling and Cluster Sampling

Table 4.7 Probability Sampling Methods with Examples

Probability sampling method	Examples
Simple random sampling (selecting individuals on a numbered list using either a table of random numbers or an online random sample generator) OR *Systematic random sampling* (selecting every *n*th individual from a list after a random start point)	Leong, Madden, Gray, Waters, and Horwath (2011) used a self-administered mail survey to collect data about the speed of eating and degree of obesity in New Zealand women aged 40 to 50 years old (*target population*). This age bracket was chosen because of high prevalence of obesity and also because women often gained weight at this time. The *accessible population* was female residents who were eligible to vote. A sample of 2,500 New Zealand women were randomly selected from the national electoral rolls (the *sampling frame*) using either simple or systematic random sampling (the study does not say which). The survey's response rate was 65.8%. Results showed that as body mass index (BMI) significantly increased, so did self-reported speed of eating.
Stratified random sampling (dividing the accessible population into groups or strata, and then using simple random sampling to select from each group)	Ritchie et al. (2015) conducted an online and mail survey of child care sites in California (*target population*) in 2012. The purpose was to determine if policies (one federal and one Californian) enacted since their prior survey (2008) had improved the quality of the beverages served to children aged 2 to 5 years. State databases of all licensed childcare centers and family homes in California served as the *sampling frame*. The researchers randomly picked 1,484 childcare sites, equal numbers from each of six categories (or *strata*): Head Start, state preschool, and so on. The survey's response rate was 31%. Results showed improvements in the serving of healthy beverages from 2008 to 2012.
Cluster random sampling (dividing the population into clusters, such as geographic clusters, randomly picking some of the clusters, and then randomly sampling within each of those clusters)	A researcher wants to learn if Latinos in an urban setting use and understand the Nutrition Facts label. The Latino area of the city is split into 16 clusters that are of similar population size. Five of the clusters are randomly chosen. Next, 150 households are randomly selected within each cluster. Interviewers ask for the adult who is most involved in food purchasing and preparation to be surveyed in each household. (This is a simple two-stage cluster sample.)
Multistage cluster sampling (using cluster sampling that is carried out in stages using smaller and smaller sampling units at each stage)	NHANES (2011–2014) used a four-stage sample design. In the first stage, counties are randomly chosen (in some cases, counties are combined to keep them big enough). In the second stage, a random selection is made of census blocks (or combinations of blocks) within the selected counties. In the third stage, households (or dwelling units) are selected, and in the fourth stage a person within the household was selected. In each stage, the rates required for sampling individuals were based on sex, age, race, Hispanic origin, and income. Hispanics were oversampled because more reliable information was needed for this population group (Johnson, Dohrmann, Burt, & Mohadjer, 2014).

- **Quota sampling** is the same as convenience sampling but there are also quotas (limits) put on the number of people in the sample of a particular gender, age, race, or other characteristic. Often the quotas are based on the proportions found within the population, such as 50% male, 50% female. So the researchers first identify the groups within the population and figure out how many should be drawn from each group, much like in stratified random sampling, only these respondents are not being drawn randomly.

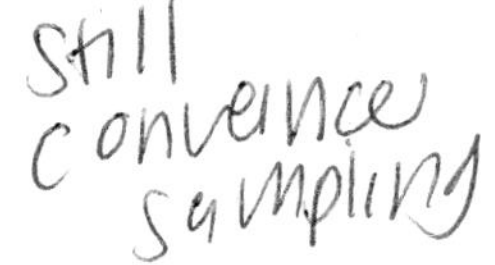

- **Purposive or judgment sampling** is also a convenience sample, but in this case the researchers choose respondents specifically based on whether the respondent is a good representative of the population.

- **Network (snowball) sampling** is used when locating respondents with the needed characteristics is difficult. Basically, when the researcher finds a few respondents who are appropriate for the study, they ask to be directed to further potential respondents. So the first few respondents are picked using purposive sampling, then the remaining respondents are picked using network or snowball sampling. This method is used more often in qualitative than quantitative studies.

The data from nonprobability sampling may not be representative of the population and is usually prone to selection bias and sampling error. **Table 4.8** lists examples of each type of nonprobability sampling.

It is important to discuss various errors and biases that prevent an accurate picture of the population from your sample. First, **sampling variance** (also called **sampling error**) happens when a characteristic from your sample, such as sugar intake in adolescents does not match the sugar intake in adolescents in the population. In any sample, even when appropriately chosen, there will be chance variation. The best way to control

Table 4.8 Nonprobability Sampling Methods with Examples

Nonprobability sampling method	Examples
Convenience sampling (members of the population are chosen simply because they are easy to reach and the researcher may have a comfort level asking them to complete a survey)	Algert, Baameur, and Renvall (2014) surveyed 83 gardeners using community gardens in San Jose, California, including what vegetables they grew in their gardens. The gardeners were recruited from four community gardens. Ten of the 83 gardeners also weighed the output of their gardens from spring through summer. Results showed that their crop yields were higher than conventional agriculture, and the gardeners saved about $435/plot on vegetable purchases (after expenses for seed, etc.).
Quota sampling (determine the groups within the population and figure out how many should be drawn from each group, which is done using convenience sampling)	Iglesia et al. (2015) conducted a cross-sectional survey in 13 countries to describe total fluid intake in children and adolescents and how it varies by age and sex. In some countries, the sample was selected using quota sampling. The quotas were based on age, sex, region of the country, habitat, and socioeconomic characteristics. Results showed that many children and adolescents are at risk of inadequate fluid intake, especially males and adolescents.
Purposive sampling (researchers choose respondents based on whether or not the respondent is a good representative of the population)	Patel, Kennedy, Blickem, Reeves, and Chew-Graham (2016) conducted interviews with British South Asian adults with diabetes living in Greater Manchester, UK. The purpose was to explore their beliefs and practices on managing diabetes when they spent the holidays (often several months) on the Indian subcontinent. Some of the respondents were purposely recruited from mosques, religious classes, and Muslim day centers to obtain a broad sample. Results showed that some respondents did not continue their medication on holiday, which suggests a poor understanding of diabetes.
Network or snowball sampling (researchers find a few good respondents and then ask them for referrals to other potential respondents)	Doub, Small, and Birch (2015) examined child feeding beliefs and practices, types of recipes, and their associations in food blogs written by mothers of preschoolers. They used an initial sample of 100 blogs to find further blog recommendations: a snowball sample of 168 blogs, of which 8 were included in the study. Results showed that blogs often described involving children in food preparation and preparing foods that children readily accept. (Note: This example shows how snowball sampling was used to find blogs that were evaluated using a survey tool, not to find respondents.)

for sampling error is to make sure you use a large enough sample size. Larger samples have a better chance of producing results closer to the real population.

Sample bias happens when the members of your sample are systematically different from the population in some way. It can occur for a variety of reasons:

- **Coverage bias** A segment of the population is excluded from the sample. For example, if an online survey is being used to collect data, and a segment of your population does not have computers or computer skills (such as the older or low-income individuals), you will be missing this segment in your results.
- **Selection bias** Some groups in the population have a higher or lower chance of being selected than others.
- **Nonresponse bias** In survey sampling, the percentage of people who do not respond to the survey varies among the different groups in the sample.

Sample bias does not improve if you increase the sample size. Getting the right information from the right people is more important than how many people are in your sample. To get the right people, you need to select a sample that fairly represents the entire population and obtain data from as much of the sample as possible.

APPLICATION 4.4

In the study by Rajkumar, Karthikeyan, Manwar, Sistla, and Kate (2013) in Appendix A, how were the participants selected? What sampling method was used?

SAMPLE SIZE

Power refers to the ability of a study to detect statistically significant differences or relationships in the groups when they really do exist. In other words, the power of a hypothesis test is the probability of rejecting the null hypothesis when you should reject it. To have enough power in a study, you need to do a **power analysis** to calculate the minimum sample size needed to detect the difference you are looking for. In general, *increasing sample size increases power*. A power analysis can be used for experimental, quasi-experimental, and correlational studies.

First, let's review a few key statistical concepts:

- Alpha (α) is the probability of a type I error.
- Beta (β) is the probability of a type II error.
- The quantity $1-\beta$ is the power of a test (the probability of *avoiding* a type II error).

In a power analysis, power is normally set at 80%, meaning that we have a 20% chance of *failing to observe a difference when there is one* (a type II error).

Power analysis uses the relationships among the following factors to determine sample size (Grove et al., 2013):

- *The level of significance you are using* (the alpha level). Often the alpha level is set at 0.05 or lower, meaning that the chance of making a type I error is 1 in 20 or lower. If you want to use a level of 0.01, you will need a much larger sample size.
- *The power level* (usually set at 0.80, so there is a 20% chance of a type II error). You may wonder why the type I error is set a lot lower than the type II error. A type I error is more serious because you claim that an intervention worked when in fact it didn't.

- *The expected effect size* (the magnitude or size of the difference between the groups). For example, if a study showed that the Healthy Eating Index of the experimental group was 65/100 and the control group was 54/100, the difference between the groups is 11. The effect size is often estimated by taking the difference between the two groups and dividing it by the standard deviation of the participants. If the result is between 0.3 and 0.5, the effect size would be considered moderate (although it varies depending on the context and other factors). For a power analysis, you need to look at previous studies (if available) to see what the difference might be between the groups. The smaller the effect size, the larger the necessary sample size because it will be harder to detect. If the effect size is fairly large, you do not need as large of a sample. Researchers often use a value of 0.5 for effect size because it indicates a moderate to large difference.
- *The sample size.*

When working with a statistician or using a power or sample size program, you will be expected to provide information on the effect size as well as the level of type I and type II error you are willing to accept. Other factors considered are the type of study, number of variables, expected standard deviation, method of data analysis, and sample design.

Doing a power analysis enables you to determine whether the available sample is adequate to answer your research questions and to detect important effects or associations. When sample size is too small, you run the risk of concluding that the groups were not different when in fact they were (type II error). One last thing to keep in mind is that if you need a sample of, let us say 1,100 people, you need to include more than that in your initial sample to account for attrition.

To determine sample size, consulting a statistician is definitely recommended. For more information on calculating sample size, consult Boushey (2008) and Hulley, Cummings, Browner, and Grady (2013). Sample size calculators are available online, and some are noted at the end of the chapter under "Suggested Readings and Activities."

INSTRUMENTS AND MEASUREMENT

Nutrition research uses a variety of methods and instruments to measure variables, from self-reported dietary recalls and food frequency questionnaires to anthropometric, laboratory, and clinical measurements. Once you know exactly what you want measured in a study, you can assess which instruments to use and how they are to be used, taking into account factors such as each instrument's advantages and disadvantages, the budget, time frame, and number of participants.

Measuring variables accurately is not as simple as it may sound. For example, the objective in a study conducted by Rehm, Peñalvo, Afshin, and Mozaffarian (2016) was "to characterize trends in overall diet quality and multiple dietary components related to major diseases among U.S. adults, including by age, sex, race/ethnicity, education, and income" (p. 2543). They used diet data from the National Health and Nutrition Examination Survey (NHANES) and chose the American Heart Association (AHA) primary diet score for measuring the quality of the diet. The primary diet score measures consumption of five categories of food—fruits and vegetables, whole grains, fish and shellfish, sugar-sweetened beverages, and sodium—and each category carries equal weight.

The problem the researchers ran into was that NHANES only had one 24-hour diet recall for each participant during the early years the researchers wanted to cover, and the AHA diet score for two categories (fish and shellfish, sugar-sweetened beverages) looks at weekly (not daily) intake. So if a participant did not eat fish during the 24-hour diet recall period, then they ate no fish at all for the week, even though that person may have eaten fish on several other days of that week. This, of course, could be a source of bias, so the researchers only used data after 2003 when two consecutive 24-hour recalls were performed.

Bias can affect measurements in many ways. Errors in measurement may be due to the study participant (**response bias**), the instruments being used to make the measurement, such as weighing scales (**instrument bias**), or other factors. Here are some examples of response bias:

- **Recall bias** occurs when participants are asked to recall something from their past, such as their eating habits, and the ability to recall accurately differs between the groups.
- **Social desirability bias** occurs when participants choose responses to questions that they believe will be viewed favorably by others.
- **Extreme response set bias** happens when participants pick the most extreme answers, even when it is not accurate. Sometimes this happens when a participant is indifferent about filling out a questionnaire for instance.
- **Acquiescence bias** is a form of response bias in which respondents are more likely to agree with a list of statements than to disagree.

In assessing the quality of an instrument, consider both its reliability (consistency in measuring under similar circumstances) and validity (the instrument is measuring what it is supposed to measure). Here are some ways to test whether an instrument is reliable or consistent over time.

1. **Test-retest reliability** (also known as stability reliability) is measured by, for example, having the same respondents take the *same test at two different times* to see how consistent or stable their answers are. In the case of body weight, you may have the participants weighed twice to assess the reliability of the process. Performing test-retest reliability is not always possible, especially when it involves a lot of time and money or the second measurement is influenced by the first measurement.
   For measures with interval or ratio answers, such as weight, Pearson's correlation coefficient can be used to correlate the two measurements. A correlation coefficient (*r* value, can range from 0.00 to 1.00) of at least 0.70–0.80 is generally considered good. You can also assess the test-retest reliability of a continuous variable by using a paired *t*-test.
   For ordinal answers, such as ranking something, the Spearman nonparametric rank correlation coefficient could be used. For categorical variables, you could simply calculate the percentage of time the test-retest scores are in agreement.
2. **Inter-rater reliability** measures the *consistency of two or more raters* who, for example, have to categorize answers to open-ended questions on a survey or observe and record an event (as in a qualitative study). Inter-rater reliability is used to test how similarly raters (or observers) categorize, score, or simply measure something. You can use the same statistical tools to measure inter-rater reliability that were used in measuring test-retest reliability. Some researchers like to use an intraclass correlation coefficient (ICC) to determine inter-rater reliability (as well as test-retest reliability). A rating closer to 0.90 (or 90%) is desirable for inter-rater reliability.
3. **Internal consistency reliability** (or inter-item reliability) looks at *how well different questions measuring the same construct produce similar results*. Testing internal

consistency requires less money and time than test-retest. To use it, you administer the questions to a group of people on one occasion. Each question measuring the same construct should be highly correlated to show internal consistency. Cronbach's alpha coefficient is the most common internal consistency reliability coefficient, and it is used for interval and ratio level data. It ranges from 0.00 (no internal consistency) to 1.00 (perfect internal consistency). The higher the coefficient, the more internally consistent the questions. If Cronbach's alpha coefficient is 0.80, it indicates the test is 80% reliable with 20% random error (DeVon et al., 2007). A coefficient of 0.80 or higher is desirable, and a reliability coefficient less than 0.60 is considered low.

Validity for an instrument looks at whether the instrument accurately measures what it is intended to measure. There are various types of validity. Face and content validity are the assessments used most often, in part because they are easier to accomplish. However, criterion and construct validity are also critical.

1. **Face validity** is a first step toward establishing an instrument's credibility. In the case of a survey, the survey questions could be reviewed by untrained judges, such as people like your potential respondents. They are asked to judge (subjectively) whether the format, questions, and procedures are clear and easy to use, and whether the instrument appears to measure what it is supposed to measure.
2. **Content validity** is also subjective. Content validity looks at whether the instrument covers all the dimensions it is supposed to measure.
3. **Criterion validity** measures *how well an instrument stacks up against another instrument or predicts something*. Criterion validity can be subdivided into concurrent and predictive validity. **Concurrent validity** refers to the degree to which your instrument correlates with another previously established and valid instrument, perhaps a gold standard. For example, a tool to assess nutrition status in the elderly may be tested against the Mini-Nutritional Assessment, a validated nutrition assessment tool used to identify patients age 65 and above who are malnourished or at risk of malnutrition (Marshall, Young, Bauer, & Isenring, 2015). **Predictive validity** evaluates how well your instrument predicts a specific outcome, such as a survey asking adults about their attitudes toward healthy eating, which may predict the quality of their diets.
4. *Construct validity* can be difficult to assess but is very valuable. Basically construct validity is when you *experimentally test the quality of an instrument to determine whether it is measuring the concept it is intended to measure.* **Factor analysis** can be used to determine an instrument's construct validity when the instrument is a survey, scale, or test. To use factor analysis, the instrument must first be administered to a large, representative group. Factor analysis is a statistical technique that looks at interrelationships among many variables to identify clusters of variables that are most closely linked. In exploratory factor analysis each factor or cluster is identified. For example, if a 20-item questionnaire is a valid measure of the construct "nutrition literacy," a factor analysis on the scores of the questionnaire should result in one factor that can explain most of the variances in these 20 items. If an item is not included in a factor, meaning it does not correlate well with other items, the item may be removed. Then the researcher can develop models and use confirmatory factor analysis for statistical hypothesis testing on these proposed models.

Reliability and validity are important for evaluating quantitative instruments, but if you are using any screening or diagnostic instruments, they should be evaluated for sensitivity and specificity. **Sensitivity** tells you how well an instrument can screen or diagnose a condition; in other words, how well does it find true positives? A measure that has 65% sensitivity will screen or diagnose correctly 65 out of every 100 people who have the condition. **Specificity** tells you how well an instrument finds true negatives, so a measure with 81% specificity means it finds every 81 out of 100 people who do not have the condition.

APPLICATION 4.5

Using the study by Rajkumar, Karthikeyan, Manwar, Sistla, and Kate (2013) in Appendix B, answer the following questions about measurements.

1. What were the primary and secondary outcomes?
2. How was each outcome measured?
3. What baseline characteristics were measured on patients?

ANATOMY OF A RESEARCH ARTICLE

Table 4.9 lists the parts of a research article. By looking carefully at the title, you may be able to figure out quickly whether this study is qualitative or quantitative, and if it is quantitative, whether it has an intervention. After the title is the listing of authors. Most journals will include affiliations for the authors as well as any possible conflicts of interest and sources of research funding (either at the beginning or end of the article). You may look at the research articles in Appendix A or Appendix B for examples.

In the title of an article by McAleese and Rankin (2007), "Garden-Based Nutrition Education Affects Fruit and Vegetable Consumption in Sixth-Grade Adolescents," you see the word "affects." Often you will see the words "affects" or "associated with" in an article title; they give clues about the independent and dependent variables. If garden-based nutrition education affects fruit and vegetable consumption, then "education" is the independent variable (in this case an intervention) and "fruit and vegetable consumption" are the dependent variables. Keep in mind that the dependent (or outcome) variable "depends" on something, such as an intervention, for any change.

Let's look at an article titled "Sociodemographic and Behavioral Factors Associated with Added Sugars Intake Among U.S. Adults" (Park, Thompson, McGuire, Pan, Galuska, & Blanck, 2016). The researchers looked at which sociodemographic factors (such as income and education) or behavioral factors (such as alcohol intake and physical activity level) are *associated* with higher levels of added sugars intake. This type of study looks at an associative relationship, not cause and effect, and there is no intervention.

Table 4.9 Format of a Research Article
Title/Authors
Abstract
Introduction
Methods
Results
Discussion
Conclusions
References
Author Information and Possible Sponsorship/Conflict of Interest*

*This may appear at the beginning or end of the article.

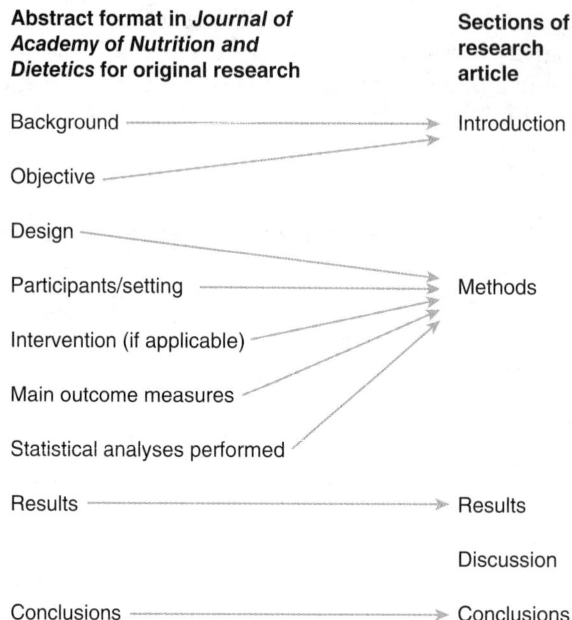

FIGURE 4.8 Where Parts of Abstract Appear in a Research Article

But the sociodemographic factors are independent variables because we are looking at how they influence someone's intake of added sugars (dependent variable). Park et al. (2016) found that adults with higher levels of added sugars intake were more likely to be younger and less educated, had lower family income, were smokers, and had less physical activity.

Depending on the journal and the type of research, the **abstract** (summary) of the article may follow a specific format. **Figure 4.8** shows how an abstract for an original research article in the *Journal of the Academy of Nutrition and Dietetics* is structured. This figure also ties each part of the abstract to the place in the article where it is discussed.

INTRODUCTION

The introduction of a research article begins with a review of relevant research already completed: the **literature review**. Prior research provides the foundation of what is known on the topic. The literature review in a research article is quite concise and brief and has two purposes. It summarizes the state of knowledge in its particular area, which will be compared to the results of the study later in the Discussion section, and it sets up the **research problem**. The research problem is where there is a knowledge gap or conflicting results in the current research.

In the introduction, the researchers need to show not just what the research problem is, but why it is *important* for patients, clients, families, nutritionists, and the health care system. The statement of the problem identifies the specific gap or problem into which the researchers want to gain further insight.

Toward the end of the introduction, usually the last paragraph, the authors clearly state the **objective** (or purpose) of the study. A research objective tells you what the researcher intends to focus on in the study, and it is usually just one sentence long.

The objective identifies the variables being studied and indicates the type of relationship being examined. The research objective should be feasible, ethical, and important.

A hypothesis may also be stated in the introduction, usually after the objective, especially if the study has an intervention. The hypothesis describes the predicted relationship between the variables, the population being studied, and sometimes other information such as the time frame. Let's look at some examples of problem statements, objectives, and hypotheses from two research studies (**Table 4.10**).

APPLICATION 4.6

Use Table 4.10 to answer these questions.

1. Which of the studies included an intervention?
2. Which objective do you like better? Why?
3. Which study has a causal hypothesis? Which has an associative hypothesis?
4. Is either hypothesis a directional hypothesis?
5. What is the null hypothesis for each study?

Table 4.10 Examples of Problem Statements, Objectives, and Hypotheses

STUDY TITLE: "Low-fat dietary pattern intervention and health-related quality of life: The Women's Health Initiative Randomized Controlled Dietary Modification Trial." Assaf, A. R., Beresford, S. A. A., Markham Risica, P., Aragaki, A., Brunner, R. L., Bowen, D. J., Naughton, M., Rosal, M. C., Snetselaar, L., & Wenger, N.		
Problem statement	**Objective**	**Hypothesis**
"Relatively few studies have examined the effect of long-term dietary interventions on quality of life or functional health status." (p. 260)	"We proposed to study changes in quality-of-life measures among women enrolled in the dietary modification trial of the Women's Health Initiative." (p. 260)	"Our specific hypotheses include intervention-associated positive changes in global quality of life, eight subscales of health-related quality of life, overall self-reported health, depression symptoms, sleep quality, and cognitive functioning at Year 1." (p. 260)
STUDY TITLE: "No association between dietary patterns and risk for cognitive decline in older women with 9-year follow-up: Data from the Women's Health Initiative Memory Study." Haring, B., Wu, C., Mossavar-Rahmani, M., Snetselaar, L., Brunner, R., Wallace, R. B., Neuhouser, M. L., & Wassertheil-Smoller, S.		
Problem statement	**Objective**	**Hypothesis**
"The effects of following a healthy diet reflected in the Healthy Eating Index (HEI) 2010, the Alternate Healthy Eating Index (AHEI) 2010, or the Dietary Approach to Stop Hypertension (DASH) score in relation to cognitive health have not been thoroughly investigated and comprehensive analyses are sparse." (p. 922)	"The purpose of this study was to compare healthy dietary patterns assessed by the aMED, HEI-2010, AHEI-2010, and DASH diet score on the risk of cognitive decline in post-menopausal women aged 65 to 79 years. Second, we examined whether adherence to a healthy dietary pattern modified the risk for decreased cognitive performance in women with hypertension." (p. 922)	"We hypothesized that a healthy dietary pattern would be associated with a decreased risk for cognitive decline. Furthermore, we anticipated that a healthy dietary pattern would be related to a decreased risk for cognitive decline in women with hypertension." (p. 922)

METHODS

The Methods section explains all the steps and tools that the researchers are going to use in their study, including the following.

1. Research design
2. Study population and how it will be chosen (sampling)
3. Setting
4. Instruments and measurement
5. Procedures
6. Statistical analysis

Sampling and measurement have already been discussed, so let's take a look at research designs.

Once a problem statement, research question(s) and hypothesis have been formulated, the researcher will work on a detailed research plan that states precisely what data are required, where the data will come from, which methods will be used to collect the data, and how the data will be analyzed. This series of decisions is called research design, and it focuses on the end-product: getting the evidence required to adequately and accurately answer the research question(s). Research design, such as a randomized controlled trial, is like a blueprint for a house. The blueprint can be used for a number of homes, but most blueprints will be changed to meet the specific needs of the new homeowner. A good research design will ensure that the results answer the research question as accurately as possible. Remember that some research questions cannot be tested.

Quantitative research designs are used to look at causal relationships as well as associations or relationships between variables. We have categorized quantitative research into five categories. First are **experimental designs** with an intervention, control group, and randomization of participants into groups. In experimental studies, the participants are randomly placed into the experimental or control groups (this is not the same as random sampling when you randomly select participants for a study). Next are **quasi-experimental designs** with an intervention but no randomization of participants into groups. **Descriptive designs** do not have an intervention or treatment and are considered nonexperimental. They usually aim to provide information about relevant variables, but they do not test hypotheses or examine cause and effect. Good descriptive studies provoke the "why" questions of analytic (cause-and-effect) research.

The last two categories of quantitative designs include **epidemiologic designs** and **predictive correlational designs**. These designs are observational in nature. In an observational study, there is no intervention, and researchers observe natural relationships between risk factors and outcomes.

Epidemiology is a discipline within public health that looks at the rates of health-related states (such as disease) in different groups of people and why they occur. Epidemiologists, sometimes called disease detectives, try to connect the dots between risk factors (called "exposures" by epidemiologists) and health or disease outcomes. Exposure can mean any factor that is associated with an outcome of interest, such as a risk factor, a dose of a drug, a surgical procedure, or a certain diet. For example, in the study "No Association Between Dietary Patterns and Risk for Cognitive Decline in Older Women with 9-Year Follow-Up: Data from the Women's Health Initiative Memory Study," Haring et al. (2016) looked at the effect of the quality of a woman's diet (exposure) on cognitive decline (outcome).

Predictive correlational designs use **regression**, a statistical technique. Regression quantifies the relationship between two variables; regression finds out *how much influence is exerted by the independent variable(s) on the dependent variable*. Regression designs are also used to predict the value of a dependent variable. For example, in this article by Park et al. (2016), "Sociodemographic and Behavioral Factors Associated with Added Sugars Intake Among U.S. Adults," they used regression to determine that adults with higher levels of added sugars intake were more likely to be younger and less educated, have lower family income, were smokers, and had less physical activity.

Sometimes you will see a term such as "cross-sectional" or "prospective" in a study title. These are not names of research designs; they simply give you an idea of the time dimension of the study. If data are collected at just one point in time, this is referred to as a **cross-sectional study**. In a **longitudinal study**, participants are observed and measurements taken usually over a long period of time. Longitudinal studies either go forward in time (**prospective**) or backward in time (**retrospective**).

Often the last section of Methods identifies the statistical analysis that will be done. According to Brase and Brase (2017), statistics is "the study of how to collect, organize, analyze, and interpret numerical information from data" (p. 4). Statistics enables us to take information from a sample of people and make *inferences* about a larger group of people—the population. In addition to making inferences, statistics help us describe or convey understanding of data, as well as test hypotheses.

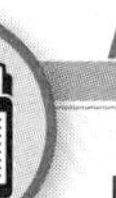

APPLICATION 4.7

Use the Methods section of the gardening education study in Appendix A to answer these questions.

1. Who were the participants in the study? How many were there in the beginning of the study? What sampling method was used?
2. How were the participants split up into groups? How many groups were there?
3. Is this an experimental or quasi-experimental design?
4. Describe the intervention(s). What happened to the control group?
5. What was measured in this study? Describe how it was measured and when.
6. How many participants were included in the statistical analysis?
7. The researchers used one-way ANOVA as the statistical test to compare which variables before and after the intervention?

Results, Discussion, and Conclusion

The Results and Discussion sections are normally separate. Some, but not all, articles also have a separate Conclusion section after the Discussion. Otherwise the conclusion is at the end of the Discussion section.

The Results section is limited to the actual data generated by this study; *any interpretation of the data is put in the Discussion section*. For human subjects studies, the first paragraph(s) and chart(s) in the Results section give you basic demographics and other pertinent characteristics of the participants, such as their pretest data. Pretest data, sometimes called baseline data, and demographic data are evaluated to see whether the groups are similar. If there are differences between the kinds of people in one group as opposed to the other group(s), the differences observed between the groups on the dependent variable may be due to the nonequivalence of the groups. Differences between the groups at the beginning of the study is a threat to internal validity, so researchers always do statistical tests to compare groups.

The Results section is sequenced to present key findings in a logical order. Tables and figures show the results, and the text highlights and explains each table and figure in order. When interpreting information in tables and figures, be sure to read all labels, headings, and footnotes carefully. If some of the results talk about differences between groups on a dependent measure, look for information on statistical significance as well as on the direction and size of differences between the groups.

TIP

According to Lipman (2013), "the critical reader concentrates on the Methods and the Results sections. The Methods section is one of the two most important parts of an article, because it is here that the authors define how they have approached answering the question that they asked. . . . Once the reader is finished with the Methods and the Results section, he or she should be able to draw his or her own conclusions" (p. 159).

When reading through the Results section, you will see examples of means with **confidence intervals**, such as a mean for systolic blood pressure of 121.6 (118.4 to 124.8). The numbers in the parentheses are the confidence intervals. Confidence intervals can be informative because they represent a range of values within which the population parameter (such as the real mean in the population from which your sample was drawn) would be expected to fall. Confidence intervals are usually created at a 95% confidence level. If you use a 95% confidence level and sample the same population on numerous occasions and develop confidence intervals each time, the resulting intervals would contain the true population parameter in approximately 95% of the cases.

What is interesting to note at this point has to do with the *width* of the confidence interval. You are going to see a lot of confidence intervals in the Results sections of research articles, so keep these concepts in mind. If the confidence interval is relatively narrow (e.g., 6.53 to 6.91), the population parameter is known quite *precisely*. If the confidence interval is really wide, then it is much less precise.

In the Discussion section, the authors give their understandings and explanations of the results in light of what is already known about the topic. The major goal of this section is to show how the study results fit into the bigger picture of research in this area. The Discussion section generally includes this information and may follow this sequence.

1. First, the results are summarized.
2. The authors compare their results to other studies, usually already mentioned in the introduction, and try to explain any agreements and differences.

APPLICATION 4.8

Use the gardening education study in Appendix A to answer these questions.

1. Which group significantly increased their consumption of fruits and vegetables from pretest to posttest?
2. Did the children in Experimental School 1 increase their consumption of fruits or vegetables by the end of the study?
3. Did any significant changes occur in fruit or vegetable consumption in the children in Experimental School 1 or the control school?
4. The children in Experimental School 2 significantly increased their intake of which three nutrients?
5. What were three limitations of this study?
6. Were any ideas for future research stated?
7. What did the authors conclude?

Table 4.11 Conclusion Statement from "Regional Differences in Sugar-Sweetened Beverage Intake Among US Adults"

"Our findings show that sugar-sweetened beverage intake among US adults remains high, and patterns of consumption by sugar-sweetened beverage type vary by region. Intervention efforts to reduce obesity and diabetes incidence by reducing sugar-sweetened beverage intake among adults could consider the regional difference in sugar-sweetened beverage intake, particularly when local-level data are not available."

3. After considering their study results and other studies, the authors explain their new understanding of the problem.
4. Limitations (and sometimes strengths) of the study are mentioned.
5. Ideas for future research are stated.

Each research article has its own unique findings, so the Discussion section can differ a lot in terms of length and structure.

The Conclusion section is a general statement of the answer to the original research question along with its scientific implications. The conclusion may also include some practical advice, as seen in **Table 4.11**.

TIP

Reading a research study for understanding is not a quick process. You can certainly read the Abstract quickly and gain a few ideas about the study; however, reading a study is like reading a chapter in a textbook, different sections build on each other. Take your time reading studies. Underline the sentences that hold key ideas, and put question marks next to the sections you are not sure about.

RESEARCHER INTERVIEW Outcomes Research

Geoffrey Greene, PhD, RD, LDN
Professor and Dietetic Internship Director, University of Rhode Island, Department of Nutrition and Food Sciences, Kingston, RI

1. **Briefly describe the areas in which you do research.**
   In general, my research is based on the Transtheoretical Model of Behavior Change (TTM) with a focus on dietary change for health promotion. I am working with young adult populations to increase fruit and vegetable intake and physical activity as well as to increase sustainable eating behaviors. I am also working with school-aged children to improve dietary and exercise behaviors in both community and school-based interventions. Finally, I have worked with older adults to improve dietary and physical activity behaviors and with general adult populations to improve dietary intake.
2. **With your experience in outcomes research, what should students/practitioners know about this area of research?**
   In general, outcomes research is hypothesis driven: hypotheses are tested using validated instruments, reliable data collection methods, and appropriate statistical techniques. I have

been involved with three randomized controlled trials in young adults to increase fruit and vegetable intake and one to increase sustainable eating behaviors. My work with school-aged children generally involves quasi-experimental designs, although a pediatric obesity prevention program is a nonexperimental design. My work with older adults has utilized randomized controlled designs.

Students and practitioners should know that instruments used to assess outcomes need to be validated, and, regardless of design, research protocols must be rigorously defined and carefully followed. I teach a graduate course, Methods in Nutrition Research, that reviews different designs and has students define research as descriptive, nonexperimental, or experimental. The key difference is whether there in an investigator-controlled intervention with clear hypotheses operationalized using validated instruments.

3. **What do you enjoy most about the research process?**
I enjoy the creativity of working with my research team to develop experiments that will answer research questions. I want to know if this intervention will work, and, perhaps more important, what are the mechanisms associated with effective behavior change.

4. **What tip(s) do you have for practitioners who want to do practice-based research?**
Research is critical for the advancement of our field. All dietitians can participate in research, but they need to be systematic, base research on previous literature, and develop research designs that will answer their research questions. It is useful to work as part of a multidisciplinary team with individuals who have the skills to provide design and statistical expertise.

SUMMARY

1. A concept or construct is called a variable in a quantitative study once it has been operationally defined.
2. In quantitative research, researchers are generally looking for a difference among the groups or an association or relationship among the variables.
3. Extraneous or confounding variables need to be controlled through methods such as random sampling and randomization.
4. In practice, theories, models, and research frameworks are often used interchangeably because they overlap a lot and the definitions are not standardized. They describe relationships among constructs to explain or predict related phenomena such as behavior change.
5. Figure 4.3 shows the dynamic relationships between theory, research, and practice.
6. A hypothesis can be categorized as causal or associative, directional or nondirectional, simple or complex, and research or null.
7. The null hypothesis always states that there is no difference between the groups. Inferential statistics tests the null hypothesis.
8. In hypothesis testing, if the P-value of the test is less than or equal to the level of significance (0.05) you set, then the results are statistically significant and you reject the null hypothesis and accept the research hypothesis. On the other hand, if the P-value is greater than the level of significance, then you accept the null hypothesis.
9. A type I error (alpha [α] error) is when you reject the null hypothesis when it is true (*the groups are truly no different from each other*). A type II error (beta [β] error) is when you accept the null hypothesis when it is false (*the groups are truly different from each other*).
10. Statistical significance can tell you whether the findings are due to chance or not, but they do not tell you if the findings are necessarily clinically important, nor do they tell you about the effect size (size or strength of the difference or relationship between two variables).
11. If the confidence interval is relatively narrow, the population parameter is known quite precisely.
12. Reliability focuses on repeatability of research findings or testing results, whereas validity looks at the degree to which conclusions drawn from a study are accurate and whether

instruments and measurements truly measure what they are intended to measure.

13. Each type of validity (internal, external, statistical conclusion, and construct) can be threatened in different ways. For example, threats to internal validity include history, maturation, selection, attrition, testing, and instrumentation.
14. All errors are either random or systematic. A random error can be due to the normal variability in people. Systematic errors, also called bias, are not due to chance and can appear in any part of a research study (Table 4.6).
15. Using probability sampling, each person in the population has an equal probability, or chance, of being selected. Examples include simple random sampling, systematic random sampling, stratified random sampling, and cluster random sampling (Table 4.7).
16. Nonprobability sampling is based on respondents being selected by convenience or judgment and is less likely to produce representative samples. Examples include convenience sampling, quota sampling, purposive or judgment sampling, and network (snowball) sampling (Table 4.8).
17. A power analysis may be used to determine sample size and requires information such as expected effect size, power level, and level of significance.
18. To assess the quality of an instrument, various tests for reliability (test-retest, inter-rater reliability, internal consistency reliability) and validity (face validity, content validity, criterion validity, and construct validity) need to be considered.
19. The Introduction section of a research article contains a brief literature review, description of the research problem, study objective or purpose, and hypothesis (if used).
20. The Methods section includes the research design, study population and sampling method, setting, instruments and measurements, procedures, and statistical analysis.
21. Research designs in this textbook are categorized as experimental (randomization required), quasi-experimental, descriptive, epidemiologic, and predictive correlational designs.
22. The Results section is limited to the actual data generated by this study; any interpretation of the data is put in the Discussion section. For human subjects studies, the first paragraph(s) and chart(s) in the Results section give you basic demographics and other pertinent characteristics of the participants, such as their pretest data. Pretest data, sometimes called baseline data, and demographic data are evaluated to see if the groups are similar.
23. The Discussion section summarizes the results, compares results to previous studies, explains limitations, and gives ideas for future research. Conclusions may appear next or at the end of the Discussion.

REVIEW QUESTIONS

1. Diet quality is an example of a/an:
   A. concept
   B. construct
   C. operational definition
   D. dichotomous variable
2. A variable is the theoretical definition of a construct.
   A. true
   B. false
3. Weight is measured at which level of measurement?
   A. ratio
   B. interval
   C. ordinal
   D. nominal
4. A Likert scale is an example of which level of measurement?
   A. ratio
   B. interval
   C. ordinal
   D. nominal
5. Research forms the basis for evidence-based practice and documents the impact of nutrition care on health outcomes.
   A. true
   B. false

6. In an associative hypothesis, one variable:
   A. causes the other variable
   B. confounds the independent variable
   C. is correlated with another variable
   D. is multidirectional
7. If you accept the null hypothesis when it is false, it is a:
   A. type I error
   B. type II error
   C. bias
   D. random error
8. _________ validity is the extent to which the independent variable actually accounted for the study outcome.
   A. internal
   B. external
   C. statistical conclusion
   D. construct
9. Which of these are threats to internal validity?
   A. maturation
   B. selection
   C. history
   D. testing
   E. all of the above
10. Dividing the accessible population into groups and then using simple random sampling for each group is which type of sampling?
    A. systematic random sampling
    B. strategic random sampling
    C. cluster random sampling
    D. stratified random sampling
11. The weakest form of sampling is:
    A. network sampling
    B. random sampling
    C. convenience sampling
    D. quota sampling
12. The quantity $1-\beta$ is the probability of *avoiding* a ___________.
    A. type I error
    B. type II error
    C. bias
    D. random error
13. Cronbach's alpha is used to test:
    A. internal consistency reliability
    B. test-retest reliability
    C. construct validity
    D. all of the above
14. Factor analysis is used to test:
    A. internal consistency reliability
    B. test-retest reliability
    C. construct validity
    D. content validity
15. Interpretation of the study results are done in which section?
    A. Results
    B. Discussion
    C. Conclusion
    D. Methods
16. In quantitative research, researchers are generally trying to answer one of two types of questions. What are the two questions?
17. Name three extraneous variables that come up often in nutrition research.
18. Explain what power is and what it is dependent upon.
19. Define bias and give five examples of bias.
20. Briefly describe five categories of research designs.

CRITICAL THINKING QUESTIONS

1. Answer questions about each of these research articles from looking at their titles.
   A. "The Effect of Mineral Water on Cardiometabolic Risk Biomarkers: A Crossover Randomized Controlled Trial in Adults with Hypercholesterolemia" Is there an intervention in this study? Is this an experimental or quasi-experimental study? What is/are the independent variable(s)? What is/are the dependent variable(s)?
   B. "Trends in Breastfeeding Initiation and Duration Among U.S. Children 1999–2014" Is there an intervention in this study? Is this an epidemiologic study or descriptive study? Is this a cross-sectional or longitudinal study?

C. "Physical Activity in Relation to Urban Environments in 14 Cities Worldwide: A Cross-Sectional Study" Is there an intervention in this study? Are the researchers looking at causal or associative relationships? What is the independent variable? What is the dependent variable? Is this an experimental study or an observational study? What does cross-sectional mean?

D. "Potato Intake and Incidence of Hypertension: Results from Three Prospective US Cohort Studies" In epidemiology a cohort is a group of individuals (usually quite a large group) who are observed over time to gather information about exposures, such as health-related habits, that can affect an outcome. What is the exposure in this study? What is the outcome? Is there an intervention in this study? Are the researchers looking at causal or associative relationships? What is the independent variable? What is the dependent variable?

2. For each hypothesis, answer these questions.
   1. Is this a causal or associative hypothesis?
   2. Is this hypothesis directional or nondirectional?
   3. Is the hypothesis simple or complex?
   4. What would be the null hypothesis?

   Hypothesis A. It was hypothesized that the eight tailored educational lessons would improve a subject's self-reported food security level compared with participants receiving no lessons.

   Hypothesis B. Adolescents who had regular family meals in middle school would have higher quality diets and eating patterns when they graduate from high school.

   Hypothesis C. A quercetin-vitamin C supplement would improve disease risk factors compared to placebo.

3. Read this article and answer the following questions.
   Parker, A.R., Byham-Gray, L., Denmark, R., and Winkle, P. J. (2014). The effect of medical nutrition therapy by a Registered Dietitian Nutritionist in patients with prediabetes participating in a randomized controlled clinical research trial. *Journal of the Academy of Nutrition and Dietetics, 114,* 1739–1748. doi: 10.1016/j.jand.2014.07.020

   A. Why was this study done? What is the "problem"?
   B. What is the purpose of the study?
   C. Is there an intervention? If so, describe it and identify the independent and dependent variables.
   D. Write a research hypothesis and null hypothesis for this study. Is the hypothesis causal or associative?
   E. How were the participants recruited? Name two inclusion and two exclusion criteria.
   F. Were the participants randomized to the experimental and usual care groups? If so, is this study experimental or quasi-experimental and how did that strengthen the internal validity of the study?
   G. How many participants started the study? How many completed the 12-week study?
   H. What were the outcome measures? Why were they chosen? Has the Diabetes Risk Score been tested for validity or reliability?
   I. Table 2 shows the demographic characteristics of each group at baseline. Did the groups vary significantly on any characteristic at the start of the study? (Hint: Look at the *P*-values.)
   J. Table 3 shows the measurements taken for each group at baseline and end point. The MNT group (compared to the usual care group) experienced significantly lower levels of which two measures at the end of the study.
   K. Name one study that was mentioned in the Discussion.
   L. What were two strengths and two limitations mentioned by the authors? Explain how its limitations affect its external validity.
   M. What did the authors conclude?

4. Read this article and answer the following questions.
   Ford, D. W., Hartman, T. J., Still, C., Wood, C., Mitchell, D. C., Bailey, R., Smicklas-Wright, H., Coffman, D. L., & Jensen, G. L. (2014). Diet quality and Body Mass Index are associated with health care resource use in

rural older Americans. *Journal of the Academy of Nutrition and Dietetics, 114,* 1932–1938. doi: 10.1016/j.jand.2014.02.016

A. Why was this study done? What is the problem?

B. What is the purpose and hypothesis of the study? What is the null hypothesis? Is the hypothesis causal or associative?

C. Is this an experimental or quasi-experimental study with an intervention?

D. What are the independent and dependent variables in this study?

E. Who are the participants? How many were included in the study results?

F. How many years of HRU data were used?

G. Was the Dietary Screening Tool tested for validity and reliability? Explain.

H. List four covariates used in the statistical analysis.

I. Table 2 looks at the *relative risk* for inpatient visits or days, ER visits, and outpatient visits *by* BMI, Dietary Screening Tool score, and fruit and vegetable scores. Relative risk (RR) is the risk of an outcome (such as an ER visit) when exposed to a factor such as a low Dietary Screening Tool score or high BMI. It expresses how many times more (or less) likely someone with a factor such as high BMI will have to go to the ER, compared to someone at a lower BMI. If the RR is more than 1, it means that the factor increases the chance of using health care resources compared to another group. If the RR is less than 1, it means that the factor decreases the chance of using health care resources compared to another group.
For example, let's look at Table 2 under ER visits at Dietary Screening tool scores. The participants with the lowest scores have a RR of 1.21 (1.00–1.46 CI) compared to the participants with the highest scores (they are the reference group). This is statistically significant with a *P*-value of 0.05. This means the participants with the lowest Dietary Screen tool scores are significantly more likely (1.21 times more likely) to go to the ER compared to the participants with the highest scores.
Were the lowest fruit and vegetables scores also associated with significantly higher ER visits than those with the highest FV scores? Explain the results for the relationship between outpatient visits and BMI.

J. Name one study that was mentioned in the Discussion.

K. What were two strengths and two limitations mentioned by the authors? Would any of its limitations affect its reliability or validity?

L. What did the authors conclude?

SUGGESTED READINGS AND ACTIVITIES

1. Boushey, C. J., Harris, J., Bruemmer, B., & Archer, S. A. (2008). Publishing nutrition research: A review of sampling, sample size, statistical analysis, and other key elements of manuscript preparation, Part 2. *Journal of the American Dietetic Association, 108*, 679–688. doi: 10.1016/j.jada.2008.01.002
2. Gleason, P. M., Harris, J., Sheean, P. M., Boushey, C. J., & Bruemmer, B. (2010). Publishing nutrition research: Validity, reliability, and diagnostic test assessment in nutrition-related research. *Journal of the American Dietetic Association, 110*, 409–419. doi: 10.1016/j.jada.2009.11.022
3. Lomangino, K. M. (2016). Countering cognitive bias: Tips for recognizing the impact of potential bias on research. *Journal of the Academy of Nutrition and Dietetics, 116*, 204–207. doi: 10.1016/j.jand.2015.07.014
4. Online Sample Size Calculators: For surveys: http://www.raosoft.com/samplesize.html For clinical trials, crossover studies, and studies to find an association: http://hedwig.mgh.harvard.edu/sample_size/size.html

REFERENCES

Algert, S., Baameur, A., & Renvall, M. (2014). Vegetable output and cost saving of community gardens in San Jose, California. *Journal of the Academy of Nutrition and Dietetics, 114*, 1072–1076. doi: 10.1016/j.jand.2014.02.030

Assaf, A. R., Beresford, S. A. A., Markham Risica, P., Aragaki, A., Brunner, R. L., Bowen, D. J. . . . Wenger, N. (2016). Low-fat dietary pattern intervention and health-related quality of life: The Women's Health Initiative Randomized Controlled Dietary Modification Trial. *Journal of the Academy of Nutrition and Dietetics, 116*, 259–271. doi: 10.1016/j.jand.2015.07.016

Beto, J. A., Champagne, C. M., Dennett, C. C., & Harris, J. E. (2016). The challenge of connecting dietary changes to improved disease outcomes: The balance between positive, neutral, and negative publication results. *Journal of the Academy of Nutrition and Dietetics, 116*, 917–920. doi: 10.1016/j.jand.2016.02.019

Boushey, C. J. (2008). Estimating sample size. In E. R. Monsen & L. Van Horn (Eds.), *Research: Successful approaches* (pp. 373–381). Chicago, IL: American Dietetic Association.

Boushey, C. J., Harris, J., Bruemmer, B., & Archer, S. A. (2008). Publishing nutrition research: A review of sampling, sample size, statistical analysis, and other key elements of manuscript preparation, Part 2. *Journal of the American Dietetic Association, 108*, 679–688. doi: 10.1016/j.jada.2008.01.002

Brase, C. H., & Brase, C. P. (2017). *Understanding basic statistics* (7th ed.) Boston, MA: Cengage Learning.

Campbell, D. T., & Stanley, J. (1966). *Experimental and quasi-experimental designs for research*. Boston, MA: Cengage Learning.

Contento, I. (2016). *Nutrition education: Linking research, theory, and practice* (3rd ed.). Burlington, MA: Jones & Bartlett Learning.

Davies, H. T., & Crombie, I. K. (2009). What are confidence intervals and p-values? (What Is? Series). Retrieved from http://www.medicine.ox.ac.uk/bandolier/painres/download/whatis/what_are_conf_inter.pdf

DeVon, H. A., Block, M. E., Moyle-Wright, P., Ernst, D. M., Hayden, S. J., Lazzara, D. J., . . . Kostas-Polston, E. (2007). A psychometric toolbox for testing validity and reliability. *Journal of Nursing Scholarship, 39*, 155–164. doi: 10.1111/j.1547-5069.2007.00161.x

Doub, A., Small, M., & Birch. L. (2015). An exploratory analysis of child feeding beliefs and behaviors included in food blogs written by mothers of preschool-aged children. *Journal of Nutrition Education and Behavior.* Advance online publication. doi: 10.1016.j.jneb.2015.09.001

Gillis, A., & Jackson, W. (2002). *Research for nurses: Methods and interpretation*. Philadelphia, PA: F. A. Davis.

Gleason, P. M., Harris, J., Sheean, P. M., Boushey, C. J., & Bruemmer, B. (2010). Publishing nutrition research: Validity, reliability, and diagnostic test assessment in nutrition-related research. *Journal of the American Dietetic Association, 110*, 409–419. doi: 10.1016/j.jada.2009.11.022

Grove, S. K., Burns, N., & Gray, J. R. (2013). *The practice of nursing research: Appraisal, synthesis, and generation of evidence*. St. Louis, MO: Elsevier Saunders.

Haring, B., Wu, C., Mossavar-Rahmani, M., Snetselaar, L., Brunner, R., Wallace, R. B., . . . Wassertheil-Smoller, S. (2016). No association between dietary patterns and risk for cognitive decline in older women with 9-year follow-up: Data from the Women's Health Initiative Memory Study. *Journal of the Academy of Nutrition and Dietetics, 116*, 921–930. doi: 10.1016/j.jand.2015.12.017

Hulley, S. B., Cummings, S. R., Browner, W. S., & Grady, D. G. (2013). *Designing clinical research* (4th ed.) Philadelphia, PA: Lippincott, Williams & Wilkins.

Iglesia, I., Guelinckx, I., De Miguel-Etayo, P., Gonzalez-Gil, E., Salas-Salvado, J., Kavouras, S., . . . Moreno, L. (2015). Total fluid intake of children and adolescents: Cross-sectional surveys in 13 countries worldwide. *European Journal of Nutrition, 54*, S57–S67. doi: 10.1007/s00394-015-0946-6

Johnson. C. L., Dohrmann, S. M., Burt, V. L., & Mohadjer, L. K. (2014). *National Health and Nutrition Examination Survey: Sample design, 2011–2014* (Vital and Health Statistics Report No. 162). Atlanta, GA: National Center for Health Statistics.

Leong, S. L., Madden, C., Gray, A., Waters, D., & Horwath. C. (2011). Faster self-reported speed of eating is related to higher body mass index in a nationwide survey of middle-aged women. *Journal of the American Dietetic Association, 111*, 1192–1197. doi: 10.1016/j.jada.2011.05.012

Lipman, T. O. (2013). Critical reading and critical thinking—Study design and methodology: A personal approach on how to read the clinical literature. *Nutrition in Clinical Practice, 28*, 158–164. doi: 10.11777/0884533612474041

Lomangino, K. M. (2016). Countering cognitive bias: Tips for recognizing the impact of potential bias on research. *Journal of the Academy of Nutrition and Dietetics, 116*, 204–207. doi: 10.1016/j.jand.2015.07.014

Lynn, M. R. (1986). Determination and quantification of content validity. *Nursing Research, 35*, 3820–3850. doi: 10.1097/00006199-198611000-00017

Marshall, S., Young, A., Bauer, J., & Isenring, E. (2015). Malnutrition in geriatric rehabilitation: Prevalence, patient outcomes, and criterion validity of the Scored Patient-Generated Subjective Global Assessment and the Mini Nutritional Assessment. *Journal of the Academy of Nutrition and Dietetics*. Advance online publication. doi: 10.1016/j.jand.2015.06.013

McAleese, J. D., & Rankin, L. L. (2007). Garden-based nutrition education affects fruit and vegetable consumption in sixth-grade adolescents. *Journal of the American Dietetic Association*, *107*, 662–665. doi: 10.1016/j.jada.2007.01.015

Park, S., Thompson, F. E., McGuire, L. C., Pan, L., Galuska, D. A., & Blanck, H. M. (2016). Sociodemographic and behavioral factors associated with added sugars intake among US adults. *Journal of the Academy of Nutrition and Dietetics*, *116*, 1–10. doi: 10.1016/j.jand.2016.04.012

Patel, N., Kennedy, A., Blickem, C., Reeves, D., & Chew-Graham, C. (2016). "I'm managing my diabetes between two worlds": Beliefs and experiences of diabetes management in British South Asians on Holiday in the East—A qualitative study. *Journal of Diabetes Research*, 1–8. doi: 10.1155/2016/5436174

Rajkumar, N., Karthikeyan, V. S., Manwar, S., Sistla, S. C., & Kate, V. (2013). Clear liquid diet vs soft diet as the initial meal in patients with mild acute pancreatitis: A randomized interventional trial. *Nutrition in Clinical Practice*, *28*, 365–370. doi: 10.1177/ 0884533612466112

Rehm, C. D., Peñalvo, J. L., Afshin, A., & Mozaffarian, D. (2016). Dietary intake among US adults, 1999–2012. *JAMA*, *315*, 2542–2553. doi: 10.1001/jama.2016.7491

Ritchie, L., Sharma, S., Gildengorin, G., Yoshida, S., Braff-Guajardo, E., & Crawford, P. (2015). Policy improves what beverages are served to young children in child care. *Journal of the Academy of Nutrition and Dietetics*, *115*, 724–730. doi: 10.1016/j.jand.2014.07.019

Shadish, W. R., Cook, T. D., & Campbell, D. T. (2002). *Experimental and quasi-experimental designs for generalized causal inference* (2nd ed.) Boston, MA: Wadsworth Cengage Learning.

Skelly, A. C., Dettori, J. R., & Brodt, E. D. (2012). Assessing bias: The importance of considering confounding. *Evidence Based Spine Care Journal*, *3*, 9–12. doi: 10.1055/s-0031-1298595

CHAPTER

5

What Do the Quantitative Data Mean?

ROSALIND M. PETERS, NOLA A. SCHMIDT, MOIRA FEARNCOMBE, KAREN EICH DRUMMOND

CHAPTER OUTLINE

- Introduction
- Levels of Measurement
- Using Frequencies to Describe Samples
- Measures of Central Tendency
- Measures of Variability
- Distribution Patterns
- Inferential Statistics: Can the Findings Be Applied to the Population?
- Reducing Error When Deciding About Hypotheses
- Using Statistical Tests to Make Inferences About Populations
- Effect Size
- Risk Statistics: Risk Ratio, Odds Ratio, and Hazard Ratio
- What Does All This Mean for Evidence-Based Practice?

LEARNING OUTCOMES

- Differentiate between descriptive and inferential statistics.
- Identify the level of measurement of a given variable.
- Identify how frequencies can be graphically depicted.
- Describe measures of central tendency and their uses.
- Describe measures of variability and their uses.
- Distinguish between data that are normally and not normally distributed, and explain the Rule of 68-95-99.7.
- Explain probability, statistical significance, and when to use inferential statistical tests.
- Distinguish between type I and type II errors.
- Identify and describe statistical tests used to determine statistically significant differences between groups and among variables.
- Assign commonly used parametric or nonparametric tests to examples based on the type of research question and level of measurement.
- Identify and interpret estimates of effect size including.
- Interpret relative risk, odds ratios, and hazard ratios.
- Differentiate between statistical significance and clinical significance.

INTRODUCTION

Originally the term *statistics* referred to information about the government because the word is derived from the Latin *statisticum*, meaning "of the state." It was given its numerical meaning in 1749 when Gottfried Achenwall, a German political scientist, used the term to designate the analysis of *data* about the *state* (Harper, 2013). Currently, there are two meanings of the term *statistics*. **Statistics**, with a capital "S," is used to describe the branch of mathematics that collects, analyzes, interprets, and presents numerical data in terms of samples and populations; **statistics**, with a lowercase "s," is used to describe the numerical outcomes and the probabilities derived from calculations on raw data.

When reporting the results of their study, researchers often present two types of statistics: descriptive and inferential. **Descriptive statistics** deal with the collection and presentation of data used to explain characteristics of variables found in a sample. As its name implies, descriptive statistics describe, summarize, and synthesize collected data. Calculations and information presented with descriptive statistics must be accurate. **Inferential statistics** involve analysis of data as the basis for predictions related to the phenomenon of interest. Inferential statistics are used to make inferences or draw conclusions about a population based on a sample. They are used to develop **population parameters** from the **sample statistics**. For example, a researcher conducted a study on the efficiency of vitamin C in preventing the common cold. Descriptive statistics would be used to report that 60% of participants in the experimental group had fewer colds than did participants receiving the placebo. The researcher would then use inferential statistics to determine whether the difference in the number of colds between the two groups was statistically significant. If it was, then it could be inferred that taking vitamin C would be advantageous. Descriptive statistics are used to provide information regarding univariate or bivariate analyses.

Univariate analysis is conducted to present organized information about only one variable at a time and includes information regarding frequency distributions, measures of central tendency, shape of the distribution, and measures of variability, sometimes known as dispersion. **Bivariate analysis** is performed to describe the relationship between two variables that can be expressed in contingency tables or with other statistical tests. **Multivariate analysis** is done when the researcher wants to examine the relationship among three or more variables.

The results of descriptive analysis are frequently presented in table format, and scientific notations are often used. Therefore, it may be helpful to review common notations used in tables as shown in **Table 5.1**.

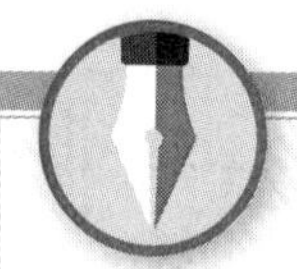

TIP

There are two types of statistics: descriptive and inferential. Descriptive statistics describe, summarize, and synthesize collected data. Inferential statistics allow a researcher to generalize about the population based on the data from the sample.

LEVELS OF MEASUREMENT

Measurement is the process of assigning numbers using a set of rules. Four categories are used to describe measurements: **nominal**, **ordinal**, **interval**, and **ratio**. These categories are more commonly known as **levels of measurement**. It is important to consider

Table 5.1 Statistical Symbols for Descriptive Statistics

Symbol/Abbreviation	Definition
f	Frequency
M	Mean
Mdn	Median
n	Number in subsample
N	Total number in a sample
%	Percentage
SD	Standard deviation
z	A standard score

the level of measurement used to measure a variable in a study because the choice of which statistic you use depends on the level of measurement.

You must be able to identify levels of measurement correctly to appraise evidence. Nominal measurement is the weakest level of measurement. The word *nominal* is derived from the word *name*. Researchers use nominal measurement to classify or categorize variables, also referred to as **categorical data**. The numbers assigned to each category are just labels and do not indicate any value. For example, responses of "yes" and "no" on a survey are often assigned numbers 1 and 2. The value of these numbers has no meaning because one cannot claim that a "no" response is higher than a "yes" response. The arbitrary numbers are assigned for the purpose of coding, recording, and entering data for collection and analysis. Questionnaires often utilize nominal measures to record a variety of categorical data and closed-ended questions with fixed responses such as gender, race, and diagnosis. **Dichotomous** is the term used when there are only two possible fixed responses, such as true or false, yes or no, and male or female.

Ordinal measurement represents the second lowest level of measurement. A continuum of numeric values is used with small numbers representing lower levels on the continuum and larger numbers representing higher values. However, although the values are ordered or ranked, the intervals are not meant to be equal. For example, in a marathon the distance and time among those who finish in first, second, and third are not equal; however, there is value to the number assigned. Many questionnaires and scales use ordinal measures.

Interval measurement is a third level of measurement and uses a continuum of numeric values, also known as **continuous data**. At this level, the values have meaning and the intervals are equal. On interval scales, the zero point is arbitrary and not absolute. The zero is not an indication of the true absence of something. The best example of this is the Celsius scale. When measuring temperature in Celsius, 0 does not mean the absence of temperature. In fact, it is quite cold. Other examples of interval scores include intelligence measures, personality measures, and manual muscle testing.

Ratio measurement is the highest level of measurement. There are equal intervals between the numbers and a true zero point. Examples include weight and height. Using ratio measurements, you can say that someone who weighs 250 pounds is twice as heavy as someone who weighs 125 pounds. You cannot do the same thing with interval data. For example, someone with an IQ of 120 is not twice as smart as someone with an IQ of 60. **Table 5.2** summarizes levels of measurement.

Table 5.2 Levels of Measurement

Level of measurement	Definition	Examples
Ratio	A continuum of numeric values with equal intervals between them and a meaningful zero point.	Weight, height, number of credits completed
Interval	A continuum of numeric values with equal intervals, but the zero point is not meaningful.	Celsius scale, standardized IQ, grade point average (GPA)
Ordinal	Using numbers to rank order an attribute. The intervals are not equal.	Student's level of standing (freshman, sophomore, junior, senior); a Likert scale such as "1. Strongly Agree, 2. Agree, 3. Neither Agree nor Disagree, 4. Disagree, 5. Strongly Disagree"
Nominal	Using numbers to categorize or label attributes into groups or categories.	Gender: Male is coded as "1" and Female as "2"

USING FREQUENCIES TO DESCRIBE SAMPLES

Information about the frequency, or how often a variable is found to occur, may be presented as either ungrouped or grouped data. Ungrouped data are primarily used to present nominal and ordinal data where the raw data represents some characteristic of the variable. In contrast, with interval- and ratio-level data, the raw data are collapsed (grouped) into smaller classifications to make the data easier to interpret. **Table 5.3** provides an example of how categorical data about a sample may be presented in ungrouped format.

Table 5.3 Example of Categorical Data Presented in Ungrouped Format

Variable	*n* (*P*)
Gender	
Men	14 (41)
Women	20 (59)
Race/Ethnicity	
White/Caucasian	190 (76.0)
Black/African American	32 (12.8)
Hispanic/Latino	12 (4.8)
Native American/Eskimo	3 (1.2)
Asian/Pacific Islander	2 (0.8)
No answer	11 (4.4)
Self-Care Behaviors	
Current smoker	7 (18)
Alcohol > 1 drink/day	0 (0)
Exercise	
No regular exercise	9 (27)
1–2 days/week	10 (29)
3–4 days/week	8 (24)
≥5 days/week	5 (15)

n = number in group; *P* = percent

Ungrouped data are rarely presented when reporting on continuous variables such as age, scores on scales, time, or physiological variables (e.g., temperature, blood pressure, cell counts). For example, if readers of an article were presented with a set of ages for 20 different participants in the study, it would be difficult to make sense of this raw data (see **Table 5.4**). However, if the numbers were arranged in a frequency distribution and graphed, they would make much more sense to the readers. Before a graph can be constructed, the researcher must create a frequency distribution table. First, the raw data are sorted, usually in ascending order. Next, the number of times each value occurs is tallied, and the frequency of each event is recorded in the table. Table 5.4 shows how the raw data can be organized to more clearly present the information, how raw data are tallied, and how the resulting frequencies and percentages are recorded. The left-hand side of the table shows the frequency with which individual age data occur. Because all possible data points are presented, it is still somewhat difficult to comprehend this presentation of the ungrouped data. The right-hand side of the table shows a grouped frequency and percentage distribution with the ages grouped in 2-year increments. It should be obvious that the grouped data are more meaningful than either the raw or ungrouped data.

Although there are few fixed rules regarding how and when to group data, it is imperative that there be no overlap of categories. Each group must have well-defined lower and upper limits so that the groups are mutually exclusive, yet the groups must include all data collected. For example, if the groupings in Table 5.4 had been 18–20 and 20–22, people who are 20 years old would have been counted in both groups, and the statistics would have been compromised. Group size also should be consistent. If the groups had been 18–20 (a 3-year span), 21–25 (a 4-year span), and older than 25 (a 3-year span), inaccurate analysis of data would occur. Although grouping data might make it easier to understand, it also results in some loss of information. The grouped data presented in Table 5.4 indicate that 30% of the participants were between 20 and

Table 5.4 Example of Frequency and Percentage Distributions of Ages

Raw data

18 18 18 19 19 19 20 21 21 21 21 21 22 22 22 23 23 25 27 28

Ungrouped data				Grouped data			
Age	**Tally**	**Frequency**	**Percentage**	**Age**	**Tally**	**Frequency**	**Percentage**
18	III	3	15	18–19	~~IIII~~ I	6	30
19	III	3	15	20–21	~~IIII~~ I	6	30
20	I	1	5	22–23	~~IIII~~	5	25
21	~~IIII~~	5	25	24–25	I	1	5
22	III	3	15	> 25	II	2	10
23	II	2	10	**Total**		20	100
25	I	1	5				
27	I	1	5				
28	I	1	5				
Total		20	100				

21 years of age; however, there is no way of knowing that most participants (five of the six) were 21, and only one participant was 20 years of age.

In addition to frequency distributions, **percentage distributions** are often used to present descriptive statistics. A percentage distribution is calculated by dividing the frequency of an event by the total number of events. For example, in Table 5.4 the three 18-year-old participants in the study represent 15% of the total number of particpants reported. Providing information about percentages is another way to group data to make results more comprehensible and allow for easier comparisons with other studies.

After data are tallied and a frequency distribution is determined, data may be converted to graphic form. Graphs provide a visual representation of data and often make it easier to discern trends. The most common types of graphs are line charts, bar graphs, pie charts, histograms, and scattergrams (or scatterplots). **Figure 5.1** depicts two different ways to present the age data from Table 5.4.

MEASURES OF CENTRAL TENDENCY

Measures of central tendency offer another way to describe raw data. These measures provide information about the "typical" case to be found in the data. The *mean*, *median*, and *mode* are the three terms most commonly used to describe the tendency of data to cluster around the middle of the data set (i.e., "averages" for the data). The mean and

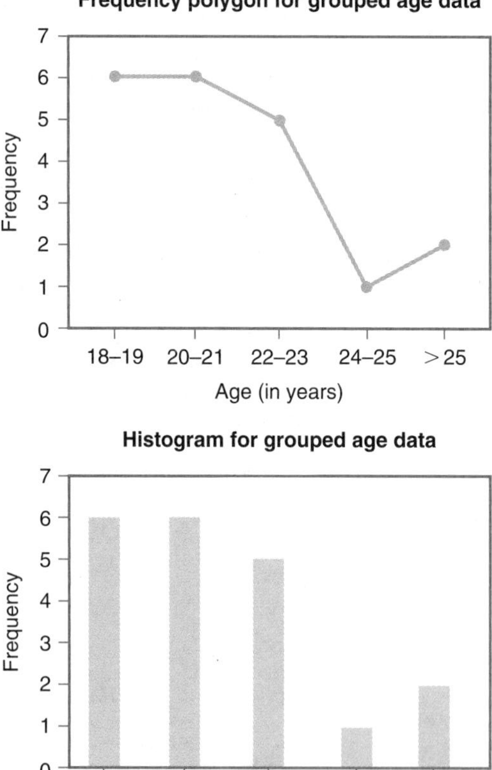

FIGURE 5.1 Frequency Polygon and Histogram of Age Data

Table 5.5 Mode

Data points	Type of mode	Location of mode
{0, 1, 2, 3}	amodal	N/A
{0, 1, 2, 2}	unimodal	2
{1, 1, 2, 2}	bimodal	1 and 2
{1, 1, 1, 2, 2}	unimodal	1
{1, 1, 1, 2, 596}	unimodal	1

median are used to describe continuous-level data; the mode is used to describe both continuous- and nominal-level data. Because the mean and median may be calculated values, they can be rounded to the nearest number; however, the mode is never rounded because it is an actual data point.

MODE

The **mode** is the easiest measure of central tendency to determine because it is the most frequently occurring value in a data set. It is the highest tally when counting and is the highest frequency in a distribution table. **Modality** refers to the number of modes found in a data distribution. Data can be **amodal** (without a mode), **unimodal** (with one mode), or **bimodal** (with two modes). There is no specific term to indicate when data have more than two modes. The mode does not mean that a data value occurs more than once in a frequency distribution because the mode is an actual data point. The mode is not affected by the existence of any extreme values in the data. **Table 5.5** demonstrates how the change in just one data point affects the modality of the data. In the age data presented in Table 5.4, note that the ungrouped data are unimodal with the mode being 21. However, when the data are grouped, they become bimodal with modes at 18–19 years as well as 20–21 years of age (**Table 5.6**). It is easy to see the modes on

Table 5.6 Mode of Age Data for 20 Participants

Ungrouped data			Grouped data		
Age	**Tally**	**Frequency**	**Age**	**Tally**	**Percentage**
18	|||	3	18–19	~~||||~~ |	6
19	|||	3	20–21	~~||||~~ |	6
20	|	1	22–23	~~||||~~	5
21	~~||||~~	5	24–25	|	1
22	|||	3	> 25	||	2
23	||	2	**Total**		20
25	|	1			
27	|	1			
28	|	1			
Total		20			

the frequency polygon and histogram in Figure 5.1 because the modes have the highest peaks and tallest bars. The mode is considered to be an unstable measure of central tendency because it tends to vary widely from one sample to the next. Given its instability, the mode is rarely presented as the sole measure of central tendency.

MEDIAN

The **median** is the center of the data set. Just as the median of the road divides the highway into two halves, the median of a data set divides data in half. If there are an odd number of data points, the median is the middle value or the score where exactly 50% of the data lie above the median and 50% of the data lie below it. If there is an even number of values in the data set, the median is the average of the two middle-most values and as such may be a number not actually found in the data set. The median refers to the average position in the data, and it is minimally affected by the existence of an outlier.

The **position of the median** is calculated by using the formula $(n + 1)/2$, where n is the number of data values in the set. It is important to remember that this formula gives only the position, and not the actual value, of the median. For example, in a study describing the number of hours that five ($n = 5$) sedentary people spent watching television last week, the following data were collected: {4, 6, 3, 38, 6} hours. To determine the median, the researcher would perform a number of easy steps.

1. Sort the data: 3 4 6 6 38
2. Determine the median's location. The median is at the (5 + 1)/2, or third, position from either end.
3. Count over three places to find that the median is 6. In this example, 6 is also the mode because it is the most frequently occurring value.

If the data set is changed to {3, 4, 6, 6}, then the position of the median would be 2.5, or halfway between the second and third sorted data points. In this example, the median is 5, and 6 is the mode. If the data set is changed again to include {3, 4, 6, 100}, the position of the median still will be 2.5, or halfway between the second and third sorted data points, and the median remains 5. This example demonstrates that the outlier value of 100 did not affect the median value. For this reason, the median is generally used to describe the average when there is an extreme value in the data.

When data are grouped, the median is determined using cumulative frequencies. In **Table 5.7** age data are reported for 20 participants. The median is located at (20 + 1)/2, the 10.5th position, and it is the average of the 10th and 11th data values. In the ungrouped data, the median is 21 years old, and the grouped median is 20–21 years.

MEAN

When people refer to an average, what they are really referring to is the **mean**. The mean is calculated by adding all of the data values and then dividing by the total number of values. The mean is the most commonly used measure of central tendency. It is greatly affected by the existence of outliers because every value in the data set is included in the calculation. The larger the sample size, the less an outlier will affect the mean. For example, using the previous data example about number of hours spent watching television, participants reported watching 4, 6, 3, 38, and 6 hours of television per week. Using these data, the mean is calculated to be 11.4 hours (57/5 = 11.4). However, 11.4 hours does not present a clear picture of the amount of television watched by most participants because the one extreme value of 38 hours skews the data. Because the mean is the measure of central tendency used in many tests of statistical significance,

Table 5.7 Median of Age Data for 20 Participants

Ungrouped data				Grouped data			
Age	**Tally**	**Frequency**	**Cumulative frequency**	**Age**	**Tally**	**Frequency**	**Cumulative frequency**
18	|	3	3	18–19	卌 |	6	6
19	|||	3	6	20–21	卌 |	6	12
20	|	1	7	22–23	卌	5	17
21	卌	5	12	24–25	|	1	18
22	|||	3	15	> 25	||	2	20
23	||	2	17	**Total**		20	
25	|	1	18				
27	|	1	19				
28	|	1	20				
Total		20					

it is imperative for researchers to evaluate data for outliers before performing statistical analyses.

When reading articles in which averages are used, Registered Dietitian Nutritionists (RDNs) must carefully examine the conclusions drawn. For example, suppose a hospital employs five staff RDNs and a clinical nutrition manager. Annual salaries of these employees are $66,500, $66,500, $67,000, $68,000, and $69,000. The clinical nutrition manager earns $133,000. During contract negotiations, RDNs indicate that they need a raise. One individual claims the "average" salary is $67,000 per year (median), and another says the "average" salary is $66,500 (the mode). When confronted by the administration, the clinical nutrition manager responds by saying the "average" salary is actually $78,333.33 (mean). So, who is correct? In fact, they are all correct. They are just using different meanings of *average*. This example demonstrates how easy it is to manipulate statistics and why careful attention must be given to the interpretation of data being presented.

When appraising evidence, it is helpful to remember that the mean is the best measure of central tendency if there are no extreme values, and the median is best if there are extreme values. Because they are calculated, the mean and median are not necessarily actual data values, whereas the mode must be an exact data point. The mean and median are unique values (again, because they are calculated), but the mode might be unique or might not exist at all, or there might be multiple modes. The mean is greatly affected

TIP

Do you have a professor who grades on a curve? When grading on a curve, the professor compares each student's grade to the class' mean score and distributes grades along a bell curve . This is known as norm-referenced testing because each student is compared to the other students. What are advantages and disadvantages of grading on a curve compared to grades that are based strictly on knowledge and proficiency?

by extreme values, the median is marginally affected, and the mode is not affected. The mean and median use continuous-level data values for their calculations, whereas the mode can use either continuous- or nominal-data values. The mean is the most stable in that if repeated samples were drawn from the same population, the mean would vary less than either the median or the mode would from sample to sample.

MEASURES OF VARIABILITY

Measures of variability provide information regarding how different the data are within a set. These can also be known as measures of dispersion because they provide information about how data are dispersed around the mean. If the data are very similar, there is little variability, and the data are considered to be **homogenous.** If there is wide variation, the data are considered to be **heterogeneous.** Common measures of variation include range, semiquartile range, percentile, and standard deviation; *z* scores and variance are used to compare the variability among data using different units of measure.

RANGE

A statistical **range** is the difference between the maximum and minimum values in a data set. Because the range is sample specific, it is considered to be an unstable measure of variability. **Table 5.8** shows the income reported for paticipants in the experimental and control groups of a study designed to evaluate health literacy. The mean for both data sets is $48,000, and the medians are each $42,000. However, the data are quite different because the data for the experimental group are more heterogeneous than for the control group. The experimental group's income varies from a minimum of $15,000 to a maximum of $103,000, with a range of $88,000. The control group's income has a minimum of $30,000 and a maximum of $73,000. Although salaries are still quite variable, they are more uniform than the experimental group's salaries because their range is $43,000. In data comparisons, the smaller the range, the more uniform the data; the greater the range, the more variable the data.

SEMIQUARTILE RANGE

Just as the median divides data into two halves, other values divide these halves in half, meaning into quarters. The **semiquartile range** is the range of the middle 50% of the data. **Figure 5.2** illustrates the semiquartile range of the age data from a previous example. The semiquartile range lies between the lower (first) and upper (third) quartile of

Table 5.8 Example of Ranges of Income

	Control	Experimental
	$30,000	$15,000
	$38,000	$23,000
	$42,000	$42,000
	$57,000	$57,000
	$73,000	$103,000
Range	$43,000	$88,000

18 18 18 19 19 | 19 20 21 21 21 | 21 21 22 22 22 | 23 23 25 27 28

$Q_1 = 19$ Median = 21 $Q_3 = 22.5$

FIGURE 5.2 Semiquartile Range of Age Data

ages. The first quartile value is the median of the lower half of the data set; one-fourth of the data lies below the first quartile and three-fourths of the data lie above it. The third quartile value is the median of the upper half of the data; three-fourths of the data lie below the third quartile and one-fourth of the data lies above it. The semiquartile range is the difference between the third and first quartile values and describes the middle half of a data distribution. In Figure 5.2, note that 50% of the data lie between 19 and 22.5, and the range is 3.5.

Percentile

A **percentile** is a measure of rank. Each percentile represents the percentage of cases that a given value exceeds. The median is the 50th percentile, the first quartile is the 25th percentile, and the third quartile is the 75th percentile score in a given data set. For example, if a newborn baby boy's weight is in the 39th percentile, he weighs more than 39% of babies tested weigh but less than 61% of the other babies.

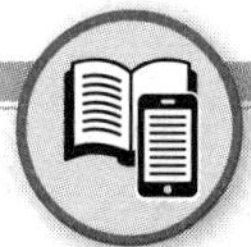

APPLICATION 5.1

Consider how your ACT or SAT scores were reported. What was your raw score? What was your percentile? What do these data indicate about your performance on these tests?

Standard Deviation

The most commonly reported measure of variability is the **standard deviation**, which is based on deviations from the mean of the data. Whereas the mean is the expectation value (the expected "average" of the data set), the standard deviation is the measure of the average deviations of a value from the mean in a given data set. Because it is a measure of deviation from the mean, a standard deviation should always be reported whenever a mean is reported. Standard deviation is based on the normal curve and is used to determine the number of data values that fall within a specific interval in a normal distribution. Understanding the standard deviation allows you to interpret an individual score in comparison with all other scores in the data set. Recall the salary example presented earlier. The data were variable because of the extreme ranges of salary values.

TIP

The most commonly reported measure of variability, the standard deviation, is the measure of the average deviations of a value from the mean in a given data set. Because standard deviations are based on the mean of the data set, information collected using different measurement scales cannot be directly compared.

Table 5.9 Standard Deviations of Income

	Control	Experimental
	$30,000	$15,000
	$38,000	$23,000
	$42,000	$42,000
	$57,000	$57,000
	$73,000	$103,000
SD	$17,073.37	$34,842.50

Calculating a standard deviation provides different information about variability. It is now apparent that the average deviation from the mean for the experimental group is $34,842.50, which is more than double that of the control group's $17,073.37 deviation (see **Table 5.9**).

COMPARING VARIABILITY WHEN UNITS OF MEASURE ARE DIFFERENT

Because standard deviations are based on the mean of the data set, information collected using different measurement scales cannot be directly compared. For example, the mean of a sample's age is reported in years, whereas the mean of a sample's weight is reported in pounds. To make comparisons among unlike data requires that all the data means be converted to standardized units called standardized or **z scores**; *z* scores are then used to describe the distance a score is away from the mean per standard deviation. A *z* score of 1.25 means that a data value is 1.25 standard deviations above the mean. A *z* score of –2.53 means that a data value is 2.53 standard deviations below the mean. Using the *z* score allows researchers to compare results of age and weight.

The coefficient of variation is a percentage used to compare standard deviations when the units of measure are different or when the means of the distributions being compared are far apart. The coefficient of variation is computed by dividing the standard deviation by the mean and recording the result as a percentage. For example, if you were to compare age and income of a sample of RDNs, you could not use range or standard deviations to discuss the variables' comparative spread because they are measured with different units. If the mean salary for RDNs is $66,000, with a standard deviation of $6,000, and the mean age is 32 years, with a standard deviation of 4 years, the coefficient of variation for the salary is 9.1%, and the coefficient of variation for age is 12.5%. Using the coefficient of variation shows that age is more variable than salaries among this group of RDNs.

APPLICATION 5.2

Do you have a professor who uses means and standard deviations, known as norm referencing, for grading exams? What are the advantages to using this approach as opposed to straight scales for grading? What are some disadvantages?

DISTRIBUTION PATTERNS

NORMAL DISTRIBUTIONS: SYMMETRICAL SHAPES

Measures of central tendencies are used to define distribution patterns. When the distribution of the data is symmetrical (that is, when the two halves of the distribution are folded over, they would be superimposed on each other and therefore be unimodal), then the mean, median, and mode are equal. In this situation, the data are considered to be normally distributed. A **normal distribution** has a distinctive bell-shaped curve and is symmetric about the mean. In **Figure 5.3**, note that the decreasing bars, or area under the curve, indicate that the data cluster at the center and taper away from the mean. A number of human traits, such as intelligence and height, are considered to be normally distributed in the population.

WHEN DATA ARE NOT NORMALLY DISTRIBUTED

Often data do not fit a normal distribution and are considered to be asymmetric or **skewed**. In asymmetric distributions, the peak of the data is not at the center of the distribution, and one tail is longer than the other. Skewed distributions are usually discussed in terms of their direction. If the longer tail is pointing to the left, the data are considered to be **negatively skewed** (**Figure 5.4**). In this situation, the mean is less

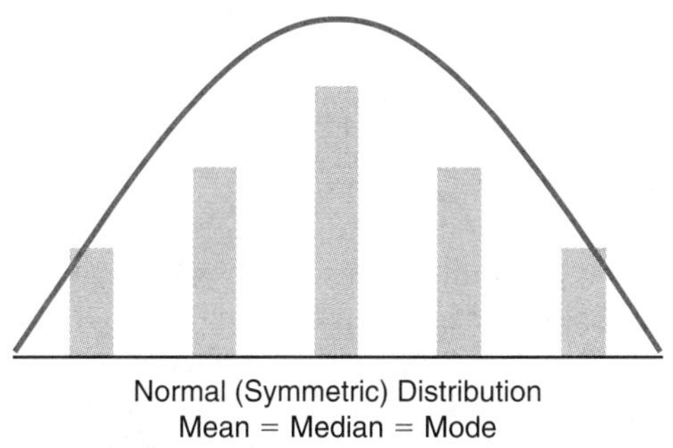

FIGURE 5.3 Example of a Normal Distribution

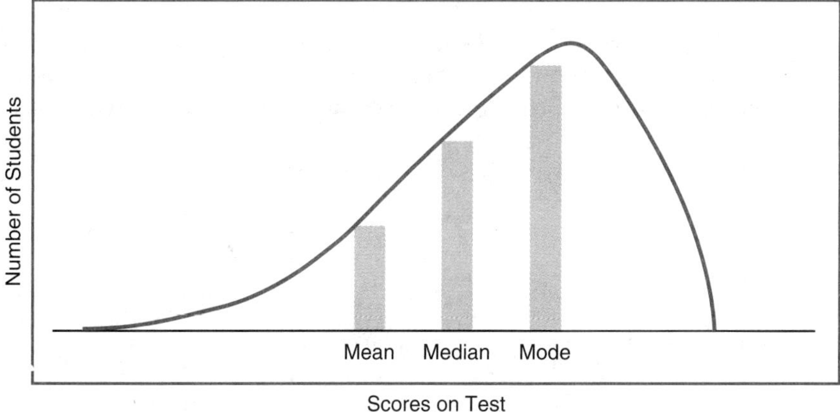

FIGURE 5.4 Example of a Negatively Skewed Distribution

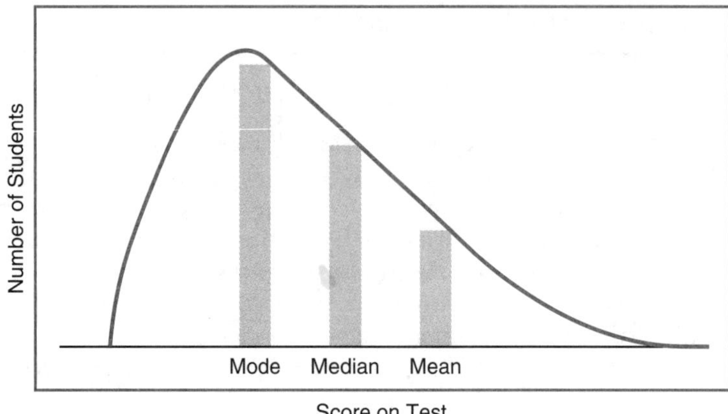

FIGURE 5.5 Example of a Positively Skewed Distribution

than the median and mode. For example, a group of students take a test for which all but one student studied. The one student, who did not study, scores very low. This low score, because it is an outlier, affects the mean because the scores of students who studied are high. This outlier contributes to a negatively skewed distribution. The low score pulls down the mean and pulls with it the tail of the distribution to the left. If the mean is greater than the median and mode, then the data are **positively skewed**, pulling the tail to the right. For example, an instructor gives a difficult test. Only one or two students scored high on the test. The rest of the students' scores were low. Most students' scores are lower than the mean because the outliers affect the mean. The distribution of these scores is positively skewed. The extremely high scores pull up the mean and pull the tail in a positive direction toward the right (**Figure 5.5**).

Attention should be given to how the data are spread, or dispersed, around the mean. Just as schoolchildren or military personnel wear uniforms to be like each other, uniform data have very little spread and look like each other. When there is greater variation in data, a wider spread results. In graphic representations of data (see **Figure 5.6**), highly uniform data have a high peak and highly variable data have a low peak. **Kurtosis** is the term used to describe the peakedness or flatness of a data set.

TAILEDNESS: THE RULE OF 68–95–99.7

The concept of **tailedness** is important to understand when reading statistical reports. Recall that a normal distribution is one in which the mean, median, and mode are all equal and the data are symmetrical. In discussing tailedness, the graph of a normal distribution is depicted as a bell-shaped curve, centered about the mean (x), with 3 standard

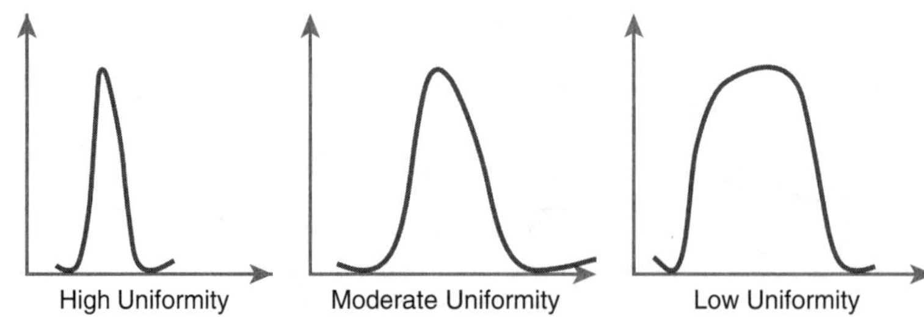

FIGURE 5.6 Example of Kurtosis

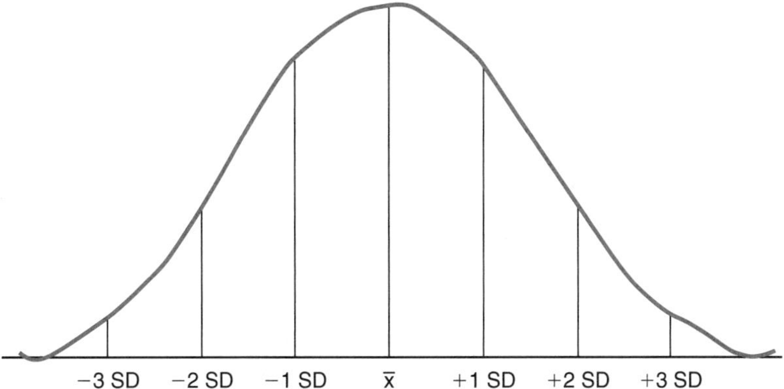

FIGURE 5.7 Normal Distribution with Standard Deviations

deviations marked to the right (positive) and also to the left (negative) (see **Figure 5.7**). Normal distributions are not shown beyond 3 standard deviations in either direction because approximately 99.7% of the data will lie within this range. Approximately 68% of all data in a normal curve lie within 1 standard deviation of the mean, and 95% of the data lie within 2 standard deviations of the mean.

Thus, the **Rule of 68–95–99.7** tells us that for every sample, 99.7% of the data will fall within 3 standard deviations of the mean. In **Figure 5.8**, note the symmetry about the mean for the standard deviations as they are divided in half for each distribution percentage. For example,1 standard deviation contains 34% of the scores above and 34% of the scores below the mean to total 68%; 2 standard deviations contain 34% plus 13.5% above and below the mean to equal 95% of the scores. On a standard deviation graph, the mean has a z score of zero. Other z-score percentages may be determined by using a table showing the area under the curve data.

Figure 5.9 shows that normal distributions may also be used to approximate percentile ranks. Actual percentile values must always be determined by using a normal distribution table to look up a given z score.

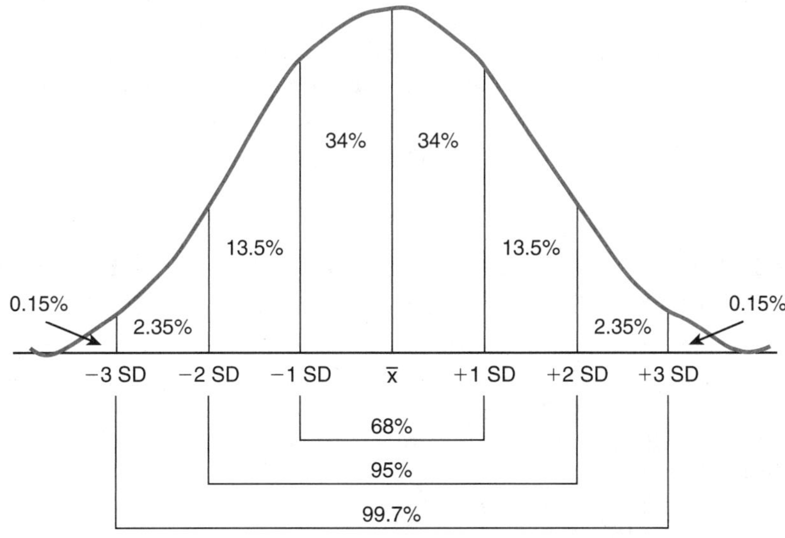

FIGURE 5.8 Standard Deviations and Percentage Distribution

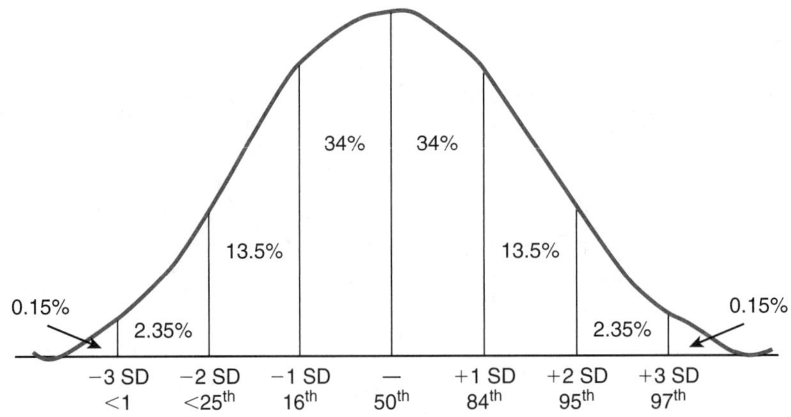

FIGURE 5.9 Percentile Rank Based on Normal Distribution

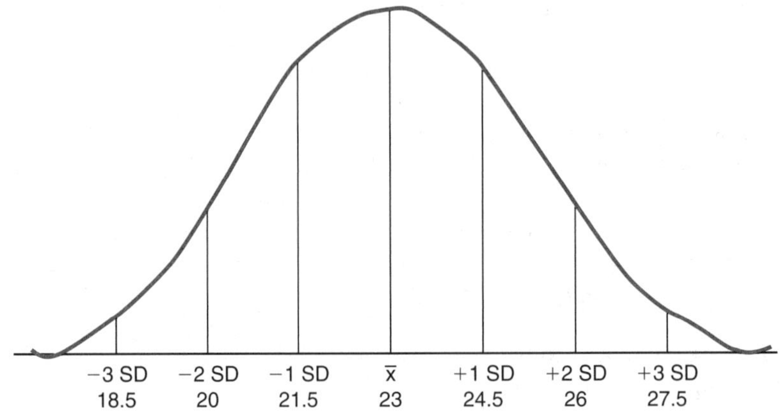

FIGURE 5.10 Standard Deviations of Age Data

The age data from previous examples do not approximate a normal distribution because the mean, median, and mode are not equal. If, however, we used data that were standardized with a mean of 23 and a standard deviation of 1.5 years, the normal curve for these data would look like the graph in **Figure 5.10**. Sixty-eight percent of these people would be between 21.5 and 24.5 years of age, and someone 26 years old would be in the 95th percentile. Half of the people would be 23 years or older, and half would be younger than 23 years.

INFERENTIAL STATISTICS: CAN THE FINDINGS BE APPLIED TO THE POPULATION?

First, samples are analyzed using descriptive statistics. Then, if appropriate, inferential statistical tests can be conducted to (1) make decisions about whether findings can be applied to the population, or in other words, to make inferences about the population based on the sample; and (2) test hypotheses. For some studies, the use of inferential statistics is not appropriate, and their use depends on the research questions being asked. Research questions that are descriptive would not require inferential statistics. For example, the research question "How often do RDNs assess the use of herbal remedies by patients?" would best be answered by using descriptive statistics, such as frequencies, means, and standard deviations.

Using parameter estimation to determine inferences to the population is becoming more popular with the emphasis on evidence-based practice (EBP) in nutrition, nursing, and medicine (Borenstein, 1997; Straus, Richardson, Glasziou, & Haynes, 2010). Most frequently, these estimates are reported as **confidence intervals** (CIs). CIs are ranges established around means that estimate the probability of being correct (American College of Physicians—American Society of Internal Medicine, 2001; Hoekstra, Johnson, & Kiers, 2012). In other words, CIs estimate the degree of confidence one can have about the inferences. Researchers typically report confidence levels of 95% or 99%.

Use of inferential statistics to test hypotheses is best suited to research questions or hypotheses that ask one of two broad questions:

- Is there a difference between the groups?
- Is there a relationship among the variables?

Most experimental and quasi-experimental designs involve questions asking if there is a difference between the groups. For example, the use of inferential statistics to test the hypothesis "Individuals who get at least 7 hours of sleep have lower body weights than do individuals who sleep less than 6 hours a night" would be appropriate. Research questions or hypotheses that ask about relationships among variables, such as "Is there a relationship between the number of hours of sleep and blood glucose levels?" can also be tested using inferential statistics.

When deciding which statistical tests to use to analyze data, researchers must take many factors into account (Hayes, 1994). After considering whether the research questions or hypotheses involve groups or variables, the next most important factor researchers consider is the level of measurement. Whether variables are nominal, ordinal, interval, or ratio is important because some tests are appropriate for interval and ratio data but not for other levels of measurement. Other factors that can influence selection of inferential statistical tests include whether (1) a probability sampling method was used, (2) the data are normally distributed, and (3) there is potential confounding of the variables. *Keep in mind that the strongest inferences can be made when the level of measurement is interval or ratio, a probability sampling method was used, the sample size is adequate, and the data are normally distributed.*

IT'S ALL ABOUT CHANCE

Regardless of the type of question being asked, the major unanswered question is, "What is the likelihood that the findings could have occurred by chance alone?" For example, suppose that you toss a coin 10 times, and each time it lands heads up. Could that happen by chance? Absolutely. Now suppose you flip it another 10 times, and it lands with heads up every time. Although it is possible that a coin could land heads up 20 times in a row, this would be a rare occurrence. Would you begin to wonder if this were happening by chance, or would you suspect that the coin is not fair? How many times would you want to toss the coin before you conclude that the coin is not fair?

Researchers ask the same types of questions when they analyze data using inferential statistics. They ask, "What is the probability that the findings were a result of chance?" **Probability** is the likelihood of the frequency of an event in repeated trials under similar conditions. Probability is the percentage of times that an event (e.g., "heads") is likely to occur by chance alone. Probability is affected by the concept of sampling error. **Sampling error** is the tendency for statistical results to fluctuate from one sample to another.

Table 5.10 Coin Toss Example

	Trial 1	Trial 2	Trial 3	Trial 4	Trial 5	Trial 6	Trial 7	Trial 8	Trial 9	Trial 10
0 Heads 10 Tails										
1 Head 9 Tails										
2 Heads 8 Tails						X				
3 Heads 7 Tails										
4 Heads 6 Tails		X					X			
5 Heads 5 Tails	X				X					X
6 Heads 4 Tails				X					X	
7 Heads 3 Tails								X		
8 Heads 2 Tails			X							
9 Heads 1 Tail										
10 Heads 0 Tails										

There is always a possibility of errors in sampling, even when the samples are randomly selected. The characteristics of any given sample are usually different from those of the population. For example, suppose a fair coin was tossed 10 times for 10 different trials. A tally of the results in **Table 5.10** shows that the trials varied; but as expected, more of the trials were nearer 50% heads than 100% heads.

Researchers determine whether the results were obtained by chance using inferential statistical tests, sometimes known as tests of significance. Mathematical calculations are performed, usually by computers, to obtain critical values. These values are plotted on a normal distribution, and determinations of whether findings are **statistically significant** or **nonsignificant** are made. Statistically significant critical values fall in the tails of the normal distributions, usually 3 standard deviations from the mean or where about only 0.3% of the data occur. Thus, when critical values are in that area, researchers believe it is appropriate to claim that the findings did not happen by chance.

REDUCING ERROR WHEN DECIDING ABOUT HYPOTHESES

Researchers do many things to reduce error so that others can have confidence in the findings. They reduce error by selecting designs that fit with research questions, controlling the independent variable, carefully measuring variables, and reducing threats to internal and external validity. They also take steps to reduce error when deciding whether a research hypothesis is supported or not supported.

When making decisions about hypotheses, researchers keep several principles in mind (Hayes, 1994). First, hypotheses are claims about the world. Second, decisions are made about null hypotheses, not research hypotheses. The purpose of inferential statistical tests is to determine whether the null hypothesis should be accepted or rejected. Third, it is important to remember that *no matter how well errors are reduced or how powerful the findings are, nothing is ever proven. The most that can be claimed is that a research hypothesis is either supported or unsupported.* Finally, it is wise to understand that an empirical view is adopted and an assumption is made that there is a single reality in the physical world and that science can be used to discover the truth about reality.

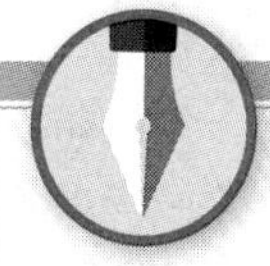

TIP

Researchers attempt to reduce error to increase confidence in their findings. Methods for reducing error include selecting designs that fit with research questions, controlling the independent variable, carefully measuring variables, and reducing threats to internal and external validity.

Type I and Type II Errors

With inferential statistics, the goal is to avoid the two kinds of errors that can be made when making decisions about null hypotheses. These errors are known as type I and type II errors. A **type I error** occurs when the researcher rejects the null hypothesis when it should have been accepted. When the null hypothesis is wrongly rejected, the usual result is that the researcher makes false claims about the research hypothesis. Usually this means that the researcher claims that some treatment works or some relationship exists, when in actuality that is not the case. This false finding could be the result of any number of errors, such as sampling bias or measurement error. The false finding could have happened by chance, just as it would be possible by chance to get 20 heads in a row when tossing a fair coin. The researcher, unaware about what is true in the world, rejects the null hypothesis based on the statistical analysis and claims that the research hypothesis is supported. This is a type I error.

A **type II error** occurs when researchers accept the null hypothesis when it should have been rejected. In nutrition, this type of error usually means that practice does not change when it should be changed. The opportunity to implement an effective treatment or claim the discovery of a relationship has been missed.

APPLICATION 5.3

Individuals make decisions every day. They make decisions based on their assumptions about the world, only to find out later that the assumptions were incorrect. Can you think of times when you have made a type I error? What about a situation when a type II error was made?

There are a few strategies for remembering type I and type II errors. One way is through the graphic representation in **Table 5.11**. One axis of the table represents whether the null hypothesis is true or false in the real world. The other axis represents the

Table 5.11 Type I and Type II Errors

	The null hypothesis is true in real world	The null hypothesis is false in real world
Researcher Accepts the Null Hypothesis	No Error	Type II Error
Researcher Rejects the Null Hypothesis	Type I Error	No Error

two decisions that can be made by researchers about the null hypothesis: to accept or to reject. The center boxes are then filled in as appropriate. No errors are made when a decision to accept a null hypothesis is made when it is true in the real world. Likewise, there is no error when a false null hypothesis is rejected. A type I error is made when researchers, obtaining statistically significant results, reject the null hypothesis when in fact it was true. A type II error occurs when researchers fail to obtain statistically significant results, and thus they accept the null hypothesis despite the fact that it is false. Another way to remember type I and type II errors is to think of the acronym RAAR (Gillis & Jackson, 2002). RAAR stands for the phrase: "*R*eject the null hypothesis when you should *a*ccept it, and *a*ccept the null hypothesis when you should *r*eject it." The first two letters, RA, stand for a type I error. The second two letters, AR, stand for a type II error.

LEVEL OF SIGNIFICANCE: ADJUSTING THE RISK OF MAKING TYPE I AND TYPE II ERRORS

In health care, type I errors are considered to be more serious than type II errors (Smith, 2012). It seems much more risky to claim that a treatment works when in reality it does not than to miss the opportunity to claim that a treatment works. For example, a researcher invents and tests a new device for measuring blood sugar. If a type I error is made, the researcher claims that the new device works when in reality it does not. Patients begin using the device, which inaccurately measures blood sugar. Because RDNs and RNs evaluate the implementation of this new device, they eventually realize that the device is not effective as the researcher claimed. The type I error could result in accusations of harming diabetics with a fraudulent measuring device. Because patients who used the device might have been harmed, they might want to sue the researcher.

However, if a type II error is made, the researcher throws away the device for measuring blood sugar even though in reality it is superior to other devices. In this situation, the researcher misses the opportunity to market the device and earn money, and diabetics miss the opportunity to benefit from the measuring device. Although neither scenario is desirable, most researchers would choose to miss the opportunity to make money rather than to harm patients and risk the legal implications.

Researchers must make decisions about how much risk they are willing to tolerate. When interventions are complex, expensive, invasive, or have many side effects, such as a new procedure for cardiac surgery, researchers are usually less willing to make type I errors. When interventions are simple, inexpensive, or noninvasive, such as a new teaching method, the tolerance for a type I error is increased.

Researchers use statistics to adjust the amount of risk involved in making type I and type II errors. It is helpful to remember that type I and type II errors have an inverse relationship. When a type I error is increased, a type II error is decreased. Risks for these errors are adjusted by selecting the **alpha level**, which is the probability of making a type I error. Alpha level is designated at the end of the tail in a distribution (see **Figure 5.11**). In nutrition research, the alpha levels are usually either 0.05 or 0.01. In

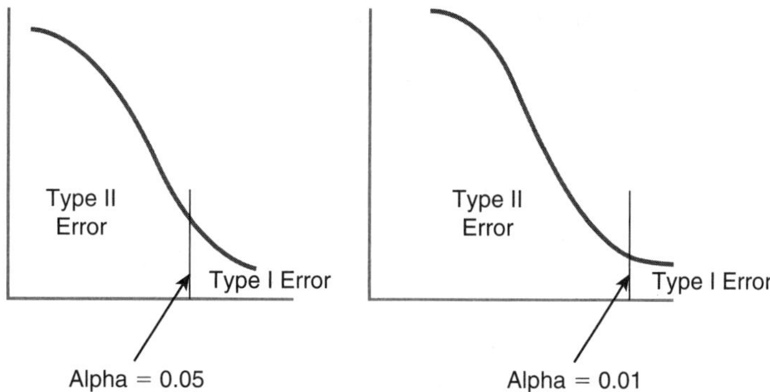

FIGURE 5.11 Placement of Alpha Level on Normal Distribution

the figure, the placement of the alpha level shows how type I and type II errors can be adjusted. In this example of a one-tailed test, the area under the curve to the left of the alpha level represents the amount of type II error. The area under the curve to the right of the line is the amount of type I error. Notice that when the alpha level is larger, there is more space to the right of the line than when the alpha level is smaller.

What are the implications of these alpha levels? When the alpha level is set at 0.05, it is likely that 5 times out of 100, the researcher would make a type I error by wrongly rejecting the null hypothesis. When 0.01 is used for the alpha level, a researcher would make a type I error only 1 time out of 100. Thus, alpha levels of 0.05 increase type I errors while reducing type II errors. In general, although alpha levels of 0.01 reduce type I errors, the likelihood of making a type II error increases. In nutrition, 0.05 is used more commonly than 0.01.

Although the mathematical difference between these alphas is miniscule, the implications for decision making are great. **Figure 5.12** provides an illustration of how the acceptance or rejection of the null hypothesis is affected by the alpha level selected. When conducting statistical tests to test hypotheses, suppose there is a chance for three possible critical values. Note in Figure 5.12 that critical value "A" falls to the left of both alpha levels. Regardless of the alpha level chosen, the results will be statistically nonsignificant, and the null hypothesis will be accepted. Critical value "B" falls to the right of both alpha levels. The results will be statistically significant regardless of the alpha level selected. Now consider the position of critical value "C." How would the decision about the null hypothesis be affected by either of these two alphas? If the alpha level is set at 0.05, the critical point would be significant and the null hypothesis would be rejected.

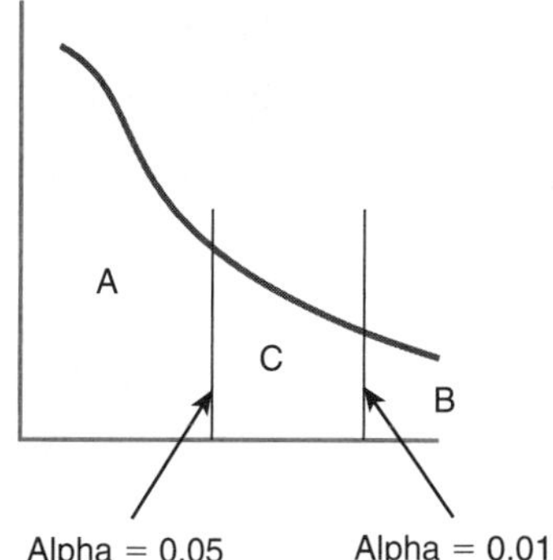

FIGURE 5.12 Relationship of Alpha Levels and Critical Values

However, if an alpha level of 0.01 is selected, the critical point would be nonsignificant, and the researcher would accept the null hypothesis. To avoid any temptation to select alpha levels that bias decision making, researchers must always state their selected alpha levels in the initial research proposal. Strong rationales for the one selected must also be provided.

USING STATISTICAL TESTS TO MAKE INFERENCES ABOUT POPULATIONS

A unique language is used by statisticians to communicate statistical data. A variety of terms and statistical symbols (**Table 5.12**) is associated with inferential statistics. Statistical tests are frequently named after the individuals who devised them, which can sometimes make the names seem arbitrary and hard to remember. The following fundamental terms are ones with which RDNs should become familiar.

Parametric tests are used to make inferences about the population when specific conditions have been met (Hayes, 1994; Plichta & Kelvin, 2013). These conditions include

1. use of probability sampling,
2. normal distribution of data,
3. measurement of variables at the interval or ratio level, and
4. reduction of error.

For example, data collected using a visual analog scale would be analyzed using parametric tests. These important conditions make parametric tests especially powerful. When parametric tests are used, you can have high levels of confidence about the conclusions made.

Table 5.12 Statistical Symbols for Inferential Statistics

Symbol/Abbreviation	Definition
ANOVA	Analysis of variance
df	Degrees of freedom
F	Fisher's *F* ratio
ns	Nonsignificant
p	Probability
r	Pearson product–moment correlation
R	Multiple correlation
R^2	Multiple correlation squared
t	Computed value of *t* test
α	Alpha; probability of type I error
β	Beta; probability of type II error
Δ	Delta; amount of change
Σ	Sigma; sum or summation
X^2	Chi-square

When all four conditions are not met, researchers must use less powerful tests known as **nonparametric** tests. Nonparametric statistics are used for interval data that do not have a normal distribution or for data that are nominal or ordinal in nature. Because these tests are considered to be less powerful, the level of confidence RDNs have about making inferences about the population is not as strong as when parametric tests are used.

Another term used when talking about statistics is **degrees of freedom**. Degrees of freedom (*df*), based on the number of elements in a sample, are used to correct for possible underestimation of population parameters when performing mathematical equations. Specifically, *degrees of freedom* refers to the freedom of a variable's score to vary given the other existing variables' score values and the sum of these score values ($df = N - 1$) (Plichta & Kelvin, 2013). For example, suppose a data set consists of four scores: 1, 4, 4, and 7. Before any of these scores were collected, the researcher did not know what these scores would be. Each score was free to vary and was independent from the other scores. Because there are four scores, there are four degrees of freedom. However, when the mean is calculated, one degree of freedom is lost because once the mean is known, along with three of the scores, the fourth score is no longer free to vary. The fourth score can be calculated, and only one value will be correct. Therefore, the data set of four scores has three degrees of freedom, $n - 1$, because one degree of freedom is lost. Many inferential statistics include degrees of freedom in their calculations.

Another concept important in the language of inferential statistics is **sampling distribution** (Nieswiadomy, 2012; Plichta & Kelvin, 2013). In theory, an infinite number of samples can be drawn from a population. Some samples are more likely to be drawn than others. For example, when sampling coin tosses, getting half heads and half tails when tossing a coin 20 times is far more likely than is tossing heads 20 times in a row. For many inferential tests, statisticians have calculated the likelihood of obtaining different samples and reported them in tables. When researchers perform certain inferential tests, they refer to these tables to find out whether their results are likely or unlikely. Results that are unlikely to occur as a result of chance are then considered to be statistically significant.

RDNs commonly see a number of inferential tests in the literature. Although the study of statistical tests can seem overwhelming to some individuals, to appraise evidence it might not be necessary to fully understand why each test is conducted and how the calculations are performed. RDNs should be able to discern that the correct tests were used to analyze data. This can be determined by focusing on two broad questions: (1) "What type of question is being asked by the researcher?" and (2) "What is the level of measurement being used to measure the variables?" Some inferential statistical tests commonly used in nursing research are listed in **Table 5.13**. Although it is beyond the scope of this text to elaborate on all the tests listed in the table, information about some of the most common tests is worth remembering. When answering questions about statistically significant differences between groups, you should be familiar with Chi-square, *t* tests, and analysis of variance (ANOVA). You should also be familiar with Pearson's *r* and multiple regression, which are tests used to determine whether there is a statistically significant correlation among the variables.

Testing for Differences Between Groups

As shown in Table 5.13, a variety of tests can be used to analyze data for the purpose of determining the statistically significant difference between the groups. When deciding which test to use, researchers must consider the number of groups to be included in the analysis and at what level variables were measured. Pilot studies frequently involve one

Table 5.13 Inferential Tests Commonly Used in Nutrition

			What is the hypothesis asking?				Is there a relationship among the variables?	
			Is there a difference between the groups?					
			1 Group	2 Groups		> 2 Groups	2 Variables	> 2 Variables
				Related	Independent			
What is the level of measurement?	**Nonparametric**	**Nominal**	Chi-square	Chi-square Fisher's exact probability test	Chi-square	Chi-square	Phi coefficient Point biserial	Contingency coefficient
		Ordinal	Kolmogorov-Smirnov	Sign test Wilcoxin matched pairs Signed rank	Chi-square Median test Mann-Whitney U	Chi-square	Kendall's Tau Spearman Rho	
	Parametric	**Interval or Ratio**	Correlated *t* (paired *t*)	Correlated *t*	Independent *t*	ANOVA ANCOVA MANOVA	Pearson's *r*	Multiple regression Path analysis Canonical correlation

Note: ANOVA = analysis of variance; ANCOVA = analysis of covariance; MANOVA = multivariate analysis of variance.

group, whereas classic experiments and quasi-experiments can include two or more groups. Before analyzing data, researchers need to consider whether the groups are dependent or independent to select the correct tests to perform.

For example, suppose a researcher is studying perceptions of health in married couples before and after a class about stress reduction. The researcher tests both men and women who are married to one another. Because individuals in a marriage have many characteristics in common, the data collected should be analyzed using inferential tests for dependent groups. Data from designs using participants as their own controls—for example, measuring blood pressures before and after exercise—are also treated as data from dependent groups. More likely than not, researchers collect data from independent groups, for example, test scores from two groups of diabetic patients.

The Chi-Square Statistic

Chi-square is a very commonly used statistic (Hayes, 1994; Plichta & Kelvin, 2013). Calculated when analyzing nominal and ordinal data, it is a nonparametric test. One reason Chi-square is used so often is because it is very useful for finding differences between the groups on demographic variables at the start of the study. For example, suppose that a researcher is studying the effect of potassium on blood pressure and randomly assigns 200 individuals to one of two groups. The experimental group contains 54 women and 46 men, and the control group has 46 women and 54 men. By performing a Chi-square test, the researcher can determine whether the groups are alike on the extraneous variable of gender. If the groups are not significantly different on gender, it can be assumed that changes in blood pressure are more likely a result of the intervention than of gender.

When Chi-square statistics are used, the frequencies that are observed during the study are compared to the frequencies that would be expected to occur if the null hypothesis were true. Observed and expected frequencies are entered into contingency tables, and a Chi-square statistic is calculated. Using the calculated Chi-square statistic, the degrees of freedom, and the alpha level, researchers consult Chi-square tables to determine the critical value and judge whether the critical value is statistically significant. In the literature, notations for Chi-square, such as $X^2 = 1.89$, $df = 1$, $p < 0.05$, appear reported with degrees of freedom and significance. Another reason Chi-squares are frequently used is because they can be calculated without the use of computers. However, the sample size must be adequate because there must be at least five or more observed frequencies in each cell of the table. If this minimum is not met, then a variation of the Chi-square, known as Fisher's exact probability test, is used.

The *t* Statistic

The ***t* statistic** is another inferential statistical test that is reported in nutrition research. Commonly known as the *t* test, or Student's *t* test, this parametric measure is used to determine whether there is a statistically significant difference between two groups (Hayes, 1994; Plichta & Kelvin, 2013).

There are two variations of the *t* test. One variation, known as the **correlated *t* test**, or paired *t* test, is used when there are only two measurements taken on the same person (one group) or when the groups are related. For example, a paired *t* test would be used to assess for differences between participants' morning and evening blood pressure readings. The other variation is known as an **independent *t* test** and is used when data values vary independently from one another.

In experimental and quasi-experimental designs, the *t* test is used to determine whether the means of two groups are statistically different. Suppose a researcher is measuring the effectiveness of applying ice for pain reduction. The mean pain intensity rating for the experimental group, which received the ice application, is 5.6, whereas for the control group, which did not get the ice, it is 6.0. As with a Chi-square test, researchers calculate the *t* statistic and consult tables using the statistic, degrees of freedom, and alpha levels to find the critical value. The critical value is obtained and a decision about its statistical significance is made. In reports, the *t* test information provided includes the number of degrees of freedom, actual *t* value obtained, and significance level, which is reported in the following manner: $t\,(2) = 2.54$, $p < 0.01$. In this case, if the researcher set a level of significance of 0.05 or even 0.01, this *t* test result shows support for the research hypothesis, that ice is effective for pain reduction.

Here's another example of using *t*-tests and also Chi-square tests. In a study involving an experimental and a control group, both Chi-square and *t*-tests were used to compare demographic and baseline characteristics of both groups (see **Table 5.14**). Note in Table 5.14 that *t* tests were used to compare the means for continuous variables such as body mass index and χ^2 tests were used for categorical variables such as medical conditions. The *P* value is listed in the right-hand column. Since the *P* values were all 0.19 or higher, the researchers can conclude that these baseline characteristics likely did not influence the study's results.

Analysis of Variance

Analysis of variance (ANOVA) is used when the level of measurement is interval or ratio and there are more than two groups or the variable of interest is measured more than

Table 5.14 Comparison of Demographic and Baseline Characteristics in a Study With Two Groups Using *t* tests and Chi-square

Variable	Intervention Group (n = 105)	Control Group (n = 110)	*P* value*
Age, mean (SD), y	46.9 (11.4)	45.3 (10.9)	.91
Weight, mean, (SD), lb	225.6 (39.2)	220.3 (38.4)	.39
Body mass index, mean, (SD)	36.2 (6.7)	36.0 (6.5)	.87
Female sex, No. (%)	69 (66)	72 (65)	.19
Medical Conditions, No. (%)			
Hypertension	61 (58.1)	66 (60.0)	.64
Diabetes	14 (13.3)	22 (20.0)	.39

* *t* tests were used for continuous variables and χ^2 tests for categorical variables.

two times (Hayes, 1994; Plichta & Kelvin, 2013). The broad question being answered is whether group means significantly differ from one another. Using ANOVA allows researchers to compare a combination of pairs of means while reducing the odds for a type I error. For example, suppose a researcher is testing three different styles of education with adolescents who have diabetes: peer, text messaging, and Web-based. Three different pairs of means would be compared: peer to text messaging, peer to Web-based, and text messaging to Web based. If *t* tests were conducted for each pair, the same null hypothesis would be tested three times, increasing the risk of a type I error. By using an ANOVA, researchers can compare the variations among the groups using one statistical test, thereby reducing the chances of making a type I error.

ANOVA and *t* tests are very closely related. When testing only two groups, the same mathematical answer would result whether an ANOVA or a *t* test were used. Using ANOVA, researchers calculate the *F* statistic, which is based on the *F* distribution using degrees of freedom. The greater the *F* statistic, the greater the variation between the means of the groups. Tables of the *F* distributions and degrees of freedom are also used. $F = 4.65$, $df = 2, 50$, $p < 0.05$ is an example of the notation that would be used to report an ANOVA. However, the *F* statistic indicates only that the null hypothesis can be rejected because there is a difference between the group means, *but the F test alone does not tell which specific group differed*. Instead, researchers have to conduct post hoc tests to determine where the significant difference occurred.

One-way ANOVA has one independent variable with more than 2 levels or conditions, as in the education example just discussed. Two-way ANOVA has two independent variables and each variable may have multiple levels.

Humphrey, Clifford, and Morris (2015) used one-way ANOVA to analyze the treatment effect in their study because their independent variable, an educational program using a nondiet approach, had two levels. In this study, the groups included students enrolled in a college course entitled "Health at Every Size: A Nondiet Approach to Wellness," a college course on nutrition with one week covering the non-diet approach instead of the traditional dieting approach, *or* a typical college nutrition course which included the dieting approach to weight management (the control group). The objective of the study was to assess intuitive eating, body esteem, dieting behaviors, and anti-fat attitudes of college students in these groups.

One of the tests that students took before and after the course was the Intuitive Eating Scale. To compare their before-and-after scores, a paired *t*-test (because it compared scores for each student) was used to determine if there was a significant change in scores for each group from pre-test to post-test. The Intuitive Eating Scale score did increase significantly from pre- to post-test for the Health at Every Size class.

Next the researchers compared the post-test scores on the Intuitive Eating Scale score for the three groups using ANOVA. ANOVA showed a significant difference in scores, but as mentioned, the researchers had to use a post hoc test to determine which groups were significantly different from each other. The post hoc tests showed that the scores for the Health at Every Size group were significantly different when compared with each of the two other groups ($P < 0.001$) (Humphrey, Clifford, and Morris, 2015).

Two variations of ANOVA, analysis of covariance (ANCOVA) and multivariate analysis of variance (MANOVA), are also used in nutrition research. ANCOVA is used to statistically control for known extraneous variables. For example, if a researcher believes that level of education affects the amount learned by the adolescents with asthma, the researcher may use ANCOVA to control for grade in school. When researchers have more than one dependent variable, they used MANOVA instead of ANOVA to analyze data.

Table 5.15 summarizes information on Chi-square, *t* tests, and ANOVA.

Table 5.15 Summary of Selected Inferential Tests

Inferential Test	Test Function	Example
Chi-Square	Simplest method to analyze variables to find differences between groups. Data is at nominal or ordinal level.	In a study involving people with diabetes, the researchers compared the number of males/females (nominal data) in the experimental and control groups to determine if the groups are alike for this extraneous variable.
t tests	A method to compare the means of two groups, and determine if there is a statistically significant difference between the groups. Data must be interval or ratio.	
Independent *t* test	A *t*-test in which the groups must be independent of one another (meaning the subjects in one group can't be members of the other group.)	In a weight control study, the mean weight loss of the experimental and control groups were compared using an independent *t*-test.
Paired or correlated *t* test	A *t*-test with one group and two measurements are taken on the same participant, such as a pretest and post-test, OR a *t*-test with two groups and each person in one group is matched to someone in the other group.	In a study looking at blood pressure, each participant's blood pressure was measured before and after a treatment, and analyzed with a paired *t* test. In a study looking at growth in vegetarian and meat-eating children, the vegetarian children were matched with meat-eating children by age, sex, and ethnic group. Mean Body Mass Index of each group was compared using paired *t* tests each time BMI was measured.
ANOVA	A method to compare and analyze the means of more than two groups *or* the variable is measured more than two times. Data must be interval or ratio.	In a study of mothers of preschoolers, the mothers were divided into four groups based upon weight status. ANOVA was used to compare mean food insecurity among the groups.

Other Tests of Significance

Table 5.13 shows that a number of other inferential statistics can be used to determine whether there are statistically significant differences between groups. These include the Kolmogorov-Smirnov test, sign test, Wilcoxin matched pairs test, signed rank test, median test, and Mann-Whitney U test (Hayes, 1994; Plichta & Kelvin, 2013). These tests are used when ordinal level data are involved; thus, they are categorized as non-parametric tests. Tests are selected based on considerations such as the number of groups being compared, the distribution pattern of the data (normal or skewed), and other nuances that can be found in the data.

TESTING FOR RELATIONSHIPS AMONG VARIABLES

To find whether there are relationships among variables, a variety of statistical tests is used to examine the relationships (see Table 5.13). Decisions about which statistical tests to use are based on the number of variables and their level of measurement. Understanding how decisions are made allows you to ascertain the quality of the findings.

Correlation and Pearson's *r*

Bivariate analyses are performed to calculate **correlation coefficients**, which are used to describe the relationship between two variables. Correlation coefficients provide information regarding the degree to which variables are related. **Correlations** are evaluated in terms of magnitude, direction, and sometimes significance. Scatterplots of data can provide hints about direction and magnitude of the correlation (**Figure 5.13**).

Direction refers to the way the two variables covary. A positive correlation occurs when an increase in one variable is associated with an increase in another, or when a decrease in one variable is associated with a decrease in the other. For example, if a researcher found that as weight increased so did systolic blood pressure, or if weight decreased so did systolic blood pressure, a "positive" relationship between weight and blood pressure exists. A negative correlation occurs when two variables covary inversely; that is, when one decreases, the other increases. For example, as exercise increases, body weight decreases.

Magnitude refers to the strength of the relationship found to exist between two variables. A correlation can range from a perfect positive correlation of 1.00 to a perfect

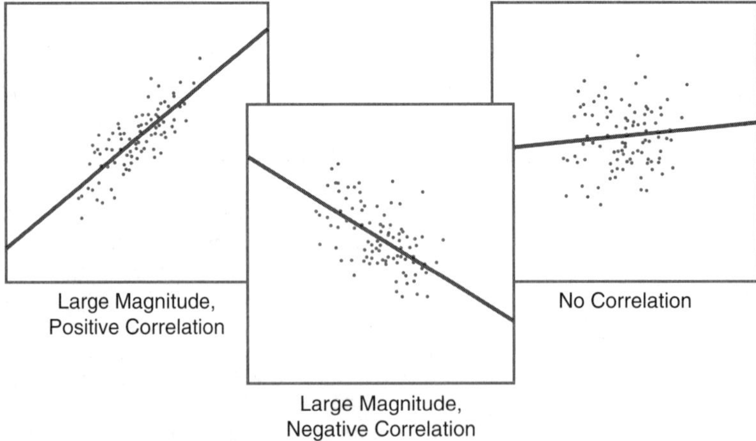

FIGURE 5.13 Scatterplots of Correlational Relationships

negative correlation of 1.00. A correlation of zero means that there is no relationship between the two variables. It is generally accepted that correlations ranging between 0.10 and 0.30 are considered to be weak, 0.30 and 0.50, moderate, and greater than 0.50, strong; however, the final determination is based on the variables being examined. It is important to remember that magnitude is not dependent on or related to the direction of the correlation.

When researchers pose hypotheses about the relationships among variables, they are testing for the significance of the correlation coefficient. When two variables are measured at the interval or ratio level, they calculate the **Pearson's** *r* statistic, also known as the Pearson product–moment correlation (Hayes, 1994; Plichta & Kelvin, 2013). The degrees of freedom for this test are always $N - 2$, which means that the correlation coefficient can be affected by the sample size. It is possible for a small correlation coefficient to be statistically significant when there is a large sample. In the literature, the notation $r = .62$, $p < .01$ is used. This notation provides three important pieces of information about the two variables. First, the variables are related at a magnitude of 0.62, which is usually considered to be a moderate—or moderately strong—relationship. Second, the two variables have a positive relationship with each other because the value is positive. Third, the correlation is statistically significant. A statistically significant correlation is one that is significantly different from zero.

Small correlations can be statistically significant because it does not take much variation to be significantly different from a correlation of zero (Nieswiadomy, 2012). Therefore, researchers can use a variation of Pearson's *r* that determines the percentage of variance shared by two variables, which provides more meaningful information. By squaring the coefficient (r^2), the overlap, or shared variance, is computed. A helpful way to think about variance is to think of a pie chart. The entire pie chart represents all the variables that can contribute to changes in the dependent variable. Each r^2 indicates how large a section of the pie chart that variable earns. With this information, knowledge of one variable can be used to predict the value of the other variable. For example, suppose that a correlation coefficient of 0.23 was obtained for the variables self-esteem and weight gain. Squaring 0.23 equals 0.0529. This is interpreted to mean that self-esteem accounts for about 5% of weight gain. Thus, the researcher would know that other variables must also contribute to weight gain.

Multiple Regression

A change in one variable is usually the result of many factors. Thus, when researchers want to study the relationship of many independent variables on one dependent variable, they use **multiple regression** analysis (Hayes, 1994; Plichta & Kelvin, 2013). Multiple linear regression is used when the dependent variable is measured at the interval or ratio level. When the dependent variable is dichotomous, you use multiple logistic regression. For example, suppose a researcher wants to determine which factors best predict an anorexic adolescent's success at maintaining a weight in the normal range. Independent variables might include self-esteem, social support, anxiety, and locus of control. In this situation, a multiple linear regression will be performed. (More examples are shown in Chapter 7.)

There are different approaches to performing multiple regression based on the way in which the predictor variables are entered into the analysis. One common approach to multiple regression is known as step-wise. This approach is used to find the smallest number of independent variables that account for the greatest proportion of variance in the outcome variable (Pedhazur, 1982). For example, in a study of adolescents with anorexia, a researcher might find that self-esteem, anxiety, and locus of control account for 24% of the variance in weight gain and that social support does not make any significant difference in weight gain.

Researchers can use another approach to multiple regression know as hierarchical regression. This approach is typically used when the importance of variables has been specified in theories. For example, suppose it is proposed in a theory about anorexia in adolescents that locus of control is the most important factor, followed by self-esteem and then anxiety. Based on this theory, the researcher would be able to specify the order the independent variables are to be entered into the equations. As in step-wise multiple regression, the amount of variance that is significant is reported.

To interpret the results of a multiple linear regression, you can use both r^2 and the regression coefficient. The r^2 number provides an estimate of the strength of the relationship between the independent and dependent variables, but it should not be used as a hypothesis test for this relationship. You also need to look at the regression coefficient. The **regression coefficient** is designated as B or β. When B is standardized, it is called beta, β. *The higher the value of β, the more the independent variable affects the dependent variable.* The value of β is tested against zero because zero means there is no significant association between the variables. *The independent variable is said to be a good predictor when β is significant* (meaning the associated *p* value is less than alpha).

The results of logistic regression includes odds ratios, which are discussed at the end of the chapter. Examples of studies using linear and logistic regression are shown in Chapter 7.

OTHER TESTS OF SIGNIFICANCE

Because all variables are not measured at interval and ratio levels, other tests of significance can be used to determine whether changes in variables are significant (Hayes, 1994; Plichta & Kelvin, 2013). When nominal data are involved, statistics such as phi coefficients, point biserials, and contingency coefficients are reported. Researchers use Kendall's Tau, Spearman Rho, and discriminate function analysis to analyze ordinal-level data. There are also very sophisticated methods for testing and predicting the strength and direction of relationships among multiple variables. These analytic methods, such as linear structural relationships or structural equation modeling, are useful ways to use data to test theories.

EFFECT SIZE

Statistical significance can tell you whether the findings are due to chance or not, *but they don't tell you:*

- *if the findings are necessarily clinically important, or*
- *anything about the size of the difference between the groups on an outcome variable, or the strength of the relationship between two variables.*

Effect size is the magnitude (or size) of an effect. It could be the size of the difference in an outcome measure between the experimental and control groups in an experimental or quasi-experimental study. It could also be the strength of the relationship between two variables, as seen, for example, in a correlation. It can be measured in a number of ways, including the following:

1. **Mean difference** (MD): When you want to examine the size of the difference in means between two groups in a study, all you have to do is subtract the means. For example, if the intervention group in a weight loss study lost 8 pounds (–8)

while the control group lost 2 pounds (–2), the difference (called the mean difference) is –6 pounds. The mean difference is an example of effect size.

2. **Standardized mean difference** (SMD): The standardized mean difference, often reported as Cohen's *d* or simply *d* in statistics, is generally calculated by taking the difference in mean outcome between the two groups (experimental minus control) and dividing it by the pooled standard deviation (a correction factor may be used). *What you end up with is a number that shows how far apart the means are in standard deviation units. So if the SMD of the experimental group is 0.8, then the score of the average person in the experimental group is 0.8 standard deviations above the average person in the control group.* As the SMD increases, the difference between the intervention and control group increases. Interpretation of *d* varies by context. If the result is about 0.5, the effect size may be considered moderate, and 0.8 may be large (although this varies depending on the context and other factors).
3. *Correlation* looks at the association (or relationship) between two continuous variables and is another example of an effect size. The correlation coefficient *r* measures both the strength and the direction of a linear relationship between two variables, from no relationship (0) to a perfect positive or negative linear relationship (+1 or 0.1). Effect size estimates, such as an *r* of 0.5 for the effect of BMI on systolic blood pressure, tell you about both the strength and the direction of the effect.

Mean difference, standardized mean difference, and correlation all use continuous variables. For categorical variables, such as has hypertension/does not have hypertension, there are other ways to measure effect size: relative risk, odds ratio, and hazard ratio. They are discussed in the next section on risk statistics.

The effect size tells you how powerful the effect of the independent variable is on an outcome variable, as well as the direction of the relationship. As mentioned, direction refers to the way the two variables covary. Both variables may increase together, decrease together, or one increases as the other decreases. If the mean difference in a weight loss study between two groups is –6 pounds, then the negative effect size indicates that the intervention decreased the mean outcome.

TIP

Statistical significance answers the question "Does it work?" whereas effect size answers the question "How well does it work?" You can also say that a *p* value tells you whether the results are real, and effect size tells you how important the results are. Use both *p* values and effect sizes to evaluate the results of a study.

RISK STATISTICS: RISK RATIO, ODDS RATIO, AND HAZARD RATIO

Researchers use statistics to determine the risk, or odds, of an outcome such as disease. This section discusses relative risk, odds ratios, and hazard ratios.

A **risk ratio**, also called **relative risk** (RR), compares the probability of an outcome in two groups. One group is exposed to something (usually a risk factor), and the other group is not. Relative risk expresses how much more (or less) likely it is for the exposed person to develop an outcome (relative to an unexposed person). *Exposure* is often a risk factor for a disease, but it could also be a treatment. Relative risk is calculated as follows.

$$\text{Relative Risk} = \frac{\text{Risk of outcome in exposed/treated group}}{\text{Risk of outcome in unexposed group}}$$

If a study's results show an RR of 1.0, there is no difference in risk between the groups: the exposure did not increase or decrease risks of an outcome. If the RR is greater than 1, it suggests an *increased* risk of that outcome (such as developing hypertension) in the exposed group (perhaps they ate a high sodium diet). If the RR is less than 1, it suggests a *reduced* risk in the exposed group.

Let's look at a study about heart disease (the outcome) in men with and without diabetes. Diabetes is the exposure or risk factor. In this study, the RR for coronary heart disease was 3.0 for men. When risk is increased, as in RR = 3.0, you can interpret it in two ways:

1. Relative risk: The men with diabetes (exposed group) have 3 times the risk of coronary heart disease compared to men without diabetes.
2. Increased risk: Men with diabetes *increase* their risk of coronary heart disease by 200% compared to men without diabetes. Increased risk is calculated as (Relative Risk – 1) × 100.

Now let's look at an example where RR is less than 1. Let's say an experiment had a group of pregnant women who were given vitamin and amino acid supplements (the exposure) and observed to see who developed pre-eclampsia (the outcome). Another group of pregnant women did not receive the supplements. Relative risk is sometimes used in randomized clinical trials where there is an intervention or treatment. The RR for this study was 0.25. This means:

1. Relative risk: Pregnant women taking the supplements had 0.25 (or one-quarter) times the risk of pre-eclampsia compared to women not taking the supplements.
2. Decreased risk: The pregnant women taking the supplements had 75% *less risk* of developing pre-eclampsia than pregnant women not taking the supplements. Decreased risk is calculated the same as just shown: (Relative Risk – 1) × 100.

As you can see, relative risk gives both direction and magnitude of the effect of the exposure on the disease or outcome. However, the data used here is considered a crude estimate because there was no adjustment for confounding variables.

When you see an RR in a study, also look at its confidence interval. The confidence interval represents the range of values in which the RR for the population is likely found. Remember that a narrower confidence interval indicates a higher precision of the RR. If the confidence interval of the RR contains 1 (meaning there is no difference between the groups), then the RR is not likely to be statistically significant, and the association between the exposure and the outcome may be due to chance.

Whereas relative risk tells you about probability, the **odds ratio** (OR) tells you about the odds of an outcome or event such as a disease. Odds and probability are not the same thing; they both express the likelihood of an outcome, but in slightly different ways. Odds ratios are used in logistic regression and in case-control studies. The odds ratio is computed as follows.

$$\text{Odds ratio} = \frac{\text{Odds of an outcome/event in experimental group}}{\text{Odds of an outcome/event in control/comparison group}}$$

An OR of 1.0 means that the odds of an event in the groups are the same. If the odds ratio for a heart attack (outcome), for example, is 2.5 for males compared to females, that means the odds of having a heart attack are 2.5 times higher for males than for females.

When you read a study using odds ratios, you may see a reference to a crude odds ratio and an adjusted odds ratio. Unlike the crude odds ratio, which does not take any other factors into account, the adjusted odds ratio controls for confounding variables.

Although odds ratios are somewhat different from relative risk ratios, an OR is often interpreted like an RR. So an OR of 3.55 would be interpreted as meaning the outcome was 3.55 times more likely to occur in the experimental group than in the control/comparison group, or risk of the outcome in the experimental group was increased by 255% compared to the control/comparison group.

The **hazard ratio** (HR) is a ratio of the hazard rate of one group to the hazard rate in another group. **Hazard** can be defined as the probability that an individual at any given time has an event (such as death) at that time (assume the individual was event-free up to then). Hazard rates answer the question, "Does a specific risk factor/treatment cause the event to occur earlier or later than without the risk factor/treatment?"

$$\text{Hazard Ratio} = \frac{\text{risk of event in treated/exposed group}}{\text{risk of event in control/comparison group}}$$

Whenever HR is 1, the event rate or risk for each group is the same. When HR = 2, it means that at any time twice as many participants in the treatment/exposed groups are having an event proportionally to the comparison group. If HR is less than 1, then fewer participants in the treatment/exposed group are having an event proportionally to the comparison group.

Hazard ratios are often interpreted like relative risk. Just keep in mind that hazard ratios look at the ratio every moment *along* the time span of the study, whereas relative risk looks at the total number of events at the *end* of the study. *In other words, hazard ratios give you instantaneous risk at a point in time, and relative risk gives cumulative risk over the time of the study.* It is best to consider the hazard ratio alongside a measure of time, such as median survival. Hazard ratios are used in survival analysis, discussed in Chapter 7.

WHAT DOES ALL THIS MEAN FOR EVIDENCE-BASED PRACTICE?

When reading research articles, RDNs must assume that mathematical calculations were done accurately because raw data are not included. What RDNs should appraise is that the correct tests were performed. **Table 5.16** is a helpful tool for appraising the analysis sections of articles.

RDNs should also appraise data presented in tables to determine whether conclusions drawn by researchers are supported by the findings. Although readers frequently skip over the tables when reading research articles, this is not a good practice. The tables contain evidence on which practice changes can be made, and for this reason they may be one of the most important components of the report. RDNs need to acquire skill at reading and interpreting tables. Some hints for doing so are presented in Table 5.16.

It is also important to differentiate between statistical significance and clinical significance;. For example, suppose a drug lowered cholesterol levels on average from 195 to 178. Analysis indicated that this decrease was statistically significant; however, because any cholesterol value below 200 is considered to be within normal range, there is no clinical

Table 5.16 Tips for Reading Statistical Tables
Be familiar with symbols used.
Read the title of the table first.
Pay attention to the labels of columns and rows.
Observe when headings for subsamples and subscales are indented.
Follow columns carefully both horizontally and vertically.
Attend to significant findings.
Alpha levels are either reported with a notation or under the table with an asterisk (*).
Pay attention to superscript or footnote markings.
Do not skip tables, because information can be clearer after studying a table.
Recognize that there can be typos and math errors.
Remember that subsamples may be omitted from the table (i.e., sample indicates total subjects and number of women, leaving reader to calculate number of men).

significance to this finding. When appraising evidence, it is wise for RDNs to keep in mind that statistically significant results must also be big enough to matter to a patient and health care provider in order to be worthwhile (Brignardello-Petersen et al., 2013).

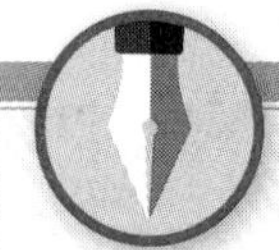

TIP

Although readers frequently skip over the tables when reading research articles, this is not a good practice. Data presented in tables may contain evidence on which practice changes can be made, and thus may be one of the most important components of a report.

Appraising the results section of research reports can be challenging. An understanding of the material presented in this chapter can assist you in meeting this challenge. **Table 5.17** lists questions that should be considered when evaluating data analysis.

Table 5.17 Questions for Appraising Analysis of Data

1. What statistics were used to describe the characteristics of the sample? What statistics were used to analyze the data that were collected? Were the statistics appropriate for the level of measurement?
2. Were measures of central tendency provided? If so, which ones were used? Are they the most appropriate? How sensitive to outliers is the measure reported?
3. Were measures of variation/dispersion provided? Were standard deviations reported for each mean that was reported?
4. What was the distribution of the data? Were data normally distributed? Was skewness or kurtosis discussed?
5. What statistics were used to determine differences between the groups? Were the results significant?
6. What statistics were used to express relationships among variables of interest? What was the magnitude and direction of the relationship? Was it significant?
7. Are all the hypotheses addressed in the analysis section of the report?
8. Is the selected level of significance appropriate for the purpose of the study and the types of analyses being conducted?
9. Do the tables and graphs agree with the text? Are they precise and do they offer economy of information?
10. Are the results understandable and presented objectively?

SUMMARY

1. Statistics are used to describe numerical outcomes and the probabilities derived from calculations on raw data.
2. There are two types of statistics: descriptive and inferential. Descriptive statistics explain characteristics of variables found in a sample. Inferential statistics are the basis for predictions about the phenomenon.
3. Univariate analysis involves only one variable at a time and includes frequency distributions, measures of central tendency, shape of the distribution, and measures of variability. Bivariate analysis is conducted to describe relationships between two variables.
4. Frequencies may be grouped or ungrouped data describing how often a variable is found to occur. Line charts, bar graphs, pie charts, histograms, and scattergrams are ways frequencies can be depicted.
5. The mode, median, and mean are measures of central tendency. In a normal distribution, they are all the same value.
6. Data with little variability are considered to be homogenous, whereas data with wide variations are considered to be heterogeneous.
7. Measures of variability include the range, semiquartile range, percentile, standard deviation, *z* scores, and coefficient of variation.
8. A normal distribution is a bell-shaped curve that is symmetric around the mean. Asymmetric distributions are known as skewed and have either positive or negative directions.
9. The Rule of 68–95–99.7 is a way of describing the percentage of scores falling within specific standard deviations of the mean.
10. Inferential statistics are used to estimate population parameters and to test hypotheses.
11. CIs describe the probability of being correct.
12. When selecting which statistical tests to use, researchers must consider the type of question being asked and the level of measurement. The null hypothesis is statistically tested and is rejected when significant findings occur. Research hypotheses are supported but never proven.
13. Probability is the likelihood of a frequency of an event in similar trials under similar conditions and indicates how probable it is that the results were obtained by chance. Sampling error is the tendency for statistics to fluctuate from one sample to another and forms the basis of probability.
14. Type I errors occur when researchers reject the null hypothesis when it should have been accepted. Type II errors occur when researchers accept the null hypothesis when it should have been rejected.
15. Alpha levels of either 0.05 or 0.01 are typically used in nursing research. Alpha levels affect the amount of risk involved for making type I and type II errors.
16. Parametric tests are more powerful than nonparametric tests because they are used with interval or ratio level data.
17. To test for differences between groups, researchers can use Chi-square, *t* test, and ANOVA.
18. Correlation coefficients are used to describe the relationship between two variables. To test for relationships among variables, Pearson's *r* and multiple regression can be used. Multiple linear regression is used when the dependent variable is at the interval or ratio level. When the dependent variable is dichotomous, you use multiple logistic regression.
19. Effect size tells you about how powerful the effect of the independent variable is on an outcome variable, as well as the direction of the relationship, and should be used with significance when interpreting study results. Examples include mean difference, standardized mean difference, correlation, relative risk, and odds ratios.
20. Researchers use risk statistics to determine the risk or odds of an outcome such as disease, including relative risk, odds ratios, and hazard ratios.
21. To apply findings to evidence-based practice, RDNs must be able to interpret statistical tables, differentiate between clinical and statistical significance, and appraise data analysis.

REVIEW QUESTIONS

1. To describe the frequency of the single variable myocardial infarction in adults aged 30–49, which of the following could be used? (Select all that apply.)
   A. descriptive statistics
   B. inferential statistics
   C. univariate analysis
   D. bivariate analysis
2. Frequency distributions are an effective way to present inferential statistics.
   A. true
   B. false
3. Categories in grouped data must be mutually exclusive.
   A. true
   B. false
4. Percentages are often used to describe characteristics of samples.
   A. true
   B. false
5. The total number of participants in a sample is represented by the symbol *n*.
   A. true
   B. false
6. The most frequent data value in a set of data is the
   A. mean
   B. median
   C. mode
   D. average
7. When data have no outliers, researchers prefer to report the
   A. mean
   B. median
   C. mode
   D. magnitude
8. If the tail of a distribution is skewed to the left, the data are negatively skewed.
   A. true
   B. false
9. In a normal distribution, the mean, median, and mode are the same value.
   A. true
   B. false
10. If data are highly uniform, a low peak will be observed in a graphic representation of the data.
   A. true
   B. false

Match the following terms:

11. Range	**A.** rank
12. Semiquartile range	**B.** difference between maximum and minimum values
13. Percentile	**C.** measure of the average deviations of a value from the mean
14. Standard deviation	**D.** percentage comparing standard deviations when units of measure are different
15. *z* score	**E.** range of the middle 50% of data
16. Coefficient of variation	**F.** converted standard deviation to a standardized unit

17. Inferential statistical tests are used to (select all that apply):
   A. make assumptions about the population
   B. describe the sample with means and standard deviations
   C. test hypotheses by asking if there are differences between the groups
   D. select a sample
   E. determine whether results occurred by chance
18. When a researcher accepts the null hypothesis when it really should have been rejected, the researcher (select all that apply):
   A. committed a type I error
   B. committed a type II error
   C. obtained significant results
   D. obtained nonsignificant results
19. The most commonly used alpha level in nutrition research is
   A. 0.001
   B. 0.0001

C. 0.005
D. 0.05

Match the following:

20.	Chi-square	**A.** uses the *F* statistic
21.	*t* test	**B.** tests for the significance of a correlation between two variables
22.	ANOVA	**C.** has independent and paired variations
23.	Pearson's *r*	**D.** tests the significance of relationships among three or more variables
24.	Multiple regression	**E.** tests for differences between groups using nonparametric data

25. A researcher is studying the relationship of amount of time spent in front of a screen and body weight. Which test would the researcher use to analyze these data?
A. Chi-square
B. Pearson's *r*
C. Phi coefficient
D. Multiple regression

26. You should determine that researchers are using the correct statistical tests to analyze data.
A. true
B. false

27. Data contained in tables are an important source of evidence for practice.
A. true
B. false

28. All statistically significant findings have clinical significance.
A. true
B. false

CRITICAL THINKING QUESTIONS

1. For the following data set, compute the measures of central tendency and these measures of variability: range and standard deviation.

   10 exam scores: 8, 6, 4, 3, 9, 5, 7, 8, 5, 5

2. What is the difference between population parameters and sample statistics? Give an example.
3. The 95% confidence interval for daily food sodium intake level in 68 nursing home patients is (2,650 mg/day, 3,150 mg/day). What does this confidence interval tell us?
4. Suppose you rejected a null hypothesis at the 1% level of significance. Would you reject the same null hypothesis at the 5% level? Explain.
5. What is the difference between statistical significance and clinical significance? Give an example.
6. A medical researcher wants to test the effectiveness of a new medicine. He did an experimental study with 80 participants split into intervention and control groups. The control group took an older medicine. Results showed that the new medicine was *not* significantly more effective than the older medicine at the 0.05 levels. Using effect size, Cohen's *d* was determined to be 0.55. Interpret the results.
7. Which of the following correlation coefficients represents the strongest relationship? Which has an inverse relationship between the variables?

   +0.14, +0.82, −0.02, −0.34, +0.56

8. The correlation coefficient between age and depression is +.85. Because this coefficient is high, can you conclude that aging will cause increasing depression? Why or why not?
9. Develop a hypothesis that could be tested with the Pearson or Spearman correlation coefficient.
10. A researcher did an experiment on how far athletes ran in 90 minutes while drinking one of two different sports drinks. On Week 1, athletes did the run, and drank one of the sports drinks for several days before and the day of the run. On Week 3, the same athletes

did the run again, and drank the alternate sports drink for several days before and the day of the run. Which *t* test should be used to compare results? If only one group of athletes did the run once, with half the group drinking one sports drink and the other half drinking the alternate sports drink, which *t* test should be used in that circumstance?

11. A study looked at patient satisfaction (dependent variable) with the independent variable being dietetics education. The independent variable had three levels: RDN with a master's degree, RDN with a bachelor's degree, and a nutrition and dietetics student doing clinical rotations in a hospital. The results showed: $F(3, 76) = 2.64, p = 0.266$. Interpret the results.

12. Calculate and interpret Cohen's *d* given the following:

    Experimental group mean: 4.5

    Control group mean: 5.57

    Pooled standard deviation: 2.85

13. A study looked at the highest diet quality versus the lowest diet quality category for Parkinson's disease. Diet quality was the exposure, and Parkinson's disease was the outcome. Interpret a relative risk of 0.75 for participants who had the highest quality diet compared to the group with the lowest quality diet.

14. What kind of statistical test would best answer each of these research questions?

    A. Is there a relationship between drinking more soda and being obese? 1,000 adults take part in the study.

    B. Are women who drink 5 ounces of red wine daily less likely to develop heart disease than women who do not? 250 women take part in the study.

    C. Do students who take dietary supplements for 12 months leading up to the GRE exam perform better than students who do not? 100 students participate in the study and grades are normally distributed.

    D. The BMI of 42 same-sex identical twins are assessed. BMI is normally distributed. Is there a difference in the BMI of the twins?

SUGGESTED READINGS AND ACTIVITIES

1. Boushey, C. J., Harris, J., Bruemmer, B., & Archer, S. A. (2008). Publishing nutrition research: A review of sampling, sample size, statistical analysis, and other key elements of manuscript preparation, Part 2. *Journal of the American Dietetic Association*, *108*, 679–688. doi: 10.1016/j.jada.2008.01.002
2. Harris, J. E., Boushey, C., Bruemmer, B., & Archer, S. L. (2008). Publishing nutrition research: A review of nonparametric methods, Part 3. *Journal of the American Dietetic Association*, *108*, 1488–1496. doi: 10.1016/j.jada.2008.06.426
3. Harris, J. E., Sheean, P. M., Gleason, P. M., Bruemmer, B., & Boushey, C. (2012). Publishing nutrition research: A review of multivariate techniques–Part 2: Analysis of variance. *Journal of the Academy of Nutrition and Dietetics*, *112*, 90–98. doi: 10.1016/j.jada.2011.09.037
4. Saracino, G., Jennings, L.W., & Hasse, J. M. (2013). Basic statistical concepts in nutrition research. *Nutrition in Clinical Practice, 28*, 182–193. doi: 10.1177/0884533613478636
5. Many videos on statistics are available at the Khan Academy website: https://www.khanacademy.org/math/statistics-probability

REFERENCES

American College of Physicians—American Society of Internal Medicine. (2001). Primer on 95% confidence intervals. *Effective Clinical Practice*, *4*, 229–231. Retrieved from http://www.vhpharmsci.com/decisionmaking/Therapeutic_Decision_Making/Fundamentals_files/ACP%20Primer%20on%2095%25%20confidence%20intervals.pdf

Boushey, C. J., Harris, J., Bruemmer, B., & Archer, S. A. (2008). Publishing nutrition research: A review of sampling, sample size, statistical analysis, and other key elements of manuscript preparation, Part 2. *Journal of the American Dietetic Association*, *108*, 679–688. doi: 10.1016/j.jada.2008.01.002

Borenstein, M. (1997). Hypothesis testing and effect size estimation in clinical trials. *Annals of Allergy, Asthma, and Immunology*, *78*, 5–11.

Brase, C. H., & Brase, C. P. (2017). *Understanding basic statistics* (7th ed.) Boston, MA: Cengage Learning.

Brignardello-Petersen, R., Carrasco-Labra, A., Prakeshkumar, S., & Azarpazhooh, A. (2013). A practitioner's guide to developing critical appraisal skills: What is the difference between clinical and statistical significance? *Journal of the American Dental Association*, *144*, 780-786.

Gillis, A., & Jackson, W. (2002). *Research for Nurses: Methods and interpretation*. Philadelphia, PA: F. A. Davis.

Harper, D. (2013). Statistics. *Online Etymology Dictionary*. Retrieved from http://www.etymonline.com/index.php?term=statistics

Harris, J. E., Boushey, C., Bruemmer, B., & Archer, S. L. (2008). Publishing nutrition research: A review of nonparametric methods, Part 3. *Journal of the American Dietetic Association*, *108*, 1488–1496. doi: 10.1016/j.jada.2008.06.426

Harris, J. E., Sheean, P. M., Gleason, P. M., Bruemmer, B., & Boushey, C. (2012). Publishing nutrition research: A review of multivariate techniques—Part 2: Analysis of variance. *Journal of the Academy of Nutrition and Dietetics*, *112*, 90–98. doi: 10.1016/j.jada.2011.09.037

Hayes, W.L. (1994). *Statistics*. Boston, MA: Wadsworth.

Hoekstra, R., Johnson, A., & Kiers, H. A. L. (2012). Confidence intervals make a difference: Effects of showing confidence intervals on inferential reasoning. *Educational and Psychological Measurement*, *72*(6), 1039–1052.

Humphrey. L., Clifford, D., & Neyman Morris, M. (2015). *Health at Every Size college course reduces dieting behaviors and improves intuitive eating, body esteem, and anti-fat attitudes. Journal of Nutrition Education and Behavior*, *47*, 354-360. doi: 10.1016/j.jneb.2015.01.008

Nieswiadomy, R. M. (2012). *Foundations of nursing research* (6th ed.). Upper Saddle River, NJ: Pearson Education.

Pedhazur, E. J. (1982). *Multiple regression in behavioral research: Explanation and prediction* (2nd ed.). Philadelphia, PA: Harcourt Brace.

Plichta, S. B., & Kelvin, E. (2013). *Munro's statistical methods for health care research* (6th ed.). Philadelphia, PA: Wolters Kluwer/Lippincott Williams & Wilkins.

Saracino, G., Jennings, L. W., & Hasse, J. M. (2013). Basic statistical concepts in nutrition research. *Nutrition in Clinical Practice*, *28*, 182–193. doi: 10.1177/0884533613478636

Smith, C. J. (2012). Type I and type II errors: What are they and why do they matter? *Phlebology*, *27*(4), 199–200.

Straus, S. E., Richardson, W. S., Glasziou, P., & Haynes, R. B. (2010). *Evidence-based medicine: How to practice and teach EBM* (4th ed.). Edinburgh, Scotland: Churchill Livingstone.

CHAPTER 6

Quantitative Research Designs: Experimental, Quasi-Experimental, and Descriptive

CHAPTER OUTLINE

- Introduction
- Experimental Study Designs
- Quasi-Experimental Designs
- Descriptive Quantitative Designs
- Additional Types of Designs
- Researcher Interview: Intervention Research, Dr. Leslie Cunningham-Sabo

LEARNING OUTCOMES

- Discuss five considerations when planning a research design.
- Explain the three essential components of experimental designs, and compare and contrast the following experimental designs: randomized controlled trials, crossover, factorial, and Solomon four group designs.
- Discuss the advantages and disadvantages of various experimental designs.
- Compare and contrast the nonequivalent control group and interrupted time series designs.
- Discuss the advantages and disadvantages of various quasi-experimental designs.
- Compare and contrast the descriptive cross-sectional, repeated cross-sectional, comparative, and descriptive correlational designs.
- Discuss the advantages and disadvantages of various descriptive designs.
- Read a research study and identify the design used and analyze study results.
- Distinguish between secondary data analysis and secondary research.

INTRODUCTION

Designing a research study requires making a number of decisions on the steps you will take to answer your research question(s). Like an architect, you need to prepare a blueprint for your project. If you have ever met with an architect before, you know that the process usually starts with a lot of questions. Research design is no different. The following questions address a number of key design features that must be considered.

1. *What is the research question? Will there be an intervention?* Testing the effects of an intervention is the hallmark of experimental and quasi-experimental research. If there is an intervention with human participants, the researcher will assign participants to be exposed to the independent variable, such as a modified diet or nutrient supplement, or be part of the control group. Experimental and quasi-experimental designs are used to test a hypothesis.
2. *Instead of an intervention, will researchers observe study participants and take measurements?* For example, researchers might observe a group over a longer period of time to see if exposure to certain factors (such as a diet high in fruits and vegetables) affects their risk of disease. This type of design is called a cohort study design. It is commonly used in the field of **epidemiology**, a discipline within public health that looks at the rates of health-related states (such as disease) in different groups of people and why they occur, and then looks at how this information can be used to control health problems. Study designs used in epidemiology are discussed in Chapter 7.
3. *What are the variables?* What comparisons are going to be made between or within groups? Comparisons are needed to examine relationships between the independent and the dependent variable.
4. *When and how often will data be collected or measurements taken?* Many experimental studies measure the dependent variable at least before and after the intervention. Weight loss studies, for example, often take measurements for a year or more to see whether participants kept the weight off. Data may be collected at just one point in time, such as in a **cross-sectional study**, or more frequently. In a **longitudinal study**, participants are observed and measurements are taken over a long period of time. Longitudinal studies either go forward in time (prospective) or backward in time (retrospective).
5. *What will the setting be for the study?* The setting could be a hospital, community center, or other location. Some studies use multiple sites.
6. *In an intervention study with at least two groups, will the participants be randomly assigned to a group?* True experimental research involves random assignment to groups so participants each have an equal chance of receiving any of the treatments (including no treatment) under study. Quasi-experimental research does not have randomization of participants to groups.
7. *In a human intervention study, will participants, researchers, and staff be blinded from knowing to which group a participant was assigned?* Blinding helps to prevent or minimize sources of bias, such as expectation bias. **Expectation bias** is when researchers' expectations of what they believe the study results should be get in the way of accurately taking measurements and reporting results.
8. *What controls will be put in place to reduce the influence of extraneous variables?* **Extraneous variables** are factors outside of the variables being studied that might influence the outcome of a study and cause incorrect conclusions. A good quantitative design identifies and rules out as many of these competing explanations as possible.

A good research design helps you answer the research question while effectively reducing threats to design validity.

Quantitative research designs are often used to look at causal relationships, but they can also be used to look at associations or relationship between variables. Quantitative research studies can be placed into one of five categories, although some categories do vary a bit from book to book. First are **experimental designs** with an intervention, control group, and randomization of participants into groups. Next are **quasi-experimental designs** with an intervention but no randomization. **Descriptive designs** do not have an intervention or treatment and are considered nonexperimental. They usually aim to provide information about relevant variables but do not test hypotheses. Good descriptive studies provoke the "why" questions of analytic (cause-and-effect) research. Two additional categories are epidemiologic and predictive correlational designs.

When you read about designs in this chapter, examples of studies are given to illustrate the design. The examples include some discussion of the results of statistical tests, as well as sample tables from the studies. In a quantitative study, statistics are often used to answer one of these questions:

1. Is there a *difference* among the groups?
   Example: "LA Sprouts: A Garden-Based Nutrition Intervention Pilot Program Influences Motivation and Preferences for Fruits and Vegetables in Latino Youth" (*Journal of the Academy of Nutrition and Dietetics*, 2012)
2. Is there an *association* or relationship among the variables?
   Example: "Preventable Incidence and Mortality of Carcinoma Associated With Lifestyle Factors Among White Adults in the United States" (*JAMA Oncology*, 2016)

You can often tell from the title of an article whether the study is looking at differences among groups or an association among variables.

Experimental and quasi-experimental designs have an intervention, so they involve questions about differences—often the difference between an outcome measured in the experimental and control groups. Correlational studies look at associations. **Table 6.1** shows examples of statistics that may be used to answer these two questions.

TIP

When you read a study, first read the abstract to determine whether there is an intervention. If so, the study is either experimental or quasi-experimental. If not, the study will fit into one of the other categories. If you see the word "association" in the title, the study is likely to be a descriptive, epidemiological, or predictive correlation design.

EXPERIMENTAL STUDY DESIGNS

To be considered an experimental design, the following must be present.

1. *An intervention or treatment*. The researcher manipulates the independent variable by, for example, requiring the intervention group to eat a diet that has been modified, take a supplement containing a nutrient or phytochemical, or take part in an educational program.
2. *Control for extraneous variables*. Various control techniques, such as randomization and having a control group, are used. Having a control group allows the researcher to compare and evaluate the performance of the experimental group on the outcome (dependent) variable.
3. *Randomization*. The researcher randomly assigns each participant to a group so that each person has an equal chance of being in either group. This removes the problem of selection bias so that comparable, balanced groups of similar size are

Table 6.1 Statistics That Look at Differences and Statistics That Look at Associations

Statistics That Look at Differences				
Name	**Test statistic**	**Purpose**	**Number of groups**	**Measurement level of dependent variable**
Independent samples *t*-test	t	To test the difference between the means of two independent groups.	2	Interval/ratio
Paired samples *t*-test (or dependent *t*-test)	t	To test the difference between the means from two paired groups (such as before-and-after observations on the same subject).	2	Interval/ratio
One-way analysis of variance (ANOVA)	F	To test the difference among means of more than two independent groups for one independent variable (with more than one level).	More than two groups	Interval/ratio
Two-way analysis of variance (ANOVA)	F	To test the difference among means for two independent variables, of which each can have multiple levels.	More than two groups	Interval/ratio
Repeated measures ANOVA (one-way within-subjects)	F	To test the difference among three or more means in the same group over time. (Extended design of dependent samples *t*-test).	One group	Interval/ratio
Chi-square	χ^2	To analyze nominal and ordinal data to find differences between groups.	Two or more groups	Nominal/Ordinal

Statistics That Look at Associations			
Name	**Test statistic**	**Purpose**	**Measurement level of dependent variable**
Pearson product-moment correlation	r	To measure the strength and direction of the relationship between two variables.	Interval/ratio
Spearman rank-order correlation	ρ	To measure the strength and direction of the relationship between two variables. (Nonparametric version of Pearson product-moment correlation)	Ordinal, interval, or ratio
Linear regression		To predict the value of a dependent variable and measure the size of the effect of the independent variable on a dependent variable while controlling for covariates.	Interval/ratio
Logistic regression		Same as linear regression; used when dependent value is binary.	Binary/dichotomous

formed. Randomization also forms the basis for statistical testing. To randomize participants, researchers first generate random numbers (using either computer software or a random number table) and use them to assign each participant to a group. This is referred to as **simple randomization**.

In a **randomized block design**, the participants are first split into homogeneous groups, or blocks, before being randomly assigned to either the treatment or control group within the block. Blocks are used to decrease the variability of the sample and to control the effects of a characteristic that could influence the outcome, such as sex, age, weight, or severity of disease. Each block generally needs at least 20 participants (Grove, Burns, & Gray, 2013). For example, a study of the effect of omega-3 fatty acids on adults with a history of heart disease may be randomized by age (see **Figure 6.1**).

Random assignment means that the groups will be comparable, and differences between the groups at the end of the experiment can be deduced as being a result of the intervention. Without randomization of participants into groups, a study is considered to be quasi-experimental.

TIP

Randomization into the treatment or control group is essential to an experimental study, but it is *not* essential that the participants be randomly selected from a target population *before* being randomly assigned to a group. Most randomized controlled trials do *not* use random sampling to pick who is in the study, but all do use random assignment to groups.

When reading research, you will come across two similar terms—control group and comparison group—and probably will wonder what the difference is. The terms are often used interchangeably, but there is a difference. Technically, a control group is chosen by random sampling of the target population, and a comparison group is chosen using

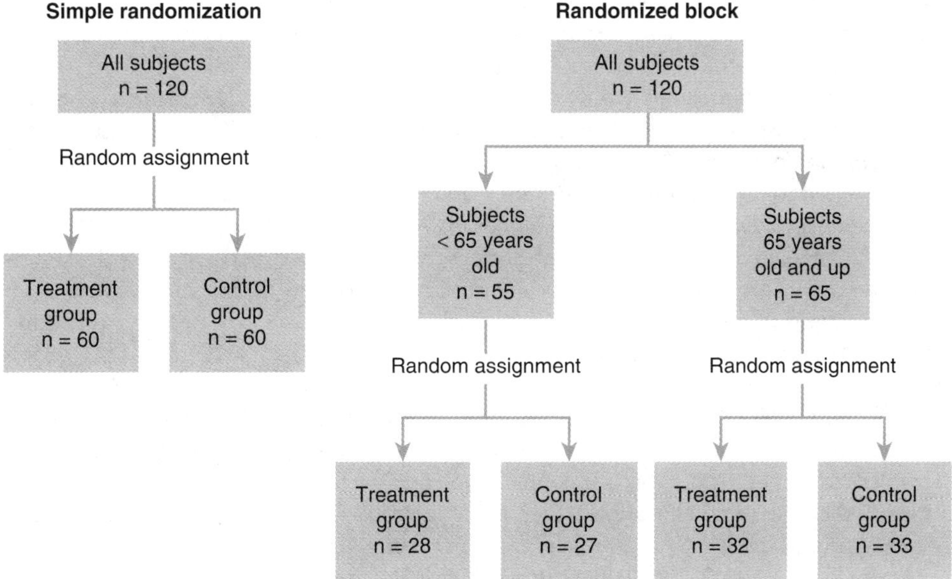

FIGURE 6.1 Simple Randomization and Randomized Block

a convenience sample. In much experimental research, the preference is for "control group." In some areas of epidemiology the preference is for "comparison group," in part because the studies do not have an intervention but do have groups they want to compare. We will use the terms *control group* and *comparison group* interchangeably unless noted.

Whether called a control or a comparison group, the researcher has a number of options to choose for this group:

1. *No intervention or treatment.*
2. *A* **placebo**. A placebo is an intervention with no effect, such as a dummy pill.
3. *Standard or usual health care*. In nursing studies, for example, patients in the control group typically receive "usual care" because no care would be unethical.
4. *A lower dose of treatment or an alternative treatment*. For example, in an experimental study examining the effectiveness of high-dose vitamin D in reducing falls and increasing lower extremity function, the control group received a low-dose of vitamin D_3, and the two experimental groups received higher doses (Bischoff-Ferrari et al., 2016).

When the control group receives no treatment, you will see a greater difference between the groups than with a placebo, usual care, or some treatment. This also makes it easier to show statistical significance.

Experimental designs are most useful with questions about therapy, such as "Which treatment options are most effective?" They can also help answer some questions about prevention, such as "Will a vitamin supplement prevent a condition?" But experimental designs are not useful for prognosis (likely course of a disease) questions. Cohort studies are much better at answering that type of question.

Keep in mind that in some situations experimental designs either cannot be used or would be unethical. Now we will look at specific experimental designs including randomized controlled trials and clinical trials, crossover designs, factorial designs, and Solomon four-group designs.

RANDOMIZED CONTROLLED TRIALS AND CLINICAL TRIALS

Randomized controlled trials (RCTs) are considered the "gold standard" for evaluating the effect of an intervention, treatment, or program. Participants are randomly assigned to the intervention or control group, and then followed forward in time (prospective) to compare the outcomes. Randomization, when done properly, creates equivalent groups so that differences between the groups can be attributed to the independent variable(s). RCTs are most often categorized as efficacy studies because they are designed to test hypotheses under ideal and controlled circumstances (as opposed to effectiveness studies, which are done under real-world conditions).

In an RCT, researchers need to carefully define how the participants will be randomized, the intervention, what the control group will do (if anything), what other research controls will be implemented, and other aspects of the experiment. Procedures for an RCT are normally documented in a study protocol. The **study protocol** explains the purpose of the study as well as all the details involved in carrying it out.

Random allocation of participants into groups involves implementing the random sequence in a way that conceals the sequence from anyone who enters participants in a study to prevent selection bias. If people who enter participants in a study know, or can detect, the upcoming allocations (such as the next participant will go into the experimental group), they may channel certain participants to a certain group. For example, a researcher may want a participant with a better prognosis to get into the experimental group. This type of practice in a study may bias the estimate of the treatment effect by 30 to 40% (Moher et al., 1998; Schulz, Chalmers, Hayes, & Altman, 1995).

Pretest data, sometimes called baseline data, is useful along with demographic data to evaluate whether randomization really produced equivalent groups. Normally, this comparison of baseline data is discussed right at the beginning of the Results section and is displayed in one or more tables.

Randomization facilitates blinding, another feature of RCTs. *The Cochrane Handbook* defines **blinding** as follows:

> In general, blinding (sometimes called masking) refers to the process by which study participants, health providers and investigators, including people assessing outcomes, are kept unaware of intervention allocations after inclusion of participants into the study. Blinding may reduce the risk that knowledge of which intervention was received, rather than the intervention itself, affects outcomes and assessments of outcomes. (Higgins & Green, 2011, Box 8.11.a)

Appropriate blinding can help reduce sources of bias such as performance bias (systematic differences between groups in the care provided).

In a **single-blind study**, participants are not told whether they are in the experimental or the control group. In a **double-blind study**, two groups have been blinded—normally the participants and one or all of these groups: health care providers, data collectors, data analysts, and the researchers themselves (who may have a number of roles in the study such as data collector). Because the term *double-blind* lacks a standard definition, you will need to read the study to see who was really blinded.

When someone involved in a research study is responsible for assessing participant outcomes and knows which intervention a participant received, that person could bias how the outcome was measured (usually reporting greater effects in the treatment group). Lack of blinding in RCTs has been shown to inflate the effect of the intervention by 9% (Pildal et al., 2007).

Blinding is possible in some, but not all, studies. In a drug study, both groups can take pills as long as they look and taste the same. In a diet study where the intervention group follows a modified diet and the control group eats their usual diet, blinding is not possible. Also keep in mind that even when a researcher can use blinding, it is not a simple procedure and it does not always work perfectly.

Attrition is another concern when conducting RCTs. If dropouts and noncompliant participants are excluded from the data, it can cause a number of problems: it reduces sample size and may disrupt the balance of characteristics in each group, thereby biasing the results. For example, if more participants in the experimental group drop out than from the control group (perhaps the intervention caused some of this), this creates an imbalance. A technique called **intention-to-treat analysis** is used to prevent biases due to participant attrition. Intention-to-treat is the principle that all participants *are used in the statistical analysis,* regardless of whether they dropped out, did not receive all the treatments, or did not comply with the treatments. Intention-to-treat has both supporters and detractors and advantages and disadvantages, but it is generally preferred. Some researchers modify intention-to-treat by, let us say, excluding certain participants.

When reading results of an RCT, examine how the study handles the following to determine possible sources of bias:

1. Power calculation to determine sample size.
2. Randomization and allocation to groups.
3. Type(s) of blinding used (if any).
4. Follow-up of participants and intention-to-treat analysis (if used).

5. Data collection.
6. Precise, complete results.

In a **clinical trial**, researchers test new treatments, drugs, or medical devices with human participants to assess efficacy and safety. Clinical trials are intervention studies that often use an RCT design. Sometimes you also hear the term **controlled clinical trials** (CCT). Controlled clinical trials do use a control group but may not assign participants to the intervention or control group in a strictly random manner, making them quasi-experimental studies.

The FDA requires (and regulates) clinical trials before a new drug, medical products such as vaccines, or medical device is sold in the United States. Clinical trials are often done in stages or phases, each designed to answer a different research question (National Institutes of Health, 2008).

Phase I: Researchers test a new drug or treatment in a small group of people for the first time to evaluate its safety, determine a safe dosage range, and identify side effects.

Phase II: The drug or treatment is given to a larger group of people to see if it is effective and to further evaluate its safety.

Phase III: The drug or treatment is given to large groups of people to confirm its effectiveness, monitor side effects, compare it to commonly used treatments, and collect information that will allow the drug or treatment to be used safely.

Phase IV: Studies are done after the drug or treatment has been approved and marketed to gather information on the drug's effect in various populations and any side effects associated with long-term use.

Clinical trials may be carried out in multiple locations simultaneously. There are a number of advantages to such multicenter studies: increased sample size, a more representative sample, more cost-effective, and increased generalizability of results. Coordination and communication in multicenter studies is, of course, more challenging than a single-center trial.

TIP

The U.S. National Institutes of Health maintains ClinicalTrials.gov, a Web site that is a registry of more than 200,000 public and privately supported clinical studies of human participants in the United States and around the world. The Web site also contains results and is used by patients, researchers, students, and study record managers.

Most RCTs use a pretest-posttest design, as shown in **Table 6.2**. The pretest and posttest are designated respectively as "O_1" and "O_2." Think of "O" as an observation in which data are collected and measurements taken. Many RCTs are simply variations of these designs; some may use multiple experimental groups, perhaps receiving treatment that varies by intensity, frequency, or duration. Sometimes there may be more than one comparison group, such as one comparison group that receives no treatment and another comparison group that receives a placebo (as in a drug study).

Table 6.2 Randomized Controlled Trial Design with Pretest-Posttest

Random assignment	Experimental group	O_1	Treatment	O_2
	Control group	O_1		O_2

Let's take a look at a research study using the randomized controlled trial design. Ramly, Ming, Chinna, Suboh, and Pendek (2014) completed an RCT, which was also a Phase II clinical trial, about the effect of vitamin D supplements (independent variable) on cardiometabolic risks and health-related quality of life (dependent variables) with urban premenopausal women in Malaysia.

1. *Participants*. A power analysis using 80% power revealed that 88 participants would be required for each group. Participants were recruited, screened, and given baseline clinical and other measurements. One group was randomized and started the study in October 2012 (n = 93), and the second cohort was randomized and started in January 2013 (n = 99). A total of 171 participants completed the 12-month follow-up, but because the researchers followed an intention-to-treat protocol, the data from all 192 were used in the statistical analysis.
2. *Measurements*. The cardiometabolic risk factors that were measured included blood pressure, insulin resistance, triglyercides, and HDL. Additional data was collected such as BMI and blood levels of vitamin D as serum 25(OH)D. Baseline measurements were taken, as well as measurements at 6 months and 12 months (end of study). Participants completed a health-related quality-of-life questionnaire as part of the baseline data and again at 12 months.
3. *Intervention*. The experimental group received 0.5 grams of cholecalciferol powder taken orally by diluting the powder in warm water once a week for 8 weeks (equivalent to 7142 IU/day) and then once a month for 10 months (equivalent to 1667 IU/day). The control group received 0.5 grams of placebo taken orally exactly like the experimental group. The placebo group was provided with cholecalciferol for four months *after* the trial was done.
4. *Randomization and blinding*. The randomization sequence was created using software. The participants' names were matched with the random number sequence and printed on tubes filled with vitamin D powder or placebo. The tubes were identical and not labeled with their contents to maintain allotment concealment. Allocation of the participants into groups was only known by one staff member with no other involvement in the trial. Outcome measurements were concealed from the researchers, staff, and participants. Because many of the outcomes being measured involved blood work analyzed in a university hospital, there were not many ways for someone to change results.
5. *Statistical analysis*. Comparison of *baseline characteristics* of the participants used independent t-tests (with normally distributed data) or Mann–Whitney tests (with non-normally distributed data) for continuous variables, and chi-square tests for categorical variables.

   The *outcome measurements* were examined statistically using a linear mixed effects model. This model is an extension of a linear regression model, and it works well here because there are multiple measurement points and some data was missing. The linear mixed effects model provides the **mean difference**, which shows the absolute difference between the groups, and estimates how much the intervention changed the outcome on average compared with the control group. Probability is used to determine whether the means are significantly different.
6. *Results*. **Table 6.3** shows some of the results. The first column shows the mean value of the outcome (such as systolic blood pressure) for the intervention group, and then for the placebo group. The third column shows the mean difference, which is simply the mean for the intervention group minus the mean for the placebo group. For example, the mean systolic blood pressure for the intervention group at 12 months was 125.8, and 123.9 for the placebo group. The mean

Table 6.3 Summary of Selected Outcome Measurements Over Time Using Linear Effects Model

	Intervention (*n* = 93) Mean (95% CI)	Placebo (*n* = 99) Mean (95% CI)	Mean difference (95% CI) between treatment groups
Systolic BP			
Baseline	121.6 (118.4 to 124.8)	118.9 (115.8 to 121.9)	2.71 (−1.71 to 7.13)
6 months	126.3 (122.9 to 129.6)	123.9 (120.7 to 127.2)	2.38 (−2.27 to 7.04)
12 months	125.8 (122.6 to 128.9)	123.9 (120.8 to 126.9)	1.89 (−2.56 to 6.35)
Diastolic BP			
Baseline	77.77 (75.56 to 79.99)	76.79 (74.65 to 78.94)	0.976 (−2.107 to 4.059)
6 months	79.74 (77.38 to 82.10)	79.23 (76.97 to 81.55)	0.508 (−2.805 to 3.820)
12 months	77.52 (75.22 to 79.81)	76.76 (74.53 to 78.99)	0.757 (−2.441 to 3.954)
Se Glucose (mmol/l)			
Baseline	5.07 (4.88 to 5.25)	4.93 (4.75 to 5.12)	0.13 (−0.13 to 0.39)
6 months	5.14 (4.97 to 5.32)	5.07 (4.89 to 5.24)	0.07 (−0.17 to 0.32)
12 months	5.04 (4.83 to 5.26)	5.11 (4.90 to 5.32)	−0.07 (−0.37 to 0.23)
Se insulin (mU/L)			
Baseline	13.81 (10.38 to 17.24)	11.07 (7.74 to 14.39)	2.74 (−2.04 to 7.51)
6 months	13.11 (11.18 to 15.04)	12.17 (10.27 to 14.06)	0.943 (−1.75 to 3.65)
12 months	13.93 (11.47 to 16.38)	12.74 (10.36 to 15.12)	1.19 (−2.23 to 4.61)
HOMA-Insulin Resistance			
Baseline	3.72 (2.25 to 5.19)	2.47 (1.04 to 3.91)	1.25 (−0.81 to 3.31)
6 months	3.12 (2.57 to 3.67)	2.84 (2.29 to 3.38)	0.28 (−0.49 to 1.05)
12 months	3.19 (2.61 to 3.78)	2.99 (2.42 to 3.56)	0.21 (−0.61 to 1.03)
TG (mmol/l)			
Baseline	1.15 (1.03 to 1.26)	1.17 (1.06 to 1.29)	−0.03 (−0.19 to 0.14)
6 months	1.38 (1.25 to 1.51)	1.19 (1.07 to 1.32)	0.19 (0.01 to 0.37)*
12 months	1.36 (1.23 to 1.49)	1.22 (1.09 to 1.35)	0.14 (−0.33 to 0.33)
HDL-C (mmol/l)			
Baseline	1.45 (1.36 to 1.54)	1.44 (1.35 to 1.52)	0.01 (−0.11 to 0.13)
6 months	1.43 (1.36 to 1.49)	1.50 (1.44 to 1.57)	−0.08 (−0.18 to 0.02)
12 months	1.52 (1.44 to 1.59)	1.53 (1.43 to 1.58)	0.02 (−0.09 to 0.13)

* Significant at $P < 0.05$

Data from "Effect of Vitamin D Supplementation on Cardiometabolic Risks and Health-Related Quality of Life among Urban Premenopausal Women in a Tropical Country – A Randomized Controlled Trial," by M. Ramly, M.F. Ming, K. Chinna, S. Suboh, and R. Pendek, 2014, *PLOS ONE, 9,* e110476, Table 2.

difference is 1.89. In this table, if these means were statistically significant, the authors would place an asterisk next to the mean difference.

There was no significant effect of vitamin D on blood pressure, insulin resistance, triglycerides, or HDL between the groups (all $P > 0.05$) except for the effect on triglycerides at 6 months. The results from the health-related quality-of-life questionnaire showed small but significant improvement in vitality (mean difference: 5.041; 95% CI: 0.709 to 9.374) and mental component score (mean difference: 2.951; 95% CI: 0.573 to 5.329) in the intervention group compared to the placebo group.

The CONSORT 2010 checklist (see Appendix C) describes information to include when reporting a randomized trial. (CONSORT stands for Consolidated Standards of Reporting Trials.) The CONSORT group, a panel of experts, developed this checklist to increase the transparency of RCTs and to reveal when there are deficiencies (Schulz, Altman, & Moher, 2010).

Advantages of RCTs include good internal validity and the use of powerful statistical tests, such as analysis of variance (ANOVA), to analyze data. RCTs often can be used in meta-analysis. RCTs are the most appropriate research design to answer research questions on treatment or therapy. As for disadvantages, randomized experiments do tend to be costly and time-consuming. RCTs often suffer from noncompliance and dropouts (sometimes due to side effects), and participants may respond differently because they know they are being observed and assessed (known as the **Hawthorne effect**). As in many research studies, their external validity (ability to generalize results) may have limitations. Threats to external validity are minimized when a broadly representative sample is used and the setting is not too controlled.

Crossover Designs

In a crossover design, each participant acts as a member of both the experimental and the control group. Studies designed to compare two different groups of participants are referred to as **between-groups design**. Crossover designs are **within-groups design** because the researcher is making comparisons within the same participants.

The most common crossover design is the two-period, two-treatment design. Participants are randomly assigned to receive either the treatment in period 1 and the control in period 2, or the reverse. For example, in a drug study, one participant initially received the active drug and then later received the placebo. To avoid **carryover effects** (when exposure to a treatment affects outcomes in a later period), researchers build in a period of time—called a **washout period**—between treatments for the effect of the treatment to disappear.

Crossover studies include a design feature known as **repeated measures**. When you see "repeated measures" in a study, it means multiple, repeated measurements are being taken, not just a pretest and posttest.

Troup et al. (2015) used a crossover design to study the effects of black tea intake (specifically the flavonoids in tea) on blood cholesterol levels on participants with mild hypercholesterolemia. Participants were block-randomized by sex to drink either 5 cups/day of black tea or 5 cups/day of the placebo for the first 4 weeks. The placebo was a caffeinated beverage that looked and tasted like tea but contained no flavonoids. After the 3-week washout period, participants switched assignments. **Figure 6.2** shows the design for this study.

During the treatment periods, participants were provided and consumed a low-flavonoid diet. During the run-in periods (13 days each), participants drank the tea-like placebo. Participants were allowed to add sugar, but not milk, to either beverage (milk reduces the antioxidant capacity of tea).

The study did not show that black tea significantly changed the lipid profile of the participants. As in the study just mentioned, the researchers here also looked at the mean difference of an outcome, such as LDL-C. None had a *p*-value below 0.05, the level of significance.

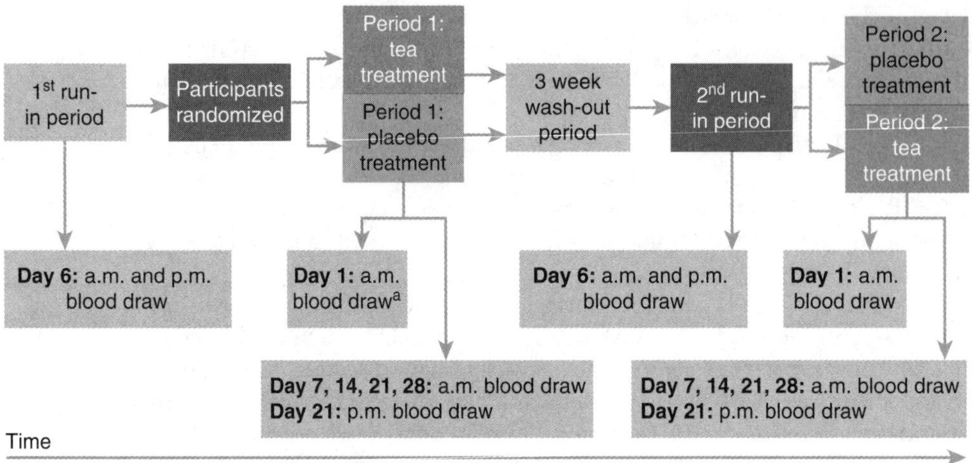

FIGURE 6.2 Crossover Study Design Overview, including timing of Biological Sample Collection Points, in a Study of the Effect of 5 Cups Per Day of Black Tea on Serum Cholesterol Concentrations (n = 57).

APPLICATION 6.1

What might have happened if the placebo was not caffeinated (the black tea, of course, had some caffeine)? What might have happened if the participants could tell the difference between the regular tea and the placebo? Could this have affected the results?

One advantage of the crossover design is that you do not have to worry about the comparability of two groups as you would in a parallel-group experiment (experimental and control groups), so this improves internal validity. Because each participant acts as his or her own control, you minimize the effect of confounding variables. You also can use smaller groups than in parallel-group studies.

FACTORIAL DESIGNS

In real life, variables rarely exist in isolation, so some designs include more than one independent variable. One design that manipulates two or more independent variables (or treatments) is a **factorial design**. In this design, the independent variables are referred to as **factors**. The simplest factorial design includes two factors, and each factor has two levels, resulting in a 2 × 2 factorial design. The first number "2" refers to the number of levels of the first independent variable, and the second number "2" refers to the number of levels for the second independent variable.

For example, a factorial, double-blind design was used to test the effect of zinc and multivitamins supplements on growth of infants in Tanzania (Locks et al., 2016). The two independent variables, or factors, were zinc supplements and multivitamin supplements. The two levels of the zinc supplements were administration of just the zinc supplement *or* administration of the zinc supplement with the multivitamin supplement. The two levels of the multivitamin supplements were administering just the multivitamin *or* administering it with the zinc supplement. Because one level of each variable is identical (infants

	Zinc Supplement (Independent Variable)	
Multivitamin Supplement (Independent Variable)	Zinc supplement + Multivitamin supplement	Zinc supplement only
	Multivitamin supplement only	Control group (placebo)

FIGURE 6.3 Example of a 2 × 2 Factorial Design

receiving both the zinc and multivitamin supplements), you can use three groups and a control group as shown in **Figure 6.3**. Locks et al. found that daily zinc supplements starting in infancy had small but significant improvement in weight for age.

This was an example of a simple factorial design. You could, for example, design a diet/exercise study with four diets and three exercise programs. That would result in 12 combinations of diet/exercise, leading to a 4 × 3 factorial design.

Solomon Four-Group Design

The **Solomon four-group design** (**Table 6.4**) is a combination of the pretest-posttest design and the posttest only design. In this design, participants are randomly assigned to one of two intervention groups or one of two control groups. Both intervention groups receive the same intervention; the only difference is that one of these groups receives the pretest, the other does not. Likewise, only one of the control groups receives the pretest. Posttest measures are collected on all four groups to assess the effect of the independent variable. Some researchers modify this design and use just one control group, which receives both the pretest and the posttest.

Atlantis, Salmon, and Bauman (2008) used a Solomon four-group design to explore the effects of television advertisements (independent variable) promoting physical activity on children's preferences for physical or sedentary activities (dependent variables). The children were randomized to one of two treatment groups or one of two control groups. The treatment groups watched a television show with standard advertisements and also advertisements promoting more physical activity instead of sedentary activity. The control groups watched the same show but without the advertisements promoting physical activity. One experimental group and one control group were assessed before *and* after watching the television show for their choices, preferences, and ratings of physical and sedentary activities. The other groups were only assessed after watching the television show. The study did not show any significant differences between groups.

This type of design is useful when a researcher thinks the outcomes could be biased by exposure to the pretest. In general, the Solomon four-group design is considered a very rigorous design that strengthens both internal and external validity. As you can

Table 6.4 Solomon Four-Group Design

Random assignment	Experimental group 1	O_1	Treatment	O_2
	Control group 1	O_1		O_2
	Experimental group 2		Treatment	O_2
	Control group 2			O_2

imagine, this design is more time consuming for researchers and also requires a large sample due to the four groups.

QUASI-EXPERIMENTAL DESIGNS

Quasi-experimental designs have an intervention and manipulation of the independent variable, but they lack a key feature of experimental studies—randomization. Because we are unsure if the groups are truly equivalent, quasi-experimental designs are ranked lower than experimental studies as sources of evidence.

Two of the most popular quasi-experimental designs are nonequivalent control group and time series designs. Be cautious when you see a quasi-experimental study that does not have a control group. Without a control group, a study has little, if any, external or internal validity.

NONEQUIVALENT CONTROL GROUP DESIGNS

In most cases, a **nonequivalent control group design** is similar to the classic experimental design except that participants are not randomly assigned to groups. Often researchers use natural groups or assign participants to groups using a nonrandom method. Sampling is still going on in terms of choosing the study's participants. It is just that participants do not have the same chance of being in either the experimental or control group, and as a result, the groups are not necessarily equivalent.

Some researchers match participants at the group level based on demographic or other possible confounding variables. The more similar the groups are, the closer the design approximates an experimental study. Researchers confirm whether two groups are comparable (especially on the dependent variable) at baseline by collecting and analyzing pertinent data, but that may not include all baseline differences in active variables.

Table 6.5 shows a nonequivalent control group design with a pretest and posttest. There are a number of variations on this design, such as posttest only with a control group (sometimes a pretest is not possible or would flaw the results) or pretest and posttest with two comparison treatments and a routine care comparison group.

McAleese and Rankin (2007) carried out a nonequivalent control group study to "determine whether adolescents who participated in a garden-based nutrition intervention would increase their fruit and vegetable consumption more than those participating in a nutrition education intervention without any garden activities (McAleese & Rankin, 2007, p. 662). This study appears in Appendix A.

1. *Participants*: A convenience sample of 99 sixth-grade students in three different schools were the participants. Two schools had the experimental groups and one school had the control group.
2. *Measurements*: All students took pretests (three 24-hour food recalls) and posttests (three 24-hour food recalls).
3. *Intervention*: Both experimental groups participated in a 12-week nutrition education curriculum, "Nutrition in the Garden." Experimental school 2 also participated in gardening activities, maintaining and harvesting a garden with vegetables, herbs, and strawberries. The control group received no intervention.

Table 6.5 Nonequivalent Control Group Pretest/Posttest Design

Experimental group	O_1	Treatment	O_2
Control group	O_1		O_2

4. *Results*: Using repeated measures ANOVA, results showed that students in experimental school 2 ate significantly more fruits, vegetables, vitamin A, vitamin C, and fiber after the intervention compared to before the intervention. For example, fruit consumption increased by 1.13 servings ($P < 0.001$) for students in experimental school 2. They also ate more fruits and vegetables than the other experimental group or the control group.

This design is not as strong in controlling for threats to internal and external validity as is a true experimental design. However, the hallmark of a good quasi-experimental study is that the researchers have instituted controls and sometimes a more natural setting is advantageous. This design can show the effect of an intervention, as well as associations and trends. When randomization is impractical or unethical, a nonequivalent control group design can be useful.

APPLICATION 6.2

In the results table for the McAleese and Rankin study (Appendix A), did the control school or experimental school 1 increase consumption of fruits or vegetables? What does the column marked "F" mean? Which additional statistical test was done (in addition to repeated measured ANOVA) to pinpoint which groups were significantly different from each other?

INTERRUPTED TIME SERIES DESIGNS

An interrupted time series design includes several waves of observation in which the dependent variable is measured before *and* after an intervention (which is the "interruption"). The **simple interrupted time series design** is shown in **Table 6.6**, and you can see that this design does not include a control/comparison group. The use of multiple observations/measurements does strengthen this design. It can also help assess trends in scores and decrease the chance of regression to the mean. **Regression to the mean** occurs when very high or low pretest scores of participants move closer to the mean on the posttest (due to natural variability), which may lead to an inaccurate conclusion that the intervention resulted in a treatment effect. Having several posttest scores is helpful because it is unlikely that small differences will be maintained if the treatment really has no effect.

Repeated measurements can create concerns about testing effects, instrumentation, and consistency in measurements. You also need to consider whether some unanticipated events occurred during this time and whether attrition will be more of an issue due to the multiple points of measurement over a longer time frame than many other designs.

The addition of a control group to this design strengthens the validity of the findings. Researchers can now look for differences in trends between the groups and control

Table 6.6 Times Series Designs

Simple Interrupted Time Series Design	
Experimental group	$O_1\ O_2\ O_3\ X\ O_4\ O_5\ O_6$
Interrupted Time Series Design with Control Group	
Experimental group	$O_1\ O_2\ O_3\ X\ O_4\ O_5\ O_6$
Control group	$O_1\ O_2\ O_3\ O_4\ O_5\ O_6$

Table 6.7 Abstract of a Study Using a Simple Interrupted Time Series Design	
Objectives	We examined changes in meal selection by patrons of university food-service operations when nutrition labels were provided at the point of selection.
Methods	We used a quasi-experimental, single-group, interrupted time-series design to examine daily sales before, during, and after provision of point-of-selection nutrition labels. Piecewise linear regression was employed to examine changes in the average energy content of entrees and a paired *t* test was used to detect differences in sales across the periods.
Results	The average energy content of entrees purchased by patrons dropped immediately when nutrition labels were made available at point of selection and increased gradually when nutrition information was removed. There was no significant change in number of entrees sold or in revenues between the two periods.
Conclusions	Use of nutrition labels reduced the average energy content of entrees purchased without reducing overall sales. These results provide support for strengthening the nutrition labeling policy in food-service operations.

Reproduced from "Improving Patrons' Meal Selections Through the Use of Point-of-Selection Nutrition Labels," by Y. H. Chu, E. A. Frongillo, S. J. Jones, & G. L. Kaye, 2009, *American Journal of Public Health, 99*, p. 2001. Reprinted with permission.

more for the history effect. Table 6.6 shows the **interrupted time series design with control group**. Some researchers also call this a *multiple time series design*. Basically a *multiple* time series design has more than one group.

Interrupted time series designs are flexible and can be used in a number of situations. This type of design is especially useful in the evaluation of community interventions when RCTs are impractical and too expensive, and you want to focus on measuring changes in behaviors and outcomes over time.

Table 6.7 contains an abstract of a study using a simple interrupted time series design (Chu, Frongillo, Jones, & Kaye, 2009). **Figure 6.4** displays the results of the study.

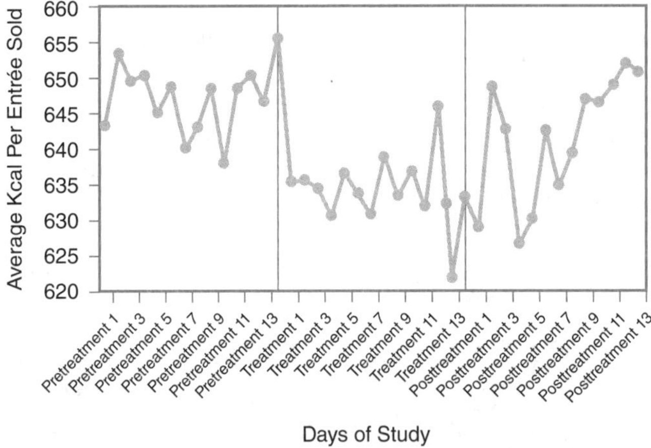

FIGURE 6.4 Average Energy Content of Entrées Sold Per Day in a Food-Service Operation Before, During, and After Provision of Nutrition Information at Point of Selection: Columbus, Ohio, October 25–December 8, 2004.

Reproduced from "Improving Patrons' Meal Selections Through the Use of Point-of-Selection Nutrition Labels," by Y. H. Chu, E. A. Frongillo, S. J. Jones, & G. L. Kaye, 2009, *American Journal of Public Health, 99*, p. 2003. Reprinted with permission.

TIP

When reading a study with an interrupted time series design, you want to take a good look at the chart (such as Figure 6.4) that shows the trend of the measurements before, during, and after the intervention. The graph is split into the three segments. The average kcalories per entrée sold was high before the intervention, and then went down during the intervention. It is also interesting that once the intervention stopped, the average kcalories slowly moved back to the preintervention numbers. Looking at a graph such as this can give you a quick mental picture of what happened during a study.

DESCRIPTIVE QUANTITATIVE DESIGNS

Descriptive designs collect information about variables without changing the environment or manipulating any variables, so they do not look at possible cause and effect. They are different from observational designs in that they do not include comparison groups. According to Grove, Burns, and Gray (2013), descriptive designs "may be used to develop theory, identify problems with current practice, justify current practice, make judgments, or determine what others in similar situations are doing" (p. 215).

Descriptive designs range from cross-sectional surveys (at one or multiple points in time) to comparative designs (comparing two groups) to correlations (relationships between two variables). You can think of many descriptive designs as creating a snapshot. We now take a look at three common descriptive designs.

DESCRIPTIVE CROSS-SECTIONAL AND REPEATED CROSS-SECTIONAL DESIGN

In a cross-sectional study, data is collected at one point in time. A purely **descriptive cross-sectional study** provides basic information about prevalence (number of existing cases of a disease or health condition in a population) and distribution, as you can see in these examples.

- Using data from the National Health and Nutrition Examination Survey (2009–2012), researchers reported that men consumed an average of 14.6 cups of water per day, and women consumed 11.6 cups of water per day (Rosinger & Herrick, 2016). This indicates that Americans seem to be taking in adequate fluids.
- You hear frequent media reports about how American adults and children are managing their weight. Using data from the National Health and Nutrition Examination Survey (2013–2014), a group of researchers announced that 16% of children and adolescents (ages 2–19 years) are overweight and 17% are obese (Skinner, Perrin, & Skelton, 2016).
- If you ever wondered how many people really use menu labeling at fast-food or chain restaurants, researchers found that of adults who noticed nutrition labeling at fast-food or chain restaurants, 25% reported frequent use of the information, 32% reported moderate use, and 43% reported they never used it (Lee-Kwan, Pan, Maynard, McGuire, & Park, 2016). The data came, again, from a national survey: the Behavioral Risk Factor Surveillance System. In this study, data from 17 states was used.

A repeated cross-sectional study generally collects the same data at multiple points in time, and usually includes both descriptive and inferential statistics (to look at the differences over time). Repeated cross-sectional studies can tell us about trends, patterns, or stages of development. For example, Larson, Story, Eisenberg, and Neumark-Sztainer (2016) used a repeated cross-sectional design to examine meal and snack patterns in adolescents in the Minneapolis/St. Paul secondary schools from 1999 to 2010. Food frequency questionnaires and surveys were the instruments used to gather data.

Selected results showed modest but significant changes: the frequency of eating breakfast and lunch increased over time, and the adolescents consumed fewer snacks with high kcalories and few nutrients (i.e., empty kcalorie foods/drinks). The total sample results row in **Table 6.8** shows how the frequency of eating breakfast and lunch changed from 1999 to 2010. For example, breakfast frequency went from 3.7 mean days/week to 4.2 mean days/week ($p < 0.001$). The P-values were calculated using two-sample t tests. (The 1999 sample was weighted so that you can see the trends over time independent of demographic shifts in the population.)

Advantages of cross-sectional studies include that they are relatively inexpensive, can estimate prevalence of an outcome of interest as well as assess risk factors, and do not have loss to follow-up. Cross-sectional studies are useful for generating hypotheses and for public health planning. Because they are only a snapshot, you cannot use this type of design to make causal inferences.

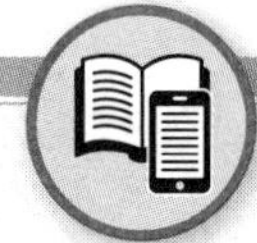

APPLICATION 6.3

Using Table 6.8, for which groups (such as male or black) did the frequency of eating breakfast change significantly (assume $P < 0.05$) between 1999 and 2010?

Comparative Design

In a comparative design, the researchers measure the dependent variable in two or more groups, but they do not manipulate the independent variable. Descriptive and inferential statistical tests can be used to look at the differences between the groups.

For example, Mathias, Jacquier, and Eldridge (2016) looked at two groups of children aged 4 to 18 years old: those who ate lunch and those who didn't eat lunch on a given day. Using data from a 24-hour recall administered as part of the National Health and Nutrition Examination Surveys, the researchers compared the dietary intakes of the children who ate lunch with those who did not eat lunch to see if not eating lunch affected nutrient and kcalorie intake for the day. The independent variable, whether the child did or did not eat lunch, was not manipulated because this is not an experimental or quasi-experimental study. The dependent variable, the nutrient and kcalorie content of the children's diets, was measured for everyone in both groups.

TIP

As you can see from the studies just discussed, descriptive studies do not just provide descriptive statistics. Descriptive studies can compare groups and use inferential statistics such as t-tests to look at the relationship between variables. The next topic, correlation, also looks at the relationship between variables.

Table 6.8 Secular Trends from 1999 to 2010 in Adolescent Meal Patterns by Sociodemographic Characteristics: Minneapolis-St. Paul, MN, Project EAT (Eating and Activity in Teens)

			Breakfast frequency (mean days/wk)			Lunch frequency (mean days/wk)		
Characteristic	**1999[a] (n)**	**2010 (n)**	**1999[a]**	**2010**	***P* value[b]**	**1999[a]**	**2010**	***P* value[b]**
Total Sample	2,598	2,540	3.7	4.2	<0.001	5.6	5.8	<0.001
Sex								
Male	1,181	1,175	4.1	4.4	0.001	5.9	5.9	0.49
Female	1,348	1,365	3.4	4.0	<0.001	5.4	5.7	<0.001
School Level[c]								
Middle school	1,148	1,136	4.1	4.3	0.20	5.9	6.0	0.25
High school	1,335	1,404	3.4	4.1	<0.001	5.4	5.7	<0.001
Ethnicity/Race[d]								
White	540	499	4.3	4.7	0.005	5.6	6.0	<0.001
Black	638	706	3.5	4.3	<0.001	5.4	5.7	0.002
Hispanic	414	435	3.2	4.0	<0.001	5.5	5.8	0.07
Asian	546	520	3.8	3.8	0.94	6.0	5.9	0.32
Native American	98	92	3.5	4.1	0.10	5.2	5.7	0.05
Mixed/Other	293	288	4.0	4.0	0.96	5.7	5.6	0.50
Socioeconomic Status[e]								
Low	936	973	3.4	3.9	0.002	5.7	5.8	0.36
Low middle	560	556	3.4	4.0	<0.001	5.4	5.9	<0.001
Middle	436	430	3.7	4.4	<0.001	5.5	5.8	0.03
High middle	335	320	4.3	4.6	0.16	5.7	5.8	0.65
High	199	193	4.9	5.0	0.63	5.8	6.1	0.16

[a] The 1999 sample was weighted to allow for an examination of secular trends in meal patterns independent of demographic shifts in the population. For example, estimates of weekly breakfast frequency within the low socioeconomic status group in 1999 and 2010 are mutually controlled so that sex, school level, and ethnicity/race makeup are the same in the low socioeconomic status group in the 1999 sample as in the 2010 sample.

[b] *P* values represent testing to examine weighted mean differences in meal frequency between 1999 and 2010.

[c] Middle school represents students enrolled in 6th to 8th grades and high school represents students enrolled in 9th to 12th grades.

[d] Adolescents could choose >1 ethnic/racial category; those responses indicating multiple categories were coded as "Mixed/Other." Because there were few participants who identified themselves as Hawaiians or Pacific Islanders, these participants were also included in the "Mixed/Other" category.

[e] The prime determinant of socioeconomic status was the higher education level of either parent with adjustments made for student eligibility for free/reduced-price school meals, family public assistance receipt, and parent employment status.

Reproduced from: "Secular Trends in Meal and Snack Patterns among Adolescents from 1999 to 2010," by N. Larson, M. Story, M. E. Eisenberg, & D. Neumark-Sztainer, 2016, *Journal of the Academy of Nutrition and Dietetics, 116*, 243. Reprinted with permission.

Descriptive statistics were used to show the percentage of children and adolescents who did not eat lunch: 7% ± 1% (standard error) for 4- to 8-year-olds, 16% ± 2% for 9- to 13-year-olds, and 17 ± 1% for 14- to 18-year-olds. Linear regression was used to show that missing lunch was associated with significantly lower intake of many micronutrients for the day in all age groups.

DESCRIPTIVE CORRELATIONAL DESIGN

Correlation is a statistical procedure used to measure and describe the relationship or association between two variables. The researcher may not know whether the variables are related, or may suspect that one influences the other. In either case, no attempt is made to manipulate an independent variable in correlational designs, so you cannot conclude that the relationship is causal simply based on correlation.

Before a correlation coefficient can be calculated, you need to draw a **scatterplot** with the quantitative data, as seen in **Figure 6.5**. Each dot in the scatterplot represents one variable (*x* or *y*) from one person or observation. The values for the *x* variable are placed on the *x*-axis (horizontal axis), and the values for the *y* variable are on the *y*-axis (vertical axis).

The variable for the *y*-axis should be the **outcome variable**, which may also be called the response or dependent variable. The variable for the *x*-axis should be the **predictor variable**, which also may be called the explanatory or independent variable. For example, in a study on carbohydrate intake and dental caries, the researcher wants to see if increasing carbohydrate intake (predictor or independent variable) increases the number of cavities (outcome or dependent variable). So the number of cavities should be on the *y*-axis and carbohydrate intake should be on the *x*-axis. This way, when you look at the scatterplot, as the carbohydrate intake (predictor variable) increases along the horizontal axis, you can see how it affects the number of cavities (outcome variable) on the vertical axis.

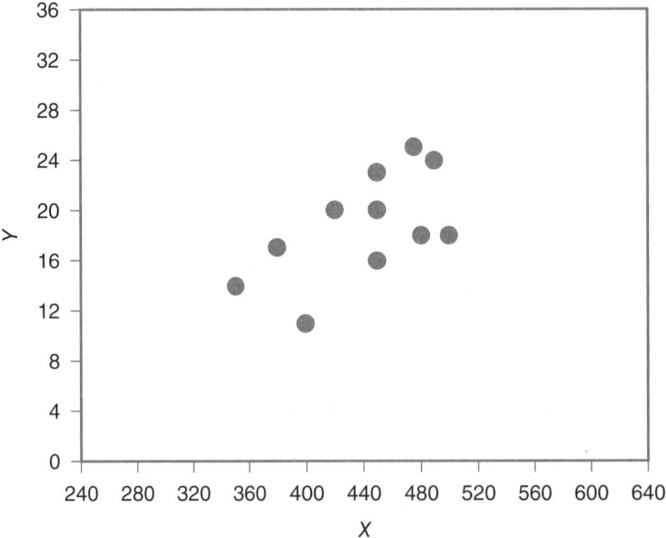

FIGURE 6.5 Example of a Scatterplot

There are several things to look for on a scatterplot: form, direction, strength, and outliers.

1. *When the dots are closely grouped along what appears to be a relatively straight line, the form is linear.* If all the points lie on a line, then we have perfect linear correlation (this is rare!). Correlation can only be used if the shape in the scatterplot is linear. The correlation coefficient tells you how well the variables fit on a straight line. Scatterplots may also be curved, curvilinear, or random.
2. **Figure 6.6** shows scatterplots with *positive and negative directions* (discussed in a moment). Sometimes you may see both a positive and a negative trend in a scatterplot, in which case you may need to split the data into subgroups.
3. *The strength of the relationship can be seen by how tightly clustered the points are along the form,* whether the form is a straight line, a curvy line, or other shaped line. The relationship is stronger when the data points are close to an imaginary line that you draw through the points. The relationship is weak when the points are all over the place, with no pattern.
4. You should also *check for outliers* because the correlation coefficient can be greatly affected by just one outlier.

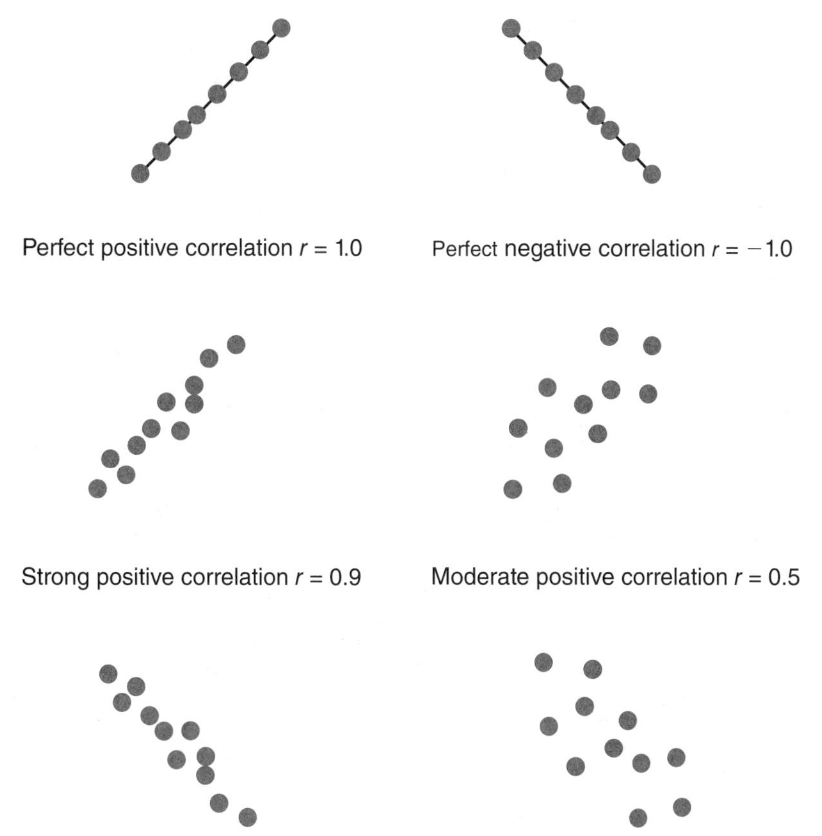

FIGURE 6.6 Scatterplots Showing Different Correlations (Positive and Negative)

Before you can use correlation, you have to be sure that there is a linear relationship and that the variables are quantitative. You also may have to make decisions about how to handle outliers.

A descriptive correlational design has the following characteristics:

1. Two variables are clearly identified and defined.
2. Data for each of the two variables are collected.
3. There is one group of participants.
4. There is no intervention or treatment going on before, during, or after data collection.
5. Data is collected at one general point in time.
6. A correlation coefficient is calculated. The correlation coefficient is a summary statistic, similar to the mean, that summarizes the strength and direction of a linear relationship.

For continuous variables that are normally distributed, a Pearson correlation coefficient (r) is calculated. If either or both variables are ordinal, the Spearman rank-order correlation (also called Spearman's rho, r_S) is used. This is a nonparametric test that has the same values as the Pearson's correlation coefficient. Correlational techniques such as Cramer's V can be used for nominal data. When researchers are trying to understand the relationship between two variables *while controlling for the effects of other variables*, they use linear regression.

The correlation coefficient r measures both the strength and the direction of the relationship between the two variables, from no relationship (0) to a perfect positive or negative linear relationship (+1 or −1). The closer a correlation coefficient is to 1.0 or −1.0, the stronger the relationship between the variables.

There are no generally accepted standards for interpreting whether a correlation is considered strong or weak, but some would say that a strong correlation should be at least ± 0.7–0.8. To interpret a correlation coefficient, you can use its statistical significance to see whether the correlation differs significantly from 0 (no correlation), although some researchers suggest paying more attention to the size of the correlation (Guyatt, Walter, Shannon, Cook, Jaeschke, & Heddle, 1995). Also, keep in mind that large sample sizes can make small correlations look significant.

The direction of the relationship can be positive or negative. When two variables are positively correlated, it means that they vary together. For example, as BMI increases, so does systolic blood pressure: this is a positive relationship in which both variables increase. If both variables decrease at the same time, that is also a positive relationship. In a negative relationship, as one variable increases, the other one decreases. So in a negative correlation, the variables move in opposite directions and are said to have an inverse relationship. For example, researchers may find that as participants in a weight loss program spend more time exercising and planning meals, their BMI decreases.

One thing to note at this point is a key difference between scatterplots and correlation. Scatterplots use the units the variables are measured in, such as BMI, whereas the formula to calculate the correlation coefficient standardizes the variables (using z scores), so changes in scale or units of measurement do not affect its value. Therefore, the correlation coefficient has no units.

Descriptive correlational studies sometimes lay the groundwork for testing a hypothesis in a later study. A common mistake with correlation is that people think a high correlation coefficient demonstrates causation. Correlation does not demonstrate cause and effect; the independent variable is not manipulated and extraneous variables (sometimes called lurking variables) are not controlled. In some cases, one variable may actually cause the other, but other research designs will be needed to prove it.

ADDITIONAL TYPES OF DESIGNS

As you read more research articles, you will find some additional types of designs.

1. *Secondary data analysis.* Researchers use data already collected in another study. Then they use a traditional research design (obviously not experimental or quasi-experimental) to answer a research question. For example, Eicher-Miller, Khanna, Boushey, Gelfand, and Delp (2016) used data from the National Health and Nutrition Examination Survey (1999–2004) to test a hypothesis. They hypothesized that the diet quality of American adults varies depending on how and when they distribute their energy/nutrient intake over the day. **Table 6.9** lists sources of data sets for NHANES and other studies. When using a national data set, be aware that they often oversample underrepresented groups, so you need to read in detail about the sampling methods.

Table 6.9 Examples of Sources of Data Sets for Secondary Data Analysis

	Centers for Disease Control and Prevention	
	Behavioral Risk Factor Surveillance System	http://www.cdc.gov/brfss/
	Youth Risk Behavior Surveillance System	http://www.cdc.gov/healthyyouth/data/yrbs/index.htm
	National Health and Nutrition Examination Survey	http://www.cdc.gov/nchs/nhanes/nhanes_questionnaires.htm
	National Health Interview Survey	http://www.cdc.gov/nchs/nhis/index.htm
	Nutrition, Physical Activity, and Obesity: Data, Trends, and Maps	https://nccd.cdc.gov/NPAO_DTM/
	National Institutes of Health	
	Clinical Trials (some include study results)	http://www.clinicaltrials.gov
	National Heart, Lung, and Blood Institute, Framingham Heart Study	http://www.framinghamheartstudy.org
	Women's Health Initiative	http://www.whi.org
	U.S. Department of Agriculture	
	Infant Feeding Practices, Study II and Its Year Six Follow Up	http://www.cdc.gov/breastfeeding/data/ifps/index.htm
	What We Eat in America	http://www.ars.usda.gov/Services/docs.htm?docid=18354
	National Collaborative on Childhood Obesity Research (A Collaboration Among CDC, NIH, USDA, and Robert Wood Johnson Foundation)	
	Catalogue of Surveillance Systems (for childhood obesity)	http://nccor.org/nccor-tools/catalogue/index
	Nurses' Health Study http://www.nurseshealthstudy.org	
	U.S. Renal Data System http://usrds.org	

2. *Methodological designs.* Methodological designs are used to test the reliability and validity of instruments used to measure variables in research. For example, Boucher et al. (2006) asked participants to take an adaptation of Block's food frequency questionnaire (FFQ). The same respondents also completed two 24-hour diet recalls via telephone. The researchers evaluated the agreement of 32 nutrient intakes between the adapted FFQ and the diet recalls for each respondent. Correlation coefficients showed moderate to high validity.
3. *Secondary research.* Original research is considered primary research, and review articles are known as secondary research because they analyze data already collected in primary research. Systematic reviews critically appraise and pool data from multiple single studies, often using meta-analysis, to answer a research question.

RESEARCHER INTERVIEW: Intervention Research

Leslie Cunningham-Sabo, PhD, RDN
Associate Professor, Department of Food Science and Human Nutrition, Colorado State University, Fort Collins, CO

1. **Briefly describe the areas in which you do research.**
My research focus is childhood obesity prevention. Most of my projects take place in public schools, but with some emphasis on families at home too.
2. **With your experience in intervention research, what should students/practitioners know about this area of research?**
Intervention research focuses on the development, implementation, and evaluation of programs or projects with the study population. You might read several different types of articles related to intervention research. For example, I recently published an article with my research team that described in detail the protocol (scientific procedures) our multicomponent study followed. It did not include any study results but focused on the design of our Fuel for Fun: Cooking with Kids Plus Parents and Play project.
Much more frequently you will find articles describing some or all of the components of an intervention study and the related results. Depending on how complex the study is, one article may describe all or just part of the intervention and results.
3. **What do you enjoy most about the research process?**
I really love the creativity of the research process. You get to answer important questions, which lead to even more questions! For example, right now we are trying to understand how best to engage parents in a school-based intervention with fourth graders. Will busy parents find it easier to connect via Facebook or through a blog? Or will they prefer materials sent home with their child that they complete together? That is just one example of the questions we try to address through our research.
Other things I enjoy about the research process are that I get to work with faculty and students from different academic disciplines (e.g., education, exercise science, public health) in addition to nutrition and dietetics. I also really enjoy mentoring students and younger professionals. I feel a sense of pride and contribution when they learn, grow professionally, and achieve their academic goals. Most important, though, is the opportunity to make a difference and improve the health and quality of life of the children and families that are part of our intervention study.
4. **What tip(s) do you have for practitioners who want to do practice-based research?**
Research can contribute to improvement in all practice settings. Think about areas where your team is struggling; it could be with delivery of client services or client outcomes, or even how your team works together. Discuss what information you need to gather to learn more about the situation. Who else do you need to involve? How will you gather the resources needed to do this work? Where are the sources of internal or external funding? Gain the necessary approvals

and move forward. Collect the information systematically, and prepare reports or presentations formatted for the audience (e.g., funder, superiors, target audience). The bottom line: identify a significant problem you want to address, find others who share your interest and commitment, gain the resources you need, and keep stakeholders apprised of your progress and results. Start small, gain experience, and achieve your initial goals. This can lead to bigger research projects in the future.

SUMMARY

1. Some research design features to consider include whether there will be an intervention, where it will take place, what comparisons will be made between or within groups, what is going to be measured, when measurements will be taken, how you will get the participants, how you will split participants up into groups if needed, and how you will control extraneous variables.
2. Quantitative research designs are often used to look at causal relationships, but they can also be used to look at associations or relationship between variables. First are experimental study designs with an intervention, control group, and randomization of participants into groups. Next are quasi-experimental designs with an intervention but no randomization. Descriptive designs do not have an intervention or treatment and are considered nonexperimental.
3. Most research questions look at either differences among groups or an association or relationship among variables.
4. Although randomization into the treatment or control group is essential to an experimental study, it is *not* essential that the participants are randomly selected from a target population *before* being randomly assigned to a group. Most randomized controlled trials do *not* use random sampling to pick who is in the study. Random assignment means the groups are comparable, so that differences between them at the end are deduced as being caused by the intervention.
5. A control or comparison group may receive no treatment, a placebo, standard or usual health care, or a lower dose of treatment or an alternative treatment.
6. Experimental designs are most useful for questions about therapy or treatment options.
7. Randomized controlled trials (RCTs) are considered the "gold standard" for assessing causality and determining efficacy in intervention research. Participants are randomly assigned to the intervention or control group, and then followed forward in time to compare the outcomes. In addition, blinding may be used. Most RCTs use a pretest-posttest design.
8. Intention-to-treat analysis is used to prevent biases due to participant attrition.
9. When reading a RCT, pay attention to how sample size was determined, how participants were randomized and allocated to groups, if blinding was used, if intention-to-treat analysis was used, how data was collected, and how complete and precise the results are.
10. Clinical trials are intervention studies that often use an RCT design. The FDA requires clinical trials before new drugs or medical products or devices are sold in the United States. Clinical trials are often done in stages or phases.
11. The most common crossover design is the two-period, two-treatment design. Participants are randomly assigned to receive either the treatment in period 1 and the control in period 2, or the reverse. To avoid carryover effects (when exposure to a treatment affects outcomes in a later period), researchers build in a period of time—a washout period—between treatments for the effect of the treatment to disappear.
12. A factorial design manipulates two or more independent variables (or treatments). In this design, the independent variables are referred to as factors. The simplest factorial design includes two factors, and each factor has two levels, resulting in a 2 × 2 factorial design. The first number "2" refers to the number of levels of the first independent variable, and

the second number "2" refers to the number of levels for the second independent variable.

13. The Solomon four-group design combines the pretest-posttest design and the posttest only design, which results in a very rigorous design.
14. Two of the most popular quasi-experimental designs are nonequivalent control group and time series designs. The nonequivalent control group design is similar to the classic experimental design except that participants are not randomly assigned to groups. An interrupted time series design includes several waves of observation where the dependent variable is measured before *and* after an intervention. This design may or may not have a control group.
15. Descriptive designs collect information about variables without changing the environment or manipulating any variables, so they do not assess cause and effect. Descriptive designs include descriptive cross-sectional (collects information at one point in time, such as the prevalence of childhood obesity), repeated cross-sectional, comparative, and descriptive correlational designs.
16. In a comparative design, the researchers measure the dependent variable in two or more groups but do not manipulate the independent variable. Descriptive and inferential statistical tests can be used to look at the differences between the groups.
17. The correlation coefficient r measures both the strength and the direction of the relationship between the two variables, from no relationship (0) to a perfect positive or negative linear relationship (+1 or −1). The closer a correlation coefficient is to 1.0 or −1.0, the stronger the relationship between the variables.
18. Two additional kinds of studies you will find in journals are those using secondary data analysis and methodological designs.

REVIEW QUESTIONS

1. A prospective longitudinal study:
   A. goes backward in time
   B. goes forward in time
   C. takes measurements only at one point in time
   D. any of the above
2. ____________ variables are factors outside of the variables being studies that could influence the outcome of a study.
   A. independent
   B. dependent
   C. extraneous
   D. extra
3. If a study has an intervention but no randomization, in which group of study designs does it belong?
   A. experimental
   B. quasi-experimental
   C. descriptive
   D. observational
4. A control or comparison group may receive:
   A. no intervention or treatment
   B. a placebo
   C. standard or usual health care
   D. a and b only
   E. a, b, and c
5. An excellent design to test treatment options is:
   A. correlational design
   B. comparative design
   C. randomized controlled trial
   D. repeated cross-sectional design
6. Most RCTs use a posttest only design.
   A. true
   B. false
7. Crossover studies use repeated measures.
   A. true
   B. false
8. Nonequivalent control group designs generally use:
   A. randomization
   B. sampling
   C. blinding
   D. repeated measures

9. A study design that is used to gather information about how much calcium Americans are taking in each day would most likely be a:
   A. clinical trial
   B. comparative design
   C. descriptive cross-sectional design
   D. analytic cross-sectional design
10. The correlation coefficient tells you about:
   A. the direction of the relationship
   B. the strength of the relationship
   C. whether the independent variable caused the dependent variable to change
   D. a and b only
   E. a, b, and c
11. What are the three main features of experimental research?
12. Explain what intention-to-treat analysis is and why it is used.
13. Why could the Solomon four-group design be more rigorous than an RCT?
14. Describe four characteristics of a descriptive correlational design.
15. Explain what secondary data analysis is and give an example.

CRITICAL THINKING QUESTIONS

1. Read this article (see Appendix B) describing a randomized controlled trial and answer the following questions.

   Rajkumar, N., Karthikeyan, V. S., Manwar, S., Sistla, S. C., & Kate, V. (2013). Clear liquid diet vs soft diet as the initial meal in patients with mild acute pancreatitis: A randomized interventional trial. *Nutrition in Clinical Practice, 28,* 365–370.

   A. What is the objective for this study?
   B. Did this study take a prospective, retrospective, or cross-sectional approach?
   C. What are the independent and dependent variables?
   D. Describe the setting and the participants.
   E. What was the primary study outcome? Were there secondary outcomes that were measured? If so, describe.
   F. What statistical test was used to compare continuous variables? What *P*-value was considered significant?
   G. What were the results?
   H. What did the researchers conclude?
   I. Discuss the generalizability of this study to the United States.
2. Read this quasi-experimental study and answer the following questions.
   Humphrey. L., Clifford, D., & Neyman Morris, M. (2015). Health at Every Size college course reduces dieting behaviors and improves intuitive eating, body esteem, and anti-fat attitudes. *Journal of Nutrition Education and Behavior, 47,* 354–360. doi: 10.1016/j.jneb.2015.01.008
   A. What is the objective for this study? If the researchers had stated a hypothesis for this study, what do you think it would be?
   B. Why is this a quasi-experimental study?
   C. What are the independent and dependent variables?
   D. Who are the participants? Describe the intervention for the experimental group and comparison groups. What did the control group do?
   E. How many students completed both pretests and posttests by group? Briefly describe each instrument.
   F. ANOVA was used to compare mean scores of posttests among the three groups. ANOVA can tell you that there are significant differences between the groups, but it cannot pinpoint which groups. So which post hoc test was used to identify groups that had significantly different scores?
   G. Table 6.3 compares the mean scores for each instrument in two ways. First, it compares the pretest and posttest score within each group (using paired sample *t*-tests). Second, it compares the posttest scores between the three groups (using ANOVA with post hoc analysis). From pretest to posttest, where did the HAES

class experience statistically significant differences? For which instruments was the HAES posttest score significantly different from *both* the comparison and control group?

H. What did this study demonstrate?

3. Read this descriptive comparative study and answer the following questions.
Zizza, C. A., Sebastian, R. S., Wilkinson, C., Isik, Z., Goldman, J. D., & Moshfegh, A. J. (2015). The contribution of beverages to intakes of energy and MyPlate components by current, former, and never smokers in the United States. *Journal of the Academy of Nutrition and Dietetics, 115,* 1939–1949. doi: 10.1016/j.jand.2015.07.015

A. What was the purpose of this study? If the researchers had stated a hypothesis, what do you think it would be?

B. Is this study an example of secondary data analysis? If so, where did the data come from?

C. What are the independent and dependent variables?

D. Why is this a descriptive study?

E. Who are the three groups being compared?

F. Table 6.2 shows mean beverage intake in grams by beverage group and smoking status for men/women. Do male current smokers drink significantly more total beverages than nonsmokers? Do female current smokers drink significantly more total beverages than nonsmokers? Compare male and female current smokers to nonsmokers in terms of coffee and alcoholic beverage consumption. Note: Within the category of men or the category of women, means with *different* superscript letters (x, y, z) differ significantly as determined by the *t*-test.

G. Interpret Figure 6.2. If you have trouble doing that, read in the article where Figure 6.2 is discussed.

H. What did the researchers conclude?

SUGGESTED READINGS AND ACTIVITIES

1. Boushey, C., Harris, J., Bruemmer, B., Archer, S. L., & Van Horn, L. (2006). Publishing nutrition research: A review of study design, statistical analyses, and other key elements of manuscript preparation, Part 1. *Journal of the American Dietetic Association, 106,* 89–96. doi: 10.1016.j.jada.2005.11.007
2. Bruemmer, B., Harris., J., Gleason, Ph., Boushey, C. J., Sheean, P. M., Archer, S., & Van Horn, L. (2009). Publishing nutrition research: A review of epidemiologic methods. *Journal of the American Dietetic Association, 109,* 1728–1737. doi: 10.1016/j.jada.2009.07.011
3. Sheean, P. M., Bruemmer, B., Gleason, P., Harris, J., Boushey, C., & Van Horn, L. (2011). Publishing nutrition research: A review of multivariate techniques–Part 1. *Journal of the American Dietetic Association, 111,* 103–110. doi: 10.1016/j.jada.2010.10.010

REFERENCES

Atlantis, E., Salmon, J., & Bauman, A. (2008). Acute effects of advertisements on children's choices, preferences, and ratings of liking for physical activities and sedentary behaviours: A randomised controlled pilot study. *Journal of Science and Medicine in Sport, 11,* 553–557.

Bischoff-Ferrari, H., Dawson-Hughes, B., Orav, E. J., Staehelin, H. B., Meyer, O., Theiler, R., . . . Egli, A. (2016). Monthly high-dose vitamin D treatment for the prevention of functional decline: A randomized clinical trial. *JAMA Internal Medicine, 176,* 175–183. doi: 10.1001/jamainternmed.2015.7148

Boucher, B., Cotterchio, M., Kreiger, N., Nadalin, V., Block, T., & Block, G. (2006). Validity and reliability of the Block98 food-frequency questionnaire in a sample of Canadian women. *Public Health Nutrition, 9,* 84–93. doi: http://dx.doi.org/10.1079/PHN2005763

Boushey, C., Harris, J., Bruemmer, B., Archer, S. L., & Van Horn, L. (2006). Publishing nutrition research: A review of study design, statistical analyses, and other key elements of manuscript preparation, Part 1. *Journal of the American Dietetic Association, 106,* 89–96. doi: 10.1016.j.jada.2005.11.007

Bruemmer, B., Harris., J., Gleason, Ph., Boushey, C. J., Sheean, P. M., Archer, S., & Van Horn, L. (2009). Publishing nutrition research: A review of epidemiologic methods. *Journal of the American Dietetic Association, 109,* 1728–1737. doi: 10.1016/j.jada.2009.07.011

Campbell, D. T., & Stanley, J. C. (1963). *Experimental and quasi-experimental designs for research*. Belmont, CA: Wadsworth Cengage.

Chu, Y. H., Frongillo, E. A., Jones, S. J., & Kaye, G. L. (2009). Improving patrons' meal selections through the use of point-of-selection nutrition labels. *American Journal of Public Health, 99,* 2001–2005. doi: 10.2105/AJPH.2009.153205

Cook, T. D., & Campbell, D. T. (1979). *Quasi-experimentation: Design & analysis issues for field settings*. Boston, MA: Houghton Mifflin Company.

Eicher-Miller, H. A., Khanna, N., Boushey, C. J., Gelfand, S. B., & Delp, E. J. (2016). Temporal dietary patterns derived among the adult participants of the National Health and Nutrition Examination Survey 1999–2004 are associated with diet quality. *Journal of the Academy of Nutrition and Dietetics, 116,* 283–291. doi: 10.1016/j.jand.2015.05.014

Forbes, D. (2013). Blinding: An essential component in decreasing risk of bias in experimental designs. *Evidence-Based Nursing, 16,* 70–71. doi: 10.1136/eb-2013-101382

Grove, S. K., Burns, N., & Gray, J. R. (2013). *The practice of nursing research: Appraisal, synthesis, and generation of evidence*. St. Louis, MO: Elsevier Saunders.

Gupta, S. K. (2011). Intention-to-treat concept: A review. *Perspectives in Clinical Research, 2,* 109–112. doi: 10.4103/2229-3485.83221

Guyatt, G., Walter, S., Shannon, H., Cook, D., Jaeschke, R., & Heddle, N. (1995). Basic statistics for clinicians: 4. Correlation and regression. *Canadian Medical Association Journal, 152*, 497–504.

Higgins, J., & Green, S. (Eds.). (2011). *Cochrane handbook for systematic reviews of intervention* (Version 5.1.0). Retrieved from http://handbook.cochrane.org

Karanicolas, P. J., Farrokhyar, F., & Bhandari, M. (2010). Blinding: Who, what, when, why, how? *Canadian Journal of Surgery, 53*, 345–348.

Larson, N., Story, M., Eisenberg. M. E., & Newmark-Sztainer, D. (2016). Secular trends in meal and snack patterns among adolescents from 1999 to 2010. *Journal of the Academy of Nutrition and Dietetics, 116,* 240–250. doi: 10.1016/j.jand.2015.09.013

Lee-Kwan, S. H., Pan. P., Maynard, L. M., McGuire, L. C., & Park, S. (2016). Factors associated with self-reported menu-labeling usage among US adults. *Journal of the Academy of Nutrition and Dietetics, 116,* 1127–1135. doi: 10.1016/j.jand.2015.12.015

Locks, L. M., Manji, K. P., McDonald, C. M., Kupka, R., Kisenge, R., Aboud, S., . . . Duggan. C. P. (2016). Effect of zinc and multivitamin supplementation on the growth of Tanzanian children aged 6–84 weeks: A randomized, placebo-controlled, double-blind trial. *American Journal of Clinical Nutrition, 103,* 910–918. doi: 10.3945/ajcn.115.120055

Mathias K. C., Jacquier, E., & Eldridge, A. L. (2016). Missing lunch is associated with lower intakes of micronutrients from foods and beverages among children and adolescents in the United States. *Journal of the Academy of Nutrition and Dietetics, 116,* 667–676. doi: 10.1016/j.jand.2015.12.021

McAleese, J. D., & Rankin, L. L. (2007). Garden-based nutrition education affects fruit and vegetable consumption in sixth-grade adolescents. *Journal of the American Dietetic Association, 107,* 662–665. doi: 10.1016/j.jada.2007.01.015

Moher, D, Pham, B., Jones, A., Cook, D. J., Jadad, A. R., Moher, M., . . . Klassen, T. P. (1998). Does quality of reports of randomised trials affect estimates of intervention efficacy reported in meta-analyses? *Lancet, 352,* 609–613. doi: 10.1016/S0140-6736(98)01085-X

National Institutes of Health. (2008). *FAQ ClinicalTrials.gov—Clinical trial phases*. Retrieved from https://www.nlm.nih.gov/services/ctphases.html

Pildal, J., Hróbjartsson, A., Jørgensen, K. J., Hilden, J., Altman, D. G., & Gøtzsche, P. C. (2007). Impact of allocation concealment on conclusions drawn from meta-analyses of randomized trials. *International Journal of Epidemiology, 36,* 847–857.

Ramly, M., Ming, M. F., Chinna, K., Suboh, S., & Pendek, R. (2104). Effect of vitamin D supplementation on cardiometabolic risks and health-related quality of life among urban premenopausal women in a tropical country—A randomized controlled trial. *PLOS ONE, 9,* e110476. doi: 10.1371/journal.pone.0110476

Rosinger, A., & Herrick, K. (2016). *Daily Water Intake Among U.S. Men and Women, 2009–2012*. (NCHS Data Brief No. 242). Retrieved from http://www.cdc.gov/nchs/products/databriefs/db242.htm

Schulz, K. F., Altman, D. G., & Moher, D. (for the CONSORT Group). (2010). CONSORT 2010 statement: Updated guidelines for reporting parallel group randomised trials. *PLoS Medicine, 7,* e1000251. doi:10.1371/journal.pmed.1000251

Schulz, K. F., Chalmers, I., Hayes, R. J., & Altman, D. G. (1995). Empirical evidence of bias: Dimensions of methodological quality associated with estimates of treatment effects in controlled trials. *JAMA, 273*, 408–412. doi:10.1001/jama.1995.03520290060030.

Shadish, W. R., Cook, T. D., & Campbell, D. T. (2002). *Experimental and quasi-experimental designs for generalized causal inference*. Belmont, CA: Wadsworth Cengage.

Sheean, P. M., Bruemmer, B., Gleason, P., Harris, J., Boushey, C., & Van Horn, L. (2011). Publishing nutrition research: A review of multivariate techniques–Part 1. *Journal of the American Dietetic Association, 111,* 103–110. doi: 10.1016/j.jada.2010.10.010

Skinner, A. C., Perrin, E. M., & Skelton, J. A. (2016). Prevalence of obesity and severe obesity in US children, 1999–2014. *Obesity, 24,* 1116–1123. doi: 10.1002/oby.21497

Troup, R., Hayes, J. H., Raatz, S. K., Thyagarajan, B., Khaliq, W., Jacobs, D. R., . . . Gross, M. (2015). Effect of black tea intake on blood cholesterol concentrations in individuals with mild hypercholesterolemia: A diet-controlled randomized trial. *Journal of the Academy of Nutrition and Dietetics, 115*, 264–271. doi: 10.1016/j.jand.2014.07.02

CHAPTER 7

Epidemiologic Research Designs and Predictive Correlational Designs

CHAPTER OUTLINE

- Introduction
- Epidemiologic Research Designs
- Causality in Epidemiological Designs
- Predictive Correlational Designs
- Researcher Interview: Epidemiology, Dr. Patricia Markham Risica

LEARNING OUTCOMES

- Explain why cohort and case-control studies are considered observational analytic study designs.
- Explain the steps taken in an epidemiologic cross-sectional study and the output statistic.
- Compare and contrast the prospective cohort, retrospective cohort, and case-control study designs, and interpret relative risk, odds ratios, and other statistics used in these studies.
- Discuss the advantages and disadvantages of the epidemiologic cross-sectional design, cohort design, and case-control design.
- Explain criteria developed by Hill (1965) to help determine if a causal relationship (or causal effect) exists between variables such as risk factors and chronic diseases in epidemiological studies.
- Compare and contrast linear regression, logistic regression, and Cox regression.
- Interpret statistics used in regression, including beta coefficients and R-squared in linear regression, odds ratios in logistic regression, and hazard ratios in Cox regression.
- Discuss the advantages and disadvantages of different predictive designs.

INTRODUCTION

Epidemiology is a discipline within public health that looks at the rates of health-related states (such as disease) in different groups of people and why they occur. Epidemiologists, sometimes called disease detectives, try to connect the dots between risk factors (called "exposures" by epidemiologists) and health or disease outcomes. **Exposure** can mean any factor that is associated with an outcome of interest, such as a risk factor, a dose of a drug, a surgical procedure, or a vaccination. The outcome is usually a disease or condition. Epidemiological studies have provided the crucial link, for example, between cholesterol and heart attacks.

Nutrition epidemiology is a subdiscipline of epidemiology. Epidemiology includes descriptive and analytic areas of study.

1. **Descriptive epidemiology** provides information about who has a disease in a population and the disease's **prevalence** (number of *existing* cases of disease in a population) and **incidence** (number of *new* cases of a disease in a population during a specified period of time). In addition, it can tell us about the pattern of the disease—meaning the time, place, and personal characteristics of those with the disease (such as age, race, socioeconomic status, or behaviors). Descriptive epidemiology is vital to assess the health of a population or community, and also to find clues about possible contributing factors and causes of diseases and other health-related states.
2. **Analytic epidemiology** digs deeper to determine the strength of the association between a risk factor and the health-related state. For example, let's look at soda drinking by obese children. Studies found that as a child drinks more soda, the risk of becoming obese increases. Finding an association does not necessarily make it a causal relationship. Epidemiologists do use some research designs, such as intervention studies, to test the association between exposure and disease.

This chapter looks at three epidemiologic designs: cross-sectional, cohort, and case-control. There are additional epidemiologic designs, such as case reports or series, but they are not included here.

This chapter also examines predictive correlational designs. These designs use regression, which, like correlation, is used to quantify the relationship between two quantitative variables. But **regression analysis** goes further than correlation by finding out how much influence is exerted by the independent variable(s) on the dependent variable. Regression designs are also commonly used to predict the value of a dependent variable.

EPIDEMIOLOGIC RESEARCH DESIGNS

The three research designs we look at here (cross-sectional, cohort, and case-control) are all observational in nature. In observational designs, researchers do not "do" anything to participants, such as tell them to jump on a treadmill every day to lose weight or take a vitamin supplement to improve their bone status. Instead, researchers observe natural relationships between risk factors and outcomes and ask participants questions, such as how much they exercise each week or if they take a vitamin D supplement daily. In brief, researchers do not manipulate an independent variable in observational studies.

Observational designs are used when researchers cannot manipulate the independent variable—when it might be impossible or unethical. For example, you cannot randomly assign people to either smoke or not smoke, and then see who develops lung cancer and who does not. But you can select current smokers and nonsmokers and move forward in time to see what develops.

Cohort and case-control studies are observational *and* analytic. They are analytic because they try to identify and quantify associations between an exposure (risk factor) and an outcome (disease), and test hypotheses. In comparison, cross-sectional studies are completely observational and descriptive.

Epidemiological studies often look at risk—the chance that an outcome will occur. Several measures of risk can be used to compare the risk of an event or outcome between groups. Measures of risk provide a measure of the strength of the association between a risk factor/exposure and an outcome. Two measures of risk that we look at are relative risk (used in cohort studies) and odds ratio (used in case-control studies). Relative risk calculations from cohort studies are generally considered stronger evidence than odds ratios calculated in case-control studies.

Cross-Sectional

In epidemiology, cross-sectional studies collect data from the population of interest *at a particular point in time* (rather than over time as seen in cohort and case-control studies) to investigate associations between exposure and outcomes. *Cross-sectional studies attempt to describe and compare the prevalence of a disease (meaning the number of existing cases of disease in a population) in an exposed group and an unexposed group.*

A cross-sectional study begins with a sample population split up as follows:

1. Participants with a disease and who have exposure (A; see Table 7.1).
2. Participants without the disease who have exposure (B).
3. Participants with the disease but without exposure (C).
4. Participants without the disease and without exposure (D).

In epidemiology, data such as this is put in to a 2 × 2 table, also known as a contingency table (**Table 7.1**). *This table is always labeled with the disease/no disease along the top and the exposure/no exposure status on the side.* In this example, we are looking at diabetes as the disease, and obesity as the exposure or risk factor. So in this study, of the 500 people who are obese, 100 have diabetes and 400 do not (see shaded line). Of the 520 people who are not obese, only 20 have diabetes.

From this table, you can calculate the **prevalence ratio** in these three steps.

1. Divide A by A + B. So divide. 100 by 500 = 0.20
2. Divide C by C + D. So divide 20 by 520 = 0.038
3. Divide 0.20 by 0.038 = 5.3 = prevalence ratio

In the first step, you are calculating the prevalence rate of diabetes in the obese group by dividing the number of people with diabetes by the total number of people. In the second step, you are calculating the prevalence rate of diabetes in the nonobese group. *The prevalence ratio of 5.3 indicates the prevalence of diabetes in the obese group relative to the unexposed (nonobese) group. In this case, people who are obese are 5.3 times more likely to have diabetes than people who are not obese.*

Although cross-sectional studies are less expensive because they are generally done at one point in time, they are not as useful as other designs. Cross-sectional studies are descriptive only and useful for identifying associations. You cannot use a cross-sectional study to validate a cause–effect relationship because you do not know if exposure *preceded*

Table 7.1 Example of a Contingency Table

	Disease	No disease	Total
Exposure (obesity)	100 (A)	400 (B)	500 (A + B)
No Exposure (not obese)	20 (C)	500 (D)	520 (C + D)
Total	120 (A + C)	900 (B + D)	1020

the disease, which is a requirement for causality. Cross-sectional studies are also prone to selection and measurement bias.

COHORT DESIGN

In epidemiology a **cohort** is a group of individuals (usually quite a large group) who share a common characteristic (such as gender or geographical location) and are observed over time to gather information about exposures, such as health-related habits or even public policies, that can affect an outcome. A **cohort design** does not include an intervention or randomization. Instead researchers form a hypothesis about the potential causes of an outcome (such as colon cancer), and then measure a variety of variables that might be relevant to the development of the outcome while also observing who in the cohort develops the disease. Cohort studies work well in situations when it would not be safe to expose participants to a factor suspected to be harmful; however, a downside is that they are long-term and expensive studies.

Cohort studies are either prospective or retrospective (**Figure 7.1**):

- A prospective study goes forward in time with the cohort. The researchers identify the population, recruit participants representative of the target population, take baseline measurements, and continue to measure exposure and diseases into the future.
- In retrospective studies, researchers go back in time to identify a cohort of individuals at a point in time *before* the individuals have developed the disease or outcome of interest. Then the researchers try to establish whether they were exposed or unexposed based on prior records or the participants themselves, and the researchers will determine each person's subsequent outcome status, such as disease/no disease or death. What distinguishes retrospective cohort studies is that the researchers identify and enroll participants after the outcomes have occurred.

Figure 7.1 illustrates both types of cohort studies. The prospective study started in 2000 and will continue until 2030. The retrospective study was conceived in 2010 and went back to 1990 to start the same process. Both studies do the same thing, just one goes forward in time and the other starts at a point in the past.

Both studies have challenges, but the retrospective study researchers are constrained by the variables available in the data sets as well as by missing data. In a prospective

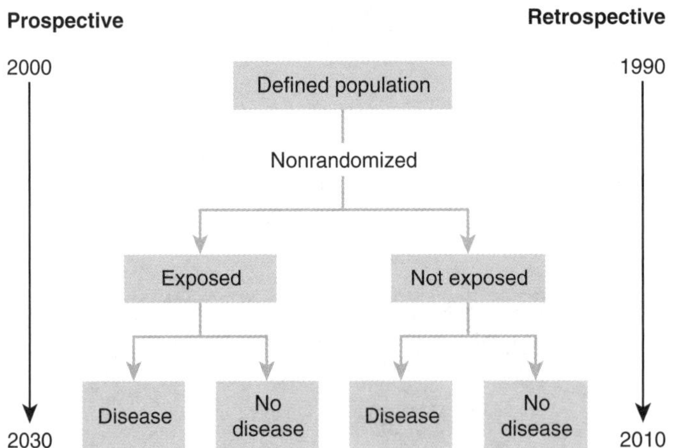

FIGURE 7.1 Prospective and Retrospective Cohort Studies

study, the researcher has many more options and control over selecting the cohort, the variables to be studied, frequency of follow-up, and so forth.

In 1948, the Framingham Heart Study (a prospective cohort study) started to study the impact of various factors or exposures on cardiovascular disease. For each exposure, researchers identified the "exposed" and "not exposed" groups, then followed these participants for the development of disease. Here are some of the exposures and outcomes that have been studied:

> Exposures: Diet, smoking, body weight, diabetes, exercise
> Outcomes: Blood pressure, coronary heart disease, stroke

The first cohort included more than 5,000 men and women (ages 30 to 62) from the town of Framingham, Massachusetts. After an initial physical exam and gathering of lifestyle data, they were asked to return every 2 years for another physical exam and medical history to evaluate risk factors and the development of cardiovascular disease. In 1971, another cohort was started; this time it included children and spouses of the first cohort. In 2002, the grandchildren of the original cohort were enrolled in a new study. The Framingham Heart Study now also includes the Omni Cohort, a group of men and women representing an ethnically diverse group. The original Omni cohort were residents of the Framingham area when the study started. In prospective cohort studies, researchers may use a fixed population in which all participants start the study at the same time (and no one can enter after that) or a dynamic population with participants entering at different times and replacing dropouts.

The goal of cohort studies is to compare the incidence of disease among the exposed to the incidence in the unexposed; this is expressed as a relative risk. Incidence is the number of *new* cases of disease in a population during a specific period of time per unit of population.

TIP

Do not confuse the terms *prevalence* and *incidence*. Prevalence describes the number of *existing cases* of disease in a population, either at one point in time or over a period of time. Incidence is the number of *new cases* of a disease in a population during a specific period of time. Incidence is useful in cohort studies because researchers are looking for new cases of a disease or outcome to crop up over time.

TIP

The cross-sectional study compared the *prevalence* of the exposed and unexposed groups, which resulted in a *prevalence ratio*. The prevalence ratio tells you about who is more likely to *have* a disease. The cohort study compares the *incidence* of the exposed and unexposed groups, which results in a *relative risk*. Relative risk tells you who is more likely to *develop* a disease.

A **risk ratio**, also called **relative risk** (RR), compares the probability of an outcome in two groups. One group is exposed to something (usually a risk factor), and the other group is not. Relative risk expresses how much more (or less) likely it is for the exposed person to develop an outcome (relative to an unexposed person). *Exposure* is usually a risk factor for a disease, but it also could be a treatment. Relative risk is calculated as follows:

$$\text{Relative Risk} = \frac{\text{Risk of outcome in exposed/treated group}}{\text{Risk of outcome in unexposed group}}$$

If a study's results show an RR of 1.0, there is no difference in risk between the groups, and the exposure did not increase or decrease risks of the outcome. If the RR is greater than 1, it suggests an *increased* risk of that outcome (such as developing hypertension) in the exposed group (perhaps they ate a high sodium diet). If the RR is less than 1, it suggests a *reduced* risk in the exposed group.

Let's look at a study about heart disease (the outcome) in men with and without diabetes. Diabetes is the exposure or risk factor. In this study, the RR for coronary heart disease was 3.0 for men. When risk is increased, as in RR = 3.0, you can interpret it in two ways:

1. Relative risk: The men with diabetes (exposed group) have 3 times the risk of coronary heart disease compared to men without diabetes.
2. Increased risk: Men with diabetes *increase* their risk of coronary heart disease by 200% compared to men without diabetes. Increased risk is calculated as: (Relative Risk – 1) × 100.

Now let's look at an example where RR is less than 1. Let's say an experiment had a group of pregnant women who were given vitamin and amino acid supplements (the exposure) and observed to see who developed preeclampsia (the outcome). Another group of pregnant women did not receive the supplements. Relative risk is used sometimes in randomized clinical trials where there is an intervention or treatment. The RR for this study was 0.25. This means that:

1. Relative risk: Pregnant women taking the supplements had 0.25 (or one-quarter) times the risk of preeclampsia compared to women not taking the supplements.
2. Decreased risk: The pregnant women taking the supplements had 75% *less risk* of developing preeclampsia than those not taking the supplements. Decreased risk is calculated the same as just shown: (Relative Risk – 1) × 100.

When you see an RR in a study, also look at its confidence interval. The confidence interval represents the range of values in which the RR for the population is likely to be found. Remember that a narrower confidence interval indicates a higher precision of the RR. If the confidence interval of the RR contains 1, then the RR is not likely to be statistically significant, and the association between the exposure and the outcome may be due to chance.

APPLICATION 7.1

A study looked at whether low-dose aspirin decreased heart attacks. The participants took either low-dose aspirin or a placebo for 5 years. The RR was 0.7. What was the exposure, and what was the outcome in this study? Interpret the RR.

In prospective cohort studies, you may also see the following statistical tests. These statistics take into account that variables are measured many times over the course of the study, which is referred to as repeated measures.

1. **Repeated measures ANOVA** or MANOVA. An ANOVA with repeated measures compares three or more group means based on a continuous dependent variable. **MANOVA** is an ANOVA with two or more continuous dependent variables. Both models assume fixed time points for the repeated measurements. Studies report the mean and the standard deviation (or standard error) for the groups at different time points.
2. **Linear mixed models**. Linear mixed models are extensions of linear regression and ANOVA. A benefit of using them is that you get a picture of the subject-level pattern of change over time, not just the population average pattern of change, which may be quite different. Also, in cohort studies, measurements may be obtained at unequal intervals or at different time points for different individuals, and measurements are sometimes missing. This can pose problems for traditional methods like ANOVA, but linear mixed models can handle participants at different time points and with incomplete measurements. Linear mixed models also provide the mean and the standard deviation (or standard error) for the groups at different time points.

For an example, let's look at a study that used data from the Framingham Heart Study to examine the association of dairy consumption on blood pressure and hypertension. Wang, Fox, Troy, Mckeown, and Jacques (2015) wanted to know if dairy consumption (independent variable) changed blood pressure or the risk of incident hypertension (dependent variables) among adults, while controlling for diet quality. Incident hypertension is the first occurrence at any follow-up examination of systolic blood pressure 140 mmHg or higher or diastolic blood pressure 90 mmHg or higher.

One part of the statistical analysis assessed the relationship between dairy consumption and changes in systolic and diastolic blood pressure using a linear mixed model. The other part of the statistical analysis used hazard rates (*which, for now, you can interpret as a relative risk [RR]*) to assess the relationship between dairy consumption and risk of incident hypertension.

1. *Participants*. The study used data from 2,636 participants in the Framingham Heart Study who underwent four examinations from 1991to 2008 and were free of hypertension at the start.
2. *Objective*. To see if dairy consumption (independent variable) changed blood pressure or the risk of incident hypertension (dependent variables) among adults, while controlling for diet quality.
3. *Measurements*. Each examination included a food frequency questionnaire, medical history, and physical exam including blood pressure measurement.
4. *Statistical analysis*. Two analyses were completed. First, a linear mixed model was used to assess the relationship between dairy consumption and changes in systolic and diastolic blood pressure. *Total* dairy consumption was categorized for each participant for each exam interval into one of three categories: <1 serving, 1 to <3 servings, and >3 servings/day. Consumption of *specific* dairy products, such as low-fat/skimmed milk or yogurt, were also categorized by serving/week.

   Second, hazard rates were calculated to assess the relationship between dairy consumption and risk of incident hypertension.

   All analyses were controlled for factors such as age, sex, lifestyle, overall diet quality using the Dietary Guidelines Adherence Index, metabolic factors, and medication use.
5. *Results*.

   A. The mean follow-up time span was 14.6 years. The linear mixed model looked at the mean annualized change in systolic blood pressure among the three categories of dairy consumption. Results showed, for example, participants who consumed ≥3 servings/day of dairy foods had 0.49 (SE 0.12) mmHg increases in systolic blood pressure every year compared with the 1.05 (SE 0.06) mmHg increase in the group who consumed <1 serving/week. The probability for this *trend* was significant ($P < 0.001$), controlling for the factors mentioned.

B. Overall, higher intakes of all dairy foods, low-fat/fat-free dairy foods, low-fat/skimmed milk, or yogurt were associated with *smaller annualized increases in systolic blood pressure* ($P < 0.05$).

C. The hazard rate (HR) of incident hypertension with each serving/day of total dairy was 0.93 (95% CI 0.86, 0.996), which means that *each additional serving of dairy/day was associated with a 7% reduced risk of incident hypertension* ($P = 0.04$). The HR of incident hypertension with each serving/week of yogurt was 0.94 (95% CI 0.90, 0.99), which means that each additional serving of yogurt/week was associated with 6% reduced risk ($P = 0.01$).

6. *Conclusion*: The researchers concluded that dairy consumption, as part of a nutritious diet, may help control blood pressure or delay the onset of hypertension (Wang et al., 2015).

A strength of cohort studies is that exposure status is determined and participants are selected *before* disease detection. Cohort studies are also quite versatile in that you can study multiple outcomes for each exposure, as well as multiple exposures on an outcome. Cohort studies are excellent for studying possible disease causes (etiology) and disease prognosis. In a narrative review, Temple (2016) summarized that "findings from randomized controlled trials are not necessarily more reliable than those from well-designed prospective cohort studies. We cannot assume that the results of RCT can be freely applied beyond the specific features of the studies" (p. 1). Limitations include that these studies are very time-consuming and expensive. As in many designs, researchers do have to spend a lot of time keeping participants active in the study to decrease loss to follow-up. If a disease is rare, a better design would be the case-control, which is described next.

CASE-CONTROL DESIGN

In a **case-control design**, we start with the outcome of interest—usually a disease (often something pretty rare)—and then work retrospectively to look at exposures (**Figure 7.2**). Participants with the disease or health-related condition are known as **cases**. All cases must have the same disease or other health-related condition, as well as meet inclusion criteria. After identifying the cases, the researchers must locate and recruit suitable controls—people without the disease but very similar to the cases. For example, if the cases are all middle-aged women, the control group should be similar.

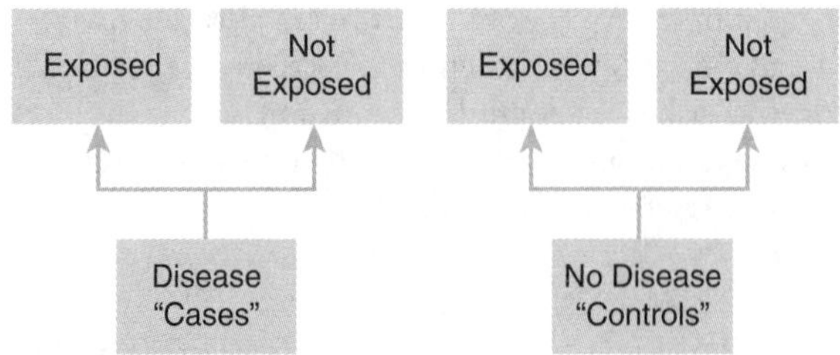

FIGURE 7.2 Case-Control Study Design

Matched pairs may be used in studies such as genetic studies where a case is matched to a genetic relative. The statistical test you use depends on whether matching is used.

Next the researchers use surveys and other techniques to determine differences in what each group was exposed to in the past. Case-control studies use **odds ratios** (OR). Odds ratios can look at the odds of an exposure (useful in case control studies) or an event (useful in logistic regression). In a case control study, you can think of an odds ratio as the odds that a case has been exposed to the risk factor of interest compared to the odds that a control has been exposed to the same risk factor.

Whereas relative risk tells you about the probability of an outcome, the odds ratio tells you about the odds. Odds and probability are not the same thing; they both express the likelihood of an outcome, but in slightly different ways.

- *Odds* is the number of times something happens *compared to the number of times it does not happen.*
- *Probability* is also the number of times something happens, but it is *compared to the number of times it could happen.*

If you know the odds, you can calculate the probability. Under some conditions, they are very similar.

Here is how to find the odds ratio in a case-control study:

$$\text{Odds Ratio} = \frac{\text{Odds of having the exposure among those with the disease (cases)}}{\text{Odds of having the exposure among those without the disease (controls)}}$$

Let's look at an example.

A researcher has exposure and outcome information from a case-control study on alcohol intake (high alcohol intake is the exposure) and esophageal cancer (disease) in which the OR is 3.55. Before we interpret an OR of 3.55, let's look at some basics on interpreting odds ratios.

- If the OR is 1, the odds of exposure are the same for cases and controls.
- If the OR is greater than 1, there is increased frequency of exposure among cases, and *exposure is positively related to disease, and could be a causal factor.* (This statistic alone does not show a cause-effect relationship.)
- If the OR is less than 1, exposure is negatively related to disease, meaning exposure is *protective.*

When an OR is calculated without controlling for any confounding variables, it is called a crude odds ratio.

An OR of 3.55 means the odds of high alcohol intake in the cases was 3.55 times higher than for the controls so *a higher alcohol intake is positively related to disease. If the odds ratio had been 0.4, then you can say that higher alcohol intake was protective against developing esophageal cancer. Although odds ratios are somewhat different from relative risk ratios, an OR in a case-control study is often interpreted in a way similar to an RR.* So an OR of 3.55 would then be interpreted as meaning the outcome (esophageal cancer) was 3.55 times more likely

TIP

Do not confuse a case-control study with a retrospective cohort even though they both go back in time. In a case-control study, the researcher says "I have 100 cases of people with Disease A, so then I found 100 people without Disease A, and compared the exposure status of the cases to the controls." In a retrospective cohort study, the researcher *separates groups by exposure and then looks at disease status.*

to occur in the cases than in the controls, or risk of the outcome in cases was increased by 255% relative to the controls.

An example of a case-control study comes from Dolwick Grieb et al. (2009). The objective of the study was to examine the effect of food groups and individual food items (the exposure) on renal cell carcinoma risk (the outcome).

1. *Participants*: Cases were identified from hospital records in three hospitals using the Florida Cancer Data System registry, if their diagnosis (renal cell carcinoma) occurred between 2000 and 2004 (this was done to allow for an adequate number of cases). Eligible cases were contacted, and 69% agreed to participate. The total sample included 335 cases and 337 controls. Controls were matched to cases by age (± 5 years), sex, and race.
2. *Objective*: To examine the effect of food groups and individual food items (the exposures or independent variables) on renal cell carcinoma risk (the outcome or dependent variable).
3. *Measurements*: All cases and controls had personal interviews where information (demographic, health and medical history. occupational history, family history, environmental and behavioral risk factors) was collected as well as calculation of BMI and completion of a 70-item block food frequency questionnaire (FFQ). Controls answered the FFQ using eating habits for the previous year. If a case had not altered his or her diet significantly since diagnosis, the FFQ was answered for the previous year. If the cases had altered their diet, they were asked to answer the FFQ for the year prior to diagnosis (so recall bias could be an issue in this study).
4. *Statistical Analysis*: For the analysis, the researchers used multiple logistic regression (discussed later in the chapter). Multiple logistic regression is used to explore relationships between two or more independent variables *and* a dichotomous dependent variable (disease/no disease). In this study, each independent variable (a food group or a food) was analyzed one at a time while also controlling for other variables such as age, sex, and income. For each independent variable, multiple logistic regression gives an odds ratio (odds of an outcome), 95% confidence intervals (CI), and its *P* value. All analyses were controlled for age, gender, race, income, BMI, and pack-years of smoking.
5. *Results*.
   A. Because the analysis controlled for these factors, the OR is called an **adjusted odds ratio** (AOR; see Table 7.2) and is more useful than a crude odds ratio, which does not control for any confounding variables. For *food groups*, the only group with significant results was the vegetable group (OR 0.56, 95% CI 0.35, 0.88). With an OR of 0.56, it showed that increased daily total consumption of vegetables *reduced* risk of renal cell carcinoma. Although the OR for fruits was less than 1, the result was not statistically significant.
   B. For *individual foods*, increased consumption of red meat significantly *increased* risk of renal cell carcinoma (OR 4.43, 95% CI 2.02, 9.75). Also increased consumption of white bread significantly *increased* risk for women only (OR 3.05, 95% CI 1.50, 6.20) as did total daily consumption of dairy (OR 2.36, 95% CI 1.21, 4.60).
   C. The results for some vegetables and potatoes are in **Table 7.2**. The frequency of eating is noted along the top of the table (from less frequent to more frequent). You will also notice that the AOR in the first column (less than once a week) is 1.00. This is because it is the reference, or denominator, in the adjusted odds ratios. For example, for tomatoes, the AOR under "5 or more times a week" is 0.50 (95% CI 0.31, 0.81), which is based on the odds ratio

Table 7.2 Adjusted Odds Ratio (AOR)[a], 95% Confidence Intervals (CIs), and Tests for Trend for Renal Cell Carcinoma by Consumption Frequency of Different Types of Vegetables and Fruits[a]

	Category of Consumption					
Vegetable or fruit item	**Less than once a week[b]**	**Once a week**	**Twice a week**	**3–4 times a week**	**5 or more times a week**	***P* for trend**
Fried potatoes[c]						
Total						
No. of cases	170	72	48	43	—	
No. of controls	213	59	27	34		
AOR (95% CI)	1.00	1.65 (1.08, 2.52)	2.40 (1.39, 4.15)	2.05 (1.19, 3.53)	—	<0.001
White potatoes (excluding fried varieties)						
Total						
No. of cases	105	79	74	58	17	
No. of controls	151	71	64	33	14	
AOR (95% CI)	1.00	1.63 (1.07, 2.50)	1.59 (1.03, 2.46)	2.56 (1.51, 4.33)	1.57 (0.70, 3.50)	0.02
Spinach and other greens (including collard greens)[c]						
Total						
No. of cases	232	48	36	17	—	
No. of controls	205	61	40	27		
AOR (95% CI)	1.00	0.71 (0.46, 1.11)	0.80 (0.48, 1.32)	0.55 (0.29, 1.07)	—	0.01
Tomatoes						
Total						
No. of cases	87	43	60	85	58	
No. of controls	82	34	44	81	92	
AOR (95% CI)	1.00	1.15 (0.65, 2.04)	1.22 (0.72, 2.07)	0.91 (0.58, 1.44)	0.50 (0.31, 0.81)	0.02

[a] Estimates from unconditional logistic regression, controlled for age at interview, sex, race, income, body mass index, and pack-years of smoking.
[b] Reference category
[c] The categories 3–4 times a week and 5 or more times a week were combined due to low numbers in the 5 or more category.
Reproduced from "Food Groups and Renal Cell Carcinoma: Results from a Case-Control Study," by S.M. Dolwick Grieb, R.P. Theis, D. Burr, D. Benardot, T. Siddiqui, and N.R. Asal, 2009, *Journal of the American Dietetic Association, 109*, p. 662-3. Reprinted with permission.

of "5 or more times a week" compared to "less than once a week." An AOR of 0.50 means that eating more tomatoes appears to be protective against renal cell carcinoma. The AOR for spinach and other greens (OR 0.55, 95% CI 0.29, 1.07) was also associated with a significant decrease in risk, but eating white potatoes (fried or not fried) was associated with a significant increase in risk (these results are in Table 7.2).

6. *Results*: The authors concluded that vegetables appear to have a protective role and meat consumption increases risk of renal cell carcinoma. They also reported new findings that white bread and white potato consumption seem to increase risk of renal cell carcinoma.

When looking at a confidence interval, keep in mind that a smaller confidence interval indicates a higher precision of the OR. Also, remember that if the confidence interval of the odds ratio contains 1, then the OR is not likely to be statistically significant.

APPLICATION 7.2

What are the OR and confidence intervals for fried potatoes and white potatoes? Were they significant? Interpret the OR for each.

Case control studies are less expensive and time-consuming than a number of other study designs, and they are efficient for studying rare diseases. They provide a potentially weaker causal investigation of an outcome, and often are not generalizable. Recall bias can be a real issue in this type of study, as participants are often asked about events, such as eating habits, from the past that cannot be confirmed in a medical chart or anywhere else. Recall bias can compromise internal validity.

Appendix D contain a checklist of items that should be included in reports of observational studies.

CAUSALITY IN EPIDEMIOLOGICAL DESIGNS

Experimental research may examine whether a cause-and-effect relationship exists between two variables. For studies (often epidemiological) looking at associations between risk factors (such as diet) and chronic diseases, researchers can use criteria developed by Hill (1965) to help determine if a causal relationship (or causal effect) exists between them. As you read the criteria in **Table 7.3**, keep in mind that one or more criteria likely will not apply or will not be met. This often happens in diet and nutrition studies because of issues such as measurement difficulties, the complexity of the disease process, and other issues noted below.

Because of some of the concerns mentioned, researchers recommend a minimum set of criteria to be used when inferring causality in associations between diet and chronic diseases (Potischman & Weed, 1999; Committee on Diet and Health, 1989). Potischman and Weed (1999) recommend using consistency of association, strength of association, dose response, biologic plausibility, and temporality (which are numbers 1–2 and 4–6 in the table). Researchers should also consider the "study design types, statistical tests, bias and confounding, and the quality of measurements" (Potischman & Weed, 1999, p. 1309S). The article by Potischman and Weed presents an insightful discussion on using causal criteria in nutrition epidemiology.

Table 7.3 Hill's Criteria for Causation

1. Strength of association	The stronger the association, the more likely the relationship is causal. Strength of association is often expressed as relative risk, which expresses how many times more (or less) likely an exposed person is to develop an outcome relative to an unexposed person. The problem with nutritional epidemiology is that associations are usually weak, with risk estimates that are considered low. However, if a dietary risk factor is common in the United States, a low risk estimate may indeed be causal and affect public health.
2. Consistency of association	If the association is seen consistently and across different research designs and statistical methods (when the studies are of high quality), the association is more likely to be causal.
3. Specificity	This criterion judges a causal relationship to be more likely if the effect has only one cause. In nutrition research, this can be very difficult to prove, as many different factors can affect one outcome (think about all the factors that influence obesity).
4. Temporality	The exposure (cause) must precede the effect or onset/progression of disease.
5. Biological gradient/ Dose response	If increased exposure increases the effect (as in smoking and lung cancer), then it increases the chance of causality. In diet and nutrition studies, dose response relationships may very well not have a linear shape. Sometimes a dose response relationship may be due to bias or confounding variables. Another problem is that if the people being studied are already exposed to levels above the threshold for the risk factor, increasing the dose may not increase the effect.
6. Plausibility	This looks at whether the cause and effect can be explained scientifically in a way that fits existing biological or medical knowledge.
7. Coherence	The cause and effect do not conflict with what is known about the disease.
8. Experimental evidence	An experimental study that backs up the cause and effect gives the strongest support for the relationship. (In nutrition research, a randomized controlled trial would have been done if it could have been done.)
9. Analogy	In some cases Hill considers judging by analogy, in other words using a more creative rather than scientific method.

Source: AB Hill, *Journal of the Royal Society of Medicine, 58(5)*, 295–300, © 1965 by SAGE. Reprinted by Permission of SAGE Publications, Ltd.

PREDICTIVE CORRELATIONAL DESIGNS

Correlation tells us about the strength and direction of the relationship between two variables, but it would be nice to know more about how much influence is exerted by the independent variable on the dependent variable, or the influence of *more than one* independent variable. You can use regression analysis, which also examines relationships among variables, to:

- Predict the value of the outcome variable from one or more predictor variables.
- Tell you if an independent variable really affects the dependent variable and the size of that effect.
- Control for extraneous variables.

Few studies just use correlation. Many studies testing for relationships use regression analysis in one of its forms. Being able to predict is important for some nutrition studies, but being able to see the size of the effect of independent variables on dependent variables while controlling for all those variables that "get in the way" is very useful.

Most regression models differ based on the type of dependent or outcome variable:

- In **linear regression** the dependent variable is continuous (such as weight or LDL).
- In **logistic regression** the dependent variable has a dichotomous outcome (such as disease/no disease).
- Cox regression is used in survival analysis when we look at time-to-event outcomes (such as time to remission).

The purpose of the following discussion on three types of regression is to give you the tools to understand and interpret the results of these studies as you read them in scientific journals. If you want to use regression in a study, it is best to consult a statistician because conditions must be met to perform each type of regression analysis, and building models involves many decisions. For example, multiple linear regression models are built gradually through a series of one variable, two variable, and multivariable methods. Decisions about which variables to include in a model, and how to code them, should also be based on expert knowledge and statistical considerations.

TIP

When you read a study using regression, identify the independent and dependent variables right from the start. In the scientific literature, you will find a number of synonyms for independent and dependent variables (see **Table 7.4**). For the discussion on regression, we will sometimes use the term "predictor" or "x" to refer to the independent variable, and "outcome" or "y" to refer to the dependent variable.

LINEAR REGRESSION

In **simple linear regression**, you predict the value of a continuous dependent variable from *one* independent variable (either continuous or categorical). In **multiple linear regression**, you can predict the value of the dependent variable from *two or more independent variables* (either continuous or categorical). To establish a relationship between the variables, linear regression always requires no more than one continuous dependent variable, a linear relationship between the variables, and normal distributions of the variables.

The first steps in a simple linear regression are to draw and evaluate a scatterplot (a graph in which the values of two variables are plotted) for form, direction, strength, and outliers (see end of Chapter 5). The next step is to calculate a correlation coefficient. Then a linear regression program is used to compute a line that "best" fits the data (**Figure 7.3**), and an equation is set up to predict the y variable from a given x variable.

Table 7.4 Terms Used for Independent and Dependent Variables in Correlation and Regression

Independent variable	Dependent variable
x	y
predictor	response
exposure	outcome
factor	disease
treatment	criterion

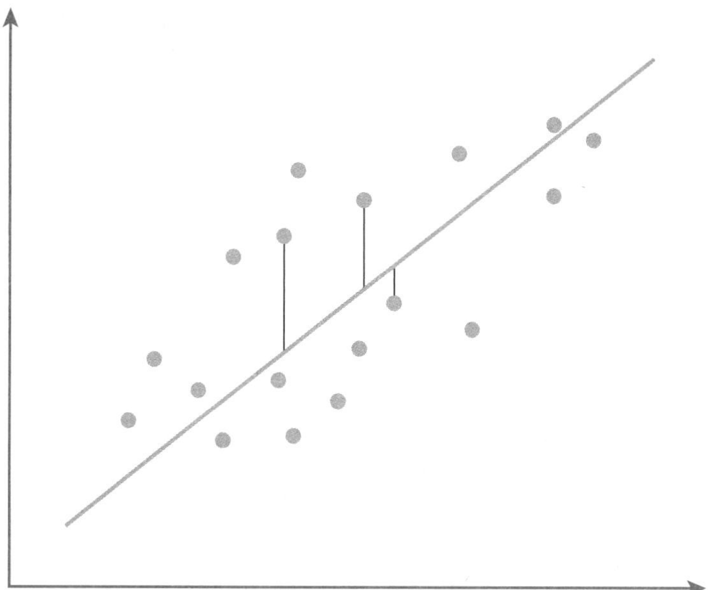

FIGURE 7.3 Linear regression analysis uses the Method of Least Squares to find the line that best fits the data with the least amount of vertical distance between the fitted line and the actual data.

Probability is used to determine whether the predictor (independent) variable significantly predicts the outcome (dependent) variable.

The square of the correlation coefficient, called **R-squared** (R^2 or r^2) is useful in linear regression because it tells you about the variance. *For example, an R-squared value of 0.59 means that 59% of the variance in the dependent variable can be accounted for by the independent variable(s).* The remaining 41% is unexplained. A helpful way to think about variance is to think of a pie chart. The entire pie chart represents all the variables that can contribute to changes in the dependent variable. Each R-squared indicates how large a section of the pie chart that variable earns. R-squared always has a value between 0 and 1, and may be called the coefficient of determination.

Evaluating R-squared requires looking at similar studies in your discipline, because values in some areas are quite low whereas others may be a good bit higher. A higher R-squared value is generally desirable, but not always necessary, especially if you have a large sample size.

R-squared provides an estimate of the strength of the relationship between the x and y, but it should not be used as a hypothesis test for this relationship. We also need to look at the regression coefficient. The **regression coefficient**, designated as B or β, is the slope of the regression line. When the slope, B, is standardized, it is called beta, β. Remember that B is in its original measurement units, while β is in standard deviation units. The slope (B or β) of the line represents how much the dependent variable changes for each 1-unit change in the independent variable (while holding other independent variables for the model constant). If B or β is negative, then for every unit increase in x, y decreases.

The higher the value of β, the more the independent variable affects the dependent variable. The value of β is tested against zero because zero means there is no significant association between the variables. *The independent variable is said to be a good predictor when β is significant* (meaning the associated *P*-value is less than alpha).

A purpose of multiple linear regression is to let you isolate the relationship between the predictor variables and the outcome variable from the effects of one or more confounding variables. Confounders are variables, such as age or income, that could influence the independent or dependent variables (**Figure 7.4**). In a study using regression, you may see the term **covariate** (also known as a **covariable**). A covariate is a variable that affects the dependent variable but is not the independent variable. *Covariates are often confounding variables*.

The process of isolating or accounting for confounding variables is called **adjustment** or **controlling**. Because adding more independent variables to the model increases R-squared, R-squared is often shown as "adjusted" R-squared in multiple linear regression to be more accurate.

In multiple regression, a problem can occur when the independent variables you are testing are highly correlated with each other. This is called **multicollinarity**. In French, *coller* means "to stick"; basically the independent variables are so highly correlated that you can think of them as sticking together. Multicollinarity is important because it can affect the reliability and stability of the regression coefficients. By doing a correlation analysis among all the independent variables, you can check on the actual correlation between each pair. If there is a problem with multicollinarity, you may have to remove one (or more) independent variables from the regression analysis, or perhaps combine them into one predictor.

TIP

Do not confuse multiple regression with multivariate regression. Multiple regression has several independent variables and one dependent variable. Multivariate regression refers to statistical models with *two or more dependent variables*. Up to this point, all the regressions we have talked about have had only one dependent variable. Any type of *multivariate* analysis always refers to the dependent variable, although researchers sometimes mistakenly call a multivariable regression a multivariate regression (Hildalgo & Goodman, 2013).

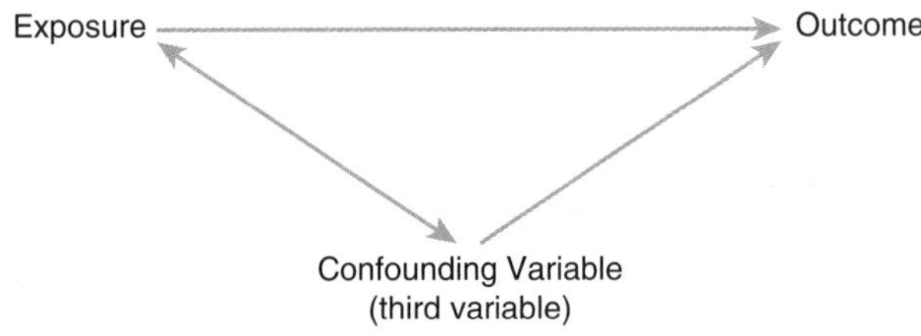

FIGURE 7.4 Relationship Between Exposure, Outcome, and the Confounder

Reproduced from "Key Concepts About Linear Regression" by Centers for Disease Control and Prevention, NHANES Web Tutorial, 2014. Retrieved from http://www.cdc.gov/nchs/tutorials/nhanes/NHANESAnalyses/LinearRegression/linear_regression_intro.htm

Let's look at a study that used multiple linear regression and see how to interpret the regression coefficients and R-squared. Robson et al. (2016) examined the relationship between the diet quality of a parent and his or her child to see if a parent's diet (independent variable) has a substantial impact on a child's diet (dependent variable).

1. *Participants*: Data was collected from 2007 to 2009 in Seattle, Washington, and San Diego, California, from 698 parent–child pairs.

2. *Objective*: To examine the relationship between the diet quality of a parent and his or her child to see if a parent's diet (independent variable) has a substantial impact on a child's diet (dependent variable).
3. *Measurements*: Using two to three 24-hour dietary recalls for each parent–child pair, diet quality was assessed using Healthy Eating Index (2010) scores and DASH scores.
4. *Statistics*: Before using multiple linear regression, the researchers used a paired *t*-test to compare the diet quality between parents and children, and they found that parent diet quality was significantly better than the child's. But the purpose of the study is really to see if a child's diet is most influenced by the parent's diet. So multiple linear regression models were used to examine *whether parent diet quality predicted (had a substantial impact on) child diet quality* after controlling for parent and child characteristics (sex, BMI, age, race), adult's highest level of education, and neighborhood type.
5. *Results*:
   A. **Table 7.5** shows the results of the multiple regression analysis. On the left are the independent variables (including parent diet quality), and the B/β (regression coefficient) is to the right for each independent variable. On the top of the chart is the dependent variable—the child's diet quality—which was measured using the Healthy Eating Index and also a DASH score. Regression coefficients are given to examine the relationship between each independent variable (controlling for other variables) and the dependent variable (the child's diet quality).
   B. The regression coefficients for each of the independent variables indicates the amount of change you could expect in the child's diet quality score given a 1-unit change in the independent variable. For example, the regression coefficient (B) for parent diet quality is 0.34 using the HEI-2010 score. This means that for every 1-unit increase in parent diet quality, child diet quality increases 0.34.
   C. The β (standardized B or *beta coefficients*) for parent diet quality is 0.39 (Healthy Eating Index), which means that for every 1 standard deviation increase in parent diet quality, child diet quality increases 0.39 standard deviations. *The higher the value of β, the more the independent variable affects the dependent variable.* Because beta coefficients are all measured in standard deviations, they can be compared. If you look at the β for the other independent variables under HEI-2010, you will see that parent diet quality has the largest β value, and it is statistically significant. It also has the lowest *P*-value (although two others are also statistically significant). The results are similar for the B/β using the DASH score.
   D. Sometimes the regression coefficient is negative, as you can see for the independent variable child age: −0.66. This means that for every 1-year increase in age, the child diet quality score *decreases* by 0.66. This study included children ages 6 to 12 years old, so older children are certainly more likely to be making more of their own food choices, for better or for worse.
   E. Table 7.5 also gives an R-squared value for the HEI-2010 and DASH scores. The R-squared is 0.17 for HEI-2010 and 0.13 for DASH. Basically, the total variance of child diet quality accounted for by all the independent variables ranges from 13 to 17%, which seems low. However, Robson et al. also calculated a different type of R-squared (semi-partial R-squared), which found that parent diet quality contributed an extra 15.1% and 10.4% of the variance in children's HEI-2010 and DASH scores (respectively) *independent* of other factors in the model.

Table 7.5 Multiple Linear Regression Models[a] Quantifying the Influence of Parent Diet Quality on Child Diet Quality by Controlling for Child Characteristics, Highest Household Education, and Neighborhood Type in a Sample of 698 Parent–Child Dyads from the Neighborhood Impact on Kids Study.

	Child Diet Quality Scores					
	Healthy Eating Index–2010			DASH Score		
Independent variables	B (β)	SE[b]	*P*-value	B (β)	SE	*P*-value
Child sex (female) (reference for sex is male)	0.84 (0.04)	0.81	0.30	0.67 (0.04)	0.62	0.28
Child BMI *z*-score	0.04 (0.00)	0.45	0.94	−0.28 (−0.03)	0.32	0.38
Child age	−0.66 (−0.09)	0.27	0.02	−0.58 (−0.10)	0.20	<0.01
Highest household education	0.83 (0.04)	0.68	0.22	0.58 (0.04)	0.52	0.26
Child race (nonwhite)	−0.00 (0.00)	1.03	1.00	−0.19 (−0.01)	0.84	0.82
High physical activity/High nutrition environment[c]	−1.77 (0.07)	1.12	0.12	−1.29 (−0.06)	0.88	0.14
High physical activity/Low nutrition environment[c]	−2.32 (0.09)	1.09	0.03	−1.59 (−0.08)	0.86	0.07
Low physical activity/High nutrition environment[c]	−1.16 (0.04)	1.15	0.32	−0.50 (−0.02)	0.87	0.57
Parent diet quality[d]	0.34 (0.39)	0.03	<0.001	0.28 (0.33)	0.03	<0.001
r^2	0.17			0.13		

Notes: [a]Maximum likelihood estimation was used to handle missing demographic data.
[b]SE is the standard error for the unstandardized beta coefficient (B).
[c]Reference for neighborhood type is low physical activity/low nutrition environment.
[d]Parent diet quality was adjusted for by parent characteristics, highest household education, and neighborhood type

6. *Conclusion*: They concluded that "Parent diet quality measures were significantly related to corresponding child diet quality measures: Healthy Eating Index-2010 (standardized β = .39; *P* < 0.001) and DASH score (standardized β = .33; *P* < 0.001)" (Robson et al., 2016, p. 984).

APPLICATION 7.3

Interpret the values of B/β for the Child BMI (independent variable).

LOGISTIC REGRESSION

When the dependent variable is continuous, you use linear regression. But what do you do if the dependent variable is dichotomous (such as disease/no disease)? Then you must use logistic regression. Logistic regression is often used to study how risk factors are associated with or predict the outcome (such as presence or absence of a disease). Unlike linear regression, logistic regression can assess relationships between independent and dependent variables that are *not* linear.

There are two types of logistic regression:

1. **Simple logistic regression** is used to explore associations between one dichotomous dependent variable and one independent variable (continuous, ordinal, or categorical). Simple logistic regression lets you answer questions like, "how does weight fluctuation affect the probability of postmenopausal breast cancer among women who gained weight as adults?" In this example, the independent variable is weight fluctuation and the dependent variable is postmenopausal breast cancer/no postmenopausal breast cancer.
2. **Multiple logistic regression** is used to explore associations between one dichotomous dependent variable and two or more independent variables (continuous, ordinal, or categorical). Multiple logistic regression lets you answer a question such as, "how do sociodemographic characteristics of Latinos affect the probability that they will read the Nutrition Facts labels while shopping for food?" Sociodemographic characteristics are the independent variables and the dependent variable is reading/not reading food labels.

Like other regression analyses, logistic regression can assess relationships between a dependent variable and several independent variables *while controlling for confounding variables.*

For each independent variable, the statistical analysis provides a regression coefficient (B), its associated P-value, and an odds ratio with confidence intervals. Logistic regression produces an odds ratio because the dependent variable only has two values, such as having diabetes/no diabetes. Remember that a smaller confidence interval indicates a higher precision of the OR.

The regression coefficient in a logistic regression does not have the same meaning as in linear regression, so to assess the effect of each independent variable, you should use the odds ratio. The odds ratio may be noted as Exp(B) on the software output. Also remember that if the confidence interval of the odds ratio contains 1, then the OR is not likely to be statistically significant.

In logistic regression, the odds ratio is the ratio of odds of an outcome (dependent variable) occurring for two groups. Let's say we are looking at the odds of a heart attack (outcome) in men and women (two groups). The outcome or dependent variable is the heart attack, and the independent variable is gender (male or female). An OR of 1.0 means that the odds of the outcome in males or females are the same.

When interpreting an OR that is greater or less than 1 for an independent variable with two or more levels, it is important to know which group appears in the numerator and the denominator of the odds ratio. The odds ratio is a fraction of the odds of the outcome in one group compared to the odds of the outcome in another group. For example, if the odds ratio for heart attacks compares males (numerator) to females (denominator), then an OR of 2.5 means that the odds of having a heart attack are 2.5 times higher for males than females. If the odds ratio compares females (numerator) to males (denominator), then an OR of 2.5 means that the odds of having a heart attack are 2.5 times higher for females than males. *Whichever independent variable is coded as "1" is in the numerator of the fraction.*

If the OR for male/female is 0.49, then males have 0.49 the odds of females. You could also say that males are 51% less likely to have a heart attack than females. You should only use percentages when the OR is close to 1.

If the independent variable is continuous, such as BMI, an odds ratio of 1.5 is interpreted as "for every 1-unit increase in BMI, the odds are 1.5 times greater to have hypertension (if hypertension is the dependent variable)." Note that in much research, BMI may not be used as a continuous variable.

TIP

Whenever you see an odds ratio, first identify the independent variable and the outcome or dependent variable. For example, a study looked at gestational diabetes outcomes in white and black pregnant women (adjusted for age). In this study, the "outcome" is whether or not the women develop gestational diabetes. Being black is treated as a "risk factor," so the odds ratio compares the odds of a black woman developing gestational diabetes to the odds of a white women developing gestational diabetes. If this odds ratio is 4.0, it means that the odds of developing gestational diabetes is 4 times higher for black mothers than for white mothers.

Knapik et al. (2016) did a survey of supplement use by U.S. Navy and Marine Corps personnel that included the use of multivariable logistic regression. The purpose of the cross-sectional study was to "investigate dietary and nutritional supplement use in Navy and Marine Corps personnel, including the prevalence, types, factors associated with use, and adverse effects" (p. 1423). This study is a good example of how you can use survey data to go beyond descriptive statistics. In this case, the authors examine the factors associated with use of dietary and nutritional supplements in a given population using logistic regression.

1. *Participants*: From a random sample of 10,000 Navy and Marine Corps personnel, the researchers obtained 1,683 questionnaires that were used for analysis.
2. *Objective*: "Investigate dietary and nutritional supplement use in Navy and Marine Corps personnel, including the prevalence, types, factors associated with use, and adverse effects" (Knapik et al., 2016, p. 1423).
3. *Measurements*: The questionnaire asked service members for personal characteristics (including physical activity) and frequency of use of specific dietary supplements (over the past 6 months) including 70 generic dietary supplements and nutritional supplements and 111 brand-name products. Dietary supplements included, for example, multivitamin/multiminerals, protein or amino acids, herbal supplements, and combination products. Nutritional supplements included sports drinks, sports bars or gels, and meal-replacement beverages. In addition, participants were asked questions about adverse effects of any of these products. *Descriptive data was collected from the survey and multivariable logistic regression was used to see which factors were most associated with dietary supplement use.*
4. *Results*:
   A. Seventy-three percent of service members reported using dietary supplements at least once a week, and the most common supplements were multivitamins/multiminerals, protein/amino acids, and combination products. Sport drinks and sport bars/gels were used by 45% and 23% of respondents.
   B. Most of the results from the logistic regression are noted in **Table 7.6**. On the left side of the chart are the independent variables being tested. As you can see, this was gathered from the personal characteristics section of the questionnaire. On the top of the chart are the dependent variables (each was tested separately). The first six columns, starting with Any Dietary Supplement, relate to whether some type of dietary supplement was taken at least once a week. The final column asked if respondents took any nutritional supplement at least once a week. Each dependent variable has two levels. For example, the

Table 7.6 Factors Associated with Dietary and Nutritional Supplement use among Navy and Marine Corps Personnel[a] (Odds Ratios with 95% CI)

		Dietary Supplements Taken 1 or More Times per Week						
Variable	**Strata**	**Any DS[b]**	**Use of ≥ 5 DSs**	**MVM[c]**	**Protein or AA[d]**	**Combination Products**	**Herbal**	**Any NS[e] taken 1 or more times/ week**
		Odds ratio (95% CI)						
Sex	Male	1.00	1.00	1.00	1.00	1.00	1.00	1.00
	Female	1.76 (1.32–2.36)	1.37 (10.4–1.81)	1.85 (1.44–2.39)	0.62 (0.46–0.83)	1.12 (0.85–1.48)	1.56 (1.11–2.18)	0.68 (0.53–0.87)
Age	18–24 y	1.00	1.00	1.00	1.00	1.00	1.00	1.00
	25–29 y	1.18 (0.84–1.67)	0.83 (0.59–1.15)	1.25 (0.92–1.70)	0.93 (0.66–1.30)	0.97 (0.69–1.34)	0.99 (0.66–1.51)	0.74 (0.54–1.00)
	30–39 y	1.36 (0.95–1.96)	0.95 (0.68–1.34)	1.58 (1.15–2.17)	0.86 (0.60–1.22)	1.45 (1.03–2.04)	0.91 (0.59–1.40)	0.78 (0.57–1.07)
	≥40 y	1.30 (0.84–2.02)	0.89 (0.58–1.37)	1.43 (0.97–2.12)	0.56 (0.35–0.87)	0.89 (0.58–1.38)	1.28 (0.77–2.14)	0.67 (0.54–1.00)
Education	Some HS[f]/HS graduate	1.00	1.00	1.00	1.00	1.00	1.00	1.00
	Some college	2.27 (1.68–3.06)	1.81 (1.33–2.45)	1.59 (1.21–2.10)	1.44 (1.06–1.97)	1.48 (1.10–1.99)	1.47 (1.00–2.17)	1.16 (0.88–1.53)
	College degree	2.23 (1.62–3.30)	1.49 (1.03–2.14)	1.77 (1.28–2.45)	1.66 (1.16–2.40)	1.10 (0.77–1.57)	1.11 (0.70–1.76)	1.16 (0.84–1.61)
Marital Status	Single	1.00	1.00	1.00	1.00	1.00	1.00	1.00
	Married	1.14 (0.87–1.49)	0.94 (0.73–1.22)	0.98 (0.77–1.25)	0.90 (0.69–1.17)	0.83 (0.64–1.07)	1.09 (0.78–1.51)	0.95 (0.75–1.21)
Body Mass Index	<25.0	1.00	1.00	1.00	1.00	1.00	1.00	1.00
	25.0–29.9	1.26 (0.98–1.63)	1.48 (1.15–1.91)	1.19 (0.95–1.49)	1.46 (1.13–1.89)	1.70 (1.32–2.19)	1.32 (0.96–1.82)	1.08 (0.86–1.36)
	>30.0	1.67 (1.06–2.63)	2.27 (1.50–3.45)	1.52 (1.03–2.25)	1.37 (0.88–2.13)	2.44 (1.61–3.69)	2.24 (1.37–3.67)	1.21 (0.82–1.79)
Aerobic exercise duration	0–100 min/wk	1.00	1.00	1.00	1.00	1.00	1.00	1.00
	101–180 min/wk	0.83 (0.60–1.16)	0.78 (0.55–1.10)	0.80 (0.59–1.08)	0.74 (0.52–1.06)	0.80 (0.57–1.11)	0.95 (0.62–1.45)	1.12 (0.83–1.51)
	181–290 min/wk	0.98 (0.70–1.37)	0.92 (0.67–1.28)	0.81 (0.60–1.09)	0.93 (0.66–1.30)	0.80 (0.58–1.10)	1.08 (0.71–1.62)	1.35 (1.01–1.82)
	>291 min/wk	0.83 (0.58–1.19)	0.89 (0.63–1.25)	0.87 (0.64–1.19)	0.75 (0.53–1.06)	0.72 (0.51–1.01)	1.30 (0.85–1.99)	1.45 (1.06–1.98)

(continues)

Table 7.6 Factors Associated with Dietary and Nutritional Supplement use among Navy and Marine Corps Personnel[a] (Odds Ratios with 95% CI) (continued)

		Dietary Supplements Taken 1 or More Times per Week						
Variable	**Strata**	**Any DS[b]**	**Use of ≥ 5 DSs**	**MVM[c]**	**Protein or AA[d]**	**Combination Products**	**Herbal**	**Any NS[e] taken 1 or more times/ week**
					Odds ratio (95% CI)			
Resistance training duration	0–45 min/wk	1.00	1.00	1.00	1.00	1.0	1.00	1.00
	46–135 min/wk	1.27 (0.94–1.74)	1.78 (1.25–2.53)	1.34 (1.00–1.79)	2.16 (1.48–3.16)	1.63 (1.16–2.29)	1.18 (0.79–1.76)	1.38 (1.04–1.83)
	136–270 min/wk	2.37 (1.65–3.40)	3.17 (2.19–4.59)	1.92 (1.40–2.65)	5.16 (3.49–7.62)	3.20 (2.23–4.59)	1.49 (0.97–2.28)	1.35 (0.99–1.86)
	>271 min/wk	2.85 (1.94–4.17)	4.90 (3.35–7.17)	2.12 (1.51–2.96)	9.15 (6.10–13.73)	4.74 (3.26–6.88)	0.92 (0.57–1.48)	1.42 (1.02–1.98)

[a] Multivariate logistic regression
[b] DS = Dietary Supplement
[c] MVM = Multivitamin/Multimineral
[d] AA= amino acid
[e] NS = nutritional supplement
[f] HS = high school

Reproduced from "Prevalence, Adverse Events, and Factors Associated with Dietary Supplement and Nutritional Supplement Use by U.S. Navy and Marine Corps Personnel." by J. J. Knapik, D. W. Trone, K. G. Austin, R. A. Steelman, E. K. Farina, & H. R. Lieberman, 2016, *Journal of the Academy of Nutrition and Dietetics, 116*, 1434–1435. Reprinted with permission of the Academy of Nutrition and Dietetics and Elsevier.

first column looks at whether the respondents took any dietary supplements at least once a week: either they did or they did not.

C. The table shows odds ratios with 95% confidence intervals. For example, let's look at the results for males/females (independent variable) using the first column (Any Dietary Supplement). First, you will notice that the OR for "Males" is 1.00 as it is for the first entry of all the independent variables listed. Since the OR looks at two groups, when you see 1.00 after "Male," that means "Male" is in the reference group and is automatically put into the denominator (bottom) of the fraction. So the OR of 1.76 for females means that odds are 1.76 times higher for a female than for a male to be taking dietary supplements one or more times a week.

D. For another example, let's look at the independent variable: resistance training. This variable has four levels, depending on how much time is spent on it each week. The first level has an odds ratio of 1; this is basically the comparison group (or bottom of the odds ratio fraction) for all the odds ratios listed below it. If someone does resistance training more than 271 minutes/week, the odds of that person taking dietary supplements at least once a week are 2.85 higher than for someone who only does up to 45 minutes of training/week.

5. *Conclusion*: Factors that were associated with using dietary supplements at least once a week were female sex (OR = 1.76, 95% CI 1.32–2.36), higher educational level (OR = 2.23, 95% CI 1.62–3.30), higher body mass index (OR =

1.67, 95% CI 1.06–2.63), and a greater amount of time spend resistance training (OR = 2.85, 95% CI 1.94–4.17). Herbal supplement use was independently associated with female sex (OR = 1.56, 95% CI 1.11–2.18) and higher BMI (OR = 2.24, 95% CI 1.37–3.67). Nutritional supplement use was associated with longer weekly duration of aerobic (OR = 1.45, 95% CI 1.06–1.98) and resistance training (OR = 1.42, 95% CI 1.02–1.98).

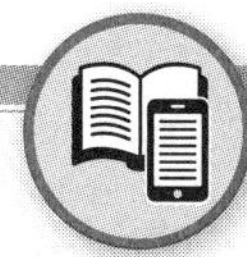

APPLICATION 7.4

Compare and interpret the odds ratios for the dependent variable "takes protein or amino acid supplements at least once a week." Which factors are most associated with taking this type of supplement?

Survival Analysis (Time-to-Event) and Cox Regression

Whereas logistic regression is useful to study risk factors for a disease, sometimes we are more interested in learning about how a risk factor, or treatment, affects the length of time until someone is diagnosed with a disease (such as diabetes) or some other event/clinical outcome such as remission. **Survival analysis** is appropriate to analyze data in which the length of time to an event is of interest. For example, a researcher may want to investigate the length of time until death occurs after a treatment intervention, or the length of time before cognitive decline occurs in older women with different dietary patterns. The event is not always death, and can indeed be positive such as recovery. The time from a defined point to the occurrence of a given event is referred to as **survival time**.

The objective of survival analysis for a study may be any of the following:

1. To estimate time-to-event for one group of individuals, such as time to type 2 diabetes diagnosis for individuals with prediabetes.
2. To compare time-to-event between two or more groups, such as remission in cancer patients receiving different chemotherapy drugs.
3. To assess the relationship of other variables to time-to-event, such as if weight or LDL levels affect survival time of patients after a myocardial infarction.

Examples of research designs that use survival analysis techniques include cohort studies (such as the Nurse's Health Study) and clinical trials that follow an exposure or risk factor (such as eating a Mediterranean diet) forward to an event or outcome (such as diagnosis of hypertension).

Regression models are used in survival analysis. **Cox's proportional hazards model**, also called **Cox regression**, is commonly used and is considered a semi-parametric test. Cox regression is useful to analyze the effect of several independent variables as it models survival rates over time. The dependent variable is always the event occurred/event didn't occur—a dichotomous variable as we saw in logistic regression. The Cox regression can also test the difference between survival times of groups while allowing covariate variables to be taken into account.

Whereas logistics regression provides odds ratios to present the relationship between the independent and dependent variables, the Cox model provides an estimate of the **hazard ratio** (HR) and its confidence interval. The hazard ratio is a ratio of the hazard rate of one group to the hazard rate in another group. **Hazard** is defined as the probability that an individual at any given time has an event at that time (assume the individual was event-free up to then). Hazard rates answer the question, "Does a specific risk factor/treatment cause the event to occur earlier or later than without the risk factor/treatment?" Here is the equation for finding the hazard ratio:

$$\text{Hazard Ratio} = \frac{\text{risk of event in treated/exposed group}}{\text{risk of event in control/comparison group}}$$

The hazard ratio may be noted as Exp(B) on the software output.

Whenever HR is 1, the event rate or risk for each group is the same. When HR = 2, it means that at any time twice as many participants in the treatment/exposed groups are having an event proportionally to the comparison group. If HR is less than 1, fewer participants in the treatment/exposed group are having an event proportionally to the comparison group.

Hazard ratios are often interpreted like relative risk. Just keep in mind that hazard ratios look at the ratio every moment *along* the time span of the study, whereas relative risk looks at the total number of events at the *end* of the study. *In other words, hazard ratios give you instantaneous risk at a point in time, and relative risk gives cumulative risk over the time of the study*. It is best to consider the hazard ratio alongside a measure of time, such as median survival.

For an example, let's look at a cohort study (not a real one!) where the event is all-cause mortality (dependent variable). The independent variables are systolic blood pressure, LDL level, and smoking. Results from the Cox regression give a hazard ratio (with 95% confidence intervals) for each independent variable, and all the independent variables are significant except LDL levels. Here is the key to interpreting HRs.

- For a continuous independent variable such as systolic blood pressure, if the HR is 1.15, it is interpreted as "for every 1-unit increase in systolic blood pressure, there is a 15% increase in all-cause mortality, holding the other variables constant." If HR is less than 1.0, as in 0.943, then the risk of all-cause mortality is reduced by 5.7% (100% − [100% × 0.943] = 5.7%) for each 1-unit increase in systolic blood pressure.
- For dichotomous independent variables, such as smoker/nonsmoker, interpret the hazard ratio directly from the output. For example, if the hazard ratio is 1.29 for a current smoker, then the risk of all-cause mortality for the current smoker is 1.29 times that of a nonsmoker, or 29% more likely, holding other variables constant. If the hazard ratio is 3.0, then the smoker was 200%, or twice, as likely to experience the event than nonsmokers. If the hazard ratio is 0.66, smokers have 0.66 the risk that nonsmokers do of all-cause mortality. You could also say that smokers are 34% less likely to experience all-cause mortality at any time than nonsmokers.

A survival analysis may also include a **Kaplan-Meier survival plot**. **Figure 7.5** is an example from a retrospective cohort study looking at time-to-medical-fall for people 65 and older (Greenwood-Hickman, Rosenberg, Phelan, & Fitzpatrick, 2015). The independent variable was exercise, and the study looked at users and nonusers of one of two different exercise programs for older adults (EnhanceFitness or Silver Sneakers). The *x*-axis represents the time of the study (in this case in days) from Day 0 to its end-point. The *y*-axis represents the probability of surviving a given time. In this study, survival means you do not have a medical fall (defined as a fall requiring medical treatment).

At the start of the study, all data points are at the upper left of the graph because the participants are all event-free. As events (medical falls) occur, the lines start to slope

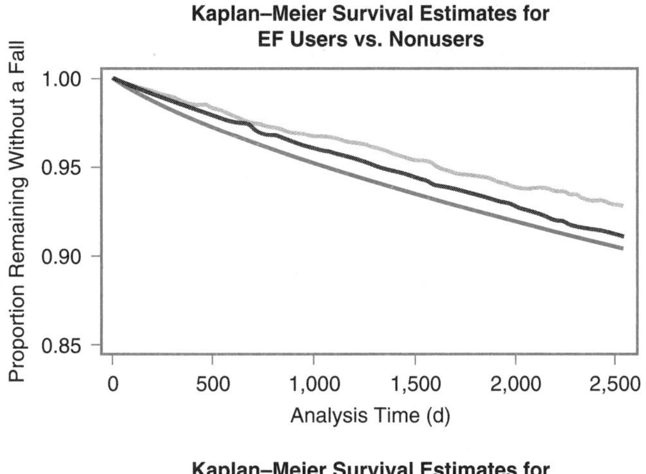

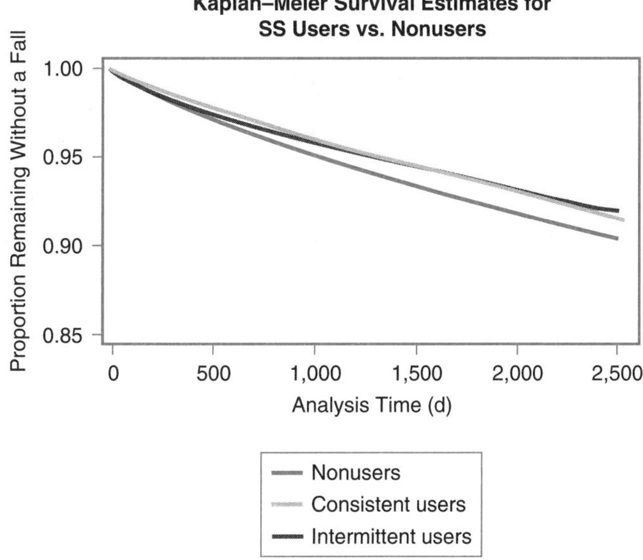

FIGURE 7.5 Kaplan-Meier survival curve of time to first medical fall for EnhanceFitness users among enrollees of the Group Health Integrated Group Practice (Seattle, Washington) by consistent, intermittent, and nonusers.

Reproduced from "Participation in Older Adult Physical Activity Programs and Risk for Falls Requiring Medical Care, Washington State, 2005 – 2011." by M. A. Greenwood-Hickman, D. E. Rosenberg, E. A. Phelan, and A. L. Fitzpatrick, 2015, *Preventing Chronic Disease, 12*, 3. Reprinted courtesy of Centers for Disease Control and Prevention.

down. A drop in the curve may reflect an event or a censored participant (such as a participant who withdraws or is lost to follow-up). A survival curve that drops sharply suggests poor survival. In Figure 7.5, each curve looks at different groups of participants: constant users, intermittent users, and nonusers of one of the exercise programs. The consistent users have the least number of medical falls when compared to the other groups.

The results from the Greenwood-Hickman et al. (2015) study are displayed in **Table 7.7**. First, you can see that there are different results shown for each of the three models used. The crude model does not adjust for covariates. The demographic model adjusts for age, race, and sex; and the full model adjusts for age, race, and sex as well as other covariates such as BMI and comorbidities (such as visual impairment). The top

Table 7.7 Risk of a Medical Fall Among EF/SS Users Compared with Nonusers, Washington State, United States, 2005–2011

	Group	*N*	Crude Model, HR (95% CI)	*P* Value	Demographic Model,[a] HR (95% CI)	*P* Value	Full Model,[b] HR (95% CI)	*P* Value
EF	Nonusers	55,127	1 [Reference]	—	1 [Reference]	—	1 [Reference]	—
	Intermittent	1,578	0.90 (0.84–0.98)	0.009	0.84 (0.77–0.91)	<0.001	0.87 (0.80–0.94)	0.001
	Consistent	517	0.73 (0.62–0.86)	<0.001	0.71 (0.60–0.84)	<0.001	0.74 (0.63–0.88)	<0.001
SS	Nonusers	55,127	1 [Reference]	—	1 [Reference]	—	1 [Reference]	—
	Intermittent	9,623	0.85 (0.82–0.88)	<0.001	0.92 (0.88–0.95)	<0.001	0.93 (0.90–0.97)	<0.001
	Consistent	3,953	0.83 (0.78–0.89)	<0.001	0.93 (0.87–0.99)	0.03	0.95 (0.89–1.02)	0.18

Abbreviations: CI, confidence interval; EF, EnhanceFitness; HR, hazard ratio; SS, Silver Sneakers.

[a] Model adjusted for age, sex, and race.

[b] Model adjusted for age, sex, race, and all covariates.

Reproduced from "Participation in Older Adult Physical Activity Programs and Risk for Falls Requiring Medical Care, Washington State, 2005 – 2011." by M.A. Greenwood-Hickman, D. E. Rosenberg, E. A. Phelan, and A. L. Fitzpatrick, 2015, *Preventing Chronic Disease*, *12*, 3. Reprinted courtesy of Centers for Disease Control and Prevention.

half of the chart shows results for EnhanceFitness (EF) and the bottom half is for Silver Sneakers (SS) users.

Let's look first at the EnhanceFitness program. The hazard ratio is given for the intermittent users and consistent users for each model. All of these hazard ratios are less than 1, which means that both groups of exercisers have a lower risk of medical falls than the nonusers (the reference group). For example, using the full model that adjusts for all covariates, the HR for consistent users of EnhanceFitness was 0.74. This means that consistent users have a 26% decreased risk of a medical fall compared with nonusers. The HR for intermittent users is 0.87, so they have a 13% decreased risk compared with nonusers. Each hazard ratio for the EnhanceFitness intermittent and consistent groups is statistically significant across models.

For the Silver Sneakers program, all of the HRs are less than 1, but one was not statistically significant. Using the full model, the HR for intermittent users was 0.93, meaning that intermittent users have a 7% decreased risk of a medical fall compared with nonusers. The HR for consistent users was actually higher, 0.95, so they have only a 5% decreased risk, and this was the only insignificant HR.

Each hazard ratio for EnhanceFitness and Silver Sneakers has a 95% confidence interval displayed. For the statistically significant hazard ratios, notice that the 95% confidence intervals do not include 1 (the null value: where there is no difference between groups). In contrast, the 95% confidence intervals for the one hazard ratio that is not statistically significant goes from 0.89 to 1.02, so it includes 1.

The authors concluded that "the magnitude of the association observed for Silver Sneakers participants was smaller than that seen with EnhanceFitness, a more structured program that includes balance and strength exercises that research suggests are critical to reducing fall risk" (Greenwood-Hickman, 2015, p. 4).

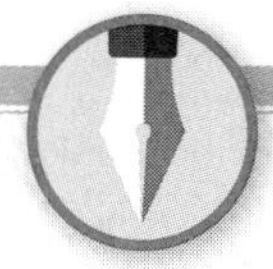

TIP

We have discussed three types of regression. Here's a summary to help you keep them straight. Remember that regression can control for covariates.

1. In simple linear regression, you predict the value of a continuous dependent variable from *one* independent variable (either continuous or categorical). In multiple linear regression, you can predict the value of the dependent variable from *two or more independent variables* (either continuous or categorical).
2. Simple logistic regression is used to explore associations between one (dichotomous) dependent variable and one (continuous, ordinal, or categorical) independent variable. Multiple logistic regression is used to explore associations between one (dichotomous) dependent variable and two or more independent variables (which may be continuous, ordinal, or categorical). Logistic regression is often used to study how risk factors are associated with the dependent variable. Logistic regression can also test relationships between independent and dependent variables that are not linear.
3. Cox's proportional hazards model, also called Cox regression, is commonly used in survival analysis. Cox regression is useful to analyze the effect of several independent variables as it models survival rates over time. The dependent variable is always the event occurred/event did not occur—a dichotomous variable.

RESEARCHER INTERVIEW: Epidemiology

Patricia Markham Risica, DrPH, RD
Assistant Professor (Research) of Epidemiology, Brown University, Providence, RI

1. **Briefly describe the areas in which you do research.**
My research has included a broad set of topics. Stemming from my work in dietetics, much of my research has focused on nutrition, food, obesity, and breast-feeding. My epidemiology work has allowed me to serve as the Epidemiologist and Evaluator for the CDC funded Initiative for a Healthy Weight at the Rhode Island Department of Health. In that role, I analyzed state level data from the Behavioral Risk Factor Surveillance System (CDC) on obesity and overweight, including behavioral risk factors such as physical activity and nutritional determinants such as consumption of fruits and vegetables, fast food, and sugar sweetened beverages. I authored reports on these data along with several other data sets pertinent to children and adolescents.

   I have also collected epidemiologic data to assess obesity-related risk factors for specific populations. This began with my work conducting house-to-house surveys of residents of four small villages in rural Alaska, which was the basis for my dissertation. We used dietary data (24- hour recall and food frequency data) and physical activity, as well as physical, clinical, and blood measurements to determine the relationships between diet and physical activity with body fatness, body fat distribution, and glucose intolerance.

   Other studies have utilized data collected for the purposes of assessment of an intervention but were analyzed to learn more about the population. For example, I have collected data prospectively, and written about the determinants of breast-feeding and infant feeding attitudes and practices. These data were available as we were able to ask about feeding intentions and practices in a study constructed to assess smoke avoidance among pregnant women. I have also studied disordered feeding behaviors among African American women, and this data was collected along with other food and physical activity data to assess a weight control intervention.

Much of my work has also involved intervention design; collaboratively I have developed many interventions designed to change dietary behavior for prevention of cardiovascular disease, diabetes, cancer or obesity, or other health behaviors such as physical activity, smoking cessation, and avoidance of environmental tobacco smoke, skin self-examination for the early detection of melanoma, or adherence to medication or other treatment regimens. As most of my work is guided by the socioecological model, my projects have also focused on environmental change, such as the food environment at home, in the workplace, or in the community, and similar environments for other health topics. My research has focused on the health needs of many different populations, including Alaska Natives, African American women, and Hispanic families.

2. **With your experience in epidemiological research, what should students/practitioners know about this area of research?**
   Evaluation of the intervention and selection of measures in epidemiology research are arguably the most important decisions when designing a study. Outcomes are health-related measures, whereas impact variables are behaviors. So in a study of a diet change intervention to influence childhood obesity, the impact measures might include the dietary change that actually occurred, but the outcome would be the measure of child weight status. Either or both might be important to include in a given study. It is important to know in any nutrition-related research that dietary intake is an incredibly complex and difficult concept to measure. One must think through very clearly what aspect of diet is of interest. For example, a research study could measure caloric intake, consumption of a particular micronutrient, or the behaviors associated with selection and preparation of a particular type of food. All of these ways of considering diet would be measured using very different techniques, so consideration of the research questions in detail is essential to selecting the right measures.
3. **What do you enjoy most about the research process?**
   The constant change in topic and challenges are my favorite parts of the research process. Boredom is rare in a world of new projects, challenging and sometimes unpredictable field research, and unexpected research findings. If you like a predictable, routine job, this might not be the occupational choice for you.
4. **What tips do you have for practitioners who want to do practice based research?**
   Find a mentor to bring you into the research world. This can be a major professor in an academic program, but it could also be an experienced researcher in your institution or in the area. Multidisciplinary teams are highly valued by many funding agencies because the varied skill sets among researchers in different professions can offset one another. Regardless, experience in working in research is very important in training to be ready for all of the unexpected events during research, especially community-based research.

SUMMARY

1. Epidemiologists try to connect the dots between risk factors (exposures, independent variables) and health or disease outcomes (dependent variables).
2. Three epidemiological research designs—cross-sectional, cohort, and case-control—are observational, and there is no manipulation of the independent variable.
3. Cross-sectional designs in epidemiology attempt to describe the prevalence of disease and nondisease of a population of which some members have been exposed to a risk factor. Using a contingency table, a prevalence ratio can be calculated.
4. In a prospective cohort study, the researchers identify the population, recruit participants representative of the target population, take baseline measurements, and continue to measure exposure and diseases into the future. In a retrospective cohort study, researchers go back in time to identify a cohort of individuals at a point in time *before* the individuals had

developed the disease or outcome of interest. Then the researchers try to establish whether they were exposed or unexposed.

5. The goal of cohort studies is to compare the incidence of disease among the exposed to the incidence in the unexposed, which is expressed as a relative risk. Relative risk (RR) is the probability or risk of an outcome (such as disease) when exposed to a risk factor. It expresses how many more (or less) times likely is an exposed person to an outcome (such as disease) relative to an unexposed person.
6. A RR of 1.0 means there is no difference between groups. If the RR is greater than 1, it suggests an increased risk of that outcome in the exposed group. If the RR is less than 1, it suggests a reduced risk in the exposed group.
7. In a case-control study, we start with the outcome (usually a disease), and then work retrospectively to look at exposures. Case-control studies use odds ratios (OR) to compare the odds of cases having had a particular exposure to controls having had that same exposure. If the OR is 1, the odds of exposure are the same for both groups. If the OR is greater than 1, exposure is positively related to disease. If the OR is less than 1, exposure is protective.
8. Whereas relative risk tells you about the probability, the odds ratio tells you about the odds. Odds and probability are not the same thing; they both express the likelihood of an outcome, but in slightly different ways.
9. Regression analysis can predict the value of the outcome variable from one or more predictor variables, tell you if an independent variable really affects the dependent variable and the size of that effect, and control for extraneous variables.
10. In linear regression the dependent variable is continuous, and in logistic regression the dependent variable has a dichotomous outcome (such as disease/no disease).
11. In linear regression, R-squared represents the percentage of the data that is closest to the fitted regression line. An R-squared value of 0.59 means that 59% of the variance in the dependent variable can be accounted for by the independent variable. The higher the value of β (standardized regression coefficient), the more the independent variable affects the dependent variable. The value of β is tested against zero because zero means there is no significant association between the variables. The independent variable is said to be a good predictor when β is significant.
12. Logistic regression produces an odds ratio because the dependent variable only has two values. The odds ratio here is defined as the ratio of odds of an outcome (not exposure as in case-control studies) occurring for two groups. You need to know which groups are in the numerator and denominator (comparison group) before you can interpret the OR.
13. Survival analysis is appropriate to analyze data in which the length of time to an event is of interest. Cox's proportional hazards model (Cox regression) is often used in survival analysis. The dependent variable is always the event occurred/did not occur. The Cox model provides an estimate of the hazard ratio (HR). The hazard ratio is a ratio of the hazard rate of one group (who usually receive an intervention or have an exposure) to the hazard rate in another group (usually a comparison group).

REVIEW QUESTIONS

1. In epidemiology, the term "exposure" can mean:
   A. a risk factor
   B. a dose of a drug
   C. a vaccination
   D. all of the above
2. The number of new cases of a disease in a population during a specific time period is:
   A. point prevalence
   B. period prevalence
   C. incidence
   D. relative risk

3. An example of a descriptive epidemiological design is:
   A. cohort study
   B. case-control study
   C. survival analysis
   D. cross-sectional

4. The Framingham Heart Study is an example of a:
   A. prospective cohort study
   B. case-control study
   C. retrospective cohort study
   D. cross-sectional

5. Relative risk is the ____________ rate of the exposed group divided by the same rate in the unexposed group.
   A. prevalence
   B. exposure
   C. incidence
   D. odds rate

6. Odds and probability are the same.
   A. true
   B. false

7. In a case-control study, if the OR is 1, the odds of exposure are the same for cases and controls.
   A. true
   B. false

8. When the dependent variable is disease/no disease, which type of regression analysis would be appropriate?
   A. linear regression
   B. logistic regression
   C. Cox regression
   D. time-to-event regression

9. In regression, the independent variable may also be referred to as the:
   A. response
   B. outcome
   C. disease
   D. predictor

10. In linear regression, the higher the level of the beta coefficient:
   A. the more the independent variable affects the dependent variable
   B. the less the independent variable affects the dependent variable
   C. the better the covariates are controlled
   D. the higher the R-squared

11. In multiple regression, if some of the independent variables are highly correlated with each other, this is called:
   A. exposure
   B. incidence
   C. multicollinarity
   D. sphericity

12. In logistic regression, you will mostly use which statistic?
   A. R-squared
   B. beta coefficient
   C. odds ratio
   D. covariation

13. In survival analysis, which form of regression is commonly used?
   A. linear regression
   B. logistic regression
   C. Cox regression
   D. time-to-event regression

14. When a hazard ratio is 2, it means that at any time twice as many participants in the treatment/exposed groups are having an event proportionally to the comparison group.
   A. true
   B. false

15. Relative risk was calculated in a cohort study that looked at the effect of drinking 4 cups of tea daily (comparison was drinking less than 1 cup of tea daily) on development of cancer. If the relative risk was 0.5, what does that mean?

16. A multiple linear regression was used to examine the relationship of waist circumference (measured in inches) and height on percentage of body fat in men. The R-squared for the regression was 71%. The regression coefficient for waist circumference was 1.77. Identify the independent and dependent variables. Interpret the R-squared and regression coefficient for waist circumference.

17. A logistic regression analysis was used to examine the relationship between age and renal insufficiency on the risk of death. All participants had had coronary bypass surgery. The odds ratio for age was 1.076. The odds ratio for renal insufficiency was 3.198. Identify the independent and dependent variables, and interpret both odds ratios.

CRITICAL THINKING QUESTIONS

1. Read this article using a prospective cohort design and answer the following questions.

   (Open Access) Borgi, L., Rimm, E. B., Willett, W. C., & Forman. J. P. (2016). Potato intake and incidence of hypertension: Results from three prospective US cohort studies. *BMJ, 353,* i2351. doi: 10.1136/bmj.i2351

   Note: This cohort study uses Cox regression to look at the time until a participant is diagnosed with hypertension. Therefore, the study reports hazard ratios, which can be interpreted similarly to relative risk. Just keep in mind that hazard ratios give you instantaneous risk at a point in time and relative risk gives cumulative risk over the time of the study.

   A. What is the objective of the study?
   B. Who were the participants in the study?
   C. What is the outcome variable? What is the independent variable(s)?
   D. What covariates are included in the analysis?
   E. What is the hazard ratio (pooled results—random effect model) for incident hypertension for total consumption of potatoes (baked, boiled, mashed, and French fries) for people who consumed at least one serving daily? Interpret this hazard ratio.
   F. Compare the answer from E to the same pooled hazard ratio in Table 5 for people who eat potato chips at least four times a week.
   G. What did the authors conclude?

2. Read this article using a case-control design and answer the following questions.

   (Open Access) Ghardirian., P., Jain, M., Ducic, Sl., Shatenstein. B., & Morisset, R. (1998). Nutritional factors in the aetiology of multiple sclerosis: A case-control study in Montreal, Canada. *International Journal of Epidemiology, 27,* 845–852.

   A. What is the objective of the study?
   B. Who were the participants in the study?
   C. What are the independent and dependent variables?
   D. Using Table 3, which nutrients had a protective effect? Which nutrients increased risk?
   E. What did the authors conclude?

3. Read this article that uses linear regression to investigate associations, and answer the following questions.

   Vollmer, R. L., Adamsons, K., Gorin, A., Foster, J. S., & Mobley, A. R. (2015). Investigating the relationship of body mass index, diet quality and physical activity level between fathers and their preschool-aged children. *Journal of the Academy of Nutrition and Dietetics, 115,* 919–926. doi: 10.1016/j.jand.2014.12.003

   A. What are the objective and hypothesis for this study?
   B. Did this study take a prospective, retrospective, or cross-sectional approach?
   C. What are the independent and dependent variables?
   D. How were the main outcomes measured?
   E. What covariates were included in the linear regression?
   F. How many participants were in this study?
   G. Table 3 gives a β value of 0.62 for vigorous intensity. What is a β value and how should this β value be interpreted?
   H. Which father–child variables were significantly related?
   I. What did the authors conclude?

4. Read this article using logistic regression and answer the following questions.

   Fulkerson, J. A., Farbakhsh, K., Lytle, L., Hearst, M. O., Dengel, D. R., Pasch, K. E., & Kubik, M. Y. (2011). Away-from-home family dinner sources and associations with weight status, body composition, and related biomarkers of chronic disease among adolescents and their parents. *Journal of the American Dietetic Association, 111,* 1892–1897. doi: 10.1016.j.jada.2011.09.035

   A. What is the objective and hypothesis for this study?

B. Did this study take a prospective, retrospective, or cross-sectional approach?
C. What are the independent and dependent variables?
D. How many participants were in this study?
E. Logistic regression models were used to examine which associations?
F. In Table 1, interpret the OR under "Adolescent overweight/obese status" for four types of away-from-home family dinner sources and also for fast-food restaurants. Do the same for "Parent overweight/obese status."
G. What did the authors conclude?

5. Read this article and answer the following questions.

   Haring, B., Wu, C., Mossavar-Rahmani, M., Snetselaar, L., Brunner, R., Wallace, R. B., Neuhouser, M. L., & Wassertheil-Smoller, S. (2016). No association between dietary patterns and risk for cognitive decline in older women with 9-year follow-up: Data from the Women's Health Initiative Memory Study. *Journal of the Academy of Nutrition and Dietetics, 116,* 921–930. doi: 10.1016/j.jand.2015.12.017

   A. What is the objective and hypothesis for this study?
   B. Did this study take a prospective, retrospective, or cross-sectional approach?
   C. What are the independent and dependent variables?
   D. How many participants were in this study?
   E. What were the covariates used in the analysis?
   F. In Table 2, interpret the hazard ratios for Q5 in each dietary pattern under mild cognitive impairment and probable dementia.
   G. What did the authors conclude?

6. Write an original abstract for this article.

   Lopez-Garcia., E., Leon-Munoz, L., Guallar-Castillon, P., & Rodriguez-Artalejo, F. (2015). Habitual yogurt consumption and health-related quality of life: A prospective cohort study. *Journal of the Academy of Nutrition and Dietetics, 115*, 31–39. doi: 10.1016/j.jand.2014.05.013

SUGGESTED READINGS AND ACTIVITIES

1. Bruemmer, B., Harris., J., Gleason, Ph., Boushey, C. J., Sheean, P. M., Archer, S., & Van Horn, L. (2009). Publishing nutrition research: A review of epidemiologic methods. *Journal of the American Dietetic Association, 109,* 1728–1737. doi: 10.1016/j.jada.2009.07.011
2. Sheean, P. M., Bruemmer, B., Gleason, P., Harris, J., Boushey, C., & Van Horn, L. (2011). Publishing nutrition research: A review of multivariate techniques—Part 1. *Journal of the American Dietetic Association, 111,* 103–110. doi: 10.1016/j.jada.2010.10.010

REFERENCES

Bruemmer, B., Harris., J., Gleason, Ph., Boushey, C. J., Sheean, P. M., Archer, S., & Van Horn, L. (2009). Publishing nutrition research: A review of epidemiologic methods. *Journal of the American Dietetic Association, 109,* 1728–1737. doi: 10.1016/j.jada.2009.07.011

Campbell, D. T., & Stanley, J. C. (1963). *Experimental and quasi-experimental designs for research.* Belmont, CA: Wadsworth Cengage.

Committee on Diet and Health. (1989). Methodological considerations in evaluating the evidence. In Food and Nutrition Board, Commission on Life Science, National Research Council (Eds.), *Diet and health: Implications for reducing chronic disease risk* (pp. 23–40). Washington, DC: National Academies Press.

Cook, T. D., & Campbell, D. T. (1979). *Quasi-experimentation: Design & analysis issues for field settings.* Boston, MA: Houghton Mifflin Company.

Dolwick Grieb, S. M., Theis, R. P., Burr, D., Benardot, D., Siddiqui, T., & Asal, N. R. (2009). Food groups and renal cell carcinoma: Results from a case-control study. *Journal of the American Dietetic Association, 109,* 656–667. doi: 10.1016/j.jada.2008.12.020

Greenwood-Hickman, M. A., Rosenberg, D. E., Phelan, E. A., & Fitzpatrick, A. L. (2015). Participation in older adult physical activity programs and risk for falls requiring medical care, Washington State, 2005–2011. *Preventing Chronic Disease, 12,* 140574. doi: 10.5888/pcd12.140574.

Gray, J. R., Grove, S. K. & Sutherland, S. (2017). *Burns and Grove's the practice of nursing research: Appraisal, synthesis, and generation of evidence* (8th ed.). St. Louis, MO: Elsevier Saunders.

Guyatt, G., Walter, S., Shannon, H., Cook, D., Jaeschke, R., & Heddle, N. (1995). Basic statistics for clinicians: 4. Correlation and regression. *Canadian Medical Association Journal, 152,* 497–504.

Hidalgo, B., & Goodman, M. (2013). Multivariate or multivariable regression? *American Journal of Public Health 103,* 39–40. doi: 10.2105/AJPH.2012.300897

Hill, Austin B. (1965). The environment and disease: Association or causation? *Proceedings of the Royal Society of Medicine, 58,* 295–300.

Knapik, J. J., Trone, D. W., Austin, K. G., Steelman. R. A., Farina, E. K., & Lieberman, H. R. (2016). Prevalence, adverse events, and factors associated with dietary supplement and nutritional supplement use by U.S. Navy and Marine Corps personnel. *Journal of the Academy of Nutrition and Dietetics, 116,* 1423-1442. doi: 10.1016/j.jand.2016.02.015

Potischman, N., & Weed, D. L. (1999). Causal criteria in nutritional epidemiology. *American Journal of Clinical Nutrition, 69,* 1309S–1314S.

Robson, S. M., Couch, S. C., Peugh, J. L., Glanz, K., Zhou, C., Sallis, J. F., & Saelens, B. E. (2016). Parent diet quality and energy intake are related to child diet quality and energy intake. *Journal of the Academy of Nutrition and Dietetics, 116,* 984–990. doi: 10.1016/j.jand.2016.02.011

Shadish, W. R., Cook, T. D., & Campbell, D. T. (2002). *Experimental and quasi-experimental designs for generalized causal inference*. Belmont, CA: Wadsworth Cengage.

Temple, N. J. (2016). How reliable are randomised controlled trials for studying the relationship between diet and disease? A narrative review. *British Journal of Nutrition, 116,* 381–389. doi: 10.1017/S0007114516002129

Wang, H., Fox, F. S., Troy, L. M., Mckeown, N. M., & Jacques, P. F. (2015). Longitudinal association of dairy consumption with the changes in blood pressure and the risk of incident hypertension: The Framingham Heart Study. *British Journal of Nutrition, 114,* 1887–1899. doi: 10.1017/S0007114515003578

Zhang, J., & Yu, K. F. (1998). What's the relative risk?: A method of correcting the odds ratio in cohort studies of common outcomes. *JAMA, 280*, 1690–1691.

CHAPTER 8

Putting It All Together: Understanding and Evaluating Quantitative Research Studies

CHAPTER OUTLINE

- Introduction
- Research Title and Authors
- Introduction of Article
- Methods
- Results
- Discussion/Conclusion
- Additional Evaluation Tools
- Researcher Interview: Food Science/Sensory Evaluation, Annette Hottenstein

LEARNING OUTCOMES

- Identify and describe the major sections and subsections found within a research paper.
- Read and understand a scientific study.
- Write an abstract for a scientific study.
- Discuss characteristics of quality research.
- Use a set of questions to appraise/evaluate quantitative research studies.

INTRODUCTION

The purpose of this chapter is to help you put together basic research concepts, research design, and statistics to truly understand and evaluate or appraise research articles. According to Burls (2009), "critical appraisal is the process of carefully and systematically examining research to judge its trustworthiness, and its value and relevance in a particular context" (p. 1). Even though most journals use a peer-review process to ensure publication of quality studies, almost all studies still have some limitations or flaws. The way an outcome is measured is sometimes imperfect, as in some self-reported data, and can prove to be a shortcoming of a study. Indeed, science itself is rarely perfect.

To help you better understand a research study, this chapter includes a series of questions to use when reading each section of a research article from the title to the conclusions. Do not just rely on the abstract to tell you everything. It may be that the authors picked the best data to present and put their "best face" on the abstract. In other words, after you read an article, you may find that the abstract is a little misleading. There is simply no substitute for reading an article from beginning to end. There will be times when you do not understand something, and that is normal. Just keep on reading and focus on the big picture and what you do understand.

To help you appraise studies, this chapter includes a different series of questions for each section of an article. Understanding and evaluating a study go hand in hand, and sometimes they overlap, so feel free to think about both sets of questions together. When you appraise studies, you are looking for strengths and weaknesses. Perhaps the researchers never did a sample size calculation, or maybe attrition was higher than anticipated. Another study may have a rigorous research design that is appropriate for the research question.

Appraising a study is necessary to ensure that the study is sound and the results and recommendations are valid. Do not be afraid to draw your own conclusions based on sound reasoning. For example, after reading the results, take a look back at the hypothesis and determine whether you think the hypothesis was supported or not. In order to appraise a study, you need to use critical thinking and evaluation skills.

In this chapter, we are going to use a research article by Eaton et al. (2016) to demonstrate how to read, understand, and appraise a study. The full study information is in the References at the end of this chapter. The study is available free online at the website of the journal *Annals of Family Medicine*. First, read the article yourself, and then continue with this chapter as we use Tables 8.1 to 8.5 to further understand and evaluate the study.

RESEARCH TITLE AND AUTHORS

When you read the research title, try to answer these key questions in this order:

1. *Is the article an example of primary, secondary, or tertiary research?* Original research articles are primary research. Secondary research includes *narrative reviews* in which authors organize, interpret, and summarize evidence from primary studies in a particular research area. *Systematic reviews* belong in the category of tertiary research because they collect and distill information from both primary and secondary sources (see Chapter 12). Narrative reviews and systematic reviews often identify themselves as such in the title.
2. *Is this a quantitative or a qualitative study?* This chapter focuses on quantitative research so make sure you have a quantitative article. Qualitative studies often have the word "qualitative" in their title. Otherwise, look for data collection methods such as focus groups, interviews, observations, and document analysis, along with a lack of statistical analysis.
3. *Is the study experimental or nonexperimental?* Does the research have an intervention and look at the differences between the groups? This is a clue to the study being experimental or quasi-experimental. Quite often studies reporting randomized controlled trials (RCT) mention that in the title; then you know the study is experimental. Or does the study lack an intervention, and instead look for an association or relationship among the variables? This study would be nonexperimental. Nonexperimental studies could be descriptive (such as descriptive

cross-sectional), observational (such as a cohort study), or predictive (as in studies using regression). In these studies, there is no manipulation of the independent variable.

4. *What are the independent and dependent variables?* You should get an idea of what the variables are from looking at the title, including which might be the independent and the dependent variables. Most studies are looking at the effect of A on B, so start hunting for what A is (the independent variable) and what B is (the dependent variable). At the same time, look for some clues about who the participants are.

By answering these questions, it will be easier to read through much of the study.

Also look at the qualifications of the researchers, if given, as well as any note about funding sources. Quite often, any funding sources are noted at the end of the article just before the references are listed.

Table 8.1 identifies questions to use to understand and evaluate the research title and authors. The title of our study is "A Randomized Clinical Trial of a Tailored Lifestyle Intervention for Obese, Sedentary, Primary Care Patients." Without reading a word of the study, we already know quite a few things. The title says it is a randomized clinical trial (research design), so it is a primary piece of research, and also a quantitative and experimental study with an intervention. Because the intervention (the independent variable) is for obese and sedentary patients, it sounds like the intervention is going to help them lose weight. The title also mentions that the intervention is a "tailored lifestyle intervention," and that gives us more clues. The dependent variables are not mentioned, but be prepared to look for weight loss and perhaps some dependent variable related to exercise. The title also mentions primary care patients, so this study will involve primary care physicians to some extent.

For this study, you can read the qualifications of all the researchers and where they work. Not everyone has a doctorate, which is normal, because there are often graduate students working on studies. Before the Reference section, mention is made of funding support from the National Institutes of Health and that one researcher is supported by grant money from the National Cancer Institute.

In terms of evaluating the title and authors, the title is clear, the author list is appropriate, and all grant money came the National Institutes of Health, which is the main source of government grants supporting nutrition research and clinical trials in the United States. The funding source does not include any special interests.

Table 8.1 Questions to Understand and Evaluate the Research Title and the Authors

Questions to understand study	Questions to evaluate study
I. Research Title and Authors	
A. What does the *title* tell you about the research design, participants, and variables?	A. Is the *title* clear and easy to understand?
B. What are the qualifications of the *researchers*? Do you suspect that some are practitioners or students? (Look for practice certifications or the lack of a doctoral degree.)	B. How many of the *researchers* have doctorates?
C. Did the researchers receive *funding* from any disclosed source? If so, name the source.	C. Does the way the study was designed and conducted reveal any bias due to its *funding* source?

INTRODUCTION OF ARTICLE

When you read the introduction of an article, focus on finding the following three elements:

1. Problem statement
2. Research objective
3. Hypothesis (if given)

Normally the introduction starts with a brief literature review that sets up the problem statement. After the problem is clearly stated, the research objective (and sometimes hypothesis) is given.

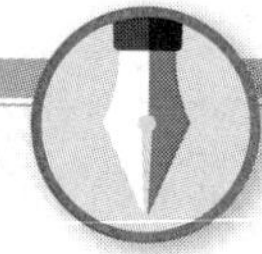

TIP

You will almost always find the objective and the hypothesis (if used) in the last paragraph of the Introduction section, just before the Methods section, and they are normally clearly labeled as such.

Table 8.2 lists questions to help you understand and evaluate the Introduction section, which we will now use to understand the Eaton et al. (2016) article. The literature review in this article is quite brief, only two paragraphs. The major theme of the first paragraph is very clear: obesity is a significant public health problem with serious health and economic implications, and it is not going away despite various efforts.

The second paragraph narrows the focus and looks at weight loss interventions in primary care, meaning interventions in which physicians are involved (even if just to

Table 8.2 Questions to Understand and Evaluate the Introduction

Questions to understand study	Questions to evaluate study
II. Introduction	
D. What are the major themes in the *literature review*? Describe two of the studies used in the literature review that are clearly cited to justify the research problem.	D. Does the *literature review* rely on primary sources and include recent research? Is the review up to date and complete? Do the authors critically appraise and compare the major references? Is the literature review organized well and does it build logically to the statement of the research problem? Do they summarize what is known and not known about the research problem?
E. What is the *research problem* (the knowledge gap or conflicting results in the current research)?	E. Is the *research problem* easy to find and clearly stated? Does the statement of the problem convince you that this study is needed? How relevant or important is the research problem?
F. What is the *objective/purpose* of the study? What variables will be studied in which population? Which is the independent variable and which is the dependent variable?	F. Is the study *objective/purpose* clearly stated and include the population? Are the variables and population described and defined? Does the study objective address the research problem? Does the study objective sound too broad or too narrow? If the study objective is carried out, will the study be ethical? Is the objective relevant in a real world setting?
G. Is a *hypothesis* given? If so, what is the predicted relationship between the variables? Is the hypothesis worded as a research or null hypothesis?	G. Is the *hypothesis* easy to find? Does the hypothesis clearly predict a relationship between the variables? Does the hypothesis flow from the research problem and objective? If there is no hypothesis, is that appropriate (such as for descriptive studies)?

refer a patient to a program and follow up with the patient). The authors make a point at the beginning of this paragraph to say that "evidence of the effectiveness of weight loss interventions delivered by primary care physicians is limited" (Eaton et al., 2016, p. 312). They attribute much of this problem to a lack of research-based programs that work in clinical practice, which is stated at the end of the first paragraph. *These two statements sum up the problem*, which basically says that physicians have *not* been very successful at treating and reducing obesity in part due to a lack of programs that have been tested in clinical practice.

Now that the problem is stated, the authors discuss the advantages of primary care physicians referring patients to other health care professionals for weight loss programs, as well as the potential for weight loss interventions that:

1. include physical activity,
2. are "tailored" to patients, and
3. use limited face-to-face meetings along with use of telephone, video, and printed materials.

The authors feel this model could be effective in primary practice.

In the third paragraph, the objective and two hypotheses are stated, and it is no surprise that they want to test a weight loss intervention. The study will look at how effective an enhanced (tailored) intervention (EI) is compared to a standard intervention (SI). Both hypotheses are undoubtedly research hypotheses (not null hypotheses) because they hypothesize that the EI group will lose more weight in 12 months, maintain the weight loss better at 24 months, and exercise more at 12 months and 24 months, compared to the standard intervention group. The independent variable is the intervention—the enhanced tailored intervention. The dependent variables are amount of weight lost and time spent in moderate/vigorous physical activity.

When evaluating the Introduction section, first we will look at the literature review.

D. *Literature Review*. The literature review includes appropriate primary sources; however, the most recent date of any of the sources is 2014, and this study was published in the middle of 2016. *The literature review could be more up to date.* Because the literature review is only two paragraphs, the authors did not appraise or compare major references other than to state that certain groups of references proved a point they were making. The literature review is organized appropriately and does a somewhat adequate job of summarizing what is known about the research problem, except for these two issues:
    a. A key statement at the end of the first paragraph, "the existing research-based programs have not been translated into clinical practice" (Eaton et al., 2016, p. 311), has no footnotes so you cannot get further clarification or substantiation. If you read the nutrition literature, it abounds with studies of weight control interventions, many with favorable results, so this is a puzzling statement. The authors needed to show documentation backing up their statement.
    b. The literature review also does not provide any background on how often primary care physicians are involved in helping patients lose weight and what methods they use. Do the majority of Americans consult and get weight loss help via their physicians, or do they just try to lose weight on their own and seek out programs such as Weight Watchers? More background and context on weight loss services in primary care would have been useful and provided more context for the study.

E. *Research Problem*. The research problem is really scattered around the Introduction section, so it is not easy to put together. The first paragraph mentions the costs of obesity and the lack of research-based interventions that work in the primary care setting. The second paragraph mentions that there is little research showing that primary practitioners have delivered effective interventions, and that translational weight loss programs have not often focused on physical activity. Although the statement of the problem is scattered around the Introduction section, it seems to be a relevant, important problem, but it could use more documentation about the lack of programs for use in primary practice and how primary practice programs are different from other community programs.

F. *Study Objective*. The study objective is clearly stated and includes the population and variables. The objective is neither too broad nor too narrow, and it does directly address the research problem. The study is definitely ethical, and the researchers did obtain institutional review board approval (mentioned at the start of the Methods section).

G. *Hypothesis*. The hypotheses are easy to find and clearly predict that the participants in the enhanced intervention will lose more weight in 12 months, maintain the weight loss better at 24 months, and exercise more at 12 months and 24 months, compared to the standard intervention group. The hypothesis clearly flows from the study objective.

Sometimes before an intervention is implemented, the authors publish a detailed description of their research plan or protocol. In this case, Hartman, Risica, Gans, Marcus, and Eaton did publish their full study protocol in 2014. What is interesting to note is that the Introduction section in their protocol does a better job of reviewing the literature and stating the problem, yet it is only a little longer. Also, the authors mention in their protocol that the objective of the study is to find an effective and *cost-effective* intervention. Eaton et al. (2016) hint about cost-effectiveness in their Introduction section when they mention using methods other than face-to-face counseling, but they should have stated that cost-effectiveness was also an important consideration.

APPLICATION 8.1

This study looks at a weight loss program to which physicians refer patients. The program is run by health care professionals who keep the physician updated on each patient's progress. Is this study similar to or different from intervention studies looking at the success of various weight loss programs? Defend your answer.

METHODS

The Methods section of a paper is usually broken down into a number of sections with headings to help you understand how the study was run. If a Methods section is poorly done, more often than not the reasons are that key information (such as how sample size was calculated) was not included, or the researchers were not clear about an aspect of the study.

To make it easier to get through the Methods section, we split it up into four major parts.

1. Study Design
2. Subjects and Setting

3. Intervention (for experimental and quasi-experimental studies)
4. Main Outcome Variables/Statistical Analysis.

You cannot skim through the Methods section (or any other part of the article), because it will undoubtedly contain a one-sentence statement somewhere that is very important. For example, toward the end of the "Statistical Analysis" section, it states: "if weight or physical activity was missing at follow-up, the value from the previous visit was used, following the last-value-carried-forward imputation method" (Eaton et al., 2016, p. 314). This is important to know because the study had just enough participants to meet the sample size requirements, and a number of participants missed one or more follow-up visits in both groups.

It is also very important to make sure you are clear about what the main outcome variables are and how they are being measured. The main outcome variables in this study are weight change (weight loss) and number of minutes/week in moderate and vigorous activity. Other variables, such as waist circumference and blood pressure, were taken at each visit, but the objective and the hypothesis of this study do not mention these variables, so we will not focus on them. Some studies are just teeming with outcome or dependent variables. You do not always need to focus on all of them. *Use the study's objective to help you key in on the main outcome variable(s).*

Table 8.3 provides questions to help you understand and evaluate the Methods section, which we will now use to understand the methods that were used in our study.

H. *Research design*. The first two paragraphs in the Methods section discuss the design.
    a. The research design is a *randomized controlled trial* (RCT), and the authors also state that it is a translational research trial. It is translational because it is applying clinical research findings in practice settings and communities (referred to as T2 translational research). Because the study is an RCT, the authors discuss the use of block randomization, allocation, and blinding in the second paragraph.
    b. The study was *prospective* in that the sample was chosen and 24 months were required to complete the intervention (12 months as active treatment and 12 months as maintenance).
    c. The independent variable is the intervention. *The main dependent variables are weight loss and moderate or vigorous exercise.* Weight loss is identified as the mean absolute change from baseline weight. Exercise is measured in how many self-reported minutes were spent per week in moderate or vigorous exercise. Moderate exercise would be the equivalent of walking at 3 to 4 mph.
I. *Sample and setting*. Starting with the third paragraph in the Methods section, the sample is described.
    a. The *sample* was drawn from the practices of 24 primary care physicians in Rhode Island and southeastern Massachusetts. Interested patients were referred by their physicians to be further screened by telephone. Predetermined inclusion criteria were used, such as 18 to 80 years old with a BMI of at least 25. Patients were excluded, for example, if they had a health condition that would make participation unsafe.
    b. Toward the end of the third paragraph, it mentions that 211 people were *randomized* to the EI group (105) or SI group (106). *Sample size calculations* required at least 104 participants in each group to detect a 5% difference in weights between the groups (last paragraph of the Methods section).
    c. This was a home-based study that required counseling sessions and data collection. The settings for counseling and data collection were not discussed.

Table 8.3 Questions to Understand and Evaluate the Methods

Questions to understand study	Questions to evaluate study
III. Methods	
H. Which *research design* will be used? Is the research design experimental, quasi-experimental, descriptive, epidemiological, or predictive correlational? Is the study cross-sectional, prospective, or retrospective?	H. Is the *research design* the most appropriate and rigorous that could be used for this research problem? For example, an RCT is best for questions about treatment, whereas cohort studies work well to examine questions about etiology or prognosis. Is the design guided by an appropriate theory or framework? Does the research design minimize biases and other threats to validity (such as by randomization, blinding, etc.)? What were limitations of the research design?
I. Describe the *sample* and *setting*, including how participants are selected (include sampling method), sample size, and how sample size is determined. How many participants withdrew from the study? In the case of a cross-sectional study, look at the response rate. If the study has more than one group, how are the participants assigned to groups?	I. Was the selection of the *sample* free from bias? Were inclusion and exclusion criteria used, and were they appropriate? Is the sample representative? Did researchers gather appropriate baseline information on all participants to be analyzed? As appropriate, was a power analysis completed and used to determine sample size? If the participants were assigned to groups, were the participants assigned randomly or without bias? If a clinical *setting* was used, was it markedly different from other clinical settings?
J. If there was an *intervention*, describe what each group experienced.	J. In the case of an *intervention*, is a protocol used to promote treatment fidelity?
K. Describe how the *main outcome variables* will be measured and the data collected. Was an intention-to-treat protocol used? Which collected data will be analyzed using statistics? List each *statistical test* that will be used for the main outcome variables, and identify the purpose for each test.	K. Are the instruments appropriate, reliable, and able to accurately measure the *main outcome variables*? Is the data collected in a consistent manner, and does it enhance valid responses? Were the number and timing of data collection points appropriate? Were data collectors carefully chosen and trained? In the case of observations, is inter-rater reliability measured and reported? Are the procedures for analyzing the data clearly described? Were appropriate *statistical tests* used, including inferential statistics? Were effect sizes (such as mean standardized difference or relative risk) reported? Were confounding variables controlled for in the statistical analysis?

J. *Intervention*. After discussing the study population, the article moves on to the intervention.

   a. *All participants met individually with a lifestyle counselor at the start of the study, and also at 6 and 12 months.* Initially they set a weight loss goal (10% over 6 months) and were given a structured meal plan based on the Diabetes Prevention Program. They were all encouraged to add 10 minutes of moderate-intensity activity most days of the week, working up to 300 minutes/week by 6 months. All participants were given blank food and exercise logs to maintain.

b. The *Standard Intervention group* received five pamphlets over the 24 months: three in the first 12 months and two in the final 12 months (maintenance phase).

c. The *Enhanced Intervention group* received phone calls from the counselor for the first 12 months, in addition to weekly mailings that included print materials, exercise DVDs, and feedback based on food and exercise logs and phone call conversations. The EI group also received monthly feedback on their exercise based on their answers to monthly questionnaires. For the maintenance phase from months 13 to 24, the EI group continued to get materials and feedback, but it did taper down in frequency.

d. Physicians were informed of their patients' progress and gave encouragement during any visits.

K. *Main outcome variables and statistical tests.* The last two paragraphs in the Methods section are about data collection and statistical analysis.

a. Blinded assessors collected various data at baseline and at the 6-, 12-, 18-, and 24-month follow-up visits, including the *main outcome variables* of weight loss and minutes/week in moderate or vigorous activity.

b. An *intention-to-treat protocol was used.* Intention-to-treat is the principle that all participants *are used in the statistical analysis,* regardless of whether they dropped out or were not compliant with follow-up visits or treatment. From 17 to 32 people from each group missed each follow-up visit (Figure 1), so researchers used their weight and physical activity numbers from the prior visit.

c. Chi-square and ANOVA were used to compare baseline characteristics. A mixed-effect model that could handle the repeated measurements and other factors in this study was used for data analysis.

TIP

Do not get overwhelmed if you do not understand parts of the statistical analysis section. When the researchers use modeling procedures, it can be hard to comprehend. But normally the modeling procedures result in *P*-values, so you can look for them. If a *P*-value was significant, the research paper will normally highlight this.

In terms of evaluating the Methods section, here are some pluses and minuses.

1. A randomized controlled trial (RCT) is an appropriate choice for testing an intervention and is a rigorous design. This study employed excellent controls via randomization, allocation, and blinding whenever possible.
2. With regard to the sample, inclusion and exclusion criteria were used, and baseline data was collected on all participants and analyzed. A power analysis was done appropriately to determine sample size.
3. A protocol was used to direct the intervention. The setting for the counseling and follow-up sessions was not described.
4. Data was collected at five points by assessors blinded to group assignment.
5. Statistical tests seem appropriate, but the authors could have been more specific on which tests they were going to run on which data. Confounding variables (such as age, sex, and race) were controlled in statistical tests involving weight. Weight loss is an example of a mean difference, an effect size, so the results were not totally based on statistical significance.

Overall, the Methods section was well done, with a couple of areas that did need more explanation (setting and statistical tests).

APPLICATION 8.2

Name three types of research designs that do not include an intervention.

RESULTS

The Results section is limited to the actual data generated by this study; *any interpretation of the data is put in the Discussion section*. For human subjects studies, the first paragraph(s) and chart(s) in the Results section provide basic demographics and other pertinent characteristics of the participants, such as their pretest data. Differences between the groups at the beginning of the study is a threat to internal validity, so researchers always do statistical tests to compare groups.

The Results section presents key findings in a logical order. Tables and figures show the results, and the text highlights and explains each table or figure in order. When interpreting information in tables and figures, be sure to read all of the labels, headings, and footnotes carefully. If the results talk about differences between groups on a dependent measure, look for information on statistical significance as well as on the direction and magnitude of differences.

TIP

You may find it easier to read and interpret the tables and figures first, and then read the text. As you read each table or figure, read the headings first so you know what information is being presented, and then read the labels and footnotes. Once you understand the results in a table or figure, look for that table or figure number in the text and compare your thoughts with what the authors have to say.

As you read the Results section, keep in mind both the research objective and the hypothesis. Sometimes researchers are selective about what data and analyses they want you to see, which encourages you to think the hypothesis was totally supported. They may try to dazzle you with statistically significant results right at the start of the section, and leave the most important results (which may not be statistically significant) until the end. You need to decide whether the results support or reject the null hypothesis, or if further testing is necessary. Ideally, the Methods section spells out how the results will be reported.

Table 8.4 provides questions to help you understand and evaluate the Results section. In this article, two tables (Tables 1 and 2) and two figures (Figures 2 and 3) show results. Let's look at Tables 1 and 2 first because they are directly related to the two hypotheses.

- Table 1 compares the *baseline characteristics* of study participants. On the right-hand side of Table 1, you can see the *P*-values—none are close to 0.05 or lower, so no differences are statistically significant, which is good. The authors also looked at the retention rate between the two groups (the EI group had better retention) and concluded that it most likely did not affect the results.

Table 8.4 Questions to Understand and Evaluate the Results

Questions to understand study	Questions to evaluate study
IV. Results	
L. Were there any important *differences between the groups* at the beginning of the study? What was the attrition/retention rate?	L. Were the *groups similar*/comparable, especially with respect to any confounding variables? Did the researchers explain why participants withdrew from the study? Was attrition excessive? Was attrition similar across groups? After taking attrition into account, are the participants still representative of the population, and are the groups still comparable?
M. What were the *results* for each statistical test? Were any of the results significant? Was effect size used for any results?	M. Are the *results* clearly described in the narrative and clearly presented in tables and figures? Was the sample size large enough to detect a difference between the groups? Were statistical significance and practical (clinical) significance discussed? Are all results presented, or just some results? Are the results accurate? Can a rival hypothesis explain some of the results?

- The left side of Table 2 looks at *average weight change from baseline* in each group. At first glance, it looks like the EI group lost about 4 to 5 pounds every 6 months, but that is not the case. First, the unit is kilograms (not pounds), and second, the weight you see at each time point is the *average change from the baseline weight.* So at 6 months, average EI group weight loss was 5 kilograms, and by 12 months, this increased to 5.4 kilograms. For the EI group, you can see that they did not lose any more weight at 18 and 24 months, and actually gained back some of the weight they had lost.
- In Table 2, you can also compare the *amount of weight lost between the two groups* at each time point. At the end of 12 months, the EI group had lost 5.4 kg, and the SI group had lost 3.8 kg. At the end of 24 months, the EI group had lost 4.1 kg, and the SI group had lost 4.0 kg; so they are basically the same. Results were not statistically significant at any time point, as is explained at the end of the "Weight Loss" discussion.
- Table 2 also shows the *average number of physical activity minutes/week* (self-reported) for each group. EI members spent more minutes/week exercising than the SI members at the four measuring points, and results were statistically significant at 12 and 18 months.
- In Table 2, an F ratio is given for a "Group by Visit Interaction" for weight loss and separately for "Physical Activity." This type of interaction occurs when the changes in weight loss or number of minutes spent exercising over time *differs by group*. The researchers used the statistical significance of the F ratio of the "Group by Visit Interactions" to state that *overall* the EI group had lost significantly more weight (group by visit, $P = 0.02$), and that *overall* the EI group reported significantly more time in physical activity (group by visit, $P = 0.04$).

In summary, Table 2 shows that the EI group did well losing weight compared to the SI group, but the total weight lost was similar at 24 months for both groups, and no results were statistically significant (except for the interaction). As for physical activity, the EI group did log more physical activity time, and these results were statistically significant at 12 and 18 months.

Keep in mind when thinking about these results that the researchers are comparing two good weight loss programs. It is going to be harder to find differences in this study than if the researchers compared the EI group to a true control group that received no intervention. Another reason it might be harder to find differences between these groups has to do with sample size. The sample size calculations recommended at least 104 people per group, and there were 105 in one group and 106 in the other group. Those group numbers are fine, except that about one-quarter of each group was missing at each follow-up visit, and data from each person's last visit was used. Would the results have been the same if fewer people missed follow-up visits?

The other results in this section (seen in Figures 2 and 3) are interesting because there is no mention of doing these tests in the Methods section. It is likely that they were added because looking at the dependent variables in a new and different way showed more statistically significant results. They do provide a different perspective on the data, and perhaps could be hypotheses for *future* studies, but they are not completely appropriate here.

- Figure 2 shows the percentage of participants losing 5% or more of their baseline weight by intervention group over the 24 months. Significantly more EI participants than SI participants lost 5% of their baseline weight at 6 and 12 months. About one-third of the EI group maintained their 5% weight loss at the end of the study.
- Figure 3 shows the percentage of participants in each group who reported at least 150 minutes/week of moderate/vigorous exercise over the 24 months. The difference was statistically significant at 12, 18, and 24 months with a higher percentage of participants attaining guidelines in the EI group.

It is notable that about one-third of the EI group maintained their 5% weight loss for 24 months.

APPLICATION 8.3

Were the research hypotheses supported? Explain your answers.

The Results section is slanted toward showing statistically significant results. In the "Weight Loss" section, the percentage of participants attaining 5% weight loss was discussed first because some of those results were statistically significant. The authors put the results in Table 8.2, which did not show statistical significance, later in the Results section. In the "Physical Activity" section, they did mention the Table 8.2 results first (some were statistically significant) and then looked at the percentage of participants attaining guideline levels of physical activity (some there were also statistically significant). The statistical significance of the "Group by Visit Interaction" effects were also woven into the Results section.

DISCUSSION AND CONCLUSION

In the Discussion section, the authors state their understandings and explanations of the results in light of what is already known about the topic. The major goal of this section is to show how the study results fit into the larger picture of research in this area, as well as to provide limitations and ideas for future research. The Conclusion section is a general statement of the answer to the original research question along with its scientific implications.

TIP

Before you read the Discussion section, take a look back at the studies mentioned in the Introduction section. The authors should be referring to those studies in the Discussion section and comparing them to results in their study. Reading the literature review again will make it easier to get through the first part of the Discussion section.

Table 8.5 provides questions to help you understand and evaluate the Discussion and Conclusion sections. In the Discussion section, the first paragraph summarizes results, which is normally done, although their summary is pretty long. The second paragraph relates their results to five other weight loss studies. The third paragraph looks at limitations and states one recommendation for future study. The fourth paragraph provides more recommendations for further study. The conclusion is clearly stated in the fifth (and final) paragraph. Following are some thoughts on the Discussion and Conclusion sections.

N. *Interpret results*. In the second paragraph, the researchers compare their results with five other trials involving referrals from primary care physicians.
   a. They note two studies in which participants maintained their weight loss during the second year (unlike this study), probably through the use of phone calls and interactions with those participants during the second year. They noted their study achieved similar (or more) weight loss compared to two other trials, without using meal replacements and medications as was done in one of those trials.

Table 8.5 Questions to Understand and Evaluate the Discussion/Conclusion

Questions to understand study	Questions to evaluate study
V. Discussion/Conclusion	
N. How do the researchers *interpret the results*? Are the results consistent with past studies?	N. Do the researchers *interpret the results* in light of the pertinent literature, study objective(s), and hypothesis? Do the researchers explain inconsistencies in results between their study and prior studies? Do the researchers explain why results were significant or not significant? Overall, are the results interpreted appropriately, and do they take into account the study's limitations?
O. What *strengths or limitations* of the study are given?	O. Did the researchers mention all *limitations* and their possible effects on the quality of the study results? Did the researchers identify the threats to validity that were not well controlled?
P. What *recommendations* for further studies are given?	P. Were *recommendations* specific, appropriate, and consistent with the research base?
Q. What is the study's *conclusion*?	Q. Are the *conclusions* clearly stated and supported by the results? Does the conclusion touch on the study objective? If the researchers generalize their findings, did they do so appropriately? Are the conclusions applicable to nutrition practice?

b. The researchers did bring up a few key studies, but they only compared parts of their results to four other studies. Many more studies were mentioned in the Introduction section (although all were at least 2 years old). Overall, they did not relate their results to many other studies or interpret their own results any further. It would have been nice to compare their results—such as 25 to 35% of their participants maintained a 5% weight loss for the full 24 months—to other studies outside of those involving a primary care physician referral.

O. *Strengths and limitations*. No strengths were mentioned. Limitations included limited geographic setting, mostly female groups, self-reporting of minutes in physical activity, and the inability to determine which methods of delivering the program were most useful. An additional limitation not mentioned by the authors relates to sample size being just adequate and an average retention of about 74%.

P. *Recommendations*. Many good recommendations for future studies were listed, such as trying out more technology to give tailored content and support, studying which methods were most effective in helping participants lose weight and which were best in the maintenance phase, as well as testing cost-effectiveness.

Q. *Conclusion*. The authors conclude that primary care physicians can support weight loss efforts by referring patients to home-based, tailored interventions to help them reach clinically significant weight loss goals and increase their exercise levels. Their conclusion does not compare the effectiveness of the EI versus the SI intervention. The authors state that *if* their study results are generalizable, only about 25 to 35% of the participants will maintain a clinically significant weight loss at 24 months. Their conclusions were reasonable.

APPLICATION 8.4

Which *type* of validity is affected by each of these study limitations?

1. Limited geographic setting
2. Mostly female groups
3. Self-reporting of minutes in physical activity
4. Average retention rate of 74%

ADDITIONAL EVALUATION TOOLS

Additional evaluation tools are available, and a number of researchers use a tool to assess risk of bias from the Cochrane Collaboration. Cochrane is a global network of researchers and others who work independently and do not accept commercial funding or any funding that creates conflicts of interest. Their mission is to provide quality information to help those involved in health make informed decisions. Their tool for assessing risk of bias looks at, for example, how randomization and blinding are accomplished, how incomplete outcome data are handled, and whether the actual results match what the researchers had initially planned (Higgins & Green, 2011). Bias *may* occur, for instance, if an outcome from the protocol is not reported at all or incompletely, or if the outcome is measured differently from how it was originally stated. A complete description of this tool, as well as criteria for grading a study on these domains, is available at www.cochrane.org.

Another evaluation tool used by Evidence Analysis Library (EAL) analysts is the Quality Criteria Checklist (QCC). EAL analysts critically appraise a study's design and methodological quality using the QCC, the Academy of Nutrition and Dietetics' risk of bias tool. The QCC includes 10 areas of validity questions (with subquestions) to assess threats that can undermine a sound study. Based on their answers to the validity questions, the analysts rate the study as positive, negative, or neutral. The QCC for each article is compiled into a Quality Rating Summary, which can be viewed on the Evidence Analysis Library. There are other Quality Criteria Checklists for other study designs. The QCC also includes four questions on the study's relevance to practice. Chapter 12 contains the QCC for primary research with human subjects.

In addition, checklists have been developed to make sure researchers performing certain types of research include all appropriate information when reporting a study.

- The CONSORT 2010 checklist provides information to include when reporting a randomized trial. CONSORT stands for Consolidated Standards of Reporting Trials. The CONSORT group, a panel of experts, developed the checklist to increase transparency of RCTs and to reveal when there are deficiencies (Schulz, Altman, & Moher, 2010). This checklist is shown in Appendix C.
- The STROBE Statement is a checklist of items that should be included in reports of observational studies. This checklist is shown in Appendix D.
- A checklist of what should be included in a systematic review was developed by the PRISMA group, an international group of clinicians and researchers who have worked to improve the quality of reporting for systematic reviews. This checklist is shown in Appendix E.

RESEARCHER INTERVIEW: Food Science/Sensory Evaluation

Annette Hottenstein, MS, RDN, LDN
President, The Food Sommelier® (www.foodsommelier.com), Baltimore County, Maryland

1. **Briefly describe the areas in which you do research.**
After completing my combined dietetic internship and master's degree in food science and technology, I decided to pursue employment in the food industry. I spent 15 years working in corporate research and development (R&D) as a sensory and consumer researcher for Pepsico and McCormick & Company. Corporate R&D is responsible for new product development as well as quality control and maintenance of existing product lines. As a sensory and consumer researcher, I was involved in the planning, execution, and interpretation of taste panels. Taste panels included working with trained "expert" tasters (descriptive panels) as well as with untrained consumers (e.g., home use tests, focus groups, and ideation sessions).

    In 2012, I left the food industry to form my own consulting company with a mission to help nutrition professionals better leverage sensory evaluation in their practice. I have coauthored seven publications in journals such as *Appetite, Food Quality and Preference,* and *The Journal of Sensory Studies.* The majority of these publications are related to food industry applications of sensory evaluation. For example, much of my research revolved around improved prediction of how much consumers will like a certain food product and how to set up laboratory conditions to make taste tests correlate to real-world consumption.

    My most recent publication allowed me to utilize my sensory evaluation skills in a clinical nutrition setting.* This was a study conducted at the Johns Hopkins School of Public Health on the effects of a behavioral intervention (which emphasized spices and herbs) on

*Anderson, C. A., Cobb, L. K., Miller, E. R., Woodward, M., Hottenstein, A., Chang, A. R., Mongraw-Chaffin, M., White, K., Charleston, J., Tanaka, T., Thomas, L., & Appel, L. J. (2015). Effects of a behavioral intervention that emphasizes spices and herbs on adherence to recommended sodium intake: Results of the SPICE randomized clinical trial. *American Journal of Clinical Nutrition, 102,* 671–679.

the maintenance of sodium intake at the recommended intake of 1,500 mg/day. Part of this research involved the use of several sensory evaluation methods to measure participants' preferred level of sodium over the course of the intervention. My role in the study was establishing the appropriate sensory methodology, working onsite to facilitate testing, and interpreting sensory results.

2. **With your experience in sensory evaluation research, what should students/practitioners know about this area of research?**

   Sensory evaluation is defined as "a scientific discipline used to evoke, measure, analyze, and interpret those responses to products that are perceived by the senses of sight, smell, touch, taste, and hearing."* The Commission on Dietetic Registration understands the value of sensory evaluation and has designated a learning need code devoted to the topic "8130: Sensory perception and evaluation of food and ingredients." However, the vast majority of learning resources for this topic are designed for applications in the food industry rather than for nutrition and dietetics.

   Sensory evaluation methodologies range from traditional methods such as the triangle test to more consumer-based research methods such as focus groups. Use of sensory methodologies in nutrition research can be broken down into several areas, as follows. An example of a research study is shown for each.

   - *Measure taste acuity in a clinical testing*

   Chapman-Novakofski, K., Brewer, M. S., Riskowski, J., Burkowski, C., & Winter, L. (1999). Alterations in taste thresholds in men with chronic obstructive pulmonary disease. *Journal of the American Dietetic Association, 99*(12), 1536–1541.

This study found that underweight COPD patients were more sensitive to bitter tastes than their normal weight counterparts. Understanding alterations in taste perception can guide nutrition professionals in their recommendations for meal plans targeting individual weight goals.

   - *Optimize the formulation of a healthy/functional food product*

   Borneo, R., Aguirre, A., & León, A. E. (2010). Chia (Salvia hispanica L) gel can be used as egg or oil replacer in cake formulations. *Journal of the American Dietetic Association, 11,* 946–949.

Sensory testing results from 75 untrained consumers indicated that a chia gel can replace as much as 25% of oil or eggs in cakes without affecting overall liking. Nutrition professionals developing healthy recipes can utilize findings such as these to formulate highly palatable recipes for clients and the general public. Likewise, they can conduct their own sensory evaluation testing to assess the palatability of recipes.

   - *Measure taste preferences in relation to dietary patterns or demographic factors*

   Drewnowski, A., Henderson, S. A., Driscoll, A., & Rolls, B. J. (1996). Salt taste perceptions and preferences are unrelated to sodium consumption in healthy older adults. *Journal of the American Dietetic Association, 96,* 471–474.

This research study investigated the link between salty taste perception and preference and sodium intake in older adults. Understanding the factors guiding salty taste preferences can help nutrition professionals tailor counseling messages to those who may benefit from a reduced sodium diet.

   - *Optimize taste preferences for different age groups*

   Zandstra, E. H., & de Graaf, C. (1998). Sensory perception and pleasantness of orange beverages from childhood to old age. *Food Quality and Preference, 9,* 5–12.

This study indicates that elderly people prefer higher concentrations of stimuli for solutions of sucrose, sodium chloride, and citric acid than younger people do. Nutrition professionals working in

---

*Stone and Sidel, 1993, p. 5.

long-term care can utilize research such as this to optimize taste preferences for older populations, many of whom suffer from poor intake and "the anorexia of aging."

- *Develop lexicon to describe foods that can be used in retail and counseling settings*

Talvera-Bianchi, M. A., Chambers, E., & Chambers, D. H. (2010). Lexicon to describe flavor of fresh leafy vegetables. *Journal of Sensory Studies, 25,* 163–183.

In this study from Kansas State University, a list of words (lexicon) was developed to describe the flavor of fresh, leafy green vegetables. The application here is that nutrition professionals can describe healthy foods such as leafy green vegetables in the same manner as a wine professional (sommelier) describes a fine wine. For instance, kale is "grassy and viney in character with moderate bitterness and faint background notes of parsley, cabbage, wood, and earth." There are many additional published lexicons, and quite a few are for healthy foods and beverages. Nutrition professionals working in retail and counseling settings could leverage this information to better engage and educate clients about healthy foods.

- *Develop nutrition education materials and programs*

Kannan, S., Smith, R., Foley, C., Del Sole, S., White, A., Sheldon, L. A., Mietlcki-Floyd, S., & Severin, S. (2011). FruitZotic: A sensory approach to introducing preschoolers to fresh exotic fruits at Head Start locations in western Massachusetts. *Journal of Nutrition Education and Behavior, 43,* 205–206.

In this educational intervention, a nutrition program involving multiple senses had a greater impact on a child's willingness to try a food than taste alone. For instance, children were exposed to the sound a coconut makes when shaken or were asked to feel the hair on the outside of a kiwi. Nutrition professionals working with children as well as adults can learn from this research by building a multisensory approach when exposing clients to new foods.

3. **What do you enjoy most about the research process?**
The part I enjoy most about the research process is analyzing and interpreting results. Most sensory scientists utilize a lot of statistics in their job function, and I have learned to appreciate this aspect of research. I enjoy finding visually interesting ways to present research findings using tables, charts, and graphs. It is fascinating that different ways of looking at the data can provide new thought-provoking outcomes.
4. **What tips do you have for practitioners who want to do practice-based research?**
For practitioners who want to do practice-based research utilizing sensory evaluation, I recommend learning more about sensory physiology and sensory methodologies. Two journals I highly recommend are *The Journal of Sensory Studies* and *Food Quality and Preference.* These journals are typically read only by sensory and consumer researchers in academia and industry, but there is much that nutrition professionals can leverage. Other favorite resources include:

- Ackerman, D. (1990). *A Natural History of the Senses.* New York: Vintage Books. (An anthropological take on the five senses.)
- Applied Sensory and Consumer Science Certificate Program. University of California Davis Extension (Training courses in sensory evaluation.)
- Civille, G. V., & Carr, B. T. (2015). *Sensory Evaluation Techniques*, 5th ed. Boca Raton, FL: CRC Press. (Excellent textbook for learning sensory methodology.)
- Society of Sensory Professionals: http://www.sensorysociety.org (professional society)
- Stucky, C. (2012). *Taste: Surprising Stories and Science About Why Food Tastes Good.* New York: Atria Paperback. (Fun sensory-focused book about food appreciation.)

At its most basic level, sensory evaluation can teach clients how to appreciate food, which is the cornerstone of good nutrition. I encourage dietetics students and nutrition professionals to seek out sensory evaluation learning opportunities. Keep in mind that these opportunities may be hiding in other fields of study, such as in food science and the culinary arts. With a little creativity, most sensory evaluation tools can be successfully leveraged for a variety of nutrition research applications.

SUMMARY

Questions to understand study	Questions to evaluate study
I. Research Title and Authors	
A. What does the *title* tell you about the research design, participants, and variables?	A. Is the *title* clear and easy to understand?
B. What are the qualifications of the *researchers*? Do you suspect that some are practitioners or students? (Look for practice certifications or the lack of a doctoral degree.)	B. How many of the *researchers* have doctorates?
C. Did the researchers receive *funding* from any disclosed source? If so, name source.	C. Does the way the study was designed and conducted reveal any bias due to its *funding* source?

Questions to understand study	Questions to evaluate study
II. Introduction	
D. What are the major themes in the *literature review*? Describe two of the studies used in the literature review that are clearly cited to justify the research problem.	D. Does the *literature review* rely on primary sources and include recent research? Is the review up to date and complete? Do the authors critically appraise and compare the major references? Is the literature review organized well and built logically to the statement of the research problem? Do they summarize what is known and not known about the research problem?
E. What is the *research problem* (the knowledge gap or conflicting results in the current research)?	E. Is the *research problem* easy to find and clearly stated? Does the statement of the problem convince you that this study is needed? How relevant/important is the research problem?
F. What is the *objective/purpose* of the study? What variables will be studied in which population? Which is the independent variable and which is the dependent variable?	F. Is the study *objective/purpose* clearly stated, and does it include the population? Are the variables and the population described and defined? Does the study objective address the research problem? Does the study objective sound too broad or too narrow? If the study objective is carried out, will the study be ethical? Is the objective relevant in a real-world setting?
G. Is a *hypothesis* given? If so, what is the predicted relationship between the variables? Is the hypothesis worded as a research or null hypothesis?	G. Is the *hypothesis* easy to find? Does the hypothesis clearly predict a relationship between the variables? Does the hypothesis flow from the research problem and objective? If there is no hypothesis, is that appropriate (such as for descriptive studies)?

Questions to understand study	Questions to evaluate study
III. Methods	
H. Which *research design* will be used? Is the research design experimental, quasi-experimental, descriptive, epidemiological, or predictive correlational? Is the study cross-sectional, prospective, or retrospective?	H. Is the *research design* the most appropriate and rigorous that could be used for this research problem? For example, an RCT is best for questions about treatment, and cohort studies work well to examine questions about etiology or prognosis. Is the design guided by an appropriate theory or framework? Does the research design minimize biases and other threats to validity (such as by randomization, blinding, etc.)? What were limitations of the research design?
I. Describe the *sample* and *setting*, including how participants are selected (include sampling method), sample size, and how sample size is determined. How many participants withdrew from the study? In the case of a cross-sectional study, look at response rate. If the study has more than one group, how are the participants assigned to groups?	I. Was the selection of the *sample* free from bias? Were inclusion and exclusion criteria used, and were they appropriate? Is the sample representative? Did researchers gather appropriate baseline information on all participants to be analyzed? As appropriate, was a power analysis completed and used to determine sample size? If the participants were assigned to groups, were the participants assigned randomly or without bias? If a clinical *setting* was used, was it markedly different from other clinical settings?
J. If there was an *intervention*, describe what each group experienced.	J. In the case of an *intervention*, is a protocol used to promote treatment fidelity?
K. Describe how the *main outcome variables* will be measured and the data collected. Was an intention-to-treat protocol used? Which collected data was analyzed using statistics? List each *statistical test* that was used for the main outcome variables, and identify the purpose for each test.	K. Are the instruments appropriate, reliable, valid, and able to accurately measure the *main outcome variables*? Is the data collected in a consistent manner that enhances valid responses? Were the number and timing of data collection points appropriate? Were data collectors carefully chosen and trained? In the case of observations, is inter-rater reliability measured and reported? Are the procedures for analyzing the data clearly described? Were appropriate *statistical tests* used, including inferential statistics? Were effect sizes (such as mean standardized difference or relative risk) reported? Were confounding variables controlled for in the statistical analysis?

(*continues*)

Questions to understand study	Questions to evaluate study
IV. Results	
L. Were there any important *differences between the groups* at the beginning of the study? What was the attrition/retention rate?	L. Were the *groups similar*/comparable, especially with respect to any confounding variables? Did the researchers explain why participants withdrew from the study? Was attrition excessive? Was attrition similar across groups? After taking attrition into account, are the participants still representative of the population, and are the groups still comparable?
M. What were the *results* for each statistical test? Were any of the results significant? Was effect size used for any results?	M. Are the *results* clearly described in the narrative and clearly presented in tables and figures? Was the sample size large enough to detect a difference between the groups? Were statistical significance and practical significance discussed? Are all results presented or just some results? Are the results accurate? Can a rival hypothesis explain some of the results?

Questions to understand study	Questions to evaluate study
V. Discussion/Conclusion	
N. How do the researchers *interpret the results*? Are the results consistent with past studies?	N. Do the researchers *interpret the results* in light of the pertinent literature, study objective(s), and hypothesis? Do the researchers explain inconsistencies in results between their study and prior studies? Do the researchers explain why results were significant or not significant? Overall, are the results interpreted appropriately, and do they take into account the study's limitations?
O. What *strengths or limitations* of the study are given?	O. Did the researchers mention all *limitations* and their possible effects on the quality of the study results? Did the researchers identify the threats to validity that were not well controlled?
P. What *recommendations* for further studies were given?	P Were *recommendations* specific, appropriate, and consistent with the research base?
Q. What are the study's *conclusions*?	Q. Are the *conclusions* clearly stated and supported by the results? Does the conclusion touch on the study objective? If the researchers generalized their findings, did they do so appropriately? Are the conclusions applicable to nutrition practice?

Additional evaluation tools, such as the EAL Quality Criteria Checklist, are mentioned toward the end of the chapter.

REVIEW QUESTIONS

Match elements of research articles to the section of a research article where they would be found.

Elements of research articles	Sections of a research article
1. How results compare to other studies	A. Introduction
2. Hypothesis	B. Methods
3. Description of participants	C. Results
4. Tables showing *P*-values	D. Discussion
5. Name of research design	E. Conclusion
6. Literature review (brief)	
7. Limitations of study	
8. Research problem	
9. Setting	
10. Recommendations for future studies	
11. Description of intervention	
12. Purpose of study	
13. How results will be analyzed	
14. Closing statement	
15. Information on randomization and blinding	

CRITICAL THINKING QUESTIONS

1. Write your own abstract for the Eaton et al. (2016) article. Try to limit each part of the abstract to five sentences. Next, compare it to the abstract at the beginning of the article. How are they different and why?
2. Use the Evidence Analysis Library's Quality Criteria Checklist to evaluate the Eaton et al. (2016) article. Compare your ratings with a classmate.
3. For the following cohort study, write your own abstract. Also write an evaluation/critique of the article using the questions in this chapter as a guide. Write a minimum of one paragraph for each of these sections: Research Title and Authors, Introduction of Article, Methods, Results, and Discussion/Conclusion.

   Song, M., Fung, T. T., Hu, F. B., Willett, W. C., Longo, V. D., Chan, A. T., & Giovannucci, E. L. (2016). Association of animal and plant protein intake with all-cause and cause-specific mortality. *JAMA Internal Medicine*, E1–E11. doi:10.1001/jamainternmed.2016.4182
4. For the following quasi-experimental study, write your own abstract. Also write an evaluation/critique of the article using the questions in this chapter as a guide. Write a minimum of one paragraph for each of these sections: Research Title and Authors, Introduction of Article, Methods, Results, and Discussion/Conclusion.

   Jacob, R., Lamarche, B., Provencher, V., Laramee, C., Valois, P., Goule, Cl., &

Drapeau, V. (2016). Evaluation of a theory-based intervention aimed at improving coaches' recommendations on sports nutrition to their athletes. *Journal of the Academy of Nutrition and Dietetics, 116,* 1308–1315. doi: 10.1016/j.jand.2016.04.005

5. Use the Evidence Analysis Library's Quality Criteria Checklist to evaluate either the article in question 3 or question 4.
6. For the following study, write your own abstract. Also write an evaluation/critique of the article using the questions in this chapter as a guide. Write a minimum of one paragraph for each of these sections: Research Title and Authors, Introduction of Article, Methods, Results, and Discussion/Conclusion.

   Barron, E., Sokoloff, N. C., Maffiazioli, G. D. N., Ackerman, K. E., Woolley, R., Holmes, T. M., Anderson, E. J., & Misra, M. 2016. Diets high in fiber and vegetable protein are associated with low lumbar bone mineral density in young athletes with oligoamenorrhea. *Journal of the Academy of Nutrition and Dietetics, 116,* 481–489. doi: 10.1016/j.jand.2015.10.022

SUGGESTED READINGS AND ACTIVITIES

1. Boushey, C. J., Harris, J., Bruemmer, B., & Archer, S. A. (2008). Publishing nutrition research: A review of sampling, sample size, statistical analysis, and other key elements of manuscript preparation, Part 2. *Journal of the American Dietetic Association, 108,* 679–688. doi: 10.1016/j.jada.2008.01.002

REFERENCES

Academy of Nutrition and Dietetics. (2012). *Evidence Analysis Manual: Steps in the Academy Evidence Analysis Process.* Retrieved from https://www.andeal.org/vault/2440/web/files/2012_Aug_EA_Manual.pdf

Boswell, C., & Cannon, S. (2017). *Introduction to nursing research: Incorporating evidence-based practice* (4th ed.). Burlington, MA: Jones & Bartlett Learning.

Burls, A. (2009). *What is critical appraisal?* (What Is? Series) Retrieved from http://www.whatisseries.co.uk/what-is-critical-appraisal/

Eaton, C. B., Hartman, S. J., Perzanowski, E., Pan. G., Roberts, M. B., Risica, P. M., ... Marcus, B. H. (2016). A randomized clinical trial of a tailored lifestyle intervention for obese, sedentary, primary care patients. *Annals of Family Medicine, 14,* 311–319. doi: 10.1370/afm.1952

Gray, J. R., Grove, S. K. & Sutherland, S. (2017). *Burns and Grove's the practice of nursing research: Appraisal, synthesis, and generation of evidence* (8th ed.). St. Louis, MO: Elsevier Saunders.

Hartman, S. J., Risica, P. M., Gans, K. M., Marcus, B. H., & Eaton, C. B. (2014). Tailored weight loss intervention in obese adults within primary care practice: Rationale, design, and methods of Choose to Lose. *Contemporary Clinical Trials, 38,* 409–419. doi: 10.1016/j.cct.2014.06.001

Higgins, J., & Green, S. (Eds.). (2011). *Cochrane Handbook for Systematic Reviews of Intervention* (Version 5.1.0). Retrieved from http://handbook.cochrane.org

Hulley, S. B., Cummings, S. R., Browner, W. S., & Grady, D. G. (2013). *Designing clinical research* (4th ed.). Philadelphia, PA: Lippincott, Williams & Wilkins.

Lipman, T. O. (2013). Critical reading and critical thinking—study design and methodology: A personal approach on how to read the clinical literature. *Nutrition in Clinical Practice, 28,* 158–164. doi: 10.11777/0884533612474041

Lomangino, K. M. (2016). Countering cognitive bias: Tips for recognizing the impact of potential bias on research. *Journal of the Academy of Nutrition and Dietetics, 116,* 204–207. doi: 10.1016/j.jand.2015.07.014

Polit, D. F., & Beck, C. T. (2014). *Essentials of nursing research: Appraising evidence for nursing practice.* Philadelphia, PA: Wolters Kluwer/Lippincott Williams & Wilkins.

Schmidt, N. A., & Brown, J. M. (2015). *Evidence-based practice for nurses: Appraisal and application of research* (3rd ed.). Burlington, MA: Jones & Bartlett Learning.

Schulz, K. F., Altman, D. G., & Moher, D., for the CONSORT Group. (2010). CONSORT 2010 Statement: Updated guidelines for reporting parallel group randomised trials. *PLoS Medicine, 7,* e1000251. doi:10.1371/journal.pmed.1000251

Stone, H., & Sidel, J. L. (1993). *Sensory evaluation practices* (2nd ed.). Cambridge, MA: Academic Press.

PART

3

How to Read, Interpret, and Evaluate Qualitative Nutrition Research

The Basics of Qualitative Research

L. SUZANNE GOODELL, PHD, RD
NATALIE K. COOKE, PHD
VIRGINIA C. STAGE PHD, RD, LDN

CHAPTER OUTLINE

- Introduction
- The Problem Statement
- Literature Review
- Methods
- Data Analysis
- Results
- Discussion and Conclusions

LEARNING OUTCOMES

- Describe the differences and similarities between qualitative and quantitative research.
- Explain the key features of a qualitative research study.
- Explain how a qualitative problem statement differs from a quantitative hypothesis.
- Compare and contrast the four types of data collection methodologies commonly used in nutrition research: focus groups, individual interviews, observations, and document analysis.
- Determine what circumstances might lend themselves to an interview rather than a focus group.
- Describe what an observation might include and when it might be used instead of, or in addition to interviews and/or focus groups.
- Explain how sample size is determined in a qualitative study.
- Given a particular study, determine what inclusion and exclusion criteria should be applied.
- Compare and contrast different sampling techniques and strategies used in qualitative research.
- Given a type of interview (semistructured, unstructured/in-depth, or structured), write an interview question that fits the interview style.
- Explain the role of summarizing and unbiased, nonjudgmental questions in reducing researcher bias.
- Describe the difference in the types of information recorded on a tool used for observation versus a tool used for document analysis.

CHAPTER 9

- ꞁs an ꞁ.
- ꞁof the ꞁdebook
- ꞁcoding and ꞁs used in data
- Describe what a memo is and what role it plays in the data analysis process.
- Differentiate between themes, theories, and models.
- Explain the role of trustworthiness in qualitative research design, data collection, analysis, and reporting.

INTRODUCTION

Quantitative research starts with hypotheses and applies statistics to find results. There are lots of numbers involved with quantitative research. In this chapter, we focus on qualitative research. In qualitative research, there are no hypotheses and no statistics, and very few numbers are presented. Instead, qualitative research focuses on words, stories, and experiences. Although some may say that qualitative and quantitative work are opposites, we like to say that they are companions, supporting and complementing each other. Although the methodologies and results appear very different, you will find that some key concepts (like how to maintain rigor) remain the same.

Researchers can use qualitative research at the beginning of a project to generate hypotheses for quantitative research or to inform the development of nutrition interventions. Researchers also can use qualitative research in the middle of a project to explain the process of quantitative research (particularly interventions). Researchers can apply qualitative research at the end of a project to bring a deeper meaning and understanding to the results of quantitative research. This is how qualitative research can be a companion to quantitative research. However, qualitative research can stand on its own, serving to expand the scientific understanding, just as quantitative research does.

In general, a qualitative study is **inductive** in nature. This means that the researcher is moving from a form of detailed data to more general ideas. Understanding this general idea will help you better understand how qualitative researchers produce broad ideas from such large, detailed databases (Creswell, 2013).

Like quantitative research designs, qualitative research also requires the investigator to follow a "blueprint" for the research project. There is not a single agreed-upon structure for how to design a qualitative study; as with quantitative designs, the design of qualitative research depends on the research question the investigator is trying to answer. With that being said, certain design principles are common in a well-designed qualitative research study and often are presented in the literature. Here are a few key features to consider:

- *Start with a problem*. Like designing a quantitative study, qualitative researchers begin with a problem. Often, researchers identify the problem through reviewing the literature on the topic along with their own knowledge of the problem that needs to be studied.
- *Ask open-ended questions*. To study the problem qualitatively, investigators ask **open-ended research questions**. Open-ended research questions allow researchers to remain "open" to understanding the participants' experiences, which keeps investigators from assuming the "researcher knows best." Open-ended questions cannot be answered with a "yes" or "no." Unlike quantitative research, additional open-ended research questions may evolve and be added

during the course of the study to help increase researchers' understanding of the problem.

- *Use of a natural setting.* Qualitative data are often collected in the setting where the individuals' being studied actually experienced the problem being studied.
- *Researchers are a "key instrument."* Qualitative researchers usually collect the data themselves by talking to individuals (e.g., interviews, focus groups), examining documents (e.g., government policy artifacts), or even observing behaviors. Generally, qualitative researchers do not rely on questionnaires or other tools alone; therefore, the human researcher acts as the "research instrument," not the tool itself.
- *Listen to participants' meanings.* In the entire qualitative research process, the researcher focuses on understanding how the individuals being studied view the problem, not how the researcher views the problem. With that being said, qualitative research does require the researcher to make an interpretation of what he or she sees, hears, and understands through the research process. It is difficult for the researcher to completely separate his or her background and prior understandings from the interpretation of the findings in a qualitative study. The final report from a qualitative study should represent the interpretation of both the individuals being studied and the researcher, as well as considering those reading the study, to allow multiple views of the problem to emerge.

THE PROBLEM STATEMENT

Just like quantitative research articles, qualitative research articles are typically presented with four distinctive parts: Introduction with Literature Review, Methods, Results, and Discussion and Conclusions. When initiating their investigations, researchers always begin with a **problem statement**. The purpose of a problem statement is to explain why the research is being conducted and why it matters to the specific population being studied. After the problem statement, researchers present the **research objective**, which often starts with "the purpose of this study was to." Following the research objective, quantitative researchers tend to present their hypothesis. However, because of the exploratory nature of qualitative research, investigators do not formulate hypotheses to include with their problem statements. *This is a key difference between qualitative and quantitative research.* Instead, they tend to include only a problem statement and a research objective. Sometimes, qualitative researchers will include an open-ended research question in place of a hypothesis.

Just as the topics in nutrition vary greatly, qualitative research questions in nutrition range in scope. Qualitative research can be used to investigate quality of patient care in inpatient settings, challenges associated with implementing behavior change in community settings, factors influencing purchasing and consumption in food service settings, and so much more.

Because our field often focuses on nutrition education and behavior change, research objectives in qualitative nutrition research often focus on barriers to and facilitators of change. For example, Bamford, Heaven, May, and Moynihan (2012) presented their research objective in this way, "Our aim was to understand facilitators and barriers to implementation of the nutrition guidelines [in residential care homes] and to use this information to optimize the implementation process" (p. 2).

However, qualitative research also can simply focus on a lived experience without purposefully seeking ways to change behavior. Research objectives associated with this kind of qualitative research often simply state the target population (who is being studied) and the experience explored (what is happening to those being studied). In "Alone at the Table: Food Behavior and the Loss of Commensality in Widowhood" (Vesnaver, Keller, Sutherland, Maitland, & Locher, 2016), the authors examined "the shifts in food behavior in widowhood" (p. 1060). They presented two research questions (rather than hypotheses): "(a) what shifts, if any, in their food behavior do widows attribute to loss of commensality and (b) how did widows experience losing commensality?" (Vensaver et al., 2016, p. 1060). Although problem statements are essential for knowing how to proceed with research, they are often not presented in an article until the end of a review of literature.

APPLICATION 9.1

If you could do a qualitative study and explore a lived experience of a certain group, who would the participants be and what lived experience would you want to study?

LITERATURE REVIEW

Every primary research article begins with a review of the scientific literature. Some may call this the "Background" or "Introduction" section. As with quantitative research articles, the main focus of the literature review is to justify to the reader why the researcher needs to conduct the study. Every researcher has a slightly different way of presenting the literature review, but four common threads are found in most articles. *First, almost all articles start by explaining broad concepts and then drill down to the specific details related to the study.* Think of this like a funnel, where the background begins with broad statements (wide part of the funnel), and then focuses in on the literature closely related to the topic (narrow part of the funnel).

For example, in an article presenting her investigation of food insecurity in children and families in the United Kingdom, Harvey (2016) began her introduction by defining food insecurity. She then presented statistics about food insecurity in the United Kingdom and general factors contributing to food insecurity. Next, she discussed the consequences of food insecurity. In the next paragraph, she highlighted the limited investigations that focused on experiences with food insecurity through direct reports from children. And finally, she contrasted the limited studies about food insecurity in the United Kingdom with those from the United States and Canada. After reading Harvey's introduction, the reader should have a clear understanding of the importance of her research and why she conducted her work.

Second, the literature review focuses on the most current published scientific research but includes seminal work published at any time in history (i.e., studies frequently cited due to their impact on the profession). There is a lot of scientific literature out in the world. With the advent of online publications, the number of research articles being published every year is soaring. It is not possible for a researcher to write a concise literature review for the background of an article that includes every article ever published about the research topic. Researchers must decide which articles to include and which to exclude. How do they do that? Researchers tend to include both recent and seminal articles in their introduction. Typically, recent articles are those published within the last 5 years, maybe 10 years if the subject matter has not been researched much. Why focus on recent literature? Nutrition knowledge and understanding are constantly changing, so it is important that researchers present the most up-to-date understanding of their research topic.

If they focused on articles from decades ago without including the more recent work, they would probably be leaving out details that could help the reader understand what we already know about the research subject. There is an important exception to this general rule: seminal articles.

Seminal articles are groundbreaking articles that made a huge impact on the field of study. They may have been the first article or series of articles ever published in a specific area of research. For example, when nutrition researchers are presenting literature related to how children learn to like new foods, they almost always cite Birch and Marlin's work from 1982 because their work is foundational to what we know about food neophobia (fear of trying new foods) and learning to like new foods. Qualitative researchers include both qualitative and quantitative studies in their literature review, as long as the work is relevant.

Third, almost all articles clearly and concisely present the gaps in the literature (e.g., research problem). Gaps in the literature are the things we do not know but would like to know. They tell the reader what research should be conducted to help the scientific community better understand a research topic or question. For example, Tanenbaum, Kane, Kenowitz, and Gonzalez (2016) explored the impact of a treatment regimen on diabetes distress in adults with type 2 diabetes. They presented the complexities of how to measure distress in patients and stated, "few studies have provided for an in-depth exploration of the relationship between the diabetes treatment regimen and the experience of emotional distress" (p. 1060). Having identified this gap, the researchers began to build the case for why they conducted their study.

TIP

Some researchers will present the gaps at the end of each paragraph in the literature review, and others will summarize the gaps in the final paragraph of the literature review. Because qualitative research is often conducted as a formative assessment, helping to determine (or form) the next steps in a project or program, researchers may have more gaps to present than if they were conducting a quantitative study.

Fourth, most researchers present their research question and a very basic overview of the study design in the last paragraph of the literature review. Unlike quantitative research articles, qualitative research articles do not contain hypotheses to be tested. Instead, qualitative researchers solely present the specific aim(s) of the study (i.e., the research objective).

METHODS

Typical subheadings found in qualitative research articles include the following:

1. Sampling and Subjects
2. Data Collection Tools
3. Data Collection
4. Data Analysis

Before discussing the contents of each subheading, we review the common data collection methods because these methods influence researchers' decisions related to all of the subheadings. As a side note, often, but not always, researchers present a brief overview of their methods under the Study Design subheading, which appears before Sampling and Subjects sections.

INTRODUCTION TO DATA COLLECTION METHODS

Depending on the research question or problem statement, researchers select one or more of the four major types of qualitative data collection methods: focus groups, individual interviews, observations, and document analysis.

1. **Focus groups** are conducted with a group of individuals who may or may not know each other but who have common characteristics. A group leader uses a semistructured group interview process to capture information such as their values, beliefs, or motivations.
2. Individual interviews are similar to focus groups, but the questions are directed to an individual rather than to a group of people.
3. Rather than interacting with an individual or a group, observations require the researcher to observe a situation as a bystander.
4. **Document analysis** involves systematically collecting, authenticating, and analyzing documents such as government press releases, pictures, or other written works.

The type of data collection method researchers choose depends on whether or not they are interested in participants' behaviors (i.e., observations) or opinions (i.e., focus groups or interviews) or the written/documented record of a topic (i.e., document analysis). Ideally, researchers provide a justification for their choice of data collection methods so the reader can better judge the quality of the research and the potential limitations of the study.

Focus Groups

Focus groups are comprised of individuals who share common experiences. This might mean, for example, that they all have children of the same age or that they are all members of the same faith-based organization, but not necessarily that they know each other in advance. There should ideally be 6 to 10 participants in a focus group, but if that is not possible based on participants' availabilities, then there should be no fewer than 4 and no more than 12. The unit of measure of a focus group is the group, not the individual, so if a researcher conducts two focus groups of 8 participants and three focus groups of 10 participants, the size is 5, *not* 46. This is because focus group data should be analyzed as one unit, a collective voice, rather than by individual voices. A researcher (or **moderator**) first establishes a set of guidelines for the conversation and then guides the participants through a series of open-ended questions. The skilled moderator asks questions that allow participants to discuss amongst themselves, limiting dialogue from the moderator. Another researcher typically serves as a notetaker to allow the moderator to focus her full attention on the progression of the conversation. Focus groups are ideal for situations in which a researcher wants individuals to feed off of each other's responses, creating a web of dialogue.

APPLICATION 9.2

What is a web of dialogue, and why is it useful in qualitative research?

As an example of using focus groups in nutrition research, Anderson et al. (2015) conducted a series of focus groups with obstetrician/gynecologists employed by a clinic that serves primarily low-income minority women and mothers, and also with the mothers who attend the clinic. The mothers did not know each other in advance, but they all were seeing obstetrician/gynecologists at that clinic. In addition to location commonalities, researchers established that participants needed to be of a certain age, health state (pregnant or within 1 year postpartum), and BMI, and eligible for WIC. The researchers developed a series of focus group questions related to barriers and facilitators to gestational weight gain, asking a different set of questions of the mothers than of the obstetrician/gynecologists.

Individual Interviews

Individual interviews are similar to focus groups, but they involve a one-on-one conversation between the interviewer and the participant rather than a conversation with a group of people. Whereas the sample size for a focus group study is equal to the number of groups, the sample size of a series of individual interviews is equal to the number of participants. Focus groups can be useful when a group discussion and exchange of ideas are beneficial. However, if the researcher is concerned that "group think" (the phenomenon in which a group influences an individual's beliefs or discourages someone from speaking up against the group) might sway individuals' opinions, an individual interview is a better option. Therefore, sensitive topics and research questions in which individual voices are needed are most suited for individual interviews.

If a researcher is exploring restrictive eating patterns in women with eating disorders, an interview is more appropriate than a focus group because of the sensitive topic but also because the researcher would not want to give other participants ideas for restrictive eating practices. Weisberg-Shapiro and Devine (2015) were interested in individual differences related to dietary acculturation in Dominican women, so they conducted a series of individual interviews with 29 Dominican women living in San Diego, California, and in New York City. Because the researchers were interested in individual behaviors, they crafted a series of interview questions to elicit participants' views on what they ate before and after moving from the Dominican Republic to the United States. They asked questions that lent themselves to individual, rather than group, conversation. For example, "Please tell me about everything you ate and drank yesterday, starting with the first thing you ate after you woke up."

When researchers are working with a population with restrictive schedules, such as physicians, it can be difficult to find a common time when participants can meet for a focus group. This is another reason researchers might choose individual interviews rather than focus groups. Therefore, interviews might be the chosen data collection method due to convenience, sensitivity of the topic, or desired depth of the interview content. For example, Carraway-Stage et al. (2014) chose individual interviews to explore the state of nutrition education in Head Start preschools, not just because the topic lends itself to individual conversation but also because finding a common time for a focus group when sampling a population of teachers and administrators can be difficult. Also, due to the topic, researchers wanted to maintain the confidentiality of teachers and administrators and avoid a situation in which teachers might not want to disclose their true opinions of nutrition education in the classroom for fear that other teachers or administrators might not support their opinions.

Observations

Because nutrition and behavior are closely linked, observations can be useful when exploring a nutrition-related research question, and they allow the researcher to observe participants' behaviors and interactions in their natural environment (Merriam, 2009).

Observations can stand alone or be combined with other methods, such as interviews or focus groups. Just like interviews and focus groups, what is recorded during an observation depends on the research question, but it can include the setting, the participants, activities and interactions, conversation, subtle factors, and the researcher's own behavior (Merriam 2009).

Bamford et al. (2012) conducted observations of staff in five residential care homes as part of a multi-method qualitative study. Interested in the process of implementing nutrition guidelines for older people in residential care homes, the researchers observed both meal preparation and interactions between the staff in meetings, using field notes to document their observations. They focused their observations on taken-for-granted work practices and routines.

Similarly, Flacking, and Dykes (2013) used a combination of observations and interviews. When conducting observations at each of the four Neonatal Intensive Care Units (NICUs), the researchers used a nine-dimensional framework that included "the physical space; people involved; related acts people do; objects present; single actions; set of related activities carried out; sequencing over time; goals people try to accomplish; and emotions felt and expressed" (p. 3). By outlining what they were going to observe, researchers were able to focus on these nine dimensions during their 300 hours of observations.

As you see with both of these studies, observations are commonly used in either a **multimethod qualitative study**, which combines multiple qualitative data collection methods, or in a **mixed methods study**, which combines both qualitative and quantitative methods. In the case of a multimethod qualitative study, researchers can compare what they observe with what participants tell them in focus groups or interviews. With mixed methods studies, the qualitative piece—observations—provides an explanation for why researchers saw certain quantitative trends. Although observations can stand alone in a study, researchers often use the time in that location to collect other data as well, which may be qualitative or quantitative.

Document Analysis

The name of this type of data collection method can be misleading because document analysis includes collection and organization of different types of documents as well as analysis. According to Bowen (2009), this includes "finding, selecting, appraising (making sense of), and synthesizing data contained in documents" (p. 28). Just as an interview, focus group, or observation involves a rigorous set of steps, so too does document analysis (**Figure 9.1**).

Researchers have to select appropriate documents to be used as part of the study, using a systematic approach to collecting these data. Documents might include public records (e.g., nutrition legislation), personal documents (e.g., personal medical records), popular culture documents (e.g., newspaper articles about nutrition trends in society), or visual documents (e.g., social media photographs of meals). The documents can be collected online or offline (Merriam, 2009).

Documents used in document analysis are classified as primary, secondary, or auxiliary. **Primary documents** are all the documents that are the main focus of your study. For example, if you are studying the federal, state, and local food laws pertaining to school gardens, the primary documents would be all the written laws found on the matter. **Secondary documents** are documents written about those primary documents. Continuing the example, secondary documents might include drafts of the laws and notes made about the laws by senators, representatives, and other federal, state, and local officials. **Auxiliary documents** are relevant but not central to the research question (Altheide & Schneider, 2013). To further illustrate the example of studying food

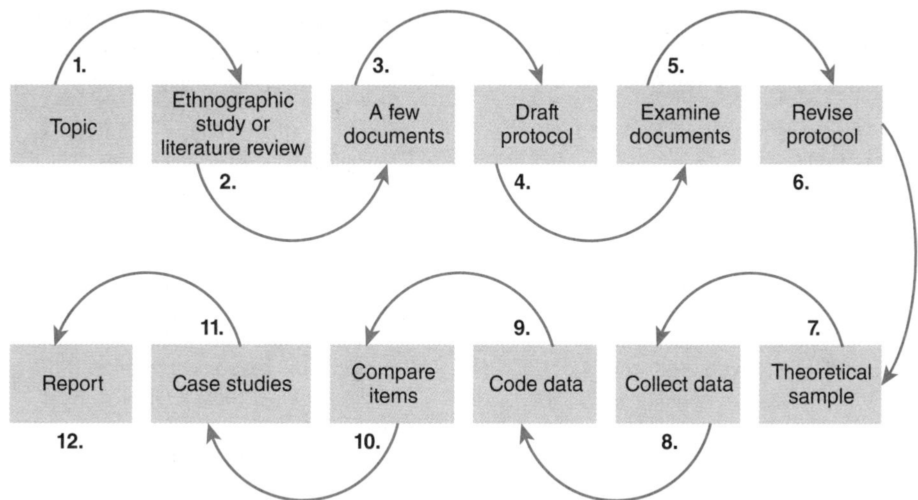

FIGURE 9.1 The Process of Qualitative Document Analysis

Republished with permission of Sage Publications, from *Qualitative Media Analysis*, D.L. Altheide & C.J. Schneider, p. 19, Copyright 2013 permission conveyed through Copyright Clearance Center, Inc.

laws pertaining to school gardens, one might obtain newspaper articles and blog posts that describe experiences about creating school gardens as part of the auxiliary documents. The lines between secondary and auxiliary documents can be blurry, so it is most important that researchers explain *all* documents analyzed in their study and their methods for analyzing each group of documents.

You might see document analysis used along with other methods, such as interviews or focus groups, in a case study methodology, or in a mixed methods study where both qualitative and quantitative methods are combined (Bowen, 2009). Document analysis can also stand alone as a study, serving as a cost-effective and comprehensive way to analyze a large volume of documents, spanning long periods of time (Bowen, 2009). Although there are many uses for document analysis, this data collection method is much less common than interviews or focus groups within nutrition research.

Because online documents are a vast and readily available source, qualitative researchers are just now beginning to determine considerations when conducting document analysis with online sources, including ethics and the impact of culture (writing style and representation of personality) on documents (Merriam, 2009). An example of online document analysis is a study in which Perrin, Goodell, Allen, and Fogleman (2014) extracted data from 954 individuals who were engaging in milk sharing via public Facebook pages. Based on their selection criteria, they were able to extract 1,492 milk sharing posts that served as the data for the qualitative part of a mixed methods study. Using traditional qualitative analysis, they determined two themes relative to requesting milk and offering milk, providing insight into the inner workings of the network of online milk sharing.

Table 9.1 lists the strengths and limitations of qualitative data collection methods.

Subjects and Sampling

As with quantitative researchers, qualitative researchers are expected to describe how they chose the sample from whom (or which) they collected data. This section may be labeled Participants and Recruitment for focus group and interview studies; it may be

Table 9.1 Strengths and Limitations of Qualitative Data Collection Methods

	Strengths	Limitations
Focus Groups	• Most time-efficient of the four data collection methods. • Group discussion may allow participants to remember information they might not otherwise recall on their own. • Ideal for decision making, product or program development, and insight into organizational principles.[1] • Combine well with other methods, including survey design.[1]	• Does not allow analysis of differences in individual voices or opinions. • Time restraints may limit the depth of the conversation. • It can be difficult to arrange a time when a group of individuals can all meet in one room to discuss an issue. • "Group think" can influence participants responses, especially if one group member is very vocal and opinionated.[1] • For fear of sounding uneducated, participants might make up responses.[1] • Quality of the data depends on the quality of the questions asked.[2]
Individual Interviews	• Participants can be honest and share opinions without fear of being judged by a group. • Because only one participant is speaking, conversation can be more in-depth and elicit more personal answers.	• Time-intensive because sample size depends on saturation. • It can be difficult to recruit participants to agree to an in-depth interview due to busy schedules. • Quality of the data depends on the quality of the questions asked.[2]
Observations	• Individuals are observed within their natural environment, so actions are natural and authentic. • Combining with interviews and focus groups, observation data can help to fully understand a phenomenon.[1]	• Time-intensive because it can be difficult to capture everything at once. • Participants might change behavior if they know they are being observed. • There might be too much to observe at once, meaning that the researcher might miss an important action due to focusing on another action.
Document Analysis	• Allows for broad-sweeping analysis of a large data set. • Much information is available online, so documents are more readily accessible now. • Allows for historical review, especially when individuals are not available for interviews.[2] • The researcher does not sway the evidence through conversation.[2] • Because they were created by individuals in the real world, for use in the real world, they are a strong representation of the realities of a topic.[2]	• Researcher cannot ask follow-up questions to elicit clarification on information presented in the document. • Information might not be useful because it was not created specifically for the research process.[2] • It can be difficult to determine whether documents or artifacts are authentic.[2] • Participants might represent themselves differently online than in real life, exhibiting different personalities in online documents.[2] • Online data changes quickly, so multiple versions may need to be analyzed.[2]

Data from: [1]Kreuger and Casey (2009), [2]Merriam (2009).

combined with the Data Collection section and labeled Data Extraction for document analysis studies. In either case, researchers should describe at least three components:

1. *Inclusion and exclusion criteria* explain the qualifications of an individual for participation in an interview or focus group or to be observed during the study. Similarly, when conducting document analysis, researcher include inclusion and exclusion criteria for choosing which documents to review, just like when choosing individuals to participate.
2. A study's *sample size* reflects how many people, groups, or documents were included in a study. Researchers should also explain how they determined when a sample size was sufficient.
3. Because recruiting participants and selecting documents can be challenging, researchers employ various *sampling techniques and strategies* to obtain their target sample size.

Inclusion and Exclusion Criteria

Inclusion criteria are the rules followed for including someone or something in a study. With focus groups, interviews, and observations, inclusion criteria typically are based on demographic variables (e.g., age, gender, socioeconomic status, job, ethnicity, race) or a common experience (e.g., breastfeeding, disease state, food insecurity). For example, if you decided to conduct a study investigating mothers' breastfeeding habits, you might want to create inclusion criteria. Would you want to include all moms or just moms who are currently breastfeeding? Do you want the moms to be breastfeeding their first child or does that matter? Do the moms need to be exclusively breastfeeding or can they be using breast milk and formula? Does the age of the child matter? All of these answers are inclusion criteria.

With document analysis, inclusion criteria might be based on dates, locations, and content. For example, Goonan, Mirosa, and Spence (2014) selected documents ("company policies and plans, production and service materials, waste records, and quality assurance tools and records" p. 64) at three hospital food service sites where observations, focus groups, and interviews were also being conducted. Time, rather than location, was used as an inclusion criterion for another study in which researchers extracted data (posts on milk sharing Facebook groups) during a 3-month period (Perrin et al., 2014). Faraji, Etemad, Sari, and Ravaghi (2015) included only relevant documents that were yielded from a PubMed and ScienceDirect search using the terms "diabetes," "policies," "programs," "processes," "strategies," "intervention," and "Iran." Lachat et al. (2008) also used certain search terms but only selected cases (countries) where both policy and secondary documents were available related to the specific nutrition policy of interest.

Exclusion criteria are the rules made about keeping someone or something out of a study, even though all of the inclusion criteria are met. These rules might be in place to prevent nonconformists or outliers from affecting your data. To clarify, let's look at the inclusion criteria from the breastfeeding example. In your study, you might choose only to include moms who are currently exclusively breastfeeding their first child, and their first child must be less than 6 months of age. However, you might find that you want to leave some of these moms out of your study. You might decide that you do not want to include moms who are breastfeeding premature infants. Why? Because premature infants have special needs that might affect a mother's breastfeeding habits. If you were to include a mom of a premature infant in your study, you would not expect her data to be similar to the data of the other mothers. Therefore, in this particular study, you would exclude mothers of premature infants.

Continuing with our examples of document analysis, Goonan et al. (2014) did not seek documents outside of the three hospitals, and Perrin et al. (2014) did not analyze any Facebook posts outside of the 3-month window. Faraji et al. (2015) did not include documents that were not related to Iran, the country of interest; and Lachat et al. (2008) excluded countries for which only policy documents or secondary documents were available. The researchers may not explicitly state exclusion criteria, but these criteria can be determined based on the inclusion criteria. This information might also be included in the Results section; for example, Lachat et al. (2008) listed all of the countries for which nutrition policy documents could not be located.

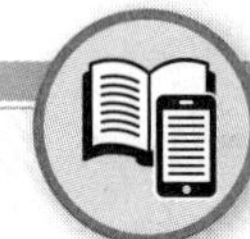

APPLICATION 9.3

How do inclusion and exclusion criteria in qualitative research sometimes differ from inclusion and exclusion criteria in quantitative research?

Sample Size

In quantitative research, sample size is often determined based on how many people are needed to determine statistical significance. In quantitative research, sample size is most often determined before data collection begins. In qualitative research, however, researchers are not looking for statistical significance.

Qualitative researchers may determine their sample size in different ways, but the most common method reported in the literature is **saturation**. "Saturation" is reached when researchers conclude they are not learning anything new from additional data collection (Creswell, 2013). Data collection and data analysis should occur simultaneously in qualitative research. As researchers develop themes or theories (discussed in the Data Analysis section), they may determine they need more data to confirm their findings or that they are missing pieces to the story they are trying to tell. When this happens, the researchers may choose to collect data from new participants or from documents. However, when the researchers believe they are not hearing anything new and are not adding anything to their findings, they will stop data collection because they have reached saturation. In nutritional biochemistry, "saturation" is used to describe a fatty acid that includes no double bonds; it is full of hydrogen atoms and nothing else can be added. Likewise, in qualitative research, saturation is reached when the research findings are full and there is nothing new to be added. Of note, **theoretical saturation** refers to when a researcher obtains saturation in theory development, and it is not a term for "presumed saturation."

Sampling Techniques and Strategies

To assist with identifying and recruiting sufficient participants for their study, researchers often employ one or more sampling techniques. There are many types of sampling techniques, but qualitative researchers often report that their sampling was purposeful or purposive, meaning they used inclusion and exclusion criteria to purposefully select their participants. Some researchers may use a **convenience sample**, which means they recruited participants in a way that saved time, money, and effort. Some may recruit participants to obtain **maximum variation** (i.e., to hear as many different ideas and experiences as possible), whereas others may recruit a homogenous population (a group of individuals as similar to one another as possible). Finally, you may also read that researchers used **snowball sampling** to recruit participants. In this method, the researcher asks original participants (or other key informants) to help identify people who might qualify for the study. The recommendations of one participant may result in the recruitment of two or three more participants. In this way, just as rolling a snowball can help gather more snow, asking participants to help identify participants can help gather more participants and grow the sample size.

APPLICATION 9.4

Are the sampling techniques mentioned based on probability or nonprobability sampling?

DATA COLLECTION TOOLS

Regardless of the type of data collection method, all types of qualitative research methodologies use a *research tool* or *guide* to maintain consistency throughout the data collection process (similar to a protocol in an intervention study). Typically, a **guide** is used for individual interviews or focus groups, and a **tool** is used for observations or document analysis. It would be irresponsible to enter into a scientific experiment and begin combining chemicals without having a protocol. Similarly, starting to conduct interviews, focus groups, or observations before having a plan would be harmful to the research process. These data collection tools are an important part of the data collection plan. The research process is informed by prior research, so the development of these research tools is based on existing knowledge and the need to better understand a topic (see Chapter 1).

Interview and Focus Group Guides

The data collection tool used with interviews and focus groups is called a guide. Because several members of the research team might be collecting data at the same time, it is important that all researchers use a standard guide to calibrate their work. When you read a qualitative research article that used interviews or focus groups, the researchers will likely describe the basic concepts about their guide. A guide is like a roadmap or GPS for how the conversation will evolve. The researcher has an idea of what the conversation will include but has to be open to detours in the conversation. This is what we call being semi-structured. Semistructured interviews differ from unstructured/in-depth interviews and structured interviews in these ways:

- **Structured interviews** are more rigid, almost resembling a survey rather than an interview. For example, in a structured interview, a researcher might ask the participant, "What was the first thing you ate when you woke up yesterday?" followed by a list of questions about that food such as how big it was, how much of it he or she ate, what he or she had with it (e.g., condiments), and so forth. The researcher would then ask the same questions of the second food the person ate, and so on.
- **Unstructured interviews** allow for the participant to guide the conversation completely. In this type of interview, a researcher might ask an empty nester, "Tell me about how family meals have changed, if at all, since your children went away to college." This conversation could go any number of ways, to talking about how the foods have changed, the time of day has changed, the location has changed, and so on.

- **Semistructured interviews** allow for structure but are not so rigid that they limit the participant from sharing tangential, and oftentimes relevant, information; they are the most common type of interview in nutrition research. In a semi-structured interview about adjusting to a new diagnosis of diabetes, a researcher might have three to five main questions like these: "What are some tactics you use to control your blood sugar." "What things prevent you from being able to control your blood sugar." These are open enough that the participant can talk about anything related to barriers and motivators; however, it is not as unstructured as "Tell me about how you are adjusting to your new diagnosis."

The guide keeps the conversation on track, allowing the researcher to bring the conversation back to the purpose of the research. The structure of a guide is therefore an important part of the research methodology. Although a researcher might not specify each section of the guide in a research article, guides typically include the following:

- An ice-breaker question to get the participant comfortable with talking
- Main interview questions with probes to encourage the participant to talk more about the subject
- Time for summarizing participant responses
- Time when the researcher repeats information to the participant to confirm, deny, or elaborate on the information discussed

Researchers may summarize the components of their guide, provide a table with main interview questions, or provide the entire guide as supplemental material. Journals have varying preferences about how this information is reported.

Regardless of the questions asked, the wording of the questions and how they are presented to the participants is crucial to the quality of data collected. Therefore, researchers often report that the language in the guide they used was open-ended, unbiased, and nonjudgmental. Because interviews and focus groups are used to describe or explore a certain topic, guide questions need to be carefully designed to encourage participants to share their perspectives through stories and examples. This means that all questions need to be open-ended to encourage participants to share their opinions and experiences. Imagine that someone asks you: "Do you eat breakfast in the morning?" You would answer "yes" or "no" because this is a **closed-ended question**. Rather, imagine that someone asks you: "What do you typically eat for breakfast?" This question would encourage you to give examples of foods you consume in the morning, perhaps leading you to tell a story about a time you and your roommates prepared a brunch or a family tradition of eating breakfast for dinner on Sunday evenings. By changing just a few words, the type of data you would collect would be much different.

As mentioned, the wording of guide questions also needs to be unbiased and nonjudgmental. Researchers bring their own perspectives about the research topic, so they have to be careful to leave their biases out of the research process, a phenomenon called **researcher bias**. This relates to the interview or focus group questions, probe, and the summary. Avoid using qualifying words such as "good" or "bad" in the interview questions. Asking a participant to "Tell me why YOU canot stick to a healthy diet" would come across as judgmental. However, rephrasing the question to "Tell me what it is like to try to stick to a healthy diet" would elicit conversation about successful tactics and barriers or challenges to healthy eating. The researcher could then probe to find out more about strategies that work and barriers that stand in the way. Similarly, when summarizing, the researcher should avoid putting words into a participant's mouth. If the researcher recognizes what the participant shares as unhealthy practices; the researcher would not call them unhealthy or bad unless the participant used those words. The way a researcher asks these questions is also important, and this style is refined during the researcher's training.

Observation and Document Analysis Tools

The generic term "tool" is typically used to describe the data collection documents used in observations and document analysis. These tools are like worksheets with categories for purposefully collecting specific areas of qualitative data. The categories are chosen by the researcher, based on the overarching research question. Because research questions differ widely between studies, there is no standard structure for this type of data collection tool. However, a well-formatted tool can help researchers, especially novice researchers, consistently record the events of an observation or key pieces of information in a document. Without a clear and consistent understanding for how data will be selected and recorded, researchers could be subject to **biased selectivity** (Bowen, 2009). Although a fresh tool is used for each observation or document extraction, the completed (filled in) tools can be compared during data analysis.

Because of the difference in research questions, researchers will record very different data for an observational study than for a document analysis study. An observation tool might include the physical setting, the participants present, activities and interactions, conversations, subtle factors, and the researcher's own behavior within the environment (Merriam, 2009). The descriptions of activities, interactions, and conversations will focus on key questions that will help answer the overarching research questions. A document analysis tool might include the medium type (e.g., newspaper, blog post, picture), date of creation, location of key information (e.g., headline versus body of text), length of document, and descriptions of the document content (Altheide & Schneider, 2013). Similar to observations, the descriptions of content will focus on key questions that will help answer the overarching research questions.

Because many research studies involving observations or document analysis are mixed method studies, often the tools used in these studies include areas for documenting both quantitative and qualitative data. **Figure 9.2** is an example of an observational tool used to collect both qualitative and quantitative data to document how mothers prepared infant formula for feeding their infant.

Piloting

To demonstrate that a guide is worded well or that a tool is designed to help the researcher observe the "right things" or to extract the right information from the documents, researchers **pilot test** their data collection tools. During the pilot, researchers typically conduct a series of interviews, focus groups, observations, or document analyses that are not intended to be included in final data set. After each round of pilot data collection, the researcher edits the data collection tool to improve the quality of the data collected. To do this, the researcher analyzes the data collected and the process of collecting the pilot data, to see if anything needs to be changed to improve the quality (the fit of the data to the research question) of the data. For uniformity, ideally the same guide or tool is used in each data collection (interview, focus group, observation, data analysis), so the editing process should happen before real data collection begins. However, in some cases, it is necessary to make adjustments part way through the study. Researchers often disclose these changes in their research article in an attempt to be transparent about their methods.

Researcher as an Instrument: Training

Researchers can also demonstrate the quality of their data through explaining researcher training. Much like you might calibrate a laboratory tool before using it, researcher training plays an important role in "calibrating" the researcher (the instrument) to collect strong qualitative research data. Without training, a researcher might unintentionally

Version: October 24, 2012 Baby Mine Phase 2A **Bottle Prep Observation**
Subject ID: P2A15

MASTER

Date: 1/10/13 **Researcher (Interviewer):** KB
Notetaker JN

1. What is your ethnicity/race?

☐ American Indian/Alaska Native ☐ Asian ☐ Black/African American
☐ Hispanic/Latino ☐ Native Hawaiian/Other Pacific Islander ☑ White/Caucasian
☐ Two or more races ☐ Other: ____

2. What is the highest grade of school you have completed?

☐ Primary (elementary) ☐ Secondary (middle & high) ☐ GED ☐ Vocational/technical
☑ Some college ☐ College ☐ Graduate school
☐ Other: ____
2 years

3. What is your current emloyment status?
a. [If working] Full-time or part-time?
b. [If NOT] Do you plan on returning to work?

☐ Currently working
☐ Full-time ☐ Part-time
☒ NOT currently working
☐ With no plan to return
☒ Planning to return to work full-time
☐ Planning to return to work part-time

	Date	Initials
Entered	1/14/13	KC
Verified	1/15/13	AD

4. What is your marital status?

☐ Single ☒ Married ☐ Divorced ☐ Separated ☐ Living with Partner ☐ Widowed
☐ Other: ____

5. Is this your first baby? ☒ No ☐ Yes

6. Including your baby, how many children are in your household? 3

7. Have you ever breastfed this or another baby? ☑ No ☐ Yes

[If YES]
a. Was it this baby that you breastfed? NA ☐ No ☐ Yes
b. For the most recent baby you breastfed, how long did you breastfeed? NA

FIGURE 9.2 Example of a Completed Observation Tool (Qualitative and Quantitative)

Printed with permission from Katherine F. Kavanagh, adapted from original source. Ellison R.G., Greer B.P., Burney J.L., Goodell L.S., Bower K.B., Nicklas J.C., Lou Z., Kavanagh K. Observations and conversations: A mixed-methods approach to describing home-preparation of infant formula among a sample of low-income mothers. Under review. Submitted to JNEB, October 2016. This study was funded by the United States Department of Agriculture (USDA, NIFA, AFRI: 2009-05111);258.

Version: October 24, 2012　　Baby Mine Phase 2A　　**MASTER**　　**Bottle Prep Observation**

Subject ID: P2A15

Date: 1/10/13　M　**Researcher Initials:** KB ☐ Interviewer　JN ☐ Note-Taker

Bottle 1. Current Formula		
	Checklist	**Notes**
Environment	1. Location: ☒ Living Room ☐ Kitchen ☐ Bedroom ☐ Other (note) 2. Distractions: ☐ TV ☐ Radio ☐ Phone ☐ Computer ☐ People ☒ None 3. Other people present: ☒ No ☐ Yes (note) 4. Suppliers from other room: ☐ No ☒ Yes (note)	1. bedroom for (N) supplies
Sanitation & Sterilization	1. Washed hands with soap and water: ☑ No ☐ Yes ☐ Not Observed 2. Bottle equipment inspected: ☑ No ☐ Yes ☐ Not Observed 3. Bottle washed with soap and water: ☑ No ☐ Yes ☐ Not Observed a. If sponge/bottle brush used, disinfected: ☑ No ☐ Yes ☐ N/A 4. Source of water: ☐ Tap ☐ Filtered ☐ Bottled ☑ Sterile baby water ☐ Other (note) 5. Water boiled: ☑ No ☐ Yes 6. Bottle warmed: ☑ No ☐ Yes	2. Nursery water purified (I)
Formula Prep	1. In bottle first: ☑ Water ☐ Formula 2. Amount of water: 4 oz a. Water leveled: ☐ Flat surface ☐ At eye level ☑ Quickly eyed ☐ Already in bottle 3. Scoop from can used: ☐ No (note) ☑ Yes a. # of scoops: 2 b. Formula scoop: ☑ Level ☐ Unleveled c. Formula leveled: ☑ Against can ☐ Tapped ☐ Used finger ☐ N/A ☐ Other (note) 4. Cereal in bottle: ☑ No ☐ Yes 5. Other additions to bottle: NO 6. Shakes bottle: ☐ No ☑ Yes a. How long: ~5–10 Sec 7. More formula added: ☑ No ☐ Yes 8. More water added: ☑ No ☐ Yes	3. Food Start Gentle, (N) usually microwaves to warm even though knows about hot spots; no microwave right now (N)

Version: October 24, 2012　　Baby Mine Phase 2A　　**MASTER**　　**Bottle Prep Observation**

Subject ID: P2A15

Bottle 1. Lab Formula		
	Checklist	**Notes**
Environment	1. Location: ☑ Living Room ☐ Kitchen ☐ Bedroom ☐ Other (note) 2. Distractions: ☐ TV ☐ Radio ☐ Phone ☐ Computer ☐ People ☑ None 3. Other people present: ☐ No ☑ Yes (note) 4. Supplies from other room: ☑ No ☐ Yes (note) 5. Read instructions on can: ☐ No ☑ Yes (note)	husband (N)
Sanitation & Sterilization	1. Washed hands with soap and water: ☑ No ☐ Yes ☐ Not Observed 2. Bottle equipment inspected: ☑ No ☐ Yes ☐ Not Observed 3. Bottle washed with soap and water: ☑ No ☐ Yes ☐ Not Observed a. If sponge/bottle brush used, disinfected: ☑ No ☐ Yes ☐ N/A 4. Source of water: ☐ Tap ☐ Filtered ☐ Bottled ☑ Sterile baby water ☐ Other (note) 5. Water boiled: ☑ No ☐ Yes 6. Bottle warmed: ☑ No ☐ Yes	nursery water (N)
Formula Prep	1. In bottle first: ☑ Water ☐ Formula 2. Amount of water: 2 oz a. Water leveled: ☐ Flat surface ☑ At eye level ☐ Quickly eyed ☐ Already in bottle 3. Scoop from can used: ☐ No (note) ☑ Yes a. # of scoops: 1 b. Formula scoop: ☐ Level ☑ Unleveled c. Formula leveled: ☐ Against can ☐ Tapped ☐ Used finger ☑ N/A ☐ Other (note) 4. Cereal in bottle: ☑ No ☐ Yes 5. Other additions to bottle: NO 6. Shakes bottle: ☐ No ☑ Yes a. How long: ~3 Sec 7. More formula added: ☑ No ☐ Yes 8. Mote water added: ☑ No ☐ Yes	2 halfish scoops (I) to equal 1

FIGURE 9.2 Example of a Completed Observation Tool (Qualitative and Quantitative) (*continued*)

Printed with permission from Katherine F. Kavanagh, adapted from original source.

ask leading questions or insert her own opinion into a focus group, or leave out a document that conflicts with his personal beliefs, thereby contaminating the data. This can be the same effect as contaminating laboratory samples.

The process of qualitative researcher training is not well-documented because there is no standard approach, and training differs based on the study design, data collection methods, and the research question. However, it is important for researchers to understand the theoretical principles of qualitative research and ethics, as well as to have a rigorous protocol for implementation of the research process. Therefore, research training should be a rigorous process, so that everyone involved in carrying out the study acts in a skilled and ethical manner.

For interviews and focus groups, one established training involves a five-phase process.

1. Ethics training
2. A review of basic qualitative research methods and data collection procedures
3. Mock interview with previously recorded interview
4. Mock interviews within the research team
5. Mock interviews within the participant or closely related population (Goodell, Stage, & Cooke, 2016).

Researcher training for observations differs from interviews and focus groups because they are focused more on the art of note-taking, rather than on facilitating a conversation with an individual or a group of people. When conducting observations for the first time, the training researcher might become overwhelmed (Merriam, 2009). Training for an observer could include (1) learning to pay attention, (2) learning to write descriptively, (3) disciplined recording of **field notes**, and (4) separating detail from trivial information (Merriam, 2009; Patton, 2002). Even fewer descriptions exist for training in document analysis because both the protocols and the media will differ so greatly. Regardless, researchers should hone their data collection skills while revising the data collection tool before final data collection.

DATA COLLECTION

Having discussed the different data collection methods, in this section we briefly discuss the information typically presented in the Data Collection section of an article. This section typically includes the steps followed on the day of data collection.

Focus Groups and Interviews

Typically, the researcher provides a brief synopsis of what was discussed when writing about the data collection for focus groups or interviews. The researcher often provides a description of the setting in which the focus groups or interviews took place. This is done to emphasize the privacy (or lack thereof) afforded to the participants, which could affect the trustworthiness of the data. Researchers often also write about the average time of a focus group or an interview to demonstrate the depth of the conversations. They may only use two or three sentences to state that during the focus group or interview the moderator/interviewer gave a brief introduction to the purpose of the research, guided participants through the consent process, and then began asking questions from the guide. The researcher will likely also include that the interviewer (interviews) or the notetaker (focus groups) took handwritten notes about what was discussed and what happened during the interview/focus group. These notes may be converted into more in-depth field notes, similar to the data collection process for observational studies.

The output of each focus group or interview is an audio recording and a field note. The audio recording is then transcribed verbatim, meaning that a trained researcher listens to the audio file and types out word-for-word exactly what he or she hears, creating a typed document of the conversation, called a **transcript**. Typically the transcript is the primary data source, and the field notes are the secondary source for analysis.

Observations

When discussing data collection, the researcher of an observational study writes about the data collection setting, just as with focus groups and interviews. They often also discuss how long each observation lasted and how many observations occurred. Similar to focus groups and interviews, researchers describe these details as one indication of the depth of the data collected. Both interviews and focus groups are audio recorded, but observations may or may not be audio or video recorded, depending on the impact a camera might have on participants' real, honest interactions. Researchers state whether the observations were recorded. Some observations are based solely on recordings. Other researchers may use the recordings as a supplement to live data collection, and still others may choose to rely solely on live observations.

Regardless of whether or not the researcher uses live or recorded observations, he or she will likely describe a two-step process for transforming the observations into something that can be analyzed. In the first step, during the observation, the researcher will take notes, or **jottings**, which serve as shorthand for more in-depth field notes that will be written later. If one exists, this is the point at which an observation tool is used. In the second step, the researcher transforms the jottings into field notes, a detailed description of what the researcher observed. The details provided in the field notes focus on the overarching research question and the key points of the observation tool and can include diagrams, lists, quotes, and narrative descriptions of the observation, including what are called **observer's comments**, editorializing in the margins (Merriam, 2009). Video recordings may or may not be transcribed, depending on the goal of the research. Video transcripts (if they exist) and field notes are used in data analysis.

Document Analysis

The data collection process in document analysis consists of physically or electronically gathering the documents and applying the data collection tool or protocol to each document. For example, merely collecting tweeted photographs featuring school lunches is not performing *document analysis*. That is merely gathering documents. To perform the data collection process of document analysis, the researcher uses a series of guidelines to extract specific types of information from the photographs for later analysis. For example, researchers might use the data collection tool to extract the date, time, and type of food included in each picture tweeted. They might also record statements made about the food and how much food was consumed from the plate. Because the data collection process is different for document analysis, researchers may not include Data Collection subheading in the article. Instead, they may use the subheading Data Extraction. In

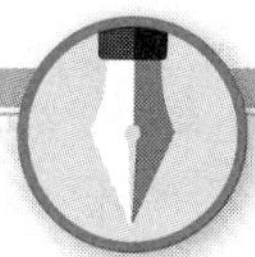

TIP

To reiterate, the unit of analysis is one document or set of documents; the data that are analyzed during data analysis are the extracted data, not the document itself.

this part of the Methods section, the researchers discuss their data extraction protocols, including who was involved in the data extraction, the steps taken to extract data from the document, and the process for handling unusual or nonconforming cases.

DATA ANALYSIS

Data analysis in quantitative research is often sequential, but this is not the case for qualitative research. In quantitative research, generally, all the data for a single study are collected, organized, analyzed, and then findings are described in a written report (Creswell, 2013). Qualitative data analysis, on the other hand, is more iterative in nature. However, researchers typically explain this iterative process in a linear fashion for ease of writing and understandability.

Researchers may not write about their analytic process in detail because they may not have room in the Methods section of the article to discuss all of nuances of their work. Typically, researchers only describe data analysis in basic terms, and then provide one example to illustrate their point. However, by doing so, they are leaving out many little details of the process. In the following sections, we discuss what is often implied by some of the common statements made in the Data Analysis section of qualitative research articles.

DATA ORGANIZATION

Researchers do not use a lot of space to explain how they organized data; however, for transparency, they most often include these two key elements of data organization:

- *Transcription*. The process of converting audio or videotape into text data is called **transcription** (Creswell, 2008). It is important that researchers maintain consistency in formatting transcripts so that data review can be done consistently. Verbatim (word-for-word) transcripts are most desirable for analysis because the researcher will be analyzing the participants' words directly and not a paraphrase created by a researcher.
- *Qualitative Software*. Researchers often use special software made just for qualitative research to organize and analyze their data. If they do, the researchers include the type of software used in their article. These types of programs include, but are not limited to, ATLAS.ti, NVivo, MAXQDA, and dedoose.

APPLICATION 9.5

Look up one of these software programs online and write a paragraph about product, including how it works and any interesting features.

THE CODING PROCESS

Regardless of the type of data collected, after carefully reviewing their data, researchers begin analyzing qualitative data with a method called **coding**. The specific task of coding is the process researchers use to segment or "chunk" (break down into smaller parts) their qualitative data. A **code** is a label a researcher uses to describe a segment of data (image, group of sentences, or even paragraphs). This is like a hashtag (#qualitatiVeresearchisawesome) or in the example used here: #nooutsidefoodordrink.

When discussing their approach to the coding process, researcher's explanations may vary based on their methodological approach (see Chapter 10). The jargon used to describe the stages of coding can be complex and overwhelming, even for an advanced qualitative researcher. However, generally speaking, the coding process can be broken into three key concepts:

1. *Initial stages of coding*. Simply put, early on in the analysis process, researchers begin the coding process. They read through the data and put labels on parts.
2. *Codebook development*. Depending on when the methodological approach calls for it, the researcher develops and eventually finalizes a codebook.
3. *Final stages of coding*. The researcher always engages in additional coding after the codebook is developed. The number of phases of coding and when they occur in the process is dependent on the methodological approach and the data collected.

In the next section, we review the coding process as one continuous process, but remember to look for these three key concepts to help you better understand the coding process.

To begin the coding process, researchers add labels (otherwise known as "codes") to the segmented data (e.g., photographs, chunks of text) to help form descriptions and identify patterns within and across their database. (See **Figure 9.3** for an overview of the process.) The researcher's ultimate goal is to reduce the total number of codes to a manageable amount (e.g., 25–30). The coding process typically begins by identifying segments of data (e.g., highlighting, underlining, or circling the data) that might be of importance to the research question. Each identified segment is then labeled with a word or phrase (i.e., a code) that describes the segmented data (Creswell, 2008). In inductive qualitative research, the individual coding the work is the individual who creates the code. Codes are created based on the overarching research questions and what is seen in the data.

To give you an idea of what this might look like, **Figure 9.4** presents a passage of text from Carraway-Stage et al. (2014), a study in which a preschool teacher describes the inability to bring outside food or drink into their classroom. In this case, the researcher decided to create and then apply a single code to this segment of text, NO OUTSIDE FOOD/DRINK. Note that other codes also may have been applicable. Other segments of data (e.g., from field notes or interview transcripts) might also relate to

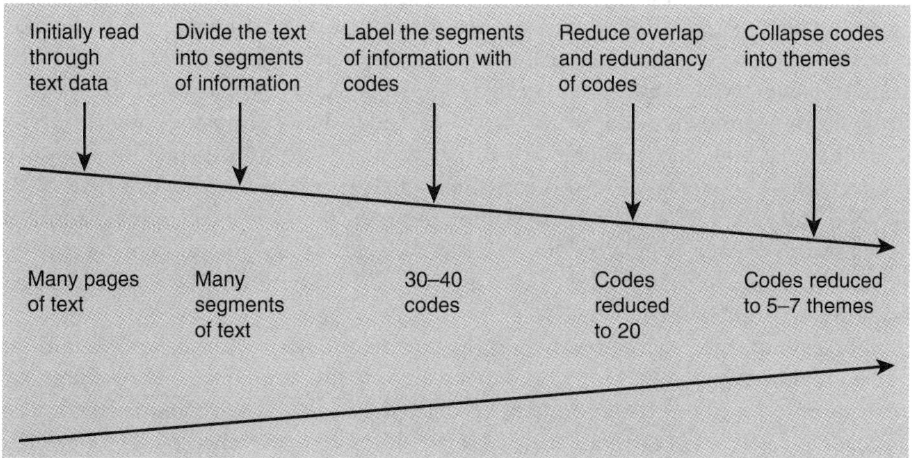

FIGURE 9.3 A Visual Model of the Coding Process in Qualitative Research

Reproduced from *Educational Research: Planning, Conducting, and Evaluating Quantitative and Qualitative Research* (3rd ed.), p. 151, by J. W. Creswell, 2008, Boston, MA: Pearson. Reprinted with permission.

["Since this is a Head Start program, we are not allowed to give the children any food that does not come from the cafeteria and is on their diet, unless it is with a lesson. Um... like this week, for instance, we are studying their senses, therefore we are going to bring in like citrus and fruits and things like that so that they can taste the way different things taste and they will be allowed to, you know, taste the different food but we are not allowed, in our program our policy is the children must only receive food from the cafeteria that is supplied by Head Start."]	**NO OUTSIDE FOOD/DRINK**

FIGURE 9.4 Section of Coded Text From Interview Transcript Discussing Nutrition Education in the North Carolina-Based Head Start Classroom

Printed with permission of Virginia C. Stage.

NO OUTSIDE FOOD/DRINK and be coded as such (Miles, Huberman, & Saldana, 2014). A few key things to notice include the following:

- The margins are left wide enough to allow for ideas to be written in the margins, such as initial codes and memos (notes on the data).
- Preliminary ideas for codes are short, only one to three words each.
- Segments of text considered important are highlighted, underlined, or circled. In this example, brackets were used to denote the start and end of the phrase associated with the NO OUTSIDE FOOD/DRINK code.

The researchers' goal for coding is to make sense of their data; therefore, coded sections of data may vary in size, and labels may be straightforward, descriptive, or even complex (Creswell, 2008; Miles et al., 2014). Codes are used to address a variety of topics such as the setting (e.g., HOME or CLASSROOM) or activities (e.g., COOKING or LEARNING). Codes also can be created using the participant's actual words (e.g., LEARN BY DOING) or by using standardized terms (e.g., EXPERIENTIAL LEARNING or MODELING) (Creswell, 2008). See **Figure 9.5** for more examples of codes.

Using a smaller number of codes helps make the codebook more manageable for the researchers, particularly when they begin to organize and reduce their identified codes into a broader set of themes (patterns). Once researchers have made an initial set of codes, they will work to group similar codes together, called *collapsing codes*. Researchers also look for redundancy and overlap between codes. For example, Figure 9.5 shows an example of how codes might change between the creation of preliminary codes and deciding on final codes. In this case, researchers combined the codes LEARN BY DOING and HANDS-ON because the intent for each code was the same, and initial coding revealed that researchers often chose to code the same segments of text with both codes. The same was found to be true about EDUCATING DURING MEAL-TIME and DISCUSSIONS AT MEALS.

Throughout the process, researchers may revise or develop new codes as additional data are reviewed and collected. Codes that were initially thought to be important may prove to be minor, and the code may be deleted or merged with another code. For example, in Figure 9.5, the code SMALL GROUPS was developed by the researchers in the initial review of data to describe how teachers organized children while providing education; however, this code was eventually deleted because it was discussed infrequently throughout the interviews and ultimately determined to be uninformative for

PRELIMINARY CODES	FINAL CODES
CODE: Child Interest	**CODE:** Child Interest
CODE: Learn by Doing	**CODE:** Learn by Doing/Hands-On
CODE: Hands-On	**CODE:** Modeling or Repeating
CODE: Modeling or Repeating	**CODE:** Integrating
CODE: Small Groups	**CODE:** Experiential Learning
CODE: Integrating	**CODE:** Cooking
CODE: Experiential Learning	**CODE:** Engaging
CODE: Cooking	**CODE:** Educating During Meal-Time/Discussions at Meals
CODE: Engaging	**CODE:** Themes
CODE: Educating During Meal-Time	**CODE:** Exposing
CODE: Discussions at Meals	**CODE:** Taste Testing
CODE: Themes	
CODE: Exposing	

FIGURE 9.5 Sample Codes Related to Nutrition Education Strategies Participants Discussed in North Carolina-Based Head Start Classrooms

Printed with permission of Virginia C. Stage.

the broader research questions for the study. Other codes may prove to be too vague and end up being applied to too many segments of data. The researcher may have to break the major code down into more descriptive subcodes to ensure the that these data are accurately reflected during analysis (Miles et al., 2014).

For example, in Figure 9.5, the code EXPOSING was originally developed to describe any situation in which children were exposed to new foods in the classroom environment. After reviewing additional data, the researchers determined that this code was too vague and added an additional code, TASTE TESTING, to allow researchers to discriminate between simply exposing children to new foods as a general concept and using taste testing as a specific teaching strategy to learn about new foods.

As researchers create and refine codes, it is important that they create and refine the definitions for each code (Miles et al., 2014). These definitions are typically recorded in a codebook. A **codebook** provides a detailed list of all codes and code definitions created for a single database. Think of this as a glossary for the transcripts, much like the one you find at the end of this textbook. **Figure 9.6** shows a single page from the codebook used in the Carraway-Stage et al. (2014) study.

Clear definitions for each code are necessary to ensure that each code is applied consistently to the database by a single person or by multiple researchers over time. Because codes are typically described using one to three words, it is easy for individuals to interpret the meaning of codes differently (Miles et al., 2014). To ensure data analysis procedures are trustworthy, code definitions must be precise and their meaning understood by all the researchers analyzing data.

Apart from a code definition, a codebook may also include any of the following:

- Exclusion or inclusion rules (when a code should be or should not be applied)
- Text examples (e.g., quotes) to support a code's rule
- Memos or thoughts about the code

STATE OF NUTRITION EDUCATION IN THE PRESCHOOL CLASSROOM

Child-Related Factors: Administrator and teacher reported factors specifically related to children within this age group that can impact the teacher's ability to teach nutrition education within the classroom.

CODE: "Cultural Diversity" (Children of other ethnicities that speak no or limited English. Impacts teacher's ability to teach all subjects, including nutrition. Includes language barrier, exposure to uncommon foods, and religious beliefs that may impact dietary intake.)

CODE: "Hyperactivity"/"Behavioral Concerns" (Children that may display behaviors that are distracting in the classroom environment such as "acting up", screaming, hyperactivity).

CODE: "Attention Span" (Children have short attention span based on their young age which may limit length of lessons.)

CODE: "Special Needs" (Specifically related to dietary needs i.e., diabetes. Includes food allergies; allergies are a concern and potential barrier to food in the classroom.)

CODE: Peers Influencing (Other children can influence a child's response to a particular food item in a positive or negative manner making other children more or less likely to try new foods that are introduced.)

CODE: Age Appropriate (Age appropriate materials & education that are on the "children's level". Age appropriate materials improves the likelihood that children will pay attention to the task at hand and retain information long term.)

CODE: Developmental Delay (Children with developmental delays and/or disabilities impacting ability to learn nutrition education.)

CODE: Child Preferences (Child has specific preferences towards a food, may be positive or negative. Preference may impact the way a teacher educates children, especially at mealtime. Includes neophobia; child hesitant to try new foods.)

Classroom-Based Factors: Classroom-related factors that can impact (positive or negative) a teacher's ability or time to teach nutrition education to children.

CODE: "Scheduling Time" (Teachers find it difficult to fit nutrition education in to their busy classroom schedule.)

Subcategory: Classroom Interruptions: Individuals or things causing classroom interruptions from within the Head Start center.

CODE: "Behavioral Concerns" (Children that may display behaviors that are distracting in the classroom environment. Control issues may or may not be related to the ratio of adults to children, behavioral concerns, language barriers, etc.)

CODE: "Classroom Control" (Ability of teacher to maintain control of their classroom considering various distractions.)

CODE: Class Attendance (Teachers may modify planned nutrition education based on how many children are present each day.)

CODE: Staff Coming In (Adults who are not the primary instructors of a classroom coming in may distract children from the lesson that is being taught. A teacher may have to stop teaching the planned lesson to deal with the person coming in which may further break children's attention span.)

CODE: "Parent Dropping By" (Parents coming in to the classroom during the course of the day and interrupting the flow of the classroom activities.)

CODE: "Consultant Coming In" (Program consultants or other outside guests coming in to the classroom during the course of the day and interrupting the flow of activities.)

CODE: Substituting (Teachers that are in the classroom temporarily and may not be familiar with the nutrition education that should be taught.)

FIGURE 9.6 Sample Codebook Page

Figure 9.7 provides example code definitions for one code. The code is accompanied by a detailed definition and inclusion or exclusion rules to help guide researchers as they code the data. As researchers proceed to analyze the data, code definitions generally become more precise through additional detail, such as inclusion or exclusion rules, being incorporated. This is especially true when multiple researchers are engaged in the data analysis process.

As researchers independently code the same data, inconsistencies in how codes are applied often arise and result in meaningful discussion about why each researcher applied codes the way he or she did. These discussions often result in an expanded or amended code definition that all researchers agree upon (Miles et al., 2014). Because multiple coders can be involved in the coding process, it is important for these researchers to be like-minded in their coding process; therefore, they need to have the same interpretation of the code definitions. As we saw in the data collection process, coders, like interviewers, must calibrate their technique with the other members of the research team.

Keep in mind, throughout the coding process (the review of data and research meetings with the research team), that researchers gain a broad perspective of their data, allowing them to see the depth of their data and the gaps that might need to be filled. This is one reason coding is an important part of the data analysis process.

Inter-Rater Reliability Versus Consensus Coding

Depending on the number of individuals working to analyze the database, coding may be completed by a single researcher or a team of researchers. When more than one person is involved in the coding process, the research team must decide how they are going to demonstrate consistency between coders and how they are going to come to an

"Integrating"	**Integration of nutrition education into other classroom topics and activities.**
✓ Inclusion:	Can include specific integration with other topics informal conversation outside of mealtime includes conversations regarding nutrition education related to colors, alphabet, countin and sorting.
✗ Exclusion:	Only including if the integration involves food that includes a tasting experience — Just talking about a food item or doing a "pretend" activity does not count.

Representative Quote: "This last week was a good one with fractions. For them to really understand the fractions I had gotten a pizza and they had got a chance to cut out a pizza so we just took the pizza apart, the bread from the bread and the cheese from the dairy, and then the other vegetables like people like peppers. And then you have the math, you cut that pizza in half and then you have half of that."

Researcher Memo: The coordinator brought up an interesting description for why teachers choose their lessons. She basically said that teachers would plan their curriculum based on a particular topic they want to teach (i.e. community helpers – grocery store) and then will integrate everything around that topic. Maybe the approach should be to find out what a preschooler teacher typically covers over a school year and then develop a piece meal nutrition curriculum that flows and integrates with those topics versus developing an independent curriculum that stands alone? It would be interesting to discover how well the existing curricular resources are actually integrated into these centers.

FIGURE 9.7 Sample Code Definition, Quote, and Memo Created to Define Nutrition Education Strategies Participants Discussed in North Carolina-Based Head Start Classrooms

agreement when coders disagree on how to code a segment of data. Ideally, researchers present their approach to obtaining consistency within the Data Analysis section of an article. Researchers typically choose between one of two approaches:

1. When a research group chooses **consensus coding** as their mode of demonstrating coding consistency, coders first independently apply a set of codes to the same data. Then the coders compare their coded data sets and meet to discuss their disagreements. In this discussion, the coders decide together (e.g., coming to consensus) the final codes that are to be applied to segments of data. When the coders cannot come to consensus through discussion, they will ask a researcher who is familiar with the study but not involved in coding to give an outside opinion and help develop consensus. Because every coding disagreement is discussed and resolved, researchers do not typically report within an article the number of disagreements that occurred with coding data.
2. **Inter-rater reliability** is a quantitative approach to demonstrating how similarly two or more coders applied a set of codes to the same data. As with consensus coding, coders first independently apply a set of codes to the same data set. However, then the coders compare their coded data sets and calculate inter-rater reliability. Typically, researchers report Cohen's Kappa, a statistic that calculates the amount of agreement between two coders while taking mere chance of agreement into consideration. This number is reported in the research article as an indication of consistency in coding. Cohen's Kappa values can range from −1.0 to +1.0. A value of +0.8 or higher is considered acceptable for the purposes of qualitatively coding data (Cohen, 1960, 1968).

Some research teams may then engage in consensus coding, but most will choose one person's coded data as the final coded data set.

MEMOING

Memoing has been described as writing an "analytic sticky note"—a piece of writing that can often fit on a small square piece of paper (Miles et al., 2014). In more specific terms, a **memo** or jotting is a short phrase, idea, concept, or even "hunch" that a researcher might think of when engaging in data analysis. Memoing can occur at any point in data analysis. Memos help researchers explore their initial ideas related to the data, and memos can be written in the margins of transcripts or field notes or underneath photographs (Creswell, 2008). **Figure 9.8** provides an example of a memo.

Memoing much like a personal diary or journal, except in this case the researcher is journaling about his or her thoughts and ideas related to the study's findings. However, it is important to know that research journals and memos are not meant to be touchy-feely diaries (a common misconception for those who think qualitative research is not rigorous enough to be considered scientific research). For example, a researcher might memo about any of the following (Miles et al., 2014):

- The participants themselves (e.g., stated words or described/observed actions)
- Data collections methods (e.g., quality of data collected or thoughts about interview questions or observation protocols)
- Ideas for future data collection
- Ideas for data analysis (e.g., compare data in one interview to data in another interview to look for similarities or differences)

When a researcher runs into examples such as these while reviewing the database, it is helpful to write a note about his or her thoughts in that moment.

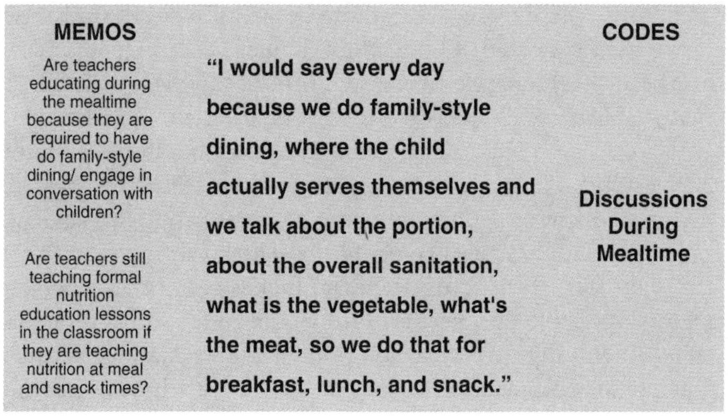

MEMOS		CODES
Are teachers educating during the mealtime because they are required to have do family-style dining/ engage in conversation with children? Are teachers still teaching formal nutrition education lessons in the classroom if they are teaching nutrition at meal and snack times?	**"I would say every day because we do family-style dining, where the child actually serves themselves and we talk about the portion, about the overall sanitation, what is the vegetable, what's the meat, so we do that for breakfast, lunch, and snack."**	**Discussions During Mealtime**

FIGURE 9.8 Sample Memos Written While Analyzing Nutrition Education Strategies in North Carolina-Based Head Start Classrooms

Reprinted with permission of Virginia C. Stage.

As previously described, researchers typically engage in memoing throughout the data analysis process. This means that coding and memoing occur in tandem. The coding process can be tedious, and often methodical. Memoing can be a useful tool to ensure the researcher remains mindful during the data analysis. As coding progresses, memoing encourages researchers to think about their ideas, reactions to, and meaning behind the data they are analyzing. These ideas are vital to the data analysis process because they suggest new leads, interpretation of findings (e.g., themes), connections to other parts of the database, and new questions to ask or issues to examine during data collection (Miles et al., 2014).

Here is another short memo written to describe one researcher's thoughts about how a school administrator described policies and regulations related to nutrition education in the Carraway-Stage et al. (2014) study.

> **MEMO:** This coordinator appeared frustrated that they did not have kitchen facilities. Because of this in combination with existing sanitation regulations, it makes any food prep difficult. Specifically, she stated it is an issue with fresh fruit. For instance, strawberries are difficult to come by due to regulations. If a banana is to be chopped up, each child has to have their own. This seems like it could be a major barrier to healthy foods in the preschool center. Explore this as an issue in other facilities with new data collection. *Code(s) relevant to this memo include*: SANITATION

Notice how the researcher writes about a single piece of data and suggests a possible new lead for future data collection.

Some memos can be longer and narrative in form. These memos are primarily conceptual and do not simply describe short pieces of data but rather help the researcher to synthesize meaning from the data. In other words, analytic memos tie pieces of data together from across the database to form a broader meaning from the findings. A researcher might write a memo about any of these ideas:

- The study's research questions
- Emergent patterns, themes, or theories within the data (see Theming and Theories sections)
- Connections (links, overlaps) between codes, themes, and theories
- New directions for the current or a future study
- Ideas for the final study report

In short, researchers use these memos to capture broad ideas about study findings as seen across all forms of data collected. Often, these longer memos represent text that will result in the first draft of a report on the study's findings (Miles et al., 2014).

Figure 9.9 is another example of a memo written to describe one researcher's thoughts about policies and regulations related to nutrition education in the Carraway-Stage et al. (2014) study. Compared to the previous shorter memo describing policies and regulations, notice how this longer memo discusses the issue as it was observed across the dataset. Additionally, it also relates the pattern to the study's research question, writes about a pattern seen across the data, makes connections between multiples codes, and suggests a possible new lead for future data collection and/or analysis.

As you can see, memoing is a crucial component of data analysis. Without memoing, researchers may miss the complexities of their data or how their own bias might be influencing their interpretation of the data. In both instances, the researcher is affecting the trustworthiness of the data by failing to memo.

THEMING

In the next phase of the qualitative analytic process, researchers must determine themes from the data that answer their major research questions and form a more in-depth understanding of the study's findings. To accomplish this goal, researchers must examine their data to identify patterns and develop broad explanations. Theming is depicted in Steps 2 and 3 of the data analysis spiral.

Theming typically occurs in tandem with coding and is facilitated through memoing. As a reminder, a **theme** is a pattern that is seen throughout the data. Each theme should be related to the research question and should generally explain part of the

MEMO: In general, administrators have stated they feel there were too many regulations in place. "There is lots that we can do, but sometimes it feels almost like there is more we can't do." This pattern in the data is an unexpected finding, but it likely has a large impact on the broader research aim to explore experiences implementing nutrition education in the Head Start setting. Are the regulations in place interfering with teacher's ability to teach nutrition in the classroom in a way appropriate for a preschool child (i.e. hands-on education)? I am getting the feeling from teachers in general that most of the policies in place regarding nutrition education are negative. They highlight things teachers CAN NOT do versus what they CAN do in regards to nutrition education. Is it possible there are more positive policies and the teachers are only focusing on the negative? Are the policies in place so complicated that teachers decide to avoid the issue all together vs. put in the effort? What kinds of policies would be helpful for clearing up this issue? If administrators feel there are too many regulations, how do teachers feel? Administrators have hinted that regulations prevent teachers from doing things they really want to do. When asked about regulations regarding nutrition education many administrators said they didn't know what they were. If anyone were to know them wouldn't it be the individual in the position as Nutrition Coordinator? Approaching this issue will be interesting. Due to the large number of regulations coming from multiple directions (e.g. Child and Adult Care Feeding Program (CACFP), Head Start, Health Department, State Childcare Licensing Regulations) administrators are very hesitant to suggest that MORE policies or regulations are needed. They have enough policies to remember and implement as it is, additionally policies may just make the environment more confusing and difficulty for all parties. This issue will need to be approached in a manner that will not make things more difficult and come down to checking a box. *Code(s) relevant to this memo include*: RULES & REGULATIONS, MULTIPLE AGENCIES REGULATING, CLEAR POLICY, NOT AWARE OF POLICY

FIGURE 9.9 Example of a Memo

Reprinted with permission of Virginia C. Stage.

phenomenon of study. Here are the themes and theme descriptions researchers identified from the Carraway-Stage et al. (2014) study:

- *Nutrition Education Strategies*. Methods teachers use to teach nutrition education to preschool children.
- *Teacher-Related Factors*. Teacher-related factors that can affect the extent, amount, and frequency of nutrition education occurring in the classroom.
- *Support for Nutrition Education*. Teacher support received for nutrition education in the form of individual, organizational, or community resources.
- *Training and Education in Nutrition*. Training and education that administrators or teachers have received related to nutrition education. Topics range from past training or education to needed or potential opportunities for training and education related to nutrition.
- *Policy and Regulations/Restrictions*. Policies and regulations/restrictions that may affect a teacher's ability to teach nutrition education in the classroom. Policies and regulations may stem from any level of administration (center, state, or federal).

Researchers typically use multiple themes to explain their findings. Similar to codes, themes represent ideas within the data. Like codes, themes are also labeled using a single word or a phrase.

One of the major goals of theming is to condense a large amount of data into smaller, more manageable units (Miles et al., 2014). Theming requires the researcher to continue to reflect on the meaning of the data. Once the final list of codes has been identified and all data have been coded, researchers review the data within each code and between codes to determine how the codes connect to each other, if at all. Because it is probably the most important concept for all of theming, we repeat the previous statement. *Researchers will review the data within each code and between codes to determine how the codes connect to each other, if at all. Researchers identify themes by examining the codes that show up most frequently in the data, have the most evidence to support them, are interesting/unique, or are an expected finding in the study* (Creswell, 2008). Remember, theming is an iterative process, just like coding. Thus initial themes will likely change over time as data analysis unfolds.

For example, the codes listed in Figure 9.5 were compiled to form the "Nutrition Education Strategies" theme. When reviewing the set of codes, researchers determined that these codes were similar in nature (all described strategies teachers discussed they used to provide nutrition education to preschool children). These similarities resulted in merging these codes together under a broader category known as a theme.

TIP

To summarize, theming is the process researchers use to help make sense of the data. If a researcher just presented codes in an article, the work often would not make sense to the reader. However, by identifying how the codes connect and beginning to explain what themes mean, researchers can begin to present the answer to their research question.

Theory Development

At times, researchers find it necessary to integrate their themes into one cohesive **theory** to adequately explain their findings. They may start out with a theory (e.g., Social Cognitive Theory or the Theory of Planned Behavior) and purposefully look for connections in their data related to the theory and its constructs. Or they may begin with themes and decide they can better explain the data with an integrated visual representation. In this case, researchers use a pictorial **model** to illustrate the findings applied to the theory. More details about theories are presented in the Results section.

TRUSTWORTHINESS

A common misconception surrounding qualitative research is that it "lacks rigor" around collecting and analyzing research data. Although some weak qualitative studies may exist in the published literature, the same can be said for quantitative studies. Rigor in quantitative research methodology is often discussed using the terms **reliability** and **validity** (see Chapter 4). Qualitative researchers are capable of similar rigor in their studies by achieving **trustworthiness**. Trustworthiness is defined as a set of criteria for judging the quality, or goodness, of a qualitative study (Lincoln & Guba, 1985). Although parallel in nature, achieving trustworthiness in a qualitative study looks very different from obtaining reliability/validity in a quantitative study. As with achieving reliability/validity, achieving trustworthiness does not rely on a single approach but rather is a combination of strategies researchers use to determine the accuracy and credibility of their findings. To emphasize the trustworthiness of their data and findings, researchers may choose to include a paragraph in the Methods section that highlights many of the steps taken to improve trustworthiness. Others may choose to include these steps throughout the Methods section at the time they occurred (e.g., recruitment, data collection).

Creswell (2008) recommends qualitative researchers implement at least two methods of trustworthiness in their study design. The most popular, cost-effective methods are:

- *Adoption of research methods*. The researcher should identify a specific research methodological "approach" or design (e.g., thematic analysis, case study, phenomenology, grounded theory) to guide the study. Using a specific approach means the researcher will identify the approach being used, and follow the specific procedures outlined for the approach when collecting and analyzing data (Shenton, 2004). See Chapter 10.
- *Detailed, thick descriptions*. It is important that a qualitative researcher provides a detailed description of the research study. Description should include, but is not limited to, sample size, geographic location, limitations on how the data were collected, data collection methods, number and length of data collection sessions (e.g., average length of focus groups), and time period over which data was collected (Cole & Gardner, 1979; Marchionini & Teague, 1987; Pitts, 1994).
- *Member checking*. This method involves checking data accuracy during data collection (e.g., during or at the end of an interview through a summarized verbal description) and at the end of data collection (e.g., providing interview transcripts for review by the participant) by giving the participant an opportunity to confirm, clarify, or correct how the researcher recorded what was said. This method is particularly useful during recorded interviews and focus groups. Mita, Gray, and Goodell (2015) describe use of this strategy when investigating teacher perceptions of the mealtime environment: "interviewers summarized participant answers at the conclusion of the interview. The interviewer then requested frequency from the participants to increase the accuracy of the interviewers' interpretation, as well as to give the interviewees an opportunity to add anything that the interviewer may have missed" (p. 39). Hall, Chai, and Albrecht (2016) describe a slightly different approach to the member checking strategy when investigating elementary teacher perceptions of nutrition education: "Final themes ... were emailed to all teacher participants for review. Teachers were asked to examine themes and reflect on accuracy" (p. 139). In this case,

researchers addressed accuracy of findings by asking participants to confirm that theme descriptions were accurate and that interpretations of the findings were representative of the teachers' actual perceptions (Creswell, 2008).

- **Triangulation**: Using this method a researcher would make use of multiple (and often times different) types of data sources (e.g., observational field notes and interviews) or methods (e.g., written policy and focus groups) to investigate and provide additional evidence for understanding the problem being studied. Another form of triangulation involves using a range of participants or supporting documents to inform the problem (Shenton, 2004). For example, Peterson, Goodell, Hegde, and Stage (2017) triangulated written federal and state policy with interview data exploring Head Start teachers' perceptions of how policies influenced their ability to provide nutrition education to preschool children in their classrooms.
- *Frequent peer review or debriefing*. Debriefing is a common strategy used to describe ongoing discussions that occur between a researcher and his or her colleague or superior (e.g., research lead, project director). In these debriefing sessions, the colleague/supervisor acts as a "sounding board" for the researcher by engaging him or her in conversations that help develop new ideas and interpretations or recognize biases throughout the research process (Shenton, 2004).

Understanding various methods of achieving trustworthiness in a qualitative study will help you recognize rigorous methods in published literature.

It is up to the qualitative researcher to employ a rigorous study design. In qualitative studies, this means employing some of the listed strategies, but it also means spending adequate time in the field to gain an understanding of the environment and context being studied, keeping a detailed record of study methods (audit trail), and adequately summarizing findings from the data collected. Researchers must use their experience, skills, creativity, and flexibility to ensure rigorous approaches are being followed throughout all phases of the study (Creswell, 2008).

RESULTS

In qualitative research, results (also called findings) can be presented in numerous ways, including as themes and theories.

- A theme is a pattern seen throughout the data that explains part of the phenomenon of the study and is related to the research question. Researchers typically use multiple themes to explain the findings.
- To better explain how themes relate to each other, researchers may use a theory to organize the results. In this case, researchers often use a pictorial model to illustrate the findings applied to the theory.

When reading the Results section, it is important to keep in mind that qualitative research is "interpretative," meaning the researcher is key to the analysis and interpretation of the data. The researcher reviews the data and makes his or her own assessment of the study findings. This interpretation may differ from the interpretation of another researcher. One interpretation is not necessarily more accurate than another, but it does mean that the researcher brings his or her own perspective to the meaning seen in the data.

THEMES

As explained in the Data Analysis section, themes are a researcher's way of summarizing the study findings in a quick yet meaningful way. To better understand themes, let's look at an excerpt (**Figure 9.10**) from an article by Goodell, Pierce, Bravo, and Ferris (2008) entitled "Parental Perceptions of Overweight During Early Childhood."

Typically, researchers include three components (name, description, quotes) for each theme in the Results section. First, researchers name a theme with a short descriptive statement that summarizes the concept of the theme. This name may be found as a subheading in the Results section. It may also be found in the introductory sentence of the full description of the theme. In the case of the example passage, the theme name "Too Big" is presented as a subheading.

After researchers name the theme, they provide a detailed description of the theme, demonstrating how the theme relates to the research question. In the example passage, the theme "Too Big" is defined in the first paragraph of the theme. In subsequent paragraphs, the researchers provide further examples of the theme "Too Big." It is hoped that after reading the excerpt you can see how the theme relates to the research question: What are parents' perceptions of early childhood overweight?

To reinforce the concepts provided in the theme's description and to provide evidence of the theme directly from the data, researchers also provide supporting quotes. These quotes may be intertwined in the description, placed at the end of the theme's description, or organized in a table along with quotes from other themes. Quotes may be short phrases, whole sentences, or whole paragraphs. Because of page limits for research articles in journals, researchers must choose quotes that concisely exemplify the theme. In our example, the researchers embedded quotes within their description of the theme "Too Big."

Sometimes researchers include subthemes to demonstrate the complexities and the range of a theme. Researchers may need to divide a theme into subthemes to provide a

Too Big

Participants became concerned about a child's weight at the point that the child was either blatantly too big or when the child experienced negative effects associated with large size. Providing a nebulous definition, one mother told us, "You can physically see it" when a child is too big. Another mother described children she had seen on a television show, stating, "Them [sic] babies are like 300, almost 300 pounds and they only about 4 years old." Parents used subjective or exaggerated examples rather than objective, measurable guidelines.

Unlike health care providers, these parents did not use scales, measuring tapes, or growth charts to determine whether a child was too big; they used their eyes. If the child looked too big to parents, then she or he was too big. If she or he did not look too big, then the child was fine. One mother stated.

> To me, if I can see what the normal, the norm is for a certain age group, not knowing about their background, just by looking. If I see a group of kids and one is way bigger than the other one, then I would say, "Well, he's overweight."

In addition, parents rejected the growth chart used by health care providers. One mother referred to the growth chart as a "foreign language to me," and said she wanted the doctor to "just talk to me about my kid." Another mother described the enigma of the growth chart:

> Because for instance, they've got this thing, this book that each time a certain age you're supposed to be weighing a certain amount of weight. So that's why they determine they're overweight, but to you, they don't look that way.

Because of the differences between parents and practitioners in determining overweight during early childhood, many parents told us that the doctor was wrong. For example, one mother said, "Some doctors say that they're overweight, but they're really not overweight." Parents disagreed with the use of the growth chart because it did not account for the uniqueness and individuality of eah child. One mother said, "That chart is just a piece of paper and it don't mean a thing . . . that's how God made him and that's just who he is." To parents, their child was more than a number, a weight and height, or a category.

Parents did recognize overweight when the weight resulted in unfavorable outcomes. Participants discussed four categories of negative effects associated with being too big as a preschooler: health, abilities, esteem, and appearance/economics.

FIGURE 9.10 Example of a Theme (Too Big)

Reproduced from "Parental Perceptions of Overweight During Early Childhood," by L. S. Goodell, M. B. Pierce, C. M. Bravo, and A. M. Ferris, 2008, *Qualitative Health Research, 18*, p. 1551. Copyright by Sage Journals. Reprinted with permission.

deeper explanation about the theme or to explain its different parts. Subthemes are typically presented using the same components as a theme (name, description, quotes). In our example, the theme "Too Big" has four subthemes: Health, Ability, Self-Esteem, and Appearance and Economics. Demonstrating the range of the theme, the researchers explain how parents define "Too Big" for each subtheme. Typically, each subtheme is presented using a subheading to identify its name, followed by a paragraph or two describing the subtheme, and including a quote to illustrate the subtheme.

Because problem statements in qualitative research are broad and nutrition is full of complexities, one theme will not fully address the research question posed in a given article. Instead, researchers describe multiple themes to present the depth and breadth of the research question. In the Goodell et al. (2008) article, the "Too Big" theme describes how parents define excessive weight in early childhood and how they view the consequences of excessive weight. However, the "Too Big" theme does not begin to address how parents view the causes, treatment, or prevention of excessive weight in early childhood. Additional themes within the article present these concepts in more detail.

Multiple themes within an article will likely be somewhat related to each other because they are all addressing a component of the central research question. However, unless the researchers are applying a theory or creating a model, the themes may not clearly connect together to form one cohesive understanding of the research question. When presenting results as themes, the themes are like beads strung loosely on a necklace. They might touch each other, but they do not have to be connected to make a necklace. Instead, a thread or string holds them together. *This thread or string is your research question.*

Theories and Models

To better explain how themes or other key elements of the findings are related to each other, researchers often use theories as a framework for study results. Typically, researchers identify the theory used to organize findings before beginning data collection and analysis. When researchers apply a theory or a model to explain how the parts of the research topic fit together, it is called **articulation**. Substituting the word "articulate" for "organize," "present," "map," or "apply" may be a helpful way to understand the concept. In nutrition research, the theories typically used to articulate findings can be grouped into two categories: qualitative methodologies and behavior change models. However, some researchers may choose to develop their own model to illustrate the results as part of their data analysis process.

TIP

Think of a theory or model like a house made out of building blocks. For the house to hold together, the building blocks need to connect with a common point. If you pull out one building block, the house loses its identity or does not hold together. Each piece is connected to the others to create the whole house. This is true with a theory or model, where each theme is like a building block that connects to another building block. If you miss one block, you are not telling the whole story.

When researchers begin with an already existing theory, they use the theory's **constructs** (parts of the theory) to organize the results. Although you may not be familiar with the theories we discuss, we hope the examples provide enough detail for you to understand the concepts behind presenting qualitative research findings in theory form.

As one example, the four main constructs of the theory of planned behavior (TPB) are (1) attitude toward behavior, (2) subjective norms, (3) perceived behavioral control, and (4) behavior intention (Ajzen, 2002). In a qualitative study exploring parents' attitudes and beliefs around feeding their preschool children, Duncanson, Burrows, Holman, and Collins (2013) articulated themes of the study to the four constructs of TPB. One of the themes included examples of how parents felt they lacked the skills to change their child's feeding behavior. Let's call this the "Lacking Skills" theme. The researchers determined this theme best fit into the "perceived behavioral control" construct of TPB. The researchers articulated all the themes of the study with one or more of the constructs of TPB. Using our example of a house made out of building blocks, the TPB is a house that has doors, walls, a roof, and windows (four constructs). The researchers analyzed their data and determined that "Lacking Skills" fit as a window in the house rather than as a door.

In all cases, researchers use the text of the Results section to explain each key construct of the final theory articulated with the research question. Most of the time, researchers present one or more themes for each construct. Regardless of the organizational strategy, researchers provide a name, description, and quotes for the key themes/constructs of the Results section. Researchers may or may not use a visual aid to help illustrate their articulation of a model to the research question. In our example, Duncanson et al. (2013) organized themes, subthemes, model constructs, and quotes into one table.

In a grounded theory-based study exploring how mothers' interactions with their infants affected their compliance to feeding recommendations, Waller, Bower, Spence, and Kavanagh (2015) used a figure to depict their final theoretical model (**Figure 9.11**). Some researchers opt not to use a figure or table to supplement the text.

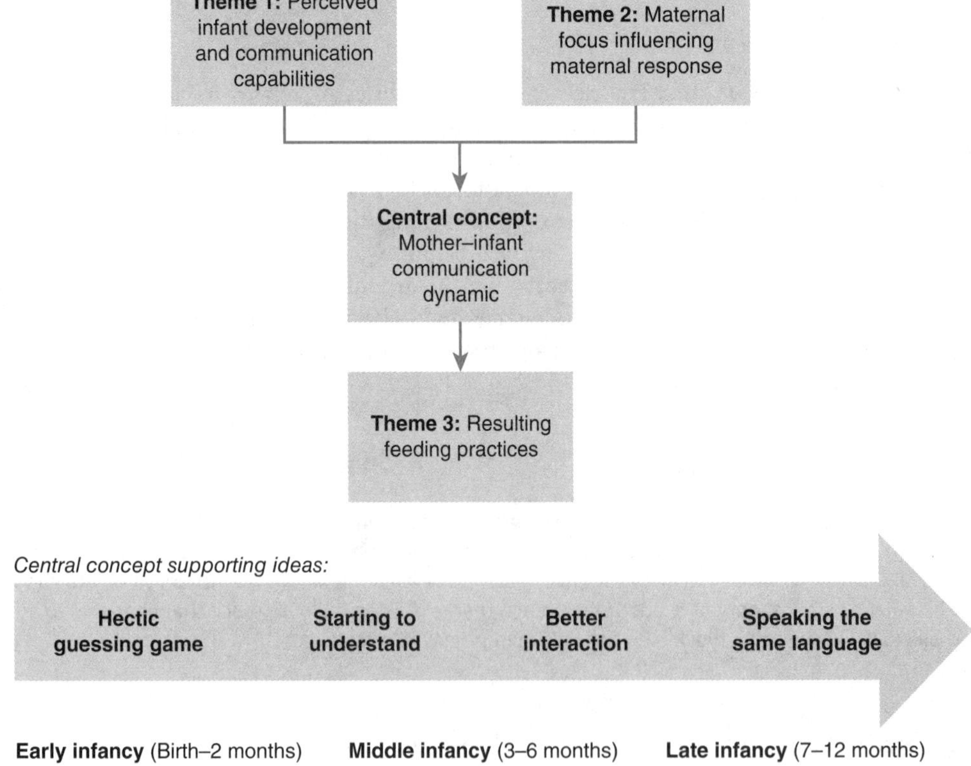

FIGURE 9.11 Theoretical Model Representing the Mother–Infant Feeding Dyad: Birth to 12 Months in a Primiparous, Low-Income, Southeastern United States Population

Reproduced from "Using Grounded Theory Methodology to Conceptualize the Mother-Infant Communication Dynamic: Potential Application to Compliance with Infant Feeding Recommendations," by J. Waller, K. M. Bower, M. Spence, and K. F. Kavanagh, 2015, *Maternal & Child Nutrition, 11*, 754.

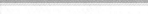

APPLICATION 9.6

Explain the theoretical model in Figure 9.11 or the conceptual framework in Figure 9.12.

Because some theories and models may be too complex to present every detail about the findings in a page-limited article, researchers may choose to present only part of a model. Furthermore, some researchers may find that modifying the theory from its original form better explains the results. For example, in the grounded theory–based study exploring preschool teachers' perceptions of a positive mealtime environment, Mita et al. (2015) originally articulated their work with the five major elements of grounded theory (central phenomenon, causal conditions, intervening conditions, strategies, consequences). However, as analysis continued and the researchers began to clarify the results, the final theory morphed into an explanatory model that looks very little like the original model (**Figure 9.12**). Therefore, if an article uses a model but the results do not look the same as the original model, reading the article's Data Analysis subsection may provide more information about changes.

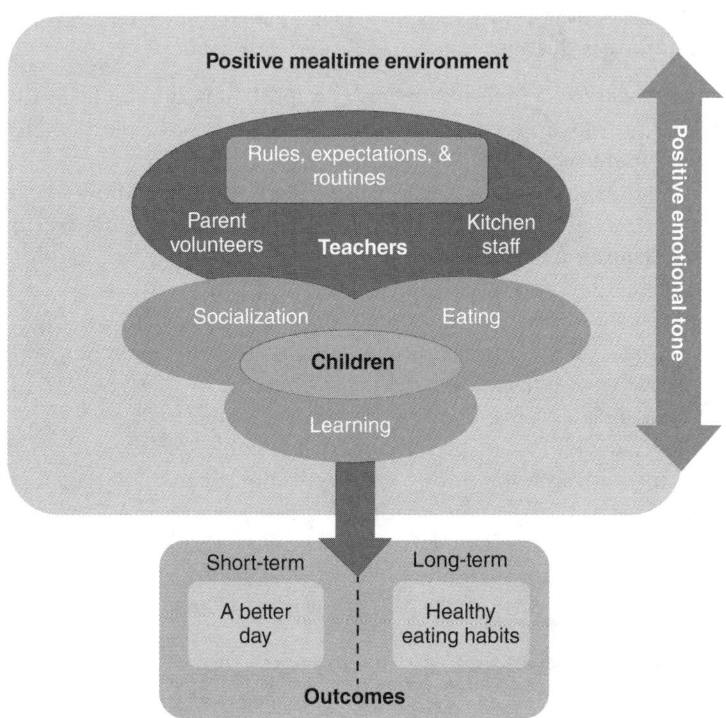

FIGURE 9.12 Conceptual Framework of Head Start Preschool Teachers' Definition of a Positive Mealtime Environment

Reproduced from "An Explanatory Framework of Teachers' Perceptions of a Positive Mealtime Environment in a Preschool Setting," by S. C. Mita, S. A. Gray, & L. S. Goodell, 2015, *Appetite, 90*, 40. Copyright by Elsevier. Reprinted with permission.

DISCUSSION AND CONCLUSIONS

The Discussion and Conclusions section of a qualitative research article should be similar to that in a quantitative research article because the goal is to weave the results together with findings from previous literature into a set of "take-aways" for the reader. An example of the typical "flow" of a discussion is Kamar, Evans, and Hugh-Jones's (2016) article about the factors that affect adolescents consuming whole grains.

First, the researchers explain how their findings compare to other research studies, both qualitative and quantitative. Kamar et al. (2016) did this with a general section summarizing the implications of the research and then specifically comparing their research to others' with respect to barriers and facilitators to whole grain consumption as well as the fit of their work within the "reasoned action approach."

Second, future work is discussed, including what the researchers plan to do next and what they suggest others should attempt in light of the findings from this study. Some do this within the body of the discussion, and others save this for the conclusion. Kamar et al. (2016) summarized their study with the following impact statement.

> The results of this study highlight the need for raising awareness of the specific health benefits of whole grain consumption among adolescents to motivate consumption. Moreover, they revealed a unique need to address issues of product appeal and the targeted tailoring of products for young people. This study has the potential to inform further research on whole grain consumption, and acts as a basis to guide public health nutritionists involved in development of programmes and strategies to improve whole grain intake in this age group. (p. 132)

This statement or set of statements is especially important because it helps to encourage future research. For students looking for a thesis topic, this is the place to look for ideas of research that can make an impact in the field.

Finally, strengths and limitations are discussed, including how the researchers attempted to decrease the impact of these limitations by improving trustworthiness. You will notice that some of the strengths and limitations we discussed in the data collection Methods section are found in these articles as well. For example, Kamar et al. (2016) discusses the need for much probing with a teen population, the impact of mixed gender focus groups, and the limited sample size affecting the representativeness of their sample. However, their strengths, which also speak to the impact of the research on the body of literature, include using an ethnically diverse sample.

Depending on the journal in which the article is published, the authors might conclude their writing with an Implications and Applications section, or they might provide a Conclusion that summarizes the findings. An Implications and Application section includes both future work and how practitioners may use the findings to affect how they interact with their clients immediately.

SUMMARY

1. A qualitative study is inductive; it goes from detailed data to more general ideas.
2. Qualitative studies start with a problem, ask open-ended research questions, use a natural setting, listen to participants' meanings, and use researchers as a "key instrument."
3. Just like quantitative research articles, qualitative research articles have four distinctive parts: Introduction with Literature Review, Methods, Results, and Discussion and Conclusions. When initiating their investigations, researchers always begin with a problem

statement and objective, but *no* hypothesis. Research objectives often focus on barriers, facilitators to change, and a lived experience.

4. In the Literature Review, the authors use a funnel approach to narrow down to the topic and details of the study. The Literature Review uses recent research and seminal works. Almost all articles clearly and concisely present the gaps in the literature (e.g., research problem).
5. The four major types of qualitative data collection methods are focus groups, individual interviews (structured, unstructured, or semi-structured), observations, and document analysis.
6. The term "document analysis" can be misleading because it includes not just analysis but also collection and organization of different types of documents. You might see document analysis used along with other methods, such as interviews or focus groups, in a case study methodology, or in a mixed methods study where both qualitative and quantitative methods are combined (Bowen, 2009). Document analysis can also stand alone as a study, serving as a cost-effective and comprehensive way to analyze a large volume of documents.
7. Table 9.1 lists the strengths and limitations of qualitative data collection methods.
8. Obtaining a sample is normally done with nonprobability sampling methods. Inclusion and exclusion criteria are often used. Researchers should explain how they determined when a sample size was sufficient. Qualitative researchers may use different methods to determine their sample size, but the most common method used in the literature is saturation. Saturation occurs when researchers are not learning anything new from additional data collection.
9. All types of qualitative research methodologies use a *research tool* or *guide* to maintain consistency throughout the data collection process (similar to a protocol in an intervention study). Typically, a guide is used for individual interviews or focus groups and a tool for observations or document analysis. They are often pilot tested.
10. A moderator or interview guide is like a roadmap or GPS for how the conversation will evolve. Regardless of the questions asked, the wording of the questions and how they are presented to participants are crucial to the quality of data collected. Therefore, researchers often report that the language in the guide they used was open-ended, unbiased, and nonjudgmental. Because interviews and focus groups are used to describe or explore a certain topic, guide questions need to be carefully designed (many are open-ended) to encourage participants to share their perspectives through stories and examples.
11. Tools are like worksheets with categories for purposefully collecting specific areas of qualitative data. The categories are chosen by the researcher, based on the overarching research question. See Figure 9.2 for an example.
12. Researchers can also demonstrate the quality of their data through explaining researcher training. Much like you might calibrate a laboratory tool before using it, researcher training plays an important role in "calibrating" the researcher (the instrument) to collect strong qualitative research data.
13. The output of each focus group or interview is an audio recording and a field note. The audio recording is then transcribed verbatim into a transcript. Typically, the transcript is the primary data source and the field notes are the secondary source for analysis.
14. During observations, the researcher takes notes, or jottings, which serve as shorthand for more in-depth field notes that are written later. If one exists, this is the point in which an observation tool is used. The details provided in the field notes are based on the focus of the overarching research question and the key points of the observation tool and can include diagrams, lists, quotes, and narrative descriptions of the observation, including what are called observer's comments.
15. The unit of analysis is one document or a set of documents. The data analyzed during data analysis are the extracted data, not the document itself.
16. Researchers often use special software made just for qualitative research to organize and analyze their data.
17. The coding process typically begins by identifying segments of data (e.g., highlighting, underlining, or circling the data) that might be of importance to the research question.

Then researchers add labels or codes to the segmented data (e.g., photographs, chunks of text) to help form descriptions and identify patterns within and across their database (see Figure 9.3). The researcher's ultimate goal is to reduce (collapse codes) the total number of codes to a manageable number (e.g., 25–30). Using a smaller number of codes helps make the codebook (which contains the codes and their definitions) more manageable for researchers, particularly when they begin to organize and reduce their identified codes into a broader set of themes (patterns).

18. Coders, like interviewers, must calibrate their technique with the other members of the research team.
19. Consensus coding and inter-rater reliability can be used to demonstrate coding consistency.
20. A memo or jotting is a short phrase, idea, concept, or even "hunch" that a researcher might think of when engaging in data analysis. Memos help researchers explore their initial ideas related to the data and can be written in the margins of transcripts or field notes. Without memoing, researchers may miss the complexities of their data or fail to realize how their own bias might be influencing their interpretation of the data. In both instances, the researcher is affecting the trustworthiness of the data by failing to memo.
21. In the next phase of the qualitative analytic process, researchers must determine themes from the data that will answer their major research questions and form a more in-depth understanding of the study's findings. Themes may be integrated into a theory.
22. Methods of achieving trustworthiness include adoption of research methods, detailed and thick descriptions, member checking, triangulation, and frequent peer review or debriefing.
23. Results may be presented as themes or theories.
24. The discussion and conclusions are similar to those found in a quantitative article.

REVIEW QUESTIONS

1. A qualitative study is deductive in nature.
   A. true
   B. false
2. Researchers are a key instrument in a qualitative study.
   A. true
   B. false
3. A qualitative study includes an Introduction (with literature review), Methods, Results, and Discussion (with conclusions).
   A. true
   B. false
4. A qualitative study almost always has a hypothesis.
   A. true
   B. false
5. Qualitative studies often use inclusion and exclusion criteria.
   A. true
   B. false
6. Qualitative researchers may receive training on how to hold interviews and focus groups if used in studies they conduct.
   A. true
   B. false
7. Which of the following is *not* a method used in a qualitative study?
   A. focus groups
   B. interviews
   C. observations
   D. intervention
8. A study that combines multiple qualitative data collection methods is a:
   A. mixed methods study
   B. multi-method study
   C. theoretical study
   D. thematic study
9. In a qualitative study, the number of participants may be determined by:
   A. saturation
   B. maximum variation

C. purposive sampling
D. snowball sampling

10. To maintain consistency in a series of focus groups, the researchers will use a:
A. GPS
B. guide
C. tool
D. coding

11. Compare the Introduction section of a qualitative article to the Introduction in a quantitative article.

12. What are the typical subheadings found in the Methods section of a qualitative article?

13. Describe each of the data collection methods and considerations when using them.

14. Compare primary, secondary, and auxiliary documents.

15. Give an example of a situation in which it would be better to use a focus group than individual interviews.

16. Compare three kinds of interviews that qualitative researchers use.

17. Why are open-ended questions used frequently in qualitative research?

18. Compare guide and tools, and describe the purpose of each.

19. Describe how the process of coding, memoing, and theming are used in qualitative studies. Are themes discussed in the Results section?

20. Describe three ways to increase trustworthiness in a study.

CRITICAL THINKING QUESTIONS

1. Read the following qualitative study and answer these questions.
Bailey-David, L., Virus, A., McCoy, T. A., Wojtanowski, A., VanderVeur, S., & Foster, G. D. (2013). Middle school student and parent perceptions of government-sponsored free school breakfast and consumption: A qualitative inquiry in an urban setting. *Journal of the Academy of Nutrition and Dietetics, 113*, 251–257.
A. What is the problem the study is going to address? What is the purpose of the study?
B. How were the participants recruited and selected?
C. How many participants took part in the study? Were participants given anything for participating?
D. Which data collection methods were used? Explain briefly how they were implemented.
E. Was a guide used? If so, describe.
F. Were moderators trained?
G. Discuss the coding process and how it was used to identify themes.
H. Were any steps taken to increase trustworthiness?
I. What were the major results?
J. Did you feel the conclusions were appropriate? Explain your answer.

2. Read the following qualitative study and answer these questions.
Schindler, J., Kiszko, K., Abrams, C., Islam, N., & Elbel, B. (2013). Environmental and individual factors affecting menu labeling utilization: A qualitative research study. *Journal of the Academy of Nutrition and Dietetics, 113*, 667–672.
A. What is the problem the study is going to address? What is the purpose of the study?
B. How were the participants recruited and selected?
C. How many participants took part in the study? Were participants given anything for participating?
D. Which data collection methods were used? Explain briefly how they were implemented.
E. Was a guide used? If so, describe.
F. Were moderators trained?
G. Discuss the coding process and how it was used to identify themes.

H. Were any steps taken to increase trustworthiness?

I. What were the major results?

J. Did you feel the conclusions were appropriate? Explain your answer.

SUGGESTED READINGS/ACTIVITIES

1. Harris, J. E., Gleason, P. M., Sheean, P. M., Boushey, C., Beto, J. A., & Bruemmer, B. (2009). An introduction to qualitative research for food and nutrition professionals. *Journal of the American Dietetic Association, 109*, 80–90. doi: 10.1016/j.jada.2008.10.018

REFERENCES

Altheide, D. L., & Schneider, C. J. (2013). *Qualitative media analysis*. Thousand Oaks, CA: Sage.

Anderson, C. K., Walch, T. J., Lindberg, S. M., Smith, A. M., Lindheim, S. R., & Whigham, L. D. (2015). Excess gestational weight gain in low-income overweight and obese women: A qualitative study. *Journal of Nutrition Education and Behavior, 47*, 404–411. doi: 10.1016/j.jneb.2015.05.01

Ajzen, I. (2002). Perceived behavioral control, self-efficacy, locus of control, and the theory of planned behavior. *Journal of Applied Social Psychology, 32*, 665–683. doi: 10.1111/j.1559-1816.2002.tb00236.x

Bamford, C., Heaven, B., May, C., & Moynihan P. (2012). Implementing nutrition guidelines for older people in residential care homes: A qualitative study using normalizing process theory. *Implementation Science*, 7(106), 1–13. doi: 10.1186/1748-5908-7-106

Birch, L. L., & Marlin, D. W. (1982). I don't like it; I never tried it: Effects of exposure to food on two-year-old children's food preferences. *Appetite, 4*, 353–360.

Bowen, G. A. (2009). Document analysis as a qualitative research method. *Qualitative Research Journal, 9*, 27–40. doi: 10.3316/QRJ0902027

Carraway-Stage, V., Henson, S. R., Dipper, A., Spangler, H., Ash, S. L., & Goodell, L. S. (2014). Understanding the state of nutrition education in the Head Start classroom: A qualitative approach. *American Journal of Health Education, 45*, 52–62. doi:10.1080/19325037.2013.853000

Cohen, J. (1960). A coefficient of agreement for nominal scales. *Educational and Psychological Measurement, 20*, 37–46.

Cohen, J. (1968). Weighted kappa: Nominal scale agreement provision for scaled disagreement or partial credit. *Psychological Bulletin, 70*, 213–220.

Cole, J., & Gardner, K. (1979). Topic work with first-year secondary pupils In E. Lunzer & K. Gardner (Eds.), *The effective use of reading* (pp. 167–192). London: Heinemann Educational Books for the Schools Council.

Creswell, J. W. (2008). *Educational research: Planning, conducting, and evaluating quantitative and qualitative Research* (3rd ed.). Boston, MA: Pearson.

Creswell, J. W. (2013). *Qualitative inquiry & research design: Choosing among five approaches*. Thousand Oaks, CA: Sage.

Duncanson, K., Burrows, T., Holman, B., & Collins, C. (2013). Parents' perceptions of child feeding: A qualitative study based on the theory of planned behavior. *Journal of Developmental and Behavioral Pediatrics, 34*, 227–236. doi: 10.1097/DBP.0b013e31828b2ccf

Faraji, O., Etemad, K., Sari, A. A., & Ravaghi, H. (2015). Policies and programs for prevention and control of diabetes in Iran: A document analysis. *Global Journal of Health Science*, 7, 187–197. doi: 10.5539/gjhs.v7n6p187

Flacking, R., & Dykes, F. (2013). 'Being in a womb' or 'playing musical chairs': The impact of place and space on infant feeding in NICUs. *BMC Pregnancy and Childbirth, 13*, 1–11. doi: 10.1186/1471-2393-13-179

Goodell, L. S., Pierce, M. B., Bravo, C. M., & Ferris, A. M. (2008). Parental perceptions of overweight during early childhood. *Qualitative Health Research, 18*, 1548–1555. doi: 10.1177/1049732308325537

Goodell, L. S., Stage, V. C., & Cooke, N. K. (2016). Practical qualitative research strategies: Training interviewers and coders. *Journal of Nutrition Education and Behavior, 48*, 578–585. doi: 10.1016/j.jneb.2016.06.001

Goonan, S., Mirosa, M., & Spence, H. (2014). Getting a taste for food waste: A mixed methods ethnographic study into hospital food waste before patient consumption conducted at three New Zealand foodservice facilities. *Journal of the Academy of Nutrition and Dietetics, 114*, 63–71. doi: 10.1016/j.jand.2013.09.022

Hall, E., Chai, W., & Albrecht, J. A. (2016). A qualitative phenomenological exploration of teacher's experience with nutrition education. *American Journal of Health Education, 47*, 136–148. doi: 10.1080/19325037.2016.1157532

Harvey, K. (2016). "When I go to bed hungry and sleep, I'm not hungry": Children and parents' experiences of food insecurity. *Appetite, 99*, 235–244. doi: 10.1016/j.appet.2016.01.004

Kamar, M., Evans, C., & Hugh-Jones, S. (2016). Factors influencing adolescent whole grain intake: A theory-based qualitative study. *Appetite, 101*, 125–133. doi: 10.1016/j.appet.2016.02.154

Krueger, R. A., & Casey, M. A. (2009). *Focus groups: A practical guide for applied research* (4th ed.). Thousand Oaks, CA: Sage.

Lachat, C., Roberfroid, D., Huybregts, L., Van Camp, J., & Kolsteren, P. (2008). Incorporating the catering sector in nutrition policies of WHO European Region: Is there a good recipe? *Public Health Nutrition, 12*, 316–324. doi: 10.1017/S1368980008002176

Lincoln, Y. S., & Guba, E. G. (1985). *Naturalistic inquiry*. Newbury Park, CA: Sage.

Marchionini, G., & Teague, J. (1987). Elementary students' use of electronic information services: An exploratory study. *Journal of Research on Computing in Education, 20*, 139–155.

Merriam, S. B. (2009). *Qualitative research: A guide to design and implementation*. San Francisco, CA: Jossey-Bass.

Miles, M. B., Huberman, A. M., & Saldana, J. (2014). *Qualitative data analysis: A methods sourcebook*. Thousand Oaks, CA: Sage.

Mita, S. C., Gray, S. A., & Goodell, L. S. (2015). An explanatory framework of teachers' perceptions of a positive mealtime environment in a preschool setting. *Appetite, 90*, 37–44. doi: 10.1016/j.appet.2015.02.031

Patton, M.Q. (2002). *Qualitative research & evaluation methods* (3rd ed.). Thousand Oaks, CA: Sage.

Perrin, M. T., Goodell, L. S., Allen, J. C., & Fogleman, A. (2014). A mixed-methods observational study of human milk sharing communities on Facebook. *Breastfeeding Medicine, 9*, 128–134. doi: 10.1089/bfm.2013.0114

Peterson, A., Goodell, L. S., Hegde, A. V., & Stage, V. C. (2017). Teacher perceptions of multilevel policies and the influence on nutrition education in North Carolina Head Start preschools. *Journal of Nutrition Education and Behavior, 49*, Accepted for publication November 2016.

Pitts, J. M. (1994). *Personal understandings and mental models of information: A qualitative study of factors associated with the information-seeking and use of adolescents* (Doctoral dissertation). Retrieved from ProQuest Dissertations Publishing (Order Number 9416154).

Shenton, A. K. (2004). Strategies for ensuring trustworthiness in qualitative research projects. *Education for Information, 22*, 63–75.

Tanenbaum, M. L., Kane, N. S., Kenowitz, J., & Gonzalez, J. S. (2016). Diabetes distress from the patient's perspective: Qualitative themes and treatment regimen differences among adults with type 2 diabetes. *Journal of Diabetes and its Complications, 30*, 1060–1068. doi: 10.1016/j.jdiacomp.2016.04.023

Vesnaver, E., Keller, H. H., Sutherland, O., Maitland, S. B., & Locher, J. L. (2015). Alone at the table: Food behavior and the loss of commensality in widowhood. *Journal of Gerontology (Series B): Psychological Sciences and Social Sciences, 71*, 1059-1069. doi:10.1093/geronb/gbv103

Vesnaver, E., Keller, H. H., Sutherland, O., Maitland, S. B., & Locher, J. L. (2015). Food behavior change in late-life widowhood: A two-stage process. *Appetite, 95*, 399-407. doi:10.1016/j.appet.2015.07.027

Waller, J., Bower, K. M., Spence, M., & Kavanagh, K. F. (2015). Using grounded theory methodology to conceptualize the mother-infant communication dynamic: Potential application to compliance with infant feeding recommendations. *Maternal & Child Nutrition, 11*, 749–760. doi: 10.1111/mcn.12056

Weisberg-Shapiro, P., & Devine, C. M. (2015). "Because we missed the way we eat at the middle of the day:" Dietary acculturation and food routines among Dominican women. *Appetite, 95*, 293–302. doi:10.1016/j.appet.2015.07.024

CHAPTER 10

Qualitative Research Study Designs

VIRGINIA C. STAGE, PHD, RD, LDN
NATALIE K. COOKE, PHD
L. SUZANNE GOODELL, PHD, RD

CHAPTER OUTLINE

- Introduction
- Thematic Analysis
- Phenomenology
- Grounded Theory
- Case Studies
- Conclusion
- Researcher Interview: Qualitative Research, Dr. L. Suzanne Goodell, Dr. Natalie K. Cooke, Dr. Virgina C. Stage

LEARNING OUTCOMES

- Compare and contrast types of qualitative research designs: thematic analysis, phenomenology, grounded theory, and case studies.
- Discuss strengths and limitations of each of the four types of qualitative research designs.
- Explain how thematic analysis can be applied to a variety of document types.
- Describe how phenomenology can be used to describe the "lived experience" or a "phenomenon of interest."
- Describe how grounded theory can be used to develop a "baby theory."
- Discuss why a case study must be bounded by a specific set of characteristics and is a special type of research design.

INTRODUCTION

In this chapter, we focus on four *approaches* or *designs* commonly used in qualitative research:

1. **Thematic analysis** focuses on organizing key ideas that emerge from the data. It is the most flexible type of qualitative research design as it can be used to collect and analyze multiple forms of data (e.g., verbal, text, sound, images).

2. **Phenomenology** is used to better understand the *common experiences* of a group of individuals (also called a **phenomenon**). This design typically uses individual interviews to collect data to better understand the "what' and "how" of participants' experiences (e.g., diabetes educators' experience with implementing a diabetes education program for newly diagnosed clients).
3. **Grounded theory** aims to better understand a *process* among the participants being studied (e.g., teachers' perceptions of a positive mealtime environment in a preschool setting). This design is one of the more difficult approaches in qualitative research, and it often results in the development of a theoretical model to explain the study's findings visually.
4. **Case studies** explore a single case, such as an individual or group (e.g., organization, community). This design often combines a variety of data collection methods to provide a deeper understanding of the case being studied, including interviews, focus groups, observations, and document analysis.

At a basic level, the different designs in qualitative research depend heavily on the research question the researcher is trying to answer. For example, if the researcher wants to better understand the common experiences among a group of individuals, such as elementary teachers' experience with implementing nutrition education in their classrooms (Hall, Chai, & Albrecht, 2016), the researcher would use a phenomenological design. If, instead, the researcher's goal was to develop a theoretical model for better understanding the interactions between mothers and infants and the influences of these interactions on feeding practices (Waller, Bower, Spence, & Kavanagh, 2015), the researcher would use a grounded theory design.

These different research designs might use common data collection methods (e.g., interviews or focus groups), but their approach to data analysis is different. For example, phenomenology and grounded theory design generally have the most detailed procedures for analysis, whereas thematic analysis and case studies data analysis requires fewer steps and is more flexible. This does not necessarily mean that thematic analysis or case study analysis will take less time, just that the steps are fewer in number.

For all research designs, trustworthiness is an integral part of qualitative research. Regardless of the level of flexibility in methods, data collection and analysis are always conducted in a rigorous way that results in a product that honors participants' voices. As we explore each of these research designs, you will better understand the complexities of each.

THEMATIC ANALYSIS

Thematic analysis, also known as content analysis, is a commonly used qualitative research method that allows researchers to draw conclusions from their data, with the ultimate goal of obtaining new knowledge or insights into the problem being studied (Krippendorff, 1980). If this description sounds broad and generic, that is because it is a fairly unstructured approach to qualitative research. Unlike other types of qualitative research designs, thematic analysis is very flexible and can be used to understand a variety of data types including written text (e.g., newspaper articles, personal reflections), images/illustration (e.g., film footage, cartoons), electronic communication (e.g., email, blog postings), and oral materials (e.g., interviews, sound clips) (Kondracki, Wellman, & Amundson, 2002; Krippendorff, 2004; Moretti et al., 2011). The primary goal of the method is to systematically reduce and organize a large amount of data into a condensed, broad description of the problem being studied (Burnard, 1996; Weber, 1990).

The product of thematic analysis is, as the name implies, a series of themes. Recall that a theme is a pattern that researchers see in the data.

For example, Abrams, Evans, and Duff (2015) used thematic analysis to explore how parents interpret verbal and visual front of the package (FOP) information when making decisions about food products to buy for their preschool-aged children. Researchers in this study used a combination of focus groups and 10 different images of a variety of fruit snack packages as visual stimuli during discussions. The packages featured a variety of marketing tactics, such as licensed cartoon characters, brand name logos, naturalness/healthfulness claims, and more. After organizing and analyzing the two data types, researchers identified five themes: (1) characters and colors cue fun for kids but "unhealthy" to parents, (2) health claims and "natural" design are meaningful, (3) visual realism means healthier options, (4) brand trust and perceived healthfulness, and (5) ignorance is bliss. To obtain these findings, the researchers in this study used both focus groups (oral materials) and images (examples of FOP marketing). The authors explicitly state in the Methods section of the article that they used thematic analysis, defining it as "an inductive analytical technique that consists of exploring the data to identify and classify recurring patterns" (p. 24). They use the term **open coding** to describe a technique used in their thematic analysis that involves first reading data and noting themes that are evident. You will see that this term is also used in grounded theory, so this term alone does not point you to the type of research design used.

A thematic analysis study may rely on multiple forms of data, as described in the Abrams et al. (2015) study, or on a single form of data. A study by Whelan and Markless (2012) also used thematic analysis (research design) along with semi-structured interviews (data collection method), to explore the factors that influence registered dietitians' research involvement as university faculty. Researchers of this study provided a more in-depth description of their data analysis process. For example, Whelan and Markless (2012) go beyond simply identifying thematic analysis as the chosen research design by describing how many times the interview transcripts were read (between five and nine times each), and the use of research meetings as a means to discuss the coding process. A second study by Lisson, Goodell, Dev, Wilkerson, Hegde, and Stage (2016) also used thematic analysis to understand the findings in their study, and similar to Whelan and Markles (2012), they relied on interviews as their main unit of data. Researchers interviewed 63 preschool administrators and teachers via telephone to gain insight into common barriers to availability and use of nutrition education resources in Head Start classrooms. Three themes were observed across the interviews: a desire for greater organization of existing nutrition education resources, the need for increased community support and professional development opportunities, and increased funding and time spent to support nutrition education efforts in the classroom. In the Data Management and Analysis section, they describe an inductive content analysis process, including the process of memoing, open coding, and the use of consensus coding via verbal agreement. In each article, these descriptions of how data was collected and analyzed provide transparency in the research process and add to the trustworthiness of findings.

Strengths and Limitations

Thematic analysis has several strengths. The flexibility of thematic analysis enables researchers to analyze a large amount of data. Further, this flexibility allows researchers to collect several types of data that can inform the research problem being studied, so the analysis is not limited just to text transcripts, for example. Compared to other qualitative research designs, thematic analysis can be inexpensive, although the ultimate cost depends on the specific techniques chosen to analyze the data, equipment and personnel costs, and the size of the study.

Although the flexibility of thematic analysis has many benefits, it can also be a weakness of the design. For example, unlike other qualitative designs (e.g., phenomenology, grounded theory), there are no specific rules for analyzing data when using thematic analysis. Therefore, it is up to the researchers to ensure that ample time is spent in the process of data analysis and that the analysis is conducted systematically and ethically. Another limitation is that having more data is not always a good thing. A thematic analysis project that has a lot of data to analyze may prove to be labor-intensive and time-consuming, especially if the data being studied vary in type, and increase in amount or become more complex as the analysis progresses. Finally, thematic analysis lacks a specific analysis procedure, making the approach more difficult and less ideal if you are new to qualitative research (Kondracki et al., 2002) and need more structure.

PHENOMENOLOGY

The purpose of phenomenological research is to describe a phenomenon, as the name implies. This type of exploratory/descriptive research is designed to help researchers explain what happens when participants experience something in common—the "lived experience" (Creswell, 2008; Flood, 2010). In nutrition research, it is important to understand the common experiences among a group of individuals to develop effective policies and practices, or simply to gain a better overall understanding of the problem being studied. For example, a researcher might want to explore the experience of food insecurity. This phenomenon might include these individuals' environmental makeup (e.g., access to a grocery store), resources (e.g., budget), motivations (e.g., wanting to avoid the cost of health problems), barriers (e.g., economic constraints), and emotions (e.g., stigma) felt during or after the experience.

Unlike thematic analysis, phenomenology often uses a more prescribed approach to guide data collection and analysis. Understanding these key features will help you recognize and understand studies using a phenomenological approach. Phenomenological studies include these common features:

- *Researchers "bracket" personal experiences.* Although it may not be described explicitly in the research article, researchers using a phenomenological approach should **bracket** (or epoche) their personal experiences with the phenomenon. In simpler terms, this means the researchers attempt to set aside any preconceived ideas or bias before beginning the study by writing about their prior experiences with the participants' or with the problem being studied; this process is similar to journaling. For example, under the Data Collection section, Hall et al. (2016) state that the lead researcher "bracketed biases before beginning data collection to assure data accuracy." It is not possible to entirely remove researchers' prior experiences, but this is a useful exercise to help investigators take a fresh perspective on the phenomenon under investigation (Moustakas, 1994). This type of bracketing might also happen verbally in conversations during research team meetings.
- *Data is collected from individuals with a "common" experience.* Researchers using a phenomenological approach generally collect data in the form of in-depth interviews from participants. Sometimes researchers conduct single interviews or a series of interviews with the same participants. Generally, researchers ask participants two broad questions: What have you experienced? How have you experienced it?

(Moustakas, 1994). For example, Hall et al. (2016) were interested in better understanding the "what" and "how" surrounding elementary teachers' experiences with nutrition education in their classroom. Researchers presented teachers with the following questions/statements: "How would you describe your role in nutrition education?" and "Tell me about your experiences teaching the *Growing Healthy Kids* curriculum" (p. 138). Other questions focused on teachers' feelings about teaching nutrition, their views about nutrition in comparison to core subjects (e.g., mathematics, science), the influence of nutrition education on students, and barriers to nutrition education in the classroom.

- *Description of the "essence" or common experience.* The final goal of a phenomenological study is to better understand the phenomenon being studied through a detailed description of the "essence" of the experiences described by participants. In a research article, this description is found in the Results or Discussion section. It may be explicitly stated as a separate paragraph or combined with an overall discussion of the study's findings. Again, using Hall et al. (2016) as an example, they described the "essence" of teachers' experiences with nutrition education as an opportunity to positively influence students' health. Teachers discussed nutrition education as being important but acknowledged internal and external conflicts that affected prioritization of core subjects, time, resources, and uncontrollable home environments that restricted classroom efforts.

Strengths and Limitations

Unlike thematic analysis, phenomenology relies solely on interviews, providing a more streamlined method of data collection. Due to the more structured approach used to guide data collection and analysis, this method may be better suited for investigators new to qualitative research. Finally, a focus on common experiences among a group of individuals allows researchers to better understand the phenomenon being studied and can inform future nutrition-related interventions and policies.

The two primary limitations in a phenomenology research design are both related to sampling. First, because participants must have a common experience with the phenomenon in question, sampling may be a challenge. Researchers should choose participants carefully so a "common" understanding of the research problem can be obtained at the end of the study. Second, bracketing all personal experiences with the participants' and the research problem may present a challenge for some investigators (Cho & Lee, 2014), but is an essential step to ensure rigor in data analysis.

GROUNDED THEORY

Grounded theory is used when the researchers are interested in broadly explaining a process, action, or interactions about a large topic. The goal of the grounded theory design is to generate a **baby theory**. This baby theory is different from large or overarching theories, such as behavior change theories or learning theories, which apply in many different contexts and to many different problems. This baby theory will have an impact on your research and on others who study your subject matter, but is unlikely to lead to major changes applicable to all of society. For example, a researcher might develop a theory that:

- Explains a process, such as how individuals with diabetes deal with challenges in the workplace (Thomas, 2011)

- Explain actions, such as how teachers implement nutrition education in their classrooms (Carraway-Stage et al., 2014)
- Explain interactions among people, such as how the interaction between mothers and infants influences the development of feeding practices (Waller et al., 2015)

Generally, grounded theory is most appropriate when no theory yet exists that explains the problem relative to the specific participants being studied. Otherwise, there would not be a reason to develop a new theory, as researchers could explore particular facets of an already existing theory. Because the theory is "grounded," or developed from the data collected, it often does a better job of explaining the participants or the situation being studied, may be more likely to work when put into practice, and may be more sensitive to the individuals in the specific setting being studied.

Similar to a phenomenological design, grounded theory researchers often use structured procedures for collecting data, identifying codes and themes in the data, and forming the theory explaining the process being studied (Glaser & Strauss, 1967). The common features of a grounded theory study include the following:

- **Theoretical sampling**. Similar to other forms of qualitative inquiry, grounded theory collects and analyzes data simultaneously. However, in a grounded theory design, the intention behind simultaneous data collection and analysis is to collect intentional and focused data that will aid in the generation of the theory being developed, a process called theoretical sampling. Following theoretical sampling, a researcher collects initial data, reviews the data for preliminary themes, and then determines what additional data would be useful to collect to help further develop the model. Clues as to what additional data to collect might include underdeveloped themes, missing information about a sequence of events, or the realization that new individuals (similar or different) may provide further insight into the problem. The researcher then returns to the field and collects more data. The process can be imaged as a "zigzag" between data collection, analysis, and developing the pieces of the theory.
- *Development of a theory*. A common goal of grounded theory is to actually develop a baby theory, drawn from multiple individuals or data sources, to explain the problem being studied. Because the theory being developed is "grounded" in the data collected, it is limited in scope and generalizability.

Mita, Gray, and Goodell (2015) sought to create a theory that could explain Head Start teachers' perceptions of a positive mealtime environment (PME) (**Figure 10.1**). The model also highlights the issues and influential factors surrounding PME. The developed model reveals (1) people; (2) positive emotional tone; (3) rules, expectations, and routines; (4) operations of PME; and (5) outcomes of PME as key constructs. Overall, teachers' perceived PME as included learning, socializing, and eating as foundational to children's growth and development. This theory describes PME, a concept that had not previously been described in the context of Head Start preschools.

In another example of a grounded theory study, Carraway-Stage et al. (2014) describe a three-phase approach to analysis: open coding, axial coding, and selective coding. The aim of this study was to gain an understanding of Head Start administrators' and teachers' perceptions of nutrition education in the preschool classroom. In the first phase of analysis, researchers describe reviewing each interview transcript, memoing, and engaging in open coding. In phase two (**axial coding**), researchers re-read transcripts and compared preliminary codes, themes, and subthemes identified in phase one. Finally, in phase three (**selective coding**), investigators focused on "telling the story" by identifying, comparing and contrasting, and describing key themes found in

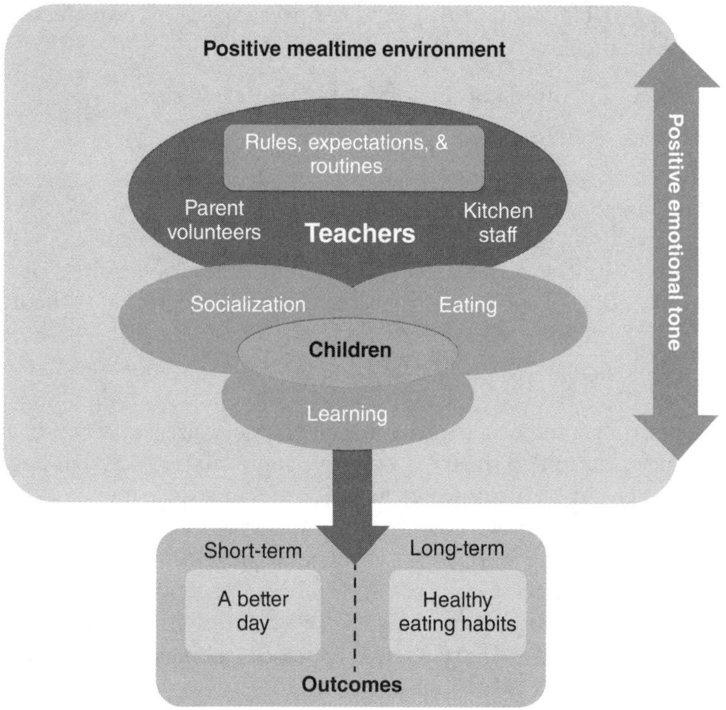

FIGURE 10.1 Theoretical Model Explaining Head Start Preschool Teachers' Definition of a Positive Mealtime Environment

Reproduced from "An Explanatory Framework of Teachers' Perceptions of a Positive Mealtime Environment in a Preschool Setting," by S.C. Mita, S.A. Gray, & L.S. Goodell, 2015, *Appetite, 90*, 40. Copyright Elsvier. Reprinted with permission.

the data. These themes were then used in the development of a visual theoretical model (**Figure 10.2**). Similar to the Mita et al. (2015) study, Carraway-Stage et al. (2014) described a concept in preschool education that had not been described previously. The theory does not always present itself as a model, as it did with these two studies.

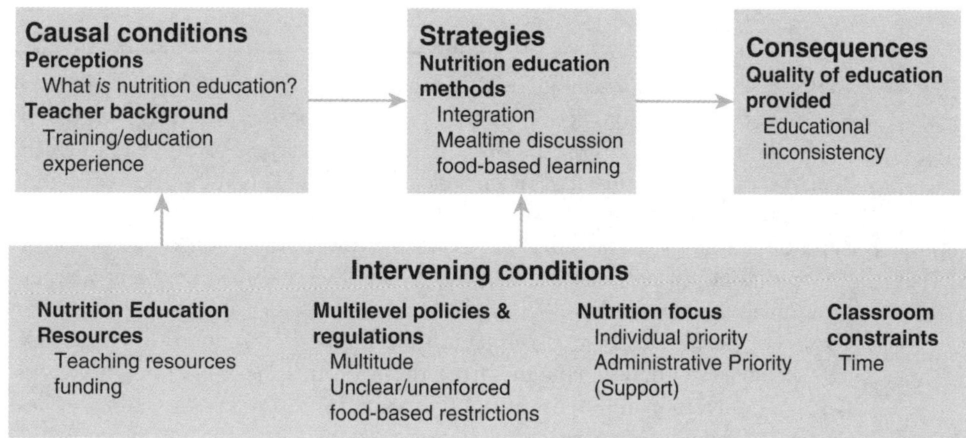

FIGURE 10.2 Theoretical Model for Understanding the State of Nutrition Education in the Head Start Preschool Classroom

Reproduced from "Understanding the State of Nutrition Education in the Head Start Classroom: A Qualitative Approach," by V. Carraway-Stage, S.R. Henson, A. Dipper, H. Spangler, S.L. Ash, and L.S. Goodell, 2014, *American Journal of Health Education, 45*, 57. Copyright by Taylor & Francis. Reprinted with permission.

When Hunt and Thomson (2016) explored peer support in breastfeeding women, the result was three themes.

1. Place, space, and timing of support
2. One way or no way
3. "It must be me"

Illustrating the concept of theoretical sampling, the researchers described how the emphasis of interview questions shifted during the process of data collection to "exhaust theoretical ideas." Similar to the previous two studies, the researchers described the iterative process of data collection and analysis, a hallmark of grounded theory research.

STRENGTHS AND LIMITATIONS

As with the previously discussed designs, grounded theory also has strengths and limitations. As a strength, grounded theory is a creative approach to understanding a research problem. Ultimately, it allows researchers to create an explanation for a process no currently existing theory can adequately explain; this has substantial implications for ensuring that nutrition interventions are effective. Grounded theory also can provide a structured approach to the research process, which can be good for a beginning qualitative researcher who needs that structure (or overwhelming if not done appropriately). Although difficult to execute, this structured approach can make data collection, analysis, and theory development easier to understand.

Despite strengths, grounded theory also presents challenges. For example, theoretical sampling can be difficult to achieve. The researchers must pay close attention to data being collected and make educated, purposeful, and timely decisions about future data collection efforts. This may be difficult for some researchers, and formal meetings with the research team or informal discussions with colleagues might help navigate this potentially "gray area." Further, due to the rigor used in this design (e.g., theoretical sampling, goal of theory development), a grounded theory study can be time- and labor-intensive compared to other approaches (Cho & Lee, 2014). Some novice researchers may find this structure beneficial in learning qualitative research; others might become overwhelmed.

CASE STUDIES

A case study is a special subset of qualitative research that researchers use to explain a "bounded case," or a concept that can be "fenced in" to have a unit of one **case** (Merriam, 2009). This means that the researcher has set parameters to define the case, such as one specific hospital or one specific school. To explore this case, the researcher uses multiple methods, which can include interviews, focus groups, documents analysis, and observations (Creswell, 2013). Of note, just because a researcher chooses to combine methods (interviews, focus groups, and observations) to explore a larger issue does not mean that the study is "fenced in" and defined as a case study. If there is no defined case, the researcher is just using multiple methods to explore the research question. Researchers might use principles from thematic analysis or phenomenology to approach analysis; therefore, although case studies are a distinct type of research method, you will often see them intertwined with another research method.

For example, Ofei, Holst, Rasmussen, and Mikkelsen (2014) used a case study approach to explore how hospital practice affects trolley food waste in one particular hospital (the case). They used a combination of site visits, using informal interviews to gain insight into hospital workflow as well as developing interview and focus group questions. In addition to conducting interviews and focus groups, they observed the actions of trolley and food service staff during a series of lunch and dinnertime meals. Although not qualitative, the researchers also weighed food to determine the degree of food waste as a quantitative measure. Because they were focused on a multifaceted understanding of the meal system in hospitals, they elected to combine interviews, focus groups, and observations in a case study. By combining the data collected from all of these methods, they were able to determine five themes: meal ordering, communication, portion sizes, monitoring, and using unserved foods. Notice that the researchers used interviews, focus groups, and observations (multiple methods) to explore a bounded case (the hospital). The researchers explain in the Methods section that they used thematic analysis to determine the themes described in the Results section.

Jara, Ozer, and Seyer-Ochi (2014) also selected a case study methodology to evaluate the impact of a 2-year food policy intervention in one middle school in California. Interested in the impact of the intervention on the school as a whole, researchers conducted interviews with students and teachers, engaged in classroom observations of the intervention curriculum, reviewed students' reflection worksheets completed as a part of the intervention, and reviewed minutes from district-level committee meetings in which they discussed school nutrition. Researchers analyzed these data and developed an explanatory model to describe the social and environmental barriers middle school students face when trying to eat healthy. The product of their study differed from that of the Ofei et al. (2014) study (it produced an explanatory model instead a list of themes); however, both studies used thematic analysis to come to their final set of themes.

Both of these research questions lend themselves to the use of multiple methods to fully understand the complexity of the issue, but they define the case as well. In these case study research designs, the researchers also used thematic analysis for data analysis.

Strengths and Limitations

Because case studies describe a special situation, their strengths and weaknesses mirror those of the other models previously discussed. The defining feature of case studies is the bounded case, which can be difficult to define. A case study is a model or example; therefore, one case may not describe all cases. As with all qualitative research designs, it is important to note the extent to which a case study is representative, but not necessarily generalizable. For example, a case study about a school lunch program in a private school in New England may offer relevant information to the literature, but school lunch administrators in a public school in the South might not see the same themes in their own school.

CONCLUSION

We have explored some of the intricacies of qualitative research designs. **Figure 10.3** highlights some of the basic similarities and differences between the four research designs discussed in this chapter. Combining this knowledge with your knowledge of qualitative research provides a solid foundation for evaluating qualitative research designs you encounter in journal articles.

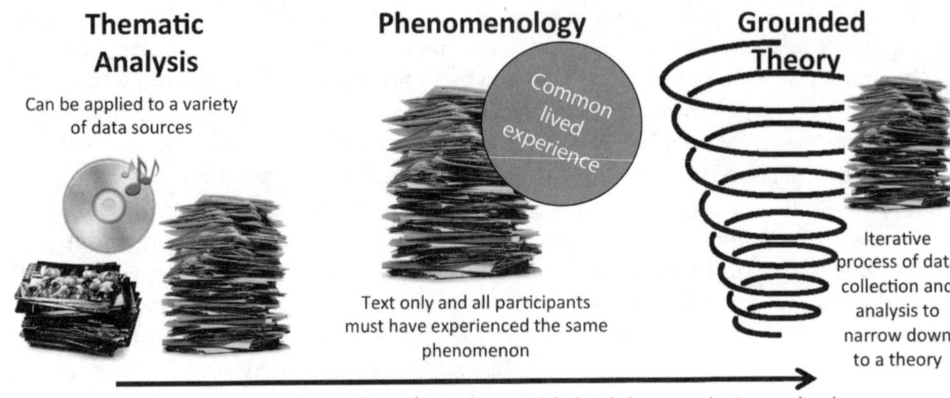

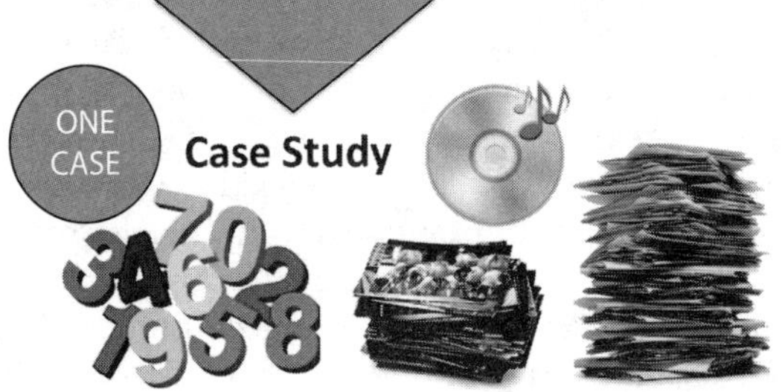

FIGURE 10.3 Summary of Characteristics of Qualitative Research Designs

RESEARCHER INTERVIEW Qualitative Research

L. Suzanne Goodell, PhD, RD
North Carolina State University;
Natalie K. Cooke, PhD
North Carolina State University;
Virginia C. Stage, PhD, RDN, LDN
East Carolina University

1. **Briefly describe the areas in which you do research.**
We are interested in several different aspects of nutrition education and behavior change. Dr. Cooke works with nutrition education in higher education, and Drs. Stage and Goodell focus their work on nutrition education and behaviors with families and teachers of Head Start preschool children. Head Start is a federally funded preschool program for 3- to 5-year-olds from low-income families.

   Dr. Goodell is most interested in the interactions between these young children and their caregivers (teachers, parents) and how that affects what the children eat.

   Dr. Stage focuses her work more on nutrition education in the preschool environment and providing nutrition education resources to these teachers. She creates nutrition education lessons that can help meet the needs of teachers and provides them with professional development (i.e., training) to help them learn how to use these nutrition education resources well.

   Dr. Cooke works primarily with preparing future nutrition education professionals through service-learning coursework. She is always looking for new ways to improve students' abilities and self-efficacy related to teaching nutrition education in the community.

2. **With your experience in qualitative research, what should students/practitioners know about this area of research? For example, how would they recognize that a published study was an example of qualitative research?**
In the past, qualitative research was not widely accepted in the nutrition field. This is partly due to the nutrition research community's lack of understanding about this branch of research, and partly due to the lack of rigor and transparency in published qualitative nutrition research. When Dr. Goodell was a graduate student, one of her professors told her that qualitative research was not research and not worth pursuing. Naively, she heard his words but did not change her interest in working in the field. She is thankful that she did not fully grasp what he was trying to say and pursued qualitative research anyway.

   Although there are still those with a basic science background who have a limited grasp of the potential impact of qualitative research, within the last 10 to 20 years qualitative research has become more broadly embraced by the nutrition research community. Many granting agencies (the places that give researchers money to do what they do) now encourage, if not require, qualitative research to be incorporated into large-scale nutrition education and behavior change projects. Clearly, these agencies are beginning to recognize the value of hearing the "why" behind the numbers (quantitative statistics), especially when it comes to understanding why interventions were or were not effective in producing nutrition-related outcomes (e.g., dietary intake, knowledge). More journals are including qualitative articles in their publications, with some (such as the *Journal of Nutrition Education and Behavior*) providing specific, unique guidelines for qualitative research, an acknowledgment that it is different from quantitative research.

   Typically, a qualitative research article uses the word "qualitative" in the last paragraph of the Introduction or in the first few paragraphs of the Methods section. However, if it does not, the data collection methods generally help readers identify that it is a qualitative study. Anything with interviews or focus groups will be a qualitative or mixed methods study. Document analyses and studies using observations can be either quantitative or qualitative in nature. To be very clear, authors typically specify that they are conducting a qualitative study.

3. **What do you enjoy most about the research process?**
Generally, we love the creativity involved in the research process. Conducting research pushes us to think deeper and more critically about a topic. We have to be prepared to see all sides of the problem: Why would we choose to collect data this way? What are the strengths and what are the limitations? How can we do it better to maximize the strengths and minimize the limitations while still remaining realistic?

   Because we often work in teams, the research process also challenges us to listen to those with differing opinions and to carefully examine and justify our own opinions. As a qualitative researcher, you are in a constant cycle of documenting your perceptions about a research topic and distancing yourself from those beliefs as you listen to the perspectives of others. Communication is so important when working in teams. We have been fortunate to find colleagues who have the same communication expectations, which makes doing research together much easier, and of course more fun! Finding a research community, whatever your specialty, is valuable, because your colleagues push you to examine research questions from a different light, and you, in turn, encourage the same in them.

   Regarding qualitative research specifically, we thoroughly enjoy hearing people's stories. We do not take for granted that participants allow us into their world and share a part of their lives with us. This openness is a gift. We are fascinated by the similarities and differences among us, and we love to learn from those who are willing to share.

   The research process does not begin and end with a "research study"; that is only one part of it. For us, the research process involves sharing ideas and disseminating results too. We are constantly striving to improve others' understanding of qualitative research and the rigorous standards of qualitative research. We enjoy sharing our experiences with other researchers and learning from them as well. We are science nerds and love hanging out with other science nerds.

4. **What tips do you have for practitioners who want to do practice-based research?**
We would suggest several things for practitioners who want to do practice-based research. First, to be published, your research methods must be approved by an ethics committee (e.g.,

a university's Institutional Review Board for Research with Human Subjects). Without this approval prior to data collection, it is unlikely that you will find a journal willing to publish your work. Some practices may have this ethics committee in-house, but you may need to partner with someone affiliated with a university to have access to one of these committees.

Second, research in isolation is almost always not as good as it would be if you were working with a team. Finding a group of collaborators, within your workplace or at a university or elsewhere, can help you find more creative and innovative solutions to research problems. If possible, work with those with whom you enjoy working. There are so many people out in the world, there is no need to be miserable while doing your job. Find people who make research enjoyable.

Third, stay organized and honor the voices of your participants. Organization is an important part not only of conducting ethical research but also maximizing your time so you can fully devote yourself to answering your research question. Qualitative research projects can be very time-consuming, especially as you immerse yourself in the data analysis. Think of the data as a puzzle that you need to put together to bring life to your participants' voices. It is a job that only you can do, and you want to be organized so you can do it well.

Fourth, and finally, always be open to learning new methodologies (ways of conducting research), strive for rigor in your work, but be open to change and accept imperfection. After all, no research study is perfect, but we can aim to do our best and learn from our experiences and from others. This is ultimately how we grow and mature as researchers, whether we are a basic scientist or a practice-based researcher.

SUMMARY

1. Thematic analysis is a qualitative design that focuses on organizing key ideas that emerge from the data. It is the most flexible type of qualitative research design because it can be used to collect and analyze multiple forms of data (e.g., verbal, text, sound, images). The product of thematic analysis is, as the name implies, a series of themes (or patterns).
2. The flexibility of thematic analysis has many benefits, but it can also be a weakness of the design. For example, there are no specific rules for analyzing data when using thematic analysis. Therefore, it is up to the researchers to ensure that ample time is spent in the process of data analysis and that the analysis is conducted systematically and ethically. Also, analyzing a lot of data is labor- and time-intensive.
3. Phenomenology is a qualitative design that is used to better understand the common experiences of a group of individuals (phenomenon). This design typically uses individual interviews to collect data to better understand the "what' and "how" of the participants' experience (e.g., diabetes educators' experience with implementing a diabetes education program for newly diagnosed clients). Researchers using a phenomenological approach should bracket their personal experiences with the phenomenon.
4. Because phenomenology relies solely on interviews, it provides a more streamlined method of data collection that enables researchers to better understand the phenomenon being studied. Sampling and bracketing all personal experiences can be difficult with this approach.
5. Grounded theory is a qualitative design that aims to better understand a process among the participants being studied (e.g., teachers' perceptions of a positive mealtime environment in a preschool setting). Similar to a phenomenological design, grounded theory researchers often use structured procedures for collecting data, identifying codes/themes in the data, and forming the theory explaining the process being studied. This design is one of the more difficult approaches in qualitative research, and it often results in the development of a theoretical model to explain the study's findings visually.

6. As a strength, grounded theory is a creative approach to understanding a research problem. Ultimately, it allows researchers to create an explanation for a process no currently existing theory can adequately explain; this has substantial implications for ensuring nutrition interventions are effective. However, theoretical sampling can be difficult, and a grounded theory study can be labor- and time-intensive.
7. Case studies explore a single "case," such as an individual or group (e.g., organization, community). This design often combines a variety of data collection methods to provide a deeper understanding of the case being studied, including interviews, focus groups, observations, and document analysis.
8. The defining feature of case studies is the bounded case, which can be difficult to define. A case study is a model or an example; therefore, one case may not describe all cases. As with all qualitative research designs, it is important to note the extent to which a case study is representative, but not necessarily generalizable.
9. These different research designs may use common data collection methods (e.g., interviews or focus groups), but their approach to data analysis is different. For example, phenomenology and grounded theory design generally have the most detailed procedures for analysis, whereas thematic analysis and case study data analysis require fewer steps and are more flexible.

REVIEW QUESTIONS

1. A qualitative design that is used to better understand the common experiences of a group is known as:
   A. thematic analysis
   B. a phenomenological approach
   C. grounded theory
   D. a case study
2. A qualitative design that uses multiple methods to explore an issue within one school is known as:
   A. thematic analysis
   B. a phenomenological approach
   C. grounded theory
   D. a case study
3. A qualitative design that focuses on organizing key ideas from the data is known as:
   A. thematic analysis
   B. a phenomenological approach
   C. grounded theory
   D. a case study
4. A qualitative design that aims to better understand a process among the participants is known as:
   A. thematic analysis
   B. a phenomenological approach
   C. grounded theory
   D. a case study
5. Develop a chart showing the key characteristics of each research design discussed in this chapter; include the strengths and limitations of each design.
6. If you are given a qualitative research study to read, what would you look for to determine which research design was being used?

CRITICAL THINKING QUESTIONS

1. Read the following qualitative study and answer these questions.
   Knoblock-Hahn, A. L., Wray, R., & LeRouge, C. M. (2016). Perceptions of adolescents with overweight and obesity for the develop of user-centered design self-management tools within the context of the Chronic Care Model: A qualitative study.

Journal of the Academy of Nutrition and Dietetics, 116, 957–967.

A. Which research design is used in this study? Support your answer.
B. What is the objective for this study?
C. Who are the participants?
D. How was data collected and analyzed?
E. What were the major results?

2. Read the following qualitative study and answer these questions.
Frerichs, L., Intolubbe-Chmil, L., Brittin, J., Teitelbaum, K., Trowbridge, M., & Huang, T. K. (2016). Children's discourse of liked, healthy, and unhealthy foods. *Journal of the Academy of Nutrition and Dietetics, 116,* 1323–1331.
A. Which research design is used in this study? Support your answer.
B. What is the objective for this study?
C. Who are the participants?
D. How was data collected and analyzed?
E. What were the major results?

3. Read the following qualitative study and answer these questions.
Handforth, B., Hennink, M., & Schwartz, M. B. (2013). A qualitative study of nutrition-based initiatives at selected food banks in the Feeding America Network. *Journal of the Academy of Nutrition and Dietetics, 113,* 411–415.
A. Which research design is used in this study? Support your answer.
B. What is the objective for this study?
C. Who are the participants?
D. How was data collected and analyzed?
E. What were the major results?

SUGGESTED READINGS AND ACTIVITIES

1. Harris, J. E., Gleason, P. M., Sheean, P. M., Boushey, C., Beto, J. A., & Bruemmer, B. (2009). An introduction to qualitative research for food and nutrition professionals. *Journal of the American Dietetic Association, 109,* 80–90. doi: 10.1016/j.jada.2008.10.018

REFERENCES

Abrams, K. M., Evans, C., & Duff, B. R. L. (2015). Ignorance is bliss. How parents of preschool children make sense of front-of-package visuals and claims on food. *Appetite, 87,* 20–29. doi: 10.1016/j.appet.2014.12.100

Burnard, P. (1996) Teaching the analysis of textual data: An experiential approach. *Nurse Education Today, 16,* 278–281.

Carraway-Stage, V., Henson, S. R., Dipper, A., Spangler, H., Ash, S. L., & Goodell, L. S. (2014). Understanding the state of nutrition education in the Head Start classroom: A qualitative approach. *American Journal of Health Education, 45,* 52–62. doi:10.1080/19325037.2013.853000

Cho, J. Y., & Lee, E. (2014) Reducing confusion about grounded theory and qualitative content analysis: Similarities and differences. *The Qualitative Report, 19,* 1–20.

Creswell, J. W. (2008). *Educational research: Planning, conducting, and evaluating quantitative and qualitative research* (3rd ed.). Boston, MA: Pearson.

Creswell, J. W. (2013). *Qualitative inquiry & research design: Choosing among five approaches.* Thousand Oaks, CA: Sage.

Flood, A. (2010). Understanding phenomenology. *Nurse Researcher, 17,* 7–15. doi: 10.7748/nr2010.01.17.2.7.c7457

Glaser, B., & Strauss, A. L. (1967). *The discovery of grounded theory: Strategies for qualitative research.* Chicago, IL: Aldine.

Hall, E., Chai, W., & Albrecht, J. A. (2016). A qualitative phenomenological exploration of teacher's experience with nutrition education. *American Journal of Health Education, 47,* 136–148. doi: 10.1080/19325037.2016.1157532

Hunt, L., & Thomson, G. (2016). Pressure and judgement within a dichotomous landscape of infant feeding: A grounded theory study to explore why breastfeeding women do not access peer support provision. *Maternal & Child Nutrition.* Advance online publication. doi: 10.1111/mcn.12279

Jara, E., Ozer, E. J., & Seyer-Ochi, I. (2014). A case study of middle school food policy and persisting barriers to healthful eating. *Ecology of Food and Nutrition, 53,* 333–346. doi: 10.1080/03670244.2014.872906

Kondracki, N. L., Wellman, N. S., & Amundson, D. R. (2002). Content analysis: Review of methods and their applications in nutrition education. *Journal of Nutrition*

Education and Behavior, 34, 224–230. doi: 10.1016/S1499-4046(06)60097-3

Krippendorff, K. (1980). *Content analysis: An introduction to its methodology*. Beverly Hills, CA: Sage.

Lisson, S., Goodell, L. S., Dev, D., Wilkerson, K., Hegde, A. V., & Stage, V. C. (2016). Nutrition education resources in North Carolina-based Head Start preschool programs: Administrator and teacher perceptions of availability and use. *Journal of Nutrition Education and Behavior, 48*, 655-663. doi: 10.1016/jneb.2016.07.016

Merriam, S. B. (2009). *Qualitative research: A guide to design and implementation*. San Francisco, CA: Jossey-Bass.

Mita, S. C., Gray, S. A., & Goodell, L. S. (2015). An explanatory framework of teachers' perceptions of a positive mealtime environment in a preschool setting. *Appetite, 90*, 37–44. doi: 10.1016/j.appet.2015.02.031

Moretti, F., van Vliet, L., Bensing, J., Deledda, G., Mazzi, M., Rimondini, M., . . . Fletcher I. (2011). A standardized approach to qualitative content analysis of focus group discussions from different countries. *Patient Education & Counseling, 82*, 420–428. doi: 10.1016/j.pec.2011.01.005

Moustakas, C. (1994). *Phenomenological research methods*. Thousand Oaks, CA: Sage.

Ofei, K. T., Holst, M., Rasmussen, H. H., & Mikkelsen, B. E. (2014). How practice contributes to trolley food waste. A qualitative study among staff involved in serving meals to hospital patients. *Appetite, 83*, 49–56. doi: 10.1016/j.appet.2014.08.001

Thomas, E. A. (2011). Diabetes at work: A grounded-theory pilot study. *Workplace Health & Safety, 59*, 213–220. doi: 10.1177/216507991105900503

Waller, J., Bower, K. M., Spence, M., & Kavanagh, K. F. (2015). Using grounded theory methodology to conceptualize the mother-infant communication dynamic: Potential application to compliance with infant feeding recommendations. *Maternal & Child Nutrition, 11*, 749–760. doi: 10.1111/mcn.12056

Weber, R. P. (1990). *Basic content analysis*. Beverly Hills, CA: Sage.

Whelan, K., & Markless, S. (2012). Factors that influence research involvement among registered dietitians working as university faculty: A qualitative interview study. *Journal of the Academy of Nutrition and Dietetics, 112*, 1021–1028. doi: 10.1016/j.jand.2012.03.002

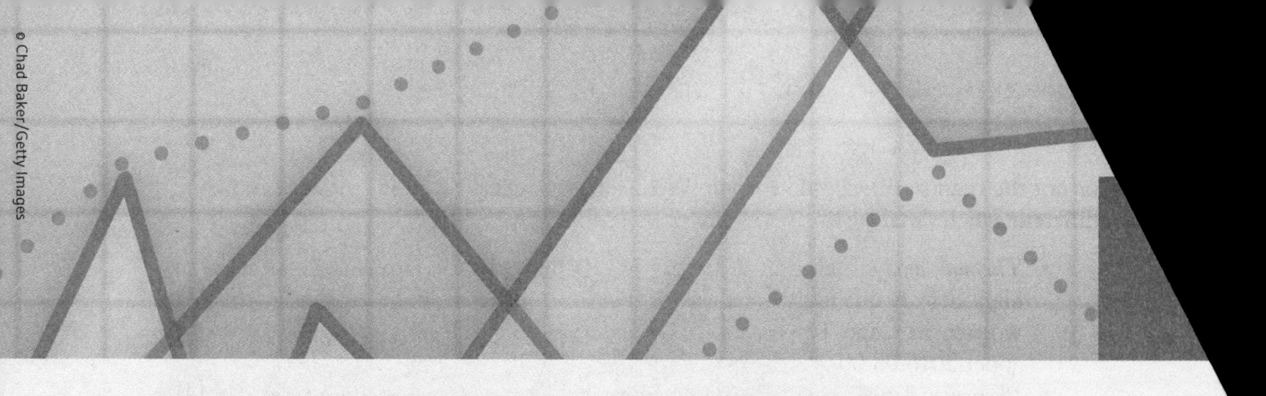

How to Evaluate Qualitative Research

NATALIE COOKE, PHD
L. SUZANNE GOODELL, PHD, RD
VIRGINIA C. STAGE, PHD, RD, LDN

CHAPTER OUTLINE

- Introduction
- Statement of the Problem
- Literature Review
- Research Design
- Subject Selection
- Data Collection
- Data Analysis
- Results
- Discussion
- Conclusions
- Trustworthiness

LEARNING OUTCOMES

- Evaluate qualitative research articles using review standards.
- Apply gained knowledge about qualitative research design to critique qualitative research articles.

INTRODUCTION

The fundamentals of qualitative research include understanding why and how qualitative research differs from quantitative research and how it can be combined with quantitative research in a mixed methods study. Different qualitative data collection methods—focus groups, individual interviews, observations, and document analysis—are available to the researcher and are chosen based on the desired outcome of the study. Four common study designs used in qualitative studies include: thematic analysis, phenomenology, grounded theory, and case studies.

This chapter focuses on evaluating and critiquing the quality of four published qualitative research studies. Think of yourself as a journal reviewer who is deciding whether

…ript should be published in your journal. You will critique four very … each employ one of these four research designs:

- …: Hunter-Adams, J., & Rother, H. A. (2016). Pregnant in a for… …tative analysis of diet and nutrition for cross-border migrant … …wn, South Africa. *Appetite, 103,* 403–410. doi: 10.1016/j. …4
- …y: Natvik, E., Gjengedal, E., Moltu, C., & Råheim, M. (2014). …odying eating: Patients' experience 5 years after bariatric surgery. *Quali… Health Research, 24,* 1700–1710. doi: 10.1177/1049732314548687
- *…rounded theory*: Lucas, C., Starling, P., McMahon, A., & Charlton, K. (2015). Erring on the side of caution: Pregnant women's perceptions of consuming fish in a risk averse society. *Journal of Human Nutrition and Dietetics, 29,* 418–426. doi: 10.1111/jhn.12353
- *Case study*: Kismul, H., Hatløy, A., Andersen, P., Mapatano, M., Van den Broeck, J., & Moland, K. M. (2015). The social context of severe child malnutrition: A qualitative household case study from a rural area of the Democratic Republic of Congo. *International Journal for Equity in Health, 14*. doi: 10.1186/s12939-015-0175-x

All of the articles, except the one on grounded theory, are open-access, so you can find them online by using the citations. Take time to read each article in full before moving on to the rest of the chapter.

As you explore each of these studies, use the Application questions in each section to evaluate the quality of the study and provide suggestions for how the researchers could have improved their research study or the reporting of their study. Recognize that some journals, but not all, provide extra space for qualitative research studies, but researchers are still limited in what they are able to present in a manuscript. Therefore, although we ask you to evaluate the strengths and limitations of each of these studies, there is a chance that the researchers actually did address that limitation in their study but did not have room to fully discuss it, due to space limitations. Each of these studies has been published in a journal, so it has made it through not only the peer review process but also "beat" many other manuscripts to "win a spot" in the journal. This is a learning exercise, and it is not meant to diminish the work of these researchers.

REVIEW CRITERIA

Some journals, such as the *Journal of Nutrition Education and Behavior*, have a checklist for researchers and reviewers that is specifically designed for qualitative studies (**Figure 11.1**). There are also checklists used across journals and disciplines, such as the Consolidated Criteria for Reporting Qualitative Research (COREQ), which is a 32-item checklist designed specifically for reporting on qualitative studies done with interviews and focus groups (**Figure 11.2**). Review each of these before moving on to the next section.

STATEMENT OF THE PROBLEM

Recall that the problem statement and objective are important because they help the reader understand the context and importance of the research study. It typically comes at the end of the literature review, after the researchers have laid a foundation of current literature. A good research objective builds on the current literature and addresses

In addition, qualitative manuscripts should also adhere to these guidelines:

Introduction
–Includes a well-articulated and defined research question and that the qualitative approach is logical

Methods
–Identifies whether and how theory informed the work (e.g. phenomenology, grounded theory, ethnography, case study, queer theory, feminist theory, narrative inquiry, participatory action research, art based inquiry, etc.) Defines which theory used.
–Describes their qualitative research approach and/or theories applied to the work (both procedural and viewpoints)
–Sampling technique(s) with justification and justification for sample size.
–If saturation was method for determining sample size, describe how saturation was determined and include group characteristics (don't just say-saturation was reached). If saturation was not reached/ used, authors need to provide explanation.
–Identifies unit of measurement versus number of participants (could be a call out for focus groups in particular)
–Describes the development of all tools/ instruments used (who was involved, what was the process of development, what informed the content, how was it pre-tested.
–If tools (e.g. interview/ moderator guides) were adapted while collecting data, discuss when, how, and why the adaptations occurred.
–Describe training (call out to article about training protocols). All interviewers were trained according to the protocols of XXX [eg, Krueger].
–Describe relationship between data collectors and participants or if data collectors are presented (states any interactions/relationship understanding that could introduce bias into answers received). If there is a relationship or potential for bias, describe.
–Describes who was involved in the process and how they were trained (training of coders)
–Describes how the code manual was developed
–Specifies use of qualitative analysis software, if any
–Specifies the extent to which independent coders agreed and how disagreements were addressed (other option- how you confirmed analysis when a single coder was involved)
–Addresses actions taken to improve trustworthiness and reduce bias throughout the methods
–Addresses what type of analysis is conducted. For example, content analysis, in a broad perspective, organizes the data into content categories. These categories represent patterns or themes that may have relationships among them or to theory used to frame the questions. Basically 3 types of content analysis may be used (Hsieh & Shannon, 2005).

Results
–Presents emergent conceptual framework (if grounded theory studies conceptual framework is presented in results)
–Provides in-depth description of main themes and subthemes

Discussion
–Discusses results in relation to theory (if theory is used)
–Specifies conclusions/generalizations or transferability and notes exceptions
–If only a convenience sample, generalizing is not appropriate nor supported by data.

FIGURE 11.1 Qualitative Reviewer Guidelines—*Journal of Nutrition Education and Behavior*

the gaps, adding a contribution to the literature in that subset of the discipline. The problem statement and objective are often intertwined, as you can see in the examples in **Table 11.1**. As a reviewer, you want to make sure that the research problem is clear, concise, and relevant and that it can be distinguished from the research objective.

Table I Consolidated criteria for reporting qualitative studies (COREQ): 32-item checklist

Numbered Items	Guide questions/description
Domain 1: Research team and reflexivity	
Personal Characteristics	
1. Interviewer/ facilitator	Which author/s conducted the interview or focus group?
2. Credentials	What were the researcher's credentials? *e.g. PhD, MD*
3. Occupation	What was their occupation at the time of the study?
4. Gender	Was the researcher male or female?
5. Experience and training	What experience or training did the researcher have?
Relationship with participants	
6. Relationship established	Was a relationship established prior to study commencement?
7. Participant knowledge of the interviewer	What did the participants know about the researcher? *e.g. personal goals, reasons for doing the research*
8. Interviewer characteristics	What characteristics were reported about the interviewer/facilitator? *e.g. Bias, assumptions, reasons and interests in the research topic*
Domain 2: Study design	
Theoretical framework	
9. Methodological orientation and Theory	What methodological orientation was stated to underpin the study? *e.g. grounded theory, discourse analysis, ethnography, phenomenology, content analysis*
Participant selection	
10. Sampling	How were participants selected? *e.g. purposive, convenience, consecutive, snowball*
11. Method of approach	How were participants approached? *e.g. face-to-face, telephone, mail, email*
12. Sample size	How many participants were in the study?
13. Non-participation	How many people refused to participate or dropped out? Reasons?
Setting	
14. Setting of data collection	Where was the data collected? *e.g. home, clinic, workplace*
15. Presence of non-participants	Was anyone else present besides the participants and researchers?
16. Description of sample	What are the important characteristics of the sample? *e.g. demographic data, date*
Data collection	
17. Interview guide	Were questions, prompts, guides provided by the authors? Was it pilot tested?
18. Repeat interviews	Were repeat interviews carried out? If yes, how many?
19. Audio/visual recording	Did the research use audio or visual recording to collect the data?
20. Field notes	Were field notes made during and/or after the interview or focus group?
21. Duration	What was the duration of the interviews or focus group?
22. Data saturation	Was data saturation discussed?
23. Transcripts returned	Were transcripts returned to participants for comment and/or correction?
Domain 3: Analysis and findings	
Data analysis	
24. Number of data coders	How many data coders coded the data?
25. Description of the coding tree	Did authors provide a description of the coding tree?
26. Derivation of themes	Were themes identified in advance or derived from the data?
27. Software	What software, if applicable, was used to manage the data?
28. Participant checking	Did participants provide feedback on the findings?
Reporting	
29. Quotations presented	Were participant quotations presented to illustrate the themes/findings? Was each quotation identified? *e.g. participant number*
30. Data and findings consistent	Was there consistency between the data presented and the findings?
31. Clarity of major themes	Were major themes clearly presented in the findings?
32. Clarity of minor themes	Is there a description of diverse cases or discussion of minor themes?

FIGURE 11.2 COREQ 32-Item Checklist

Reproduced from "Consolidated Criteria for Reporting Qualitative Research (COREQ): A 32-item Checklist for Interviews and Focus Groups," by A. Tong, P. Sainsbury, and J. Craig, 2007, *International Journal for Quality in Health Care. 19*, 352. Reprinted with permission.

APPLICATION 11.1

Using Table 11.1, evaluate each of the problem statements asking yourself these questions:

1. What is the research objective?
   - Can you distinguish between the research objective and the problem statement?
   - What, if anything, could be done to improve the research objective?
   - Which articles have research objectives intertwined with their problem statement within the last paragraph of their Introduction section?
2. Why did the researchers not include hypotheses associated with the research objective?

Table 11.1 Examples of Qualitative Problem Statements and Research Objectives

Research article	Final paragraphs of the Introduction
Hunter-Adams, J., & Rother, H. A. (2016). Pregnant in a foreign city: A qualitative analysis of diet and nutrition for cross-border migrant women in Cape Town, South Africa.	"Given the backdrop of increasing non-communicable disease and the nutrition transition, maternal nutrition may therefore be an important mechanism through which health inequalities are perpetuated. In light of the marginality of many cross-border migrant women in South Africa, we propose that exploring migrant perspectives on food during this crucial maternal period offers modest contribution to the literature pertaining to migrant health experiences in urban LMIC settings." (Hunter-Adams & Rother, 2016, p. 404)
Natvik, E., Gjengedal, E., Moltu, C., & Råheim, M. (2014). Re-embodying eating: Patients' experience 5 years after bariatric surgery.	"In a previous article, we explored essential meanings of bariatric surgery patients' lived experiences of weight loss and change for the long term. In the present article, we aim to explore meanings attached to eating after surgery. Our research questions were: How do patients experience eating and a change of eating practices in the long term after bariatric surgery? How do they describe the body in relation to eating?" (Natvik et al., 2014, p. 1701)
Lucas, C., Starling, P., McMahon, A., & Charlton, K. (2015). Erring on the side of caution: Pregnant women's perceptions of consuming fish in a risk averse society.	"The present study aimed to explore Australian women's perceptions of consuming fish and seafood during pregnancy. Barriers and motivators to consumption are explored first, in addition to perceptions and responses to fish and seafood information received during pregnancy, followed by a deeper analysis related to themes of risk aversion during pregnancy." (Lucas et al., 2015, p. 419)
Kismul, H., Hatløy, A., Andersen, P., Mapatano, M., Van den Broeck, J., & Moland, K. M. (2015). The social context of severe child malnutrition: A qualitative household case study from a rural area of the Democratic Republic of Congo.	"In small-scale agricultural communities the household is typically the unit responsible for food production and consumption. Hence, the social organisation of the household has important implications for food and nutritional security. In this paper we explore how household characteristics, access to land and inter-household cooperation affect food security and vulnerability in child malnutrition in an environment where subsistence agriculture is dominant. Using the Bwamanda area, located in a rural part of western DRC as a case, we aim to describe the social context of food production and nutrition, and explore how some households succeed to ensure that their children are well-nourished while others do not." (Kismul et al., 2015, p. 2)

LITERATURE REVIEW

The Literature Review section tells a story of what has been done previously and how it applies to a given study. Typically researchers use a "funnel" approach, starting out broad and narrowing the scope of the research to explain the significance of the research study. We illustrate the funnel approach in Natvik et al. (2014) in **Figure 11.3**.

The first sentences of a Literature Review are very broad (e.g., treatment of obesity and the fact that it is a global public health problem), and the last sentences are

APPLICATION 11.2

Read the Literature Review section of each of the four articles and answer the following questions:

1. What main points do the researchers address in the Literature Review? Using the example in Figure 11.3, fit each of the main points into a funnel to illustrate how the researchers move from broad topics to narrow focus through the Literature Review. You will have three separate funnels when you are done, one for Hunter-Adams and Rother, one for Lucas et al., and one for Kismul et al.
2. How does the Literature Review guide the reader to understand the study aims?
3. How relevant are the cited pieces of literature to the scope of the study? Consider whether the articles are current (within 5 years of when the work was published) or seminal works. (You will need to look at the references section.)
4. If the researchers are applying a preexisting theory, what definition do they provide for this theory and what justification do they use for applying the theory to their research project?

Treating obesity requires restriction and behavior change
Obesity is a global public health problem
Definition of obesity
• Most effective treatment: bariatric surgery
• Complications of bariatric surgery
• Bariatric surgery is not permanent
• Bariatric surgery is a "tool" in lifestyle change
• Behavior change might not always happen
• Bariatric surgery patients give up control to physical restriction
• Control and eating disorders
• Types of eating disorders
• Rates of eating disorders in bariatric surgery patients
• Eating disorders & poor post-surgery outcomes
• Dietary lifestyle change recommendations
• Long-term follow-up studies are limited
How do patients experience weight loss and embodied change in the long-term after bariatric surgery?

FIGURE 11.3 Example of a Literature Review Fit Into a Funnel

very specific because they focus on the specific problem being studied (e.g., long-term follow-up studies in bariatric surgery patients are limited). If the researchers are going to apply a preexisting theory to the research (e.g., behavior change theory), they will define the theory and explain its role in helping to answer the research question. As a reviewer, you want to ensure that the researchers provide adequate background information about the discipline and show multiple sides of the argument. For example, in the article on long-term follow-up with bariatric surgery patients (Natvik et al., 2014), the researchers explain the complex relationship between physical/anatomical changes to the body, emotional and behavioral implications before and after bariatric surgery, and the impact of each on the likelihood that patients will maintain weight loss through bariatric surgery. A strong Literature Review will succinctly describe the complexity of an issue, assuming that the reader knows little about the topic before reading the article.

RESEARCH DESIGN

When establishing a research design, the researchers need not only to determine the research study design type (thematic analysis, phenomenology, grounded theory, or case study) but also the technique they will use to collect the data (interviews, focus groups, observations, and document analysis). Depending on the format of the journal, this information can be included in a separate section that provides a brief summary of what was done to collect and analyze data, with further sections providing more in-depth information about specific aspects of the research design. Other times, this information is included throughout the Methods section of the article, with the information about research design and data collection methods revealed in separate sections.

None of these articles has a separate section devoted to summarizing the study; however, Natvik et al. (2014) explains the concept of phenomenology and Kismul et al. (2015) provide a geographical context before talking about the specifics of their study, making these two differ from the other two.

APPLICATION 11.3

After reading the paragraph about the research design for each study, determine the following:

1. Given the problem statement, what do you think about the appropriateness of the research study design chosen (i.e., thematic analysis, phenomenology, grounded theory, or case study)? Why did the researchers choose this design over the others?
2. Could the researchers have chosen a different research study design? If so, which one could they have chosen and why?
3. What type of data collection methods did the researchers select (i.e., interviews, focus groups, observations, or document analysis)? Is this data collection method appropriate for the study, given the problem statement?
4. Could the researchers have chosen a different data collection method? If so, which one? Which method do you think is best, given the aims of the study?

It is important to note that the Kismul et al. (2015) article is in fact a case study, even though multiple cases are presented. Recall that in a case study the case has to be "bounded" by a set of parameters. Kismul et al. bounded each case, but they had four of them. This is an established and accepted approach in qualitative research.

SUBJECT SELECTION

As you explore each of the four articles, you will notice that the headings of each Methods section are different, with three of the four having distinct sections of the methods devoted to participant selection and recruitment. Defining the participants for a study is one of the first steps to answering a research question. Researchers select a population and recruit participants who would be able to most appropriately help the researchers answer the research question. This is typically one of the first parts of the Methods section because it precedes any data collection. Recall that participants have to have something in common to be included in the study. Specific inclusion and exclusion criteria help researchers narrow the focus of their study to only the most appropriate participants.

Sometimes the number of participants and the sample size are the same number (e.g., interviews), but sometimes they are different (e.g., focus groups). Researchers will share this number, which helps the reader evaluate whether or not the sample size is appropriate to answer the research question. Recruitment techniques vary, depending on the population, and researchers may use social media with some populations and phone, mail, or word of mouth with others. A good research article discloses all of this information because it is integral to understanding the results of the study. Without knowing whose voices you are hearing, how can you truly understand what they are telling you?

APPLICATION 11.4

As you read the Methods sections of the four articles, focus on the participants and recruitment information. Fill out the following chart to help you compare and contrast methods:

	Hunter-Adams and Rother (2016)	Natvik et al. (2014)	Lucas et al. (2015)	Kismul et al. (2015)
Defining characteristic(s) of participants				
Inclusion criteria				
Exclusion criteria				
Number of participants				
Sample size				
Recruitment technique				

For sections of the chart that you did not complete because information was not provided, reflect on how sharing that information might have improved the research article.

Here are some additional questions to consider:

1. Look at the Kismul et. al article. How did the researchers define a "case"? How does the definition of a case reflect the inclusion and exclusion criteria?
2. Compare and contrast what we know about how the sample size was determined in the Natvik et al. (2014) and the Lucas et al. (2015) articles. Which article provided more details about how the final sample size was determined? What questions would you ask of the researchers to help you better understand their sample selection?
3. The sample included in the Hunter-Jones and Rother article is complex. What are some advantages to selecting this complex sample to address their research question? What are some challenges or limitations associated with this sample?

DATA COLLECTION

The Data Collection section may be named as such (see Kismul et al., 2015, and Lucas et al., 2015); carry another name, such as the data collection method (e.g., "Interviews" in Natvik et al., 2014); or be combined with other sections (e.g., Hunter-Adams & Rother, 2016). As you read the Data Collection section of a qualitative research article, you want to be able to understand exactly what steps the researchers took to collect the data, including:

- How and where the data were collected.
- Who collected the data and how they were trained.

APPLICATION 11.5

As you read the Methods section of the four articles, focus on the information about data collection. Fill out the following chart to help you compare and contrast the process of data collection:

	Hunter-Adams and Rother (2016)	Natvik et al. (2014)	Lucas et al. (2015)	Kismul et al. (2015)
Data collection method (e.g., focus groups or observations)				
How/where were data collected (e.g., by phone, in person)?				
Who collected data? What were their characteristics? How were the data collectors trained?				
How was consent obtained?				
What was included in the guide or protocol? Was it pretested?				
How did researchers decide to stop data collection, and when was saturation reached?				

For sections of the chart that you did not complete because information was not provided, reflect on how sharing that information might have improved the research article.

Here are some additional questions:

1. Kismul et al. conducted observations, along with focus groups and interviews, as part of their case study research. What was observed during the observations? What type of limitations did they put on their participant/research interactions during the observations? What additional information would you like to know about the observations?
2. In the Kismul et al. article, the researchers relied on a trained research assistant from the community to conduct interviews. In the Hunter-Adams and Rother article, researchers relied on interpreters to help facilitate data collection.
   a. What are the benefits associated with using a research assistant from the community to collect data? What are the limitations?
   b. What are the benefits associated with using an interpreter to help facilitate data collection? What are the limitations?
   c. Under what circumstances might one method be preferred over the other?
   d. Describe the characteristics of an ideal data collector. What do they know? What experience should they have? Where are they from?

- How participant consent was obtained.
- What tool was used to collect the data, and how it was developed and pretested.
- How the researchers decided to stop collecting data, and when saturation was reached.

Ask yourself if you could replicate what the researchers did, given the information described in the Data Collection sections. To save space, sometimes researchers reference another journal article where the methods are more clearly outlined or use tables or figures to show the interview/focus group questions or the observation/data analysis protocol. It is helpful when researchers include interview/focus group questions or observation/data analysis protocols because it helps future researchers in the development of their own data collection tools.

DATA ANALYSIS

Themes, theories, and models are developed through a process called coding, and data analysis differs in thematic analysis, phenomenology, and grounded theory. Case studies are a special case, and researchers use another research methodology to guide their analysis. Each of the articles you have been reviewing uses a different approach to data analysis, with some providing in-depth descriptions of what each person did, and others using more generic terms and succinct descriptions. As you read the data analysis process and consider whether or not you could replicate the study, answer these Application questions geared toward surfacing the strengths and limitations of each article.

APPLICATION 11.6

Consider the following questions as you review the four articles:

1. Looking at the terminology in the Data Analysis sections, what terms did you not understand? Look up these words to see if you can find a meaning that fits with qualitative research.
2. Practice putting what you have read into your own words. Summarize the Data Analysis section of each article. It might be helpful to read, put away the article, and then write your own summary.
   a. What was the most difficult part to put into your own words?
   b. What questions do you have about the method the researchers used to analyze data?
3. Kismul and colleagues used a case study, which is a type of research methodology. Because case studies are a special case, what type of data analysis did they use? What are the key steps they took to analyze the data?
4. Lucas and colleagues named their data analysis section Statistical Analysis, but they did conduct qualitative analysis rather than quantitative analysis.
   a. Describe what unique steps they took in analysis that demonstrate their work followed grounded theory analysis.
   b. What role did each researcher play in data analysis? Why was this important for the reader to know?
5. Using a phenomenological approach to analysis, Natvik and colleagues cite a method in which writing, reading, and rewriting are essential in the analysis process. Describe what the researchers did in each of these steps.
6. Hunter-Adams and Rother discuss the steps they took to code data and conduct thematic analysis. What details are provided? As a reviewer, what questions might you ask the researchers to further clarify their process of data analysis?

RESULTS

As you read the Results section of an article, you should ask yourself the following:

1. What were the demographics of the participants studied? Researchers might provide a summary statement of these characteristics or provide a chart describing them. For example, if the researchers conducted interviews with college students, how many were freshman? How many were seniors? What were the majors of the students? These are likely pieces of information that the researchers collected to determine inclusion/exclusion criteria but also to better tell the story of who their participants are, and why their voices are representative of the research problem.
2. What did the researchers find, and how did they present this information? There are many ways to present findings (e.g., themes, theories, or models), but is the presentation effective? It is easy to create themes from each of the major interview or focus group questions, but that is not real qualitative analysis. Telling the participants' stories should evoke creative and conclusive representations of the data.

Think about these questions as you read the Results sections of the four articles. Then, answer the Application questions.

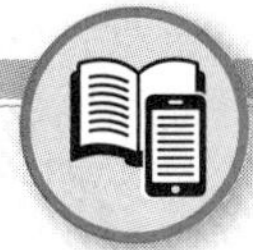

APPLICATION 11.7

In each of these articles, the researchers took a slightly different approach when presenting their results, whether through a theme, a theory, or a model.

1. How did the researchers report the demographics of the participants? Compare and contrast how this is done in each of the articles.
2. For each article, summarize the major findings. What did they discover?
3. Compare and contrast the names of the themes presented in Hunter-Adams and Rother and in Natvik et al. If you were to rename any of the themes, what names would you give them?
4. Lucas and colleagues present participant characteristics and a schematic diagram. If you were going to explain the diagram to a friend who has not read the article, what would you say?
5. In presenting their case study, Kismul and colleagues provide a description of the context and each of the cases. Describe how these findings differ from the other three articles.

DISCUSSION

As you read the Discussion section of an article, you should ask yourself the following:

1. What connections exist between what the researchers found and what others have found? Do the researchers present both sides of an argument, or just their own? The literature presented in the discussion is just as important, if not more important, than the background. Recall that researchers sought to explore this problem because there was a gap in the literature. Therefore, they should use other literature to show how their study adds to the literature.
2. What are the implications of this research in the nutrition field? Why does this matter in theory and in practice? The beauty of qualitative research is that it brings to life the voices of participants who have been previously unheard. Therefore, the themes, theories, or models often depict something that needs to happen as a result of the study. As a reader, you should understand what action should be taken after reading the article.

APPLICATION 11.8

1. Researchers must help readers understand how their work fits into the existing literature. Reread the Results section of each article. As you read, jot down the key points that stand out to you. What do you think should be included in the Discussion section?
2. Now read the Discussion section of each article. Are some things left out that you would have included? What did the researchers include that you did not think worthy of discussion? Why do you think your answers were different from theirs, if at all?

Before reading the Discussion sections again, attempt the first Application question. Then review each Discussion section with the above questions in mind and answer the other Application questions.

CONCLUSIONS

The Conclusion section of a research article is like the grand finale in a musical. It brings home the final point of the research study—namely, what the research study adds to the body of literature—and leaves the reader sure of what needs to be done next. Often, researchers use this section not only to summarize the main take-home message of the study but also to provide suggestions for future research could be conducted. Natvik et al. even include a separate section for clinical implications. The Conclusions section is often short, and it may feel like a restating of what was said earlier in the Discussion section.

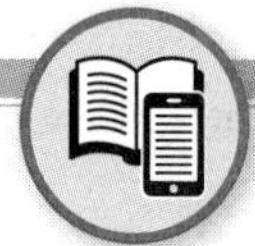

APPLICATION 11.9

After reading the conclusion of each of the four studies, determine what follow-up studies could be conducted to (1) confirm the findings, (2) compare the findings to another population, or (3) build upon the findings to conduct future research.

APPLICATION 11.10

Consider the following questions about strengths and limitations and the concept of trustworthiness:

1. For each of the articles, list the limitations and strengths. Are there more limitations or more strengths? If there are connections between the strengths and limitations, draw an arrow between them. Think about strengths and limitations that were not listed in the article, and list those in the chart as well.

Research article	Limitations	Strengths (trustworthiness)
Hunter-Adams, J., and Rother, H. A. (2016).		
Natvik, E., Gjengedal, E., Moltu, C., and Råheim, M. (2014).		
Lucas, C., Starling, P., McMahon, A., and Charlton, K. (2015).		
Kismul, H., Hatløy, A., Andersen, P., Mapatano, M., Van den Broeck, J., and Moland, K. M. (2015).		

APPLICATION 11.10 (continued)

2. Researchers must limit their descriptions of their work due to page limitations for articles in journals. Because of these restrictions, the reader is often left to wonder what the researchers did to improve the trustworthiness of their data in (1) sample selection, (2) data collection, and (3) data analysis. Review the chart you just completed.
   a. For each article, what questions did you have related to (1) sample selection, (2) data collection, and (3) data analysis. What did they leave out that you wanted to know?
   b. For each question you had, make up your own answer for how the researchers could have addressed the question. How would the trustworthiness of the data change if they had chosen to follow your method? How would the trustworthiness of the data change if the researchers did not follow your method?
   c. Explain the importance of including a detailed description of your methods for the trustworthiness of your data.

TRUSTWORTHINESS

Some qualitative researchers devote an entire section to the concept of trustworthiness; others include this information throughout the article. The limitations and methods used to improve trustworthiness are often presented together. Researchers typically use this structure: "One limitation of our study was X; however, we did Y to decrease the likelihood that this would happen and improve Z aspect of trustworthiness." Other times, the researchers list all the strengths and then all the limitations, or vice versa. Although the reader could synthesize this information through reading, explicitly stating the strengths and limitations allows the reader to consider the impact and generalizability of these findings.

SUMMARY

1. To evaluate qualitative studies, use the Qualitative Reviewer Guidelines (Figure 11.1) and the COREQ checklist (Figure 11.2).
2. A good research objective builds on the current literature and addresses the gaps, adding a contribution to the literature in that subset of the discipline. As a reviewer, you want to make sure that the research problem is clear, concise, and relevant and that it can be distinguished from the research objective.
3. A strong literature review will succinctly describe the complexity of an issue, assuming that the reader knows little about the topic before reading the article.
4. Information about research design and data collection methods may be scattered around the Methods section.
5. Sometimes the number of participants and the sample size are the same number (e.g., interviews), but sometimes they are different (e.g., focus groups). Researchers share this number, which helps the reader evaluate whether or not the sample size is appropriate to answer the research question. Researchers should also discuss recruitment techniques.
6. Data collection should include the steps taken to collect data (such as how and where data were collected), who collected the data and how they were trained, how consent was obtained, tools used to collect data, and how the researchers decided to stop collecting data.

7. As you read the Results section, ask yourself about the demographics of the participants and how the researchers presented their findings. It is easy to create themes from each of the major interview or focus group questions, but that is not real qualitative analysis. Telling the participants' stories should evoke creative and conclusive representations of the data.
8. As you read the Discussion section, look for the connections between past studies and the current study. Also consider the implications of this research in the nutrition field. The beauty of qualitative research is that it brings to life the voices of participants who have been previously unheard. The themes, theories, or models often depict something that needs to happen as a result of the study. As a reader, you should understand what action should be taken as a result of the study.
9. Researchers use the Conclusion section as a way to summarize the main take-home message of the study and to provide suggestions for future research that could be conducted.
10. Some qualitative researchers devote an entire section to the concept of trustworthiness, and others include this information throughout the article. The limitations and methods used to improve trustworthiness are often presented together. Researchers typically use this structure: "One limitation of our study was X; however, we did Y to decrease the likelihood that this would happen and improve Z aspect of trustworthiness."

REVIEW QUESTIONS

1. Match elements of research articles to the section of a research article where they would be found.

Elements of Research Articles	Sections of a Research Article
1. How results compare to other studies	A. Introduction
2. Summary statement	B. Methods
3. Subject selection	C. Results
4. Data collection	D. Discussion
5. Description of research design	E. Conclusion
6. Literature review (brief)	
7. Limitations of study	
8. Research problem	
9. Setting	
10. Recommendations for future studies	
11. Research objective	
12. How data will be analyzed	

CRITICAL THINKING QUESTIONS

1. For each of the four studies used in this chapter, why is qualitative research an appropriate approach to exploring the problem, and why did the researchers choose *not* to use quantitative research to answer their questions?

2. For each of the four studies used in this chapter, what could the researchers have done to improve the clarity of the Literature Review? What questions do you have after reading the Literature Review?
3. If multiple data collection methods were used in any of the four studies, is the study a multimethod (all qualitative) or mixed methods (qualitative and quantitative) study?
4. For each of the four studies, identify the key terms used to describe the sample or sampling technique. What are the strengths and limitations to these sampling techniques? How might the sampling affect trustworthiness of the data and the results?
5. When reviewing these four articles, data collection occurred in very different locations. Comparing and contrasting all four articles, explain why you think the researchers chose these specific methods for data collection. What might happen to the quality of the data or the ability to recruit participants if we switch data collection locations between the studies?
6. New research related to each of the four articles has likely been published since these articles were published. If you were going to publish these results today, you would need to find more up-to-date articles to include in your discussion. Choose one of the four articles, and identify one key point in the Results section. Find at least two recent (within the past 5 years) articles that would fit into a discussion on this key point. Write a new paragraph that compares and contrasts the study findings with the new articles you found.
7. Consider the concept of generalizability. For each of the four studies, to whom do the study findings apply directly? To whom might they apply (but work should be conducted to confirm the application)?

SUGGESTED READINGS AND ACTIVITIES

1. Russell, C. K., & Gregory, D. M. (2003). Evaluation of qualitative research studies. *Evidence-Based Nursing*, *6*, 36–40. doi: 10.1136/ebn.6.2.36

REFERENCES

Hunter-Adams, J., & Rother, H. A. (2016). Pregnant in a foreign city: A qualitative analysis of diet and nutrition for cross-border migrant women in Cape Town, South Africa. *Appetite*, *103*, 403–410. doi: 10.1016/j.appet.2016.05.004

Journal of Nutrition Education and Behavior. *Qualitative Reviewer Guidelines*. Retrieved from http://www.jneb.org/content/qualitative-guidelines

Kismul, H., Hatløy, A., Andersen, P., Mapatano, M., Van den Broeck, J., & Moland, K. M. (2015). The social context of severe child malnutrition: A qualitative household case study from a rural area of the Democratic Republic of Congo. *International Journal for Equity in Health*, *14*. doi: 10.1186/s12939-015-0175-x

Lucas, C., Starling, P., McMahon, A., & Charlton, K. (2015). Erring on the side of caution: Pregnant women's perceptions of consuming fish in a risk averse society. *Journal of Human Nutrition and Dietetics*, *29*, 418–426. doi: 10.1111/jhn.12353

Natvik, E., Gjengedal, E., Moltu, C., & Råheim, M. (2014). Re-embodying eating: Patients' experience 5 years after bariatric surgery. *Qualitative Health Research*, *24*, 1700–1710. doi: 10.1177/1049732314548687

Tong, A., Sainsbury, P., & Craig, J. (2007). Consolidated criteria for reporting qualitative research (COREQ): A 32-item checklist for interviews and focus groups. *International Journal for Quality in Health Care*, *19*, 349–357. doi: 10.1093/intqhc/mzm042.

PART

4

Using Research in Practice and Reporting Research

CHAPTER 12

Understanding and Using Sources of Evidence: Systematic Reviews and Evidence-Based Nutrition Practice Guidelines

CHAPTER OUTLINE

- Introduction
- Systematic Reviews
- Systematic Review Process for the Evidence Analysis Library
- Using the Evidence Analysis Library of the Academy of Nutrition and Dietetics
- Additional Sources of Systematic Reviews

LEARNING OUTCOMES

- Explain the steps taken in a systematic review, including the selection of studies, assessment of bias, and evidence synthesis results.
- Compare statistical significance with effect size, and explain how effect size is used in meta-analysis, including how to interpret a forest plot.
- Compare how systematic reviews and evidence-based nutrition practice guidelines are developed for the Evidence Analysis Library.
- Utilize the Evidence Analysis Library of the Academy of Nutrition and Dietetics to find current guidelines, recommendations, and systematic reviews.
- Use and apply other systematic review databases and resources.

INTRODUCTION

You cannot possibly keep up with the thousands of nutrition studies published every month, but thanks to **evidence analysis**, we can read excellent summaries of evidence based on evaluation of many studies and their results. This chapter helps you utilize three sources of evidence: systematic reviews, meta-analysis, and evidence-based guidelines.

Throughout your career as a nutrition professional, you will use systematic reviews and evidence-based practice guidelines in your practice with patients and the lay public. Systematic reviews are the basis for evidence-based nutrition practice guidelines, both of which can be found on the Evidence Analysis Library of the Academy of Nutrition and Dietetics. Following are key definitions from the Institute of Medicine:

> **Systematic review**: A scientific investigation that focuses on a specific question and uses explicit, planned scientific methods to identify, select, assess, and summarize the findings of similar but separate studies. It may or may not include a quantitative synthesis called a **meta-analysis**, which is a statistical technique that combines the results from separate studies. (Eden, Levit, Berg, Morton, & the Institute of Medicine, 2011, p. 21)
>
> **Clinical practice guidelines**: Statements that include recommendations intended to optimize patient care that are informed by a systematic review of evidence and an assessment of the benefits and harms of alternative care options. (Graham et al., 2011, p. 15)

Systematic reviews critically appraise and synthesize the results of primary research to answer health care–related questions such as "Does potassium intake from food sources affect blood pressure in hypertensive patients?" Systematic reviews inform and serve as the foundation for evidence-based practice guidelines. It is easy to become overwhelmed at the volume of nutrition studies being published; systematic reviews and practice guidelines help us by summarizing research and keeping us up to date in practice.

Systematic reviews normally include *quantitative* studies with similar research designs, such as randomized controlled trials. If the research studies are qualitative, researchers can do a **meta-synthesis**. A meta-synthesis involves compiling, interpreting, and integrating *qualitative* studies to possibly build a theory, explain a theory, or for some other purpose. In meta-synthesis, the researchers rigorously examine and interpret the findings of research studies using a qualitative method. **Mixed methods systematic review** is a synthesis of findings from both quantitative and qualitative studies that brings together research knowledge.

We begin with a discussion of how researchers complete systematic reviews. The systematic review process used by reviewers at the Academy of Nutrition and Dietetics (AND) Evidence Analysis Library (EAL) is also examined. Next, we address evidence-based nutrition practice guidelines and how to use the EAL to access both systematic reviews and practice guidelines to enable your participation in **evidence-based dietetics practice**. Additional sources of systematic reviews, such as the Cochrane Database of Systematic Reviews, are also discussed.

SYSTEMATIC REVIEWS

Much nutrition research is original research (also known as primary research) in which researchers define specific research objectives and try to answer questions through any number of research designs, such as a clinical trial, cohort study, or qualitative study. Systematic reviews are *not* primary research; they belong in the category of **tertiary research** because they collect and distill information from both primary and secondary sources. **Secondary research** includes **narrative reviews** in which authors evaluate, interpret, and summarize evidence from primary studies in a particular research area. Narrative review authors report inconsistencies and gaps in the literature, as well as recommend areas for further research.

Narrative reviews are different from systematic reviews in a number of ways (Cook, Mulrow, & Haynes, 1997).

- *The research question in a narrative review tends to be broad in scope; whereas in a systematic review the question is more focused.* For example, a narrative review may look at how diet affects irritable bowel syndrome (IBS) symptoms, and a systematic review may look at whether dietary fiber from whole foods and dietary supplements benefits patients with IBS.
- *Systematic reviews involve a more comprehensive literature search than narrative reviews and often including unpublished research to reduce publication bias.* **Publication bias** refers to the tendency for studies that show statistically significant findings to be published, whereas studies that do not support a hypothesis often are not published. In other words, published studies are not necessarily representative of all studies that are completed. If a study was rigorously conducted and showed no significant results, it should not be ignored. The literature selected for a systematic review is based on predetermined criteria and tends to be less biased than the literature used in a narrative review.
- *Studies used in a systematic review are more rigorously appraised than are most narrative studies.* Normally, two or more reviewers independently assess the quality of each study in a systematic review.
- *Narrative reviews include a qualitative summary, whereas systematic reviews usually include a quantitative summary of the literature.* Quantitative techniques, such as meta-analysis, are more likely than narrative reviews to identify treatment effects. Meta-analysis is a statistical technique that combines the results of a number of independent studies into a single quantitative estimate. When done correctly, a meta-analysis has greater statistical power than a single study.
- *All decisions in a systematic review, from picking to appraising studies, are more explicit and thorough than in most narrative studies.* In this way, systematic reviews are more transparent and reproducible.

To use an analogy, a narrative review is like a synopsis, whereas a systematic review is more like a synthesis. Narrative reviews have a definite place in research; they are useful when there is limited research on a topic and can provide a broad perspective on a topic. In research areas where there are many studies, systematic reviews can be useful.

Overall, a systematic review is a much more rigorous and comprehensive synthesis of research on a particular question. Because of this, it is often used to provide research evidence to promote/support an evidence-based practice. Evidenced-based practice guidelines for Registered Dietitian Nutritionists (RDNs) and nutrition professionals are based in large part on systematic reviews. First, we look at the general steps a researcher takes when conducting a systematic review.

Steps in a Systematic Review

Ten steps are used in completing a systematic review (**Table 12.1**). The review involves developing the research question to be answered, identifying all relevant literature, selecting studies for inclusion based on criteria, assessing the risk of bias in each study, synthesizing the findings in an unbiased manner, and discussing the findings. Each step is described in the left column of the table. An example from a systematic review of weight management programs is given in the right-hand column.

As you have probably noticed, a lot of time is spent on literature searching and screening in a systematic review. The PRISMA group suggests using their four-phase flow diagram (**Figure 12.1**) to show the process from identifying records to deciding

Table 12.1 Steps in a Systematic Review with an Example

Steps in a systematic review	Example of steps in a systematic review
1. *Formulate the research questions and the purpose of the review.* The research question should clearly state who the participants are, the interventions being examined, and the outcomes of interest. Systematic reviews in health care often compare an intervention or treatment with controls, standard care, or a different therapy.	*Develop Research Question* "Do behavioral weight management programs (BWMPs) involving both diet and physical activity lead to greater weight loss at 12 months (or longer) than those programs involving diet only or physical activity only?" (Johns et al., 2014, p. 1558). The purpose of the review was to identify effective ways to reduce obesity.
2. *Define inclusion and exclusion criteria for studies you will use.* These criteria should flow from the research questions. Criteria might include participant characteristics, minimum number of participants in each group, study design, sampling processes used, or how outcomes were measured. Because the research question is often about the effects of a treatment, the studies chosen are often randomized controlled trials.	*Define Criteria* • Participants: Included adults 18 years or older classified as overweight or obese using BMI (or BMI greater than or equal to 23 for Asians). Excluded pregnant women and people with a preexisting medical condition or eating disorder. • Studies: Included only randomized controlled trials; included studies of weight loss programs for general weight loss; excluded studies where weight loss was part of treatment for a medical disorder (unless losing weight was to decrease a risk factor without symptoms or to decrease medical complications of obesity when part of a mixed population). • Interventions: Included only combined BWMPs and a diet or physical activity only intervention. Included only interventions with multiple contacts and weight change documented at 12 months or more from baseline. Excluded interventions that involved any medication or surgery or that incorporated other lifestyle changes such as smoking cessation.
3. *Develop a search strategy,* including selecting relevant electronic databases and keywords to be used, as well as other strategies such as checking article reference lists, hand searching key journals, and communicating with key researchers in the research area for additional studies, some of which may not have been published. Often non-English studies and the gray literature (materials not formally published such as dissertations, technical reports, working papers, etc.) are included. A medical or other specialized librarian may be useful to help perform a comprehensive search. Identifying all studies that meet the eligibility criteria increases the external validity of the review and decreases bias.	*Develop Search Strategy* • Nine databases were chosen (such as BIOSIS and the Cochrane Database of Systematic Reviews) using these search terms (or combinations): diet, physical activity, weight loss interventions, and obese and overweight adults. • The search included studies from May 2009 to November 2012 and in any language. • References at the end of pertinent systematic reviews were checked for additional studies. • Experts were also asked for additional studies.
4. *Conduct the search of the literature using your search strategy.* Identify all possible studies (called "records" at this point). It is not unusual to have several thousand. Check the records and remove any duplicates.	*Search Literature* The search identified 2,068 records. Other sources identified 244 records. After duplicates were removed, 2,210 records remained. Thirteen studies from another systematic review were added to total 2,223 records.

Table 12.1 Steps in a Systematic Review with an Example (continued)

Steps in a systematic review	Example of steps in a systematic review
5. *Screen the records.* Using the inclusion criteria, each study gathered from the search is assessed for eligibility, usually using study titles and abstracts. This is often done independently by two reviewers and assessed to ensure that they use the criteria consistently and without bias. A log is kept of excluded studies and why studies were excluded.	*Screen Records* One reviewer screened all the records using study titles and abstracts, and a sample of them were checked by a second reviewer for consistency. Out of 2,223 records screened using the criteria, 2,016 were excluded.
6. *Assess the full text of the selected studies from the previous step for eligibility using reviewers.* The reviewers abstract key information from each study (such as sample size, whether participants were randomized to treatments, and attrition rate). Using at least two reviewers allows for assessment of inter-rater agreement. When any full-text studies are excluded at this point, the reviewers must document the rationale.	*Abstract Key Information and Check Eligibility* Of the remaining studies (207), two reviewers went through full-text articles separately and extracted key information. If they had differences, they were resolved by discussion or by bringing in a third reviewer. After assessing 207 full-text articles, 199 were excluded because the study design was not a randomized controlled trial, the study did not gather body weight at or beyond 12 months from baseline, or for other reasons.
7. *Critically assess the risk of bias in the included studies* to help determine the strength of the evidence based on the quality of the studies.	*Assess Risk of Bias* All 8 studies used in the systematic review were examined for risk of bias in four areas: randomization sequence generation, concealment of allocation, selective reporting, and attrition (described in next section). A study could be rated as high risk of bias, low risk of bias, or unclear (insufficient information) in each area.
8. *Put together the studies' findings to yield a result;* this is called **evidence synthesis**. Often a meta-analysis is used to synthesize the findings from studies, but it is not always appropriate. Results of studies with different designs or dissimilar population groups should not be pooled in a meta-analysis. A *descriptive synthesis* (exploring patterns and relationships within and between studies, identifying themes, assessing strength of the evidence) may be best when there are a limited number of studies or the primary studies are too diverse. Whether or not a meta-analysis is done, the key features and outcomes of each study are summarized in a table.	*Evidence Synthesis* Six of the studies compared BWMPs using diet and physical activity with diet only programs. The meta-analysis showed a significantly greater weight loss in the combined BWMPs at 12 months (but not at 3 to 6 months) than the diet only programs. Five studies compared BWMPs using diet and physical activity to physical activity only studies. Results showed a significantly greater weight loss in combined BWMPs at both 3 to 6 months and 12 to 18 months when compared to the physical activity only programs.
9. *Summarize and discuss the findings from the synthesis.* This includes discussing issues such as the strength of the evidence, the quality and range of studies, and applicability of the findings. Limitations of the review are discussed along with recommendations for further research and practice.	*Summarize/Discuss* Combined BWMPs involving both diet and physical activity lead to greater weight loss at 12 months (or longer) than those programs involving diet only or physical activity only. Weight loss in combined BWMPs when compared to diet only programs were similar in the short term.
10. *Finish the final report for publication.* Systematic reviews are written using a format similar to that used for primary research studies: introduction, methods, results, and discussion.	*Publish* The study was published in the *Journal of the Academy of Nutrition and Dietetics* in October 2014. It includes an introduction, methods, results, discussion, and conclusion.

From "Diet or Exercise Interventions vs Combined Behavioral Weight Management Programs: A Systematic Review and Meta-Analysis of Direct Comparisons" by Johns, Hartmann-Boyce, Jeff, & Aveyard, 2014.

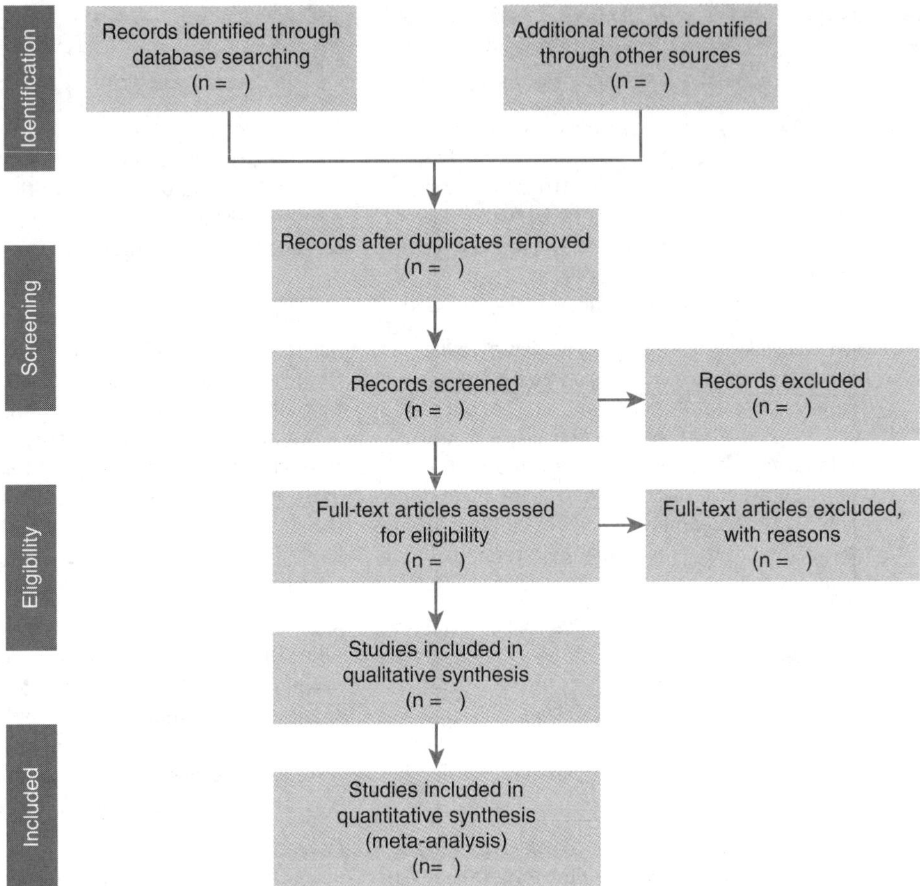

FIGURE 12.1 PRISMA 2009 Flow Diagram. Flow of information through the different phases of a systematic review.

Reproduced from "Preferred reporting items for systematic reviews and meta-analyses: The PRISMA Statement," by D. Moher, A. Liberati, J. Tetzlaff, D. G. Altman, & The PRISMA Group, 2009, *PLoS Medicine*, *6*, p. e1000097. Copyright 2009 by Moher et al. Reprinted with permission.

which studies will be used in the review. The PRISMA group is an international group of clinicians and researchers who have worked to improve the quality of reporting for systematic reviews.

You can find more information at the PRISMA group website (http://www.prisma-statement.org) as well as the articles by Moher, Liberati, Tetzlaff, Altman, and the PRISMA Group (2009) and Liberati et al. (2009). See Appendix E for a systematic review checklist developed by the PRISMA group.

Just because an article is a systematic review does not guarantee that it was conducted with appropriate rigor. You still need to evaluate the article. **Table 12.2** provides guidelines for assessing the quality of a systematic review.

ASSESSING RISK OF BIAS

A necessary step in a systematic review is to examine each of the included studies for bias. **Bias** is anything that influences a study in such a way that it distorts the findings. Bias is not a random error that shows up haphazardly; it is a systematic error. In other words, if

Table 12.2 Questions for Critiquing a Systematic Review

Table 12.2 Questions for Critiquing a Systematic Review
Research Problem and Question • Is the research problem described adequately and of significance? • Is the research question clearly expressed with variables adequately defined?
Literature Search • Were the criteria for selecting primary studies appropriate? • Did the search include appropriate databases with keywords that targeted relevant primary studies? • Did the search include additional methods to identify relevant studies, including unpublished studies and gray literature? • Was the search conducted by two people and inter-rater agreement reported? • Did reviewers try to contact authors of primary studies when additional key information was needed? • Once full-text articles were reviewed, was relevant and adequate information extracted by two or more reviewers? • Was the selection process for studies illustrated using the PRISMA flow diagram?
Risk of Bias Assessment • Were the studies assessed for risk of bias? • Was a reputable tool used to assess risk of bias? • Was the likelihood of publication bias assessed?
Evidence Synthesis • Was the decision on doing a meta-analysis or a narrative synthesis appropriate and justified? • Did the researchers explain how they pooled and integrated the study data in a meta-analysis? • Were appropriate methods used to combine the study findings? • Did the researchers assess the heterogeneity of effects? • Did the researchers explain why they chose either the random effects or fixed effects model? Was the decision appropriate? • Do tables and figures do a good job of illustrating the findings? • Were key elements of each study presented in a table? • If a narrative synthesis was performed, were relationships explored? How complete and applicable was the evidence? • Were there any potential biases in the evidence synthesis?
Discussion and Conclusions • Was the discussion section comprehensive and clear? • Were limitations noted? • Were the conclusions reasonable? • Were there recommendations for further research and practice? • Are conflicts of interest declared?

you replicate a biased study, you would continue to get the wrong answer. A study may show bias in, for example, how participants are selected (selection bias), how dropouts are handled (attrition bias), how a variable is measured (measurement bias), or how a researcher's beliefs influenced the research question or design (researcher bias).

Cochrane is a global network of researchers and others who work independently and do not accept commercial funding or any funding that creates conflicts of interest. Their mission is to provide quality information to help those involved in health make informed decisions. A number of researchers use a Cochrane Collaboration tool to assess risk of bias that includes these six domains as well as a miscellaneous domain (other sources of bias) (Higgins et al., 2011).

1. *Random sequence generation (selection bias)*. The method of assigning participants to groups should be fully described to determine if it produced comparable groups. To randomly put participants in groups first involves generating an unpredictable

random sequence. Keep in mind that for many clinical trials participants are entered into the trial over a period of time. As patients come in and are judged eligible for the study, they are assigned to a group using the random sequence.

2. *Allocation concealment (also a type of selection bias).* Random allocation concealment involves implementing the random sequence in a way that conceals group placement from anyone who enters participants in a study. If people who enter participants know, or can detect, the upcoming allocations (such as the next participant will go into the experimental group), they may channel participants to certain groups. For example, a researcher may want a participant with a better prognosis to be put into the experimental group. This type of practice may bias the estimate of the treatment effect by 30 to 40% (Moher et al., 1998; Schulz, Chalmers, Hayes & Altman, 1995).
3. *Blinding of participants and personnel (performance bias).* This looks at the measures used to blind participants and study personnel from knowing which intervention a participant received.
4. *Blinding of outcome assessment (detection bias).* If the people responsible for assessing patient outcomes know which intervention a participant received, they could bias how the outcome was measured. Blinding of outcome assessment means that the people assessing patients do not know which intervention patients received.
5. *Incomplete outcome data (attrition bias).* This domain looks at how attrition and exclusions were handled by the researchers and whether missing data (due to dropouts, etc.) could have affected the results.
6. *Selective outcome reporting (reporting bias).* A study's original protocol spells out the outcomes that will be reported and how they will be reported. Bias *may* occur if, for instance, an outcome from the protocol is not reported at all or is reported incompletely, or if the outcome is measured differently than originally stated.

A complete description of this tool, as well as criteria for grading a study on these domains, is available at www.cochrane.org.

In the study by Johns, Hartmann-Boyce, Jeff, and Aveyard (2014) described in Table 12.1, the risk of bias was assessed in four areas: random sequence generation, allocation concealment, attrition, and selective reporting. **Table 12.3** shows the results. Assessing risk of bias in the selected studies is important because it increases rigor and transparency in the systematic review process.

META-ANALYSIS AND EFFECT SIZE

Meta-analysis is a statistical technique used to *combine* the results of a number of studies, *so you can see the size of an effect of an intervention or treatment from multiple studies on a clinical outcome*, such as weight loss. Before we go into how to read and interpret the results of a meta-analysis, let's review the concept of effect size b*ecause effect size is at the heart of meta-analysis.*

Effect size is the magnitude (or size) of an effect. It could be the size of the difference in an outcome measure (such as weight loss) between the experimental and control groups in an experimental study. It could also be the strength of the relationship between two variables, as seen, for example, in correlation.

When you want to examine the size of the difference in means between two groups in a study, all you have to do is subtract the means. For example, if the intervention group in a weight loss study lost 8 pounds (−8) and the control group lost 2 pounds (−2), the difference (or effect size) is −6 pounds. This difference is called the **mean difference** and is an example of an effect size. The effect size tells you about how powerful the effect

Table 12.3 Risk of bias judgments for studies included in a systematic review and meta-analysis of direct comparisons between diet and physical activity combined behavioral weight management programs (BWMPs) and diet or physical activity only BWMPs

Study	Random sequence generation	Allocation concealment	Attrition	Selective reporting	Notes
Wadden (1988)	Unclear	Unclear	Low	Low	
Skender (1996)	Low	Unclear	Low	Low	
Wadden (1997)	Unclear	Unclear	Low	Low	
Vissers (2010)	Unclear	Unclear	High	Low	The difference in follow-up between the BWMP and the diet-only program exceeds 20%.
Rejeski (2011)	Unclear	Unclear	Low	High	Authors measured but did not report weight at 12 months.
Villareal (2011)	Low	Unclear	Low	Low	
Bertz (2012)	Low	Unclear	Low	Low	
Foster-Schubert (2012)	Low	Low	Low	Low	

"Low" indicates low risk of bias in that domain, "unclear" indicates insufficient information with which to judge, and "high" indicates high risk of bias in that domain.

Reproduced from "Diet or Exercise Interventions vs Combined Behavioral Weight Management Programs: A Systematic Review and Meta-Analysis of Direct Comparison," by D. Johns, J. Hartmann-Boyce, S. Jebb, & P. Aveyard for the Behavioural Weight Management Review Group, 2014, *Journal of the Academy of Nutrition and Dietetics, 114*, p. 1565.

of the independent variable is on an outcome variable, as well as the direction of the relationship. In the weight loss study, the larger the mean difference is, the larger is the effect of the intervention.

Correlation looks at the association (or relationship) between two continuous variables and is another example of an effect size. The correlation coefficient r measures both the strength and direction of a linear relationship between two variables, from no relationship (0) to a perfect positive or negative linear relationship (+1 or −1). For example, as the body mass index (BMI) increases, so does systolic blood pressure—that is a positive relationship. Effect size estimates, such as an r of 0.5 for the effect of BMI on systolic blood pressure, tell you about both the strength and the direction of the effect.

Effect sizes are used to compare and summarize the results of different studies in a meta-analysis. We use mean difference and standardized mean difference when comparing studies with continuous outcomes (meaning interval or ratio data such as BMI).

1. *Mean difference (MD)*. This is used when all studies in the meta-analysis measure the outcome on the *same* scale (such as pounds in a weight loss study or blood pressure in a hypertension study). The mean difference shows the absolute difference between two groups. It estimates how much the intervention changed the outcome on average compared with the control group. For example, if the intervention group in a blood pressure study had mean postintervention systolic blood pressure of 135 and the control group's mean was 140, the effect would be −5.0 (experimental mean minus control mean).

2. *Standardized mean difference (SMD)*. This is used when different scales are used to measure the same outcome in the studies. **Standardized mean difference** standardizes the results of the studies to a uniform scale so you can compare studies. The standardized mean difference, often reported as Cohen's *d* or simply *d* in statistics, is generally calculated by taking the difference in mean outcome between the two groups (experimental minus control) and dividing it by the pooled standard deviation (a correction factor may be used). *What you end up with is a number that shows how far apart the means are in standard deviation units.* So if the SMD of the experimental group is 0.8, then the score of the average person in the experimental group is 0.8 standard deviations above the average person in the control group. As the SMD increases, the difference between the intervention and control groups increases. Interpretation of *d* varies by context. If the result is about 0.5, the effect size may be considered moderate, and 0.8 may be large (although this varies depending on the context and other factors). Both MD and SMD are examples of how effect size can be measured.

To compare and summarize the results in a meta-analysis when the outcome is dichotomous (such as having diabetes or not having diabetes), researchers often use *risk ratios* (for example, in cohort studies and sometimes in randomized controlled trials) or *odds ratios* (for example, in a study using logistic regression). *Both risk ratios and odds ratios measure effect size.*

A **risk ratio**, also called **relative risk** (RR), compares the probability of an outcome (usually a disease) in two groups. One group is exposed to something, such as a risk factor, and the other group is not exposed to it. Relative risk expresses how much more (or less) likely it is for an exposed person to develop an outcome (relative to an unexposed person). *Exposure* is often a risk factor for a disease, but it could also be a treatment. Relative risk is calculated as follows:

$$\text{Relative Risk} = \frac{\text{Risk of outcome in exposed/treated group}}{\text{Risk of outcome in unexposed group}}$$

If a study's results show an RR of 1.0, that means there is no difference in risk between the groups and the exposure did not increase or decrease risks of the outcome. If the RR is greater than 1, it suggests an *increased* risk of that outcome (such as developing hypertension) in the exposed group (perhaps they were exposed to a high-sodium diet). If the RR is less than 1, it suggests a *reduced* risk in the exposed group.

For example, in a study about heart disease (the outcome) in men with and without diabetes, diabetes is the exposure or risk factor. In this study, the RR for coronary heart disease was 3.0 for men. When risk is increased, as in RR = 3.0, you can interpret that in two ways.

1. Relative risk: The men with diabetes (exposed group) have 3 times the risk of coronary heart disease compared to men without diabetes.
2. Increased risk: Men with diabetes *increase* their risk of coronary heart disease by 200% compared to men without diabetes. Increased risk is calculated as (Relative Risk − 1) × 100.

Now let's look at an example where RR is less than 1. Let's say a group of pregnant women were given vitamin and amino acid supplements (the exposure) and observed to see who developed preeclampsia (the outcome). Another group of pregnant women did not receive the supplements. Relative risk is sometimes used in randomized clinical trials in which there is an intervention or treatment. The RR for this study was 0.25. This means:

1. Relative risk: Pregnant women taking the supplements had 0.25 (or one-quarter) times the risk of preeclampsia compared to women not taking the supplements.
2. Decreased risk: The pregnant women taking the supplements had 75% *less risk* of developing preeclampsia than pregnant women not taking the supplements. Decreased risk is calculated the same as just shown: (Relative Risk − 1) × 100.

As you can see, relative risk works well as an effect size because it gives both direction and magnitude of the effect.

Whereas relative risk tells you about probability, the **odds ratio** (OR) tells you about the odds of an outcome. Odds and probability are not the same thing; they both express the likelihood of an outcome, but in slightly different ways. Odds ratios are generated in studies using logistic regression, a technique often used to study how risk factors are associated with or predict an outcome. (Odds ratios are also used in case-control studies where they are defined a little differently).

An OR of 1.0 means that the odds of an outcome in each group are the same. If the OR is greater than 1, then exposure (such as high alcohol intake) is positively related to an outcome (such as esophageal cancer) and could be a *causal factor*. If the OR is less than 1, exposure is negatively related to disease, meaning the exposure is *protective*.

Although odds ratios are somewhat different from relative risk ratios, *an OR is often interpreted the same way as an RR*. So an OR of 3.55 would be interpreted as meaning the outcome was 3.55 times more likely to occur in the exposed group than the unexposed group, or risk of the outcome in the exposed group was increased by 255% compared to the unexposed group.

When you read a study using odds ratios, you may see a reference to a crude odds ratio and an adjusted odds ratio. Unlike the crude odds ratio, which does not take any other factors into account, the adjusted odds ratio controls for confounding variables.

In meta-analysis, researchers combine the different effect size estimates from each study to give an overall best estimate of the size of the effect. The effect size is often one of the following: mean difference or standardized mean difference for continuous data, and risk ratio or odds ratio for binary data.

TIP

Of the four effect sizes used in meta-analysis, remember that only mean difference uses the raw data. Mean difference is used when all studies in the meta-analysis use the same measurement scale (such as pounds). Standardized mean difference, risk ratio, and odds ratios are all indexes of effect size. A larger value indicates a stronger effect.

How effect size may be measured in a meta-analysis with a continuous outcome	How effect size may be measured in a meta-analysis with a binary outcome
Mean difference	Risk ratio (Cohort studies)
Standardized mean difference	Odds ratio (Case control studies)

Of course every meta-analysis includes a number of studies, and the sample size of each study can vary from small to large. The effect size for studies with a larger number of participants is assumed to be a more precise estimate of the population effect than an effect size based on a smaller number of participants. In other words, larger studies should carry more weight. The method typically used in meta-analysis to weight studies is called inverse-variance weighting, which uses the standard error to calculate a weight for each study.

Another concern researchers have to address relates to the **heterogeneity** of the findings of the studies. Heterogeneity in a meta-analysis refers to the variation in the direction and magnitude of the effect size for the studies. Ideally, the results of the different studies should be similar. Researchers often do a statistical test, such as I^2, to estimate the level of heterogeneity. I^2 describes the percentage of variation across studies that is *not* due to chance. An I^2 of 50 to 90% may represent substantial heterogeneity. If results for the studies are very heterogeneous, a meta-analysis is not likely to be appropriate.

When heterogeneity is low, a fixed effects model can be used. In a fixed effects model, it is assumed that the studies have been conducted under similar conditions with similar participants. When studies are more varied, researchers often use a random effects model, which adjusts for the variability between the studies. Many researchers consider the random effects approach a more appropriate choice than fixed effects.

Interpreting Forest Plots

Reading the results of a meta-analysis can be fun because the studies and the summary estimate are often displayed using a **forest plot**, which is an interesting graphic that is easy to read. Let's take a look at each section of the forest plot in **Figure 12.2** so you can learn to read them in studies on your own.

1. Notice how each study is listed on the left-hand side along with important information. This forest plot is from the weight control study described in Table 12.1. The first author and year of study are noted to the left for each study. Then you have three columns for each group: "Mean" for mean weight loss, "SD" for standard deviation, and "Total" for the number of participants. The groups are labeled "Combined" for behavioral weight management programs (BWMPs) involving both diet and physical activity, and "Diet-only" for the programs that only included diet.

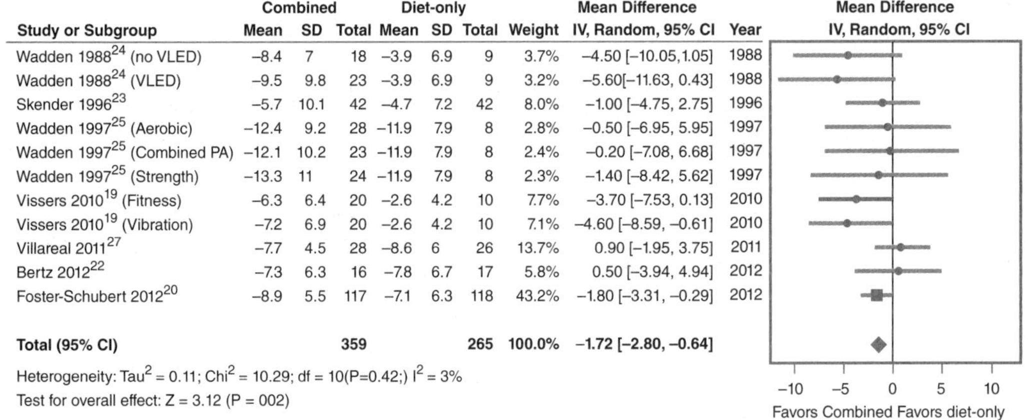

	Combined			Diet-only				Mean Difference	
Study or Subgroup	**Mean**	**SD**	**Total**	**Mean**	**SD**	**Total**	**Weight**	**IV, Random, 95% CI**	**Year**
Wadden 1988[24] (no VLED)	−8.4	7	18	−3.9	6.9	9	3.7%	−4.50 [−10.05, 1.05]	1988
Wadden 1988[24] (VLED)	−9.5	9.8	23	−3.9	6.9	9	3.2%	−5.60[−11.63, 0.43]	1988
Skender 1996[23]	−5.7	10.1	42	−4.7	7.2	42	8.0%	−1.00 [−4.75, 2.75]	1996
Wadden 1997[25] (Aerobic)	−12.4	9.2	28	−11.9	7.9	8	2.8%	−0.50 [−6.95, 5.95]	1997
Wadden 1997[25] (Combined PA)	−12.1	10.2	23	−11.9	7.9	8	2.4%	−0.20 [−7.08, 6.68]	1997
Wadden 1997[25] (Strength)	−13.3	11	24	−11.9	7.9	8	2.3%	−1.40 [−8.42, 5.62]	1997
Vissers 2010[19] (Fitness)	−6.3	6.4	20	−2.6	4.2	10	7.7%	−3.70 [−7.53, 0.13]	2010
Vissers 2010[19] (Vibration)	−7.2	6.9	20	−2.6	4.2	10	7.1%	−4.60 [−8.59, −0.61]	2010
Villareal 2011[27]	−7.7	4.5	28	−8.6	6	26	13.7%	0.90 [−1.95, 3.75]	2011
Bertz 2012[22]	−7.3	6.3	16	−7.8	6.7	17	5.8%	0.50 [−3.94, 4.94]	2012
Foster-Schubert 2012[20]	−8.9	5.5	117	−7.1	6.3	118	43.2%	−1.80 [−3.31, −0.29]	2012
Total (95% CI)			**359**			**265**	**100.0%**	**−1.72 [−2.80, −0.64]**	

Heterogeneity: $Tau^2 = 0.11$; $Chi^2 = 10.29$; df = 10(P=0.42;) $I^2 = 3\%$
Test for overall effect: Z = 3.12 (P = 002)

FIGURE 12.2 Mean difference in weight loss between behavioral weight management programs, involving both diet and physical activity and programs involving diet only at 12 months. (SD = standard deviation; IV = inverse variance; VLED = very-low-energy diet)

2. Continuing to the right are two more important columns. "Weight" tells you exactly how much weight was given to each study in the meta-analysis. That column adds up to 100%. You will notice that the largest study (by Foster-Schubert) was given the largest weight (43.2%).
3. Next is the column labeled "Mean Difference, IV, Random, 95% CI." "IV" refers to the fact that the researchers used inverse-variance weighting to weight the studies. "Random" shows that the researchers used a random effects model.
4. Now let's look at the mean difference and 95% CI. This meta-analysis uses mean difference instead of standardized mean difference because all the studies used the same measurement: pounds. You can calculate the mean difference for each study easily by subtracting the mean under "Combined" from the mean under "Diet-Only." For example, in the first study, just subtract −8.4 from −3.9 and you will get −4.5, which is listed under "Mean Difference."

   The numbers in brackets after −4.5 are the 95% confidence interval (CI) for that study: −10.05 to 1.05. The CI is a range of values within which we expect to find where the true effect lies. A wider CI means there is less certainty about the true effect size. Larger studies tend to provide more precise estimates of where the effect is, so the CI is narrower for large studies than for small studies.
5. At the bottom line of the column "Mean Difference, IV, Random, 95% CI" is the mean difference when all studies are combined in the meta-analysis (−1.72). This may be called a pooled intervention effect, pooled effect estimate, or simply a summary estimate. The standard error of the summary estimate is used to derive a confidence interval (−2.80, −0.64) and also a *P*-value. The CI of the summary estimate tells us something about the certainty, or uncertainty, of the summary estimate; a smaller interval is more precise. The *P*-value is listed at the bottom on the left; it is 0.002.
6. Now let's look at the graphic on the right. The vertical line in the graph represents the point when there is no intervention effect; in other words, it represents the null hypothesis and may be called the line of no effect. In the weight loss study, the point of no effect is labeled as "0." In the case of a risk ratio or odds ratio, the vertical line will be set at "1" because that is when the risk, or odds, are the same for both groups (see Figure 12.4). The direction of the effect is shown below the plot. For example in Figure 12.2, "Favors Combined" is on one side and "Favors Diet only" on the other side. The horizontal axis in this example is in pounds; negative pounds are pounds lost, and positive pounds are pounds gained by participants.
7. Next to each study is a horizontal line and a box that represents that study. The square on each horizontal line represents the location of the effect size for each study, and the size of the square reflects the weight of the study. Smaller squares are used for studies with smaller sample sizes. The horizontal line extends on either side of the block to depict the 95% confidence interval. So if you look at the first Wadden study, the box is at about −4.50 (the effect size), and the line extends from −10.05 to 1.05 (the CI). If the CI of a study does *not* pass through the line of no effect, the results were individually statistically significant.
8. The big diamond at the bottom represents the summary estimate. The big diamond stretches from left to right along its CI. The diamond will be spread out and thin if there is not much certainty, and squat or big when the CI is smaller and the data are stronger. If the diamond crosses over the vertical line of no effect, the difference between the groups is *not* statistically significant.
9. The next forest plot (**Figure 12.3**) uses standardized mean difference, so the horizontal axis is in standard deviations.

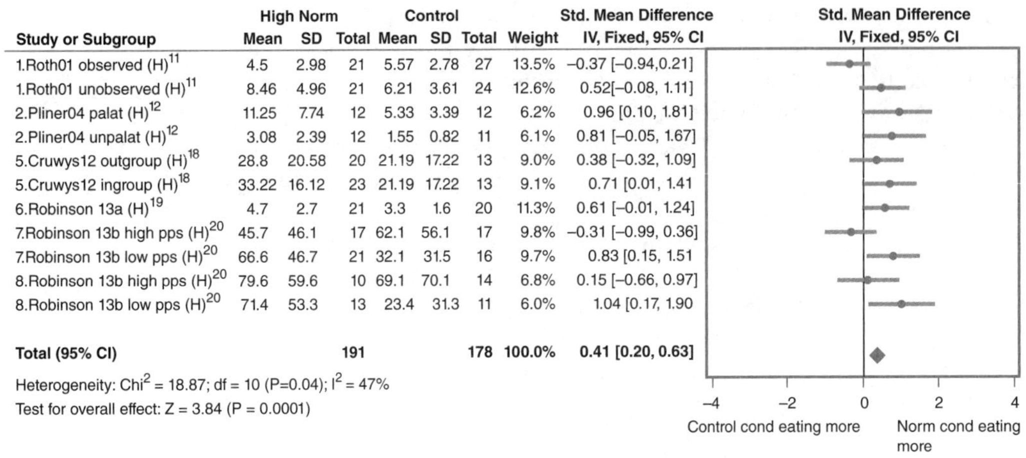

Study or Subgroup	High Norm Mean	High Norm SD	High Norm Total	Control Mean	Control SD	Control Total	Weight	Std. Mean Difference IV, Fixed, 95% CI
1.Roth01 observed (H)[11]	4.5	2.98	21	5.57	2.78	27	13.5%	−0.37 [−0.94,0.21]
1.Roth01 unobserved (H)[11]	8.46	4.96	21	6.21	3.61	24	12.6%	0.52[−0.08, 1.11]
2.Pliner04 palat (H)[12]	11.25	7.74	12	5.33	3.39	12	6.2%	0.96 [0.10, 1.81]
2.Pliner04 unpalat (H)[12]	3.08	2.39	12	1.55	0.82	11	6.1%	0.81 [−0.05, 1.67]
5.Cruwys12 outgroup (H)[18]	28.8	20.58	20	21.19	17.22	13	9.0%	0.38 [−0.32, 1.09]
5.Cruwys12 ingroup (H)[18]	33.22	16.12	23	21.19	17.22	13	9.1%	0.71 [0.01, 1.41
6.Robinson 13a (H)[19]	4.7	2.7	21	3.3	1.6	20	11.3%	0.61 [−0.01, 1.24]
7.Robinson 13b high pps (H)[20]	45.7	46.1	17	62.1	56.1	17	9.8%	−0.31 [−0.99, 0.36]
7.Robinson 13b low pps (H)[20]	66.6	46.7	21	32.1	31.5	16	9.7%	0.83 [0.15, 1.51
8.Robinson 13b high pps (H)[20]	79.6	59.6	10	69.1	70.1	14	6.8%	0.15 [−0.66, 0.97]
8.Robinson 13b low pps (H)[20]	71.4	53.3	13	23.4	31.3	11	6.0%	1.04 [0.17, 1.90
Total (95% CI)			**191**			**178**	**100.0%**	**0.41 [0.20, 0.63]**

Heterogeneity: $Chi^2 = 18.87$; df = 10 (P=0.04); $I^2 = 47\%$
Test for overall effect: Z = 3.84 (P = 0.0001)

FIGURE 12.3 Forest plot for high intake norm studies. Total refers to sample size. (SD = standard deviation; IV = independent variable)

Reproduced from "What Everyone Else Is Eating: A Systematic Review and Meta-Analysis of the Effect of Informational Eating Norms on Eating Behavior," by E. Robinson, J. Thomas, P. Aveyard, & S. Higgs, 2014, *Journal of the Academy of Nutrition and Dietetics*, *114*, p. 426. Copyright 2014 by the Academy of Nutrition and Dietetics. Reprinted with permission.

10. The final forest plot (**Figure 12.4**) uses risk ratio, so the vertical line is set at 1. This study looked at the highest diet quality versus the lowest diet quality for Parkinson's disease. Only one of the three studies was clearly under 1, and the summary statistic covers the line of no effect, so the meta-analysis did not show significance or a strong effect size (only 0.90).

APPLICATION 12.1

Using the Johns, Hartmann-Boyce, Jeff, and Aveyard (2014) study noted in Table 12.1, answer the following questions.

A. Use Figure 12.1 (the diagram showing the flow from the initial database search until the final selection of studies for the synthesis) to diagram the flow of studies in this study.
B. Using Figure 12.2, interpret the summary estimate (diamond). What is the average effect size? Does the effect size favor the combined programs or the diet-only programs for weight loss at 12 months? What does it mean that the diamond does not touch the X axis?
C. Using Figure 12.2, was heterogeneity high in this group of studies?

SYSTEMATIC REVIEW PROCESS FOR THE EVIDENCE ANALYSIS LIBRARY

The Academy's systematic reviews are the basis for evidence-based practice guidelines so practitioners make appropriate nutrition care decisions for patients. These guidelines serve as a foundation for RDNs and nutrition professionals when providing nutrition care and communicating nutrition recommendations. They also have a direct impact on third party payer reimbursement for medical nutrition therapy and public policy in dietetics practice. Utilizing professional resources such as the Evidence Analysis Library

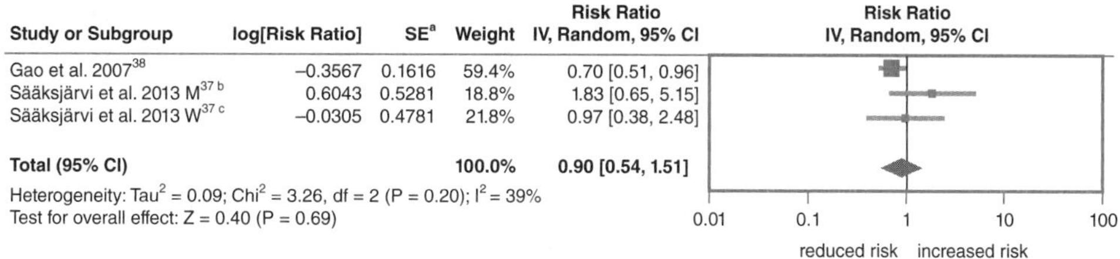

FIGURE 12.4 Forest plot showing pooled relative risks (RRs) with 95% CI for the highest diet quality (Healthy Eating Index, Alternate Healthy Eating Index, and Dietary Approaches to Stop Hypertension) vs lowest diet quality category for Parkinson's disease. (SE = standard error; I^2 = inconsistency)

Reproduced from "Diet Quality as Assessed by the Healthy Eating Index, the Alternate Healthy Eating Index, the Dietary Approaches to Stop Hypertension Score, and Health Outcomes: A Systematic Review and Meta-Analysis of Cohort Studies," by L. Schwingshackl & G. Hoffman, 2015, *Journal of the Academy of Nutrition and Dietetics, 115*, p. 797. Copyright 2015 by the Academy of Nutrition and Dietetics. Reprinted with permission.

(EAL), created by Academy members, helps us provide care that is based on evidence and free from bias.

The Evidence-Based Practice Committee oversees the EAL and the systematic review process. The committee is responsible for identifying topics, prioritizing research needs, appointing work group teams on each topic, approving new evidence-based guidelines, and overseeing policies and procedures.

The work group teams are comprised of a staff project manager, lead analyst, workgroup chair, six to eight expert work group members, and 4 to 10 evidence analysts (Handu et al., 2016). Work group members are subject matter experts in their assigned topic and must meet the following criteria to be part of an EAL work group team:

- Minimum of 5 years experience in practice and/or research.
- At least 3 years of work experience related to the topic.
- Advanced degree in the topic area or 8 years of experience.
- Willingness to volunteer their time with no compensation for their contribution to the work group project.
- Willingness to disclose potential conflicts of interest.
- Attend an Academy orientation on the systematic review process.

Each review follows a rigorous process to ensure transparency and minimize bias. In the process of creating the EAL, the Academy established guidelines for conducting systematic reviews, which generally take about 12 to 18 months to complete. The systematic review process includes the following five steps (Handu et al., 2016). Note that the steps used by the Academy to do a systematic review don't always include a meta-analysis, so they will write up an Evidence Summary.

1. *Determine the evidence analysis question*. The work group breaks down the topic into subtopics and develops research questions within each subtopic. Good quality research questions help to identify outcomes of interest. The evidence analysis question is developed using a format called PICO (Richardson, Wilson, Nishikawa, & Hayward, 1995). A well-built question should identify the population, intervention, comparison intervention, and outcomes. The nutrition care process is also used to help frame questions. Research questions are then prioritized based on criteria such as relevance to dietetics practice and potential to reduce health care costs.
2. *Gather and classify the evidence (data)*. The next step in the systematic review process is to create a plan that defines the inclusion and exclusion eligibility criteria. Specific eligibility criteria might include the study design, setting, population

size, population age, health status, ethnicity, and race. Research articles to be included must be in peer-reviewed journals, written in English, and include human patient populations because some systematic reviews will be used in evidence-based nutrition guidelines for humans.

Once the eligibility criteria are established, the work group identifies key terms and outcomes to conduct a comprehensive literature search. A medical librarian is used to help with the search, and relevant secondary research (such as review articles) are used to help identify primary articles of interest.

Next the lead analyst goes through the search results and uses the eligibility criteria to weed out citations and abstracts that do not meet the criteria. Then the included abstracts are given to work group members to further assess whther they are truly eligible for inclusion. This step yields a list of included and excluded articles. The full text of all included articles is obtained for the next step.

The literature search results are written in a search plan based on the Preferred Reporting Items for Systematic Reviews and Meta-Analyses (PRISMA) flow chart– (Figure 12.1). The search plan comprises the research question, date of literature review, inclusion and exclusion criteria, and the search terms. The search plan also identifies the articles that will be included and excluded (with rationale) from the review process.

3. *Critique each article for risk of bias*. Each study is assessed for risk of bias. Two EAL analysts critically appraise each study's design and methodological quality using the academy's risk of bias tool, the **Quality Criteria Checklist** (QCC). The QCC includes 10 areas of validity questions with subquestions (**Table 12.4**) to assess threats that can undermine a sound study. Based on answers to the validity questions, the analysts rate the study as positive, negative, or neutral (see bottom of Table 12.4 for criteria). When the analysts differ in how they rate a question, they try to resolve this through discussion, and another reviewer may be called in. The QCC for each article is compiled into a **Quality Rating Summary** that can be viewed on the Evidence Analysis Library.

   The QCC also includes four questions on the study's relevance to practice (not shown in the table). Table 12.4 is the QCC for primary research with human subjects. There are other Quality Criteria Checklists for other study designs.

4. *Summarize the evidence*. EAL analysts extract data from the research articles that meet the inclusion criteria, such as title, year of publication, journal name, study design, intervention type, and outcomes. Once the data is extracted, the lead analyst acts as the second reviewer.

   When the data extraction and risk of bias assessment are completed, the lead analyst prepares an **Evidence Summary** by research question. The Evidence Summary includes both a narrative synthesis of the studies and a chart with highlights of the studies. When appropriate, a statistical analysis may be performed, such as descriptive statistics or meta-analysis. A meta-analysis is not done if the studies show over 75% heterogeneity using the I^2 statistical test. A narrative synthesis is written when meta-analysis is not appropriate.

5. *Write the conclusion statement and assign grading*. The last step in the evidence analysis process is to write a conclusion statement that addresses the research question. The lead analyst writes a draft conclusion that answers the research question in a clear and concise manner. This is then reviewed by the work group, who may recommend changes. The group also assigns a grade to the conclusion statement. **Table 12.5** shows the criteria used to assign a grade. Conclusions statements are graded as good (I), fair (II), limited (III), expert opinion only (IV), or not assignable (V).

Table 12.4 Quality Criteria Checklist: Primary Research

VALIDITY QUESTIONS	
1. Was the <u>research question</u> clearly stated? 1.1 Was the specific intervention(s) or procedure (independent variable(s)) identified? 1.2 Was the outcome(s) (dependent variable(s)) clearly indicated? 1.3 Were the target population and setting specified?	Yes No Unclear N/A
2. Was the <u>selection</u> of study subjects/patients free from bias? 2.1 Were inclusion/exclusion criteria specified (e.g., risk, point in disease progression, diagnostic or prognosis criteria), and with sufficient detail and without omitting criteria critical to the study? 2.2 Were criteria applied equally to all study groups? 2.3 Were health, demographics, and other characteristics of subjects described? 2.4 Were the subjects/patients a representative sample of the relevant population?	Yes No Unclear N/A
3. Were <u>study groups comparable</u>? 3.1 Was the method of assigning subjects/patients to groups described and unbiased? (Method of randomization identified if RCT) 3.2 Were distribution of disease status, prognostic factors, and other factors (e.g., demographics) similar across study groups at baseline? 3.3 Were concurrent controls used? (Concurrent preferred over historical controls.) 3.4 If cohort study or cross-sectional study, were groups comparable on important confounding factors and/or were preexisting differences accounted for by using appropriate adjustments in statistical analysis? 3.5 If case control study, were potential confounding factors comparable for cases and controls? (If case series or trial with subjects serving as own control, this criterion is not applicable. Criterion may not be applicable in some cross-sectional studies.) 3.6 If diagnostic test, was there an independent blind comparison with an appropriate reference standard (e.g., "gold standard")?	Yes No Unclear N/A
4. Was method of handling <u>withdrawals</u> described? 4.1 Were follow-up methods described and the same for all groups? 4.2 Was the number, characteristics of withdrawals (i.e., dropouts, lost to follow up, attrition rate) and/or response rate (cross-sectional studies) described for each group? (Follow-up goal for a strong study is 80%.) 4.3 Were all enrolled subjects/patients (in the original sample) accounted for? 4.4 Were reasons for withdrawals similar across groups? 4.5 If diagnostic test, was decision to perform reference test not dependent on results of test under study?	Yes No Unclear N/A
5. Was <u>blinding</u> used to prevent introduction of bias? 5.1 In intervention study, were subjects, clinicians/practitioners, and investigators blinded to treatment group, as appropriate? 5.2 Were data collectors blinded for outcomes assessment? (If outcome is measured using an objective test, such as a lab value, this criterion is assumed to be met.) 5.3 In cohort study or cross-sectional study, were measurements of outcomes and risk factors blinded? 5.4 In case control study, was case definition explicit and case ascertainment not influenced by exposure status? 5.5 In diagnostic study, were test results blinded to patient history and other test results?	Yes No Unclear N/A
6. Were <u>intervention</u>/therapeutic regimens/exposure factor or procedure and any comparison(s) described in detail? Were <u>intervening factors</u> described? 6.1 In RCT or other intervention trial, were protocols described for all regimens studied? 6.2 In observational study, were interventions, study settings, and clinicians/provider described?	

(continues)

Table 12.4 Quality Criteria Checklist: Primary Research (continued)	
VALIDITY QUESTIONS	
6.3 Was the intensity and duration of the intervention or exposure factor sufficient to produce a meaningful effect? 6.4 Was the amount of exposure and, if relevant, subject/patient compliance measured? 6.5 Were co-interventions (e.g., ancillary treatments, other therapies) described? 6.6 Were extra or unplanned treatments described? 6.7 Was the information for 6.4, 6.5, and 6.6 assessed the same way for all groups? 6.8 In diagnostic study, were details of test administration and replication sufficient?	Yes No Unclear N/A
7. Were outcomes clearly defined and the measurements valid and reliable? 7.1 Were primary and secondary endpoints described and relevant to the question? 7.2 Were nutrition measures appropriate to question and outcomes of concern? 7.3 Was the period of follow up long enough for important outcome(s) to occur? 7.4 Were the observations and measurements based on standard, valid, and reliable data collection instruments/tests/procedures? 7.5 Was the measurement of effect at an appropriate level of precision? 7.6 Were other factors accounted for (measured) that could affect outcomes? 7.7 Were the measurements conducted consistently across groups?	Yes No Unclear N/A
8. Was the statistical analysis appropriate for the study design and type of outcome indicators? 8.1 Were statistical analyses adequately described the results reported appropriately? 8.2 Were correct statistical tests used and assumptions of test not violated? 8.3 Were statistics reported with levels of significance and/or confidence intervals? 8.4 Was "intent to treat" analysis of outcomes done (and as appropriate, was there an analysis of outcomes for those maximally exposed or a dose-response analysis)? 8.5 Were adequate adjustments made for effects of confounding factors that might have affected the outcomes (e.g., multivariate analyses)? 8.6 Was clinical significance as well as statistical significance reported? 8.7 If negative findings, was a power calculation reported to address type 2 error?	Yes No Unclear N/A
9. Are conclusions supported by results with biases and limitations taken into consideration? 9.1 Is there a discussion of findings? 9.2 Are biases and study limitations identified and discussed?	Yes No Unclear N/A
10. Is bias due to study's funding or sponsorship unlikely? 10.1 Were sources of funding and investigators' affiliations described? 10.2 Was there no apparent conflict of interest?	Yes No Unclear N/A
MINUS/NEGATIVE (–) *If most (six or more) of the answers to the above validity questions are "No," the report should be designated with a minus (–) symbol on the Evidence Worksheet.*	
NEUTRAL (Ø) *If the answers to validity criteria questions 2, 3, 6, and 7 do not indicate that the study is exceptionally strong, the report should be designated with a neutral (Ø) symbol on the Evidence Worksheet.*	
PLUS/POSITIVE (+) *If most of the answers to the above validity questions are "Yes" (including criteria 2, 3, 6, 7 and at least one additional "Yes"), the report should be designated with a plus symbol (+) on the Evidence Worksheet.*	

Reproduced from the *Evidence Analysis Manual*, pp. 90–92, by the Academy of Nutrition and Dietetics. © 2016. Evidence Analysis Library. Retrieved from https://www.andeal.org/evidence-analysis-manual. Reprinted with permission.

Table 12.5 Conclusion Grading Table

Strength of evidence elements	Grades				
	I Good	II Fair	III Limited	IV Expert opinion only	V Grade not assignable
Quality • Scientific rigor/validity • Considers design and execution	Studies of strong design for question. Free from design flaws, bias and execution problems.	Studies of strong design for question with minor methodological concerns OR Only studies of weaker study design for question.	Studies of weak design for answering the question OR Inconclusive findings due to design flaws, bias or execution problems.	No studies available. Conclusion based on usual practice, expert consensus, clinical experience, opinion, or extrapolation from basic research.	No evidence that pertains to question being addressed.
Consistency • Of findings across studies	Findings generally consistent in direction and size of effect or degree of association, and statistical significance with minor exceptions at most.	Inconsistency among results of studies with strong design. OR Consistency with minor exceptions across studies of weaker design.	Unexplained inconsistency among results from different studies OR single study unconfirmed by other studies.	Conclusion supported solely by statements of informed nutrition or medical commentators.	NA
Quantity • Number of studies • Number of subjects in studies	One to several good quality studies. Large number of subjects studied. Studies with negative results have sufficiently large sample size for adequate statistical power.	Several studies by independent investigators. Doubts about adequacy of sample size to avoid Type I and Type II error.	Limited number of studies. Low number of subjects studied and/or inadequate sample size within studies.	Unsubstantiated by published research studies.	Relevant studies have not been done.
Clinical Impact • Importance of studied outcomes • Magnitude of effect	Studied outcome relates directly to the question. Size of effect is clinically meaningful. Significant (statistical) difference is large.	Some doubt about the statistical or clinical significance of the effect.	Studied outcome is an intermediate outcome or surrogate for the true outcome of interest. OR Size of effect is small or lacks statistical and/or clinical significance.	Objective data unavailable.	Indicates area for future research.

(continues)

Table 12.5 Conclusion Grading Table (continued)

Strength of evidence elements	Grades				
	I Good	II Fair	III Limited	IV Expert opinion only	V Grade not assignable
Generalizability • To population of interest	Studied population, intervention and outcomes are free from serious doubts about generalizability.	Minor doubts about generalizability.	Serious doubts about generalizability due to narrow or different study population, intervention or outcomes studied.	Generalizability limited to scope of experience.	NA

Reproduced from the *Evidence Analysis Manual*, p. 105, by the Academy of Nutrition and Dietetics. © 2016. Evidence Analysis Library. Retrieved from https://www.andeal.org/evidence-analysis-manual. Reprinted with permission.

This five-step rigorous process for conducting systematic reviews makes the EAL a reliable tool for obtaining evidenced-based research. Academy members are encouraged to share their expertise by contributing to the EAL throughout the course of their dietetics or nutrition career.

APPLICATION 12.2

Complete the Quality Criteria Checklist for this study:

(Open-Access Article) Fildes, A., van Jaarsveld, C. H. M., Wardle, J., & Cookie, L. (2014). Parent-administered exposure to increase children's vegetable acceptance: A randomized controlled trial. *Journal of the Academy of Nutrition and Dietetics, 114*, 881–888. Review your ratings with another student and calculate the inter-rater agreement (the percentage of time when your ratings were the same).

USING THE EVIDENCE ANALYSIS LIBRARY OF THE ACADEMY OF NUTRITION AND DIETETICS

The Evidence Analysis Library (EAL) was designed and created specifically for nutrition professionals. Established in 2004, the EAL contains both the results of *systematic reviews*—including Evidence Summaries, Conclusions, and Grades—and *evidence-based nutrition practice guidelines*, which are defined as follows by the Academy of Nutrition and Dietetics (2016):

> **Evidence-based nutrition practice guidelines** are statements and treatment algorithms which are developed using the process of asking questions, systemically finding research evidence, and assessing its validity, applicability and importance to food and nutrition practice decisions. The guidelines are designed to assist the registered dietitian (RD) or registered dietitian nutritionist (RDN), RD or RDN/dietetic technician, registered (DTR) team and other intended users and patient/client in making decisions about appropriate nutrition care for specific disease states or conditions in typical settings. (p. 16)

Developing Evidence-Based Nutrition Practice Guidelines

We have been discussing the systematic review process, from developing a question to writing evidence summaries and assigning a grade to the conclusion. Now we need to look at a different process—using systematic reviews and the Nutrition Care Process to develop evidence-based nutrition practice guidelines. The expert work group who worked on the systematic review also develops the nutrition practice guidelines using the following process (Academy of Nutrition and Dietetics, 2012).

Step 1. Clinical Algorithm: The expert work group develops a clinical algorithm for the guideline based on the Academy's Nutrition Care Process. In this case, algorithms are illustrated in step-by-step flowcharts to illustrate how each recommendation can be used to treat patients.

Step 2. Draft Recommendations: The expert work group prepares draft recommendations for the guideline from evidence analysis using an expert consensus method. The first statement in a recommendation explains what the dietitian should do (or not do), and the next statement explains why. More than one recommendation is often needed. Each recommendation is rated based, as usual, on the strength of the evidence. **Table 12.6** shows the ratings given (Strong, Fair, Weak, Consensus, Insufficient Evidence).

Table 12.6 Criteria for Recommendation Ratings

Recommendation ratings	Explanation	Implication for practice
Strong	The benefits of the recommended approach clearly exceed the harms, and that the quality of the supporting evidence is Grade I or II.	Practitioners should follow a Strong recommendation unless a clear and compelling rationale for an alternative approach is present.
Fair	The benefits exceed the harms but the quality of evidence is not as strong (grade II or III).	Practitioners should generally follow a Fair recommendation but remain alert to new information and be sensitive to patient preferences.
Weak	The quality of the evidence is suspect or well-done studies (grade I, II, or III) show little clear advantage to one approach versus another.	Practitioners should be cautious in deciding whether to follow a Weak recommendation and should exercise judgment and be alert to emerging publications that report evidence. Patient preference should have a substantial influencing role.
Consensus	Expert opinion (Grade IV) supports the guidance recommendation even though the available scientific evidence did not present consistent results or controlled trials were lacking.	Practitioners should be flexible in deciding whether to follow a Consensus recommendation, although they may set boundaries on alternatives. Patient preference should have a substantial influencing role.
Insufficient Evidence	There is both a lack of pertinent evidence (Grade V) and/or an unclear balance between benefits and harms.	Practitioners should feel little constraint in deciding whether to follow this type of recommendation and should exercise judgment and be alert to emerging publications that report evidence that clarifies the balance of benefit versus harm. Patient preference should have a substantial influencing role.

Adapted from "Recommendation Ratings" by the Academy of Nutrition and Dietetics, Evidence Analysis Library, 2016, Retrieved from: http://www.andeal.org/recommendation-ratings. Reprinted with permission.

Each rating is also given a label: conditional or imperative. Imperative recommendations have no conditions attached to their use, but conditional recommendations use an "if, then" format so you know in which situations it can be used.

Step 3. Complete Writing Guideline: Each guideline for a specific disease has a format: Introduction, Major Recommendations, Background Information, and References/Appendices.

Step 4. Internal and External Review: The guidelines are reviewed internally and externally using a standardized evaluation tool (Appraisal of Guidelines for Research and Evaluation). EAL guidelines are reviewed for each topic every 5 years.

Step 5. Approval and Publish: The Evidence-Based Practice Committee must approve each guideline, and then it is published on the EAL.

During the early part of this process, the work group formulates a list of references that were not reviewed during the evidence analysis process but may be used at this time to support a recommendation or a component of a recommendation.

Each guideline may encompass many recommendations. For example, the guideline on the Prevention of Type 2 Diabetes includes 17 recommendations based on 108 Conclusions Statements and 108 Evidence Summaries from systematic reviews. To find this guideline on the EAL, simply click under "Projects" and find Diabetes, Type 2, Prevention. On the Diabetes Prevention Project homepage, to the left you will see a table with the most recent project at the top: Prevention of Type 2 Diabetes (PDM) Guideline (Year). Then you can read the following for this guideline.

1. Executive Summary of the Recommendations: This includes major recommendations and ratings.
2. Introduction: The Scope of the Guideline, Statement of Intent, Guidelines Methods, Implementation of the Guideline, Benefits and Risks/Harms of Implementation.
3. Major Recommendations: Include the following:
   - Recommendation, its rating and whether it is "imperative" or "conditional"
   - Risks and harms of implementing this recommendation
   - Conditions of application
   - Potential costs associated with application
   - Recommendation narrative (review of research)
   - Recommendation strength rationale (why it received the rating it did)
   - Minority opinions (listed as needed)

   Click on "Supporting Evidence" to see the evidence analysis questions on which the recommendations were developed. By clicking on a question, you can go back to the conclusion and evidence summaries of the systematic review. *All the Evidence Analysis Questions are organized using the Nutrition Care Process categories: Assessment, Diagnosis, Intervention, and Monitoring and Evaluation.* If the Evidence Analysis Questions do not fall into the Nutrition Care Process steps, they are categorized under "Basic Research."
4. Background Information
5. References

To help RDNs implement evidence-based nutrition practice guidelines, AND publishes Evidence-Based Nutrition Practice Toolkits, which contain useful tools such as medical nutrition therapy protocol, sample documentation forms, and client education resources.

TIP

The EAL contains *guidelines, recommendations,* and *evidence analysis questions with conclusions.* If you are using the EAL and are not sure whether the page you are looking at is a guideline, recommendation, or evidence analysis review, use this chart (**Figure 12.5**) to help. Also remember these facts: the results from evidence analysis review are used as the foundation for recommendations; guidelines encompass a number of recommendations; and recommendations have ratings (while evidence analysis conclusions have grades).

Guideline	Recommendation	Evidence Analysis Review
Executive Summary of Recommendations	Title of Recommendation(s)	Evidence Analysis Question
Introduction	Recommendation Rating (Strong, Fair, Weak, Consensus, Insufficient Evidence) Label (Imperative or Conditional)	Conclusion
Major Recommendations	Supporting Evidence (Evidence Analysis Questions and Reference List)	Grade - Good/strong (I), fair (II), limited/weak (III), expert opinion only (IV), or not assignable (V).
Background information		Evidence Summary
References		Search Plan and Results

FIGURE 12.5 Comparison of Structure of Guidelines, Recommendations, and Evidence Analysis Review as Found in the Evidence Analysis Library of the Academy of Nutrition and Dietetics

Navigating the EAL

Academy members can access the EAL by visiting this website: https://www.andeal.org/. This link will bring you to the EAL homepage where you can log in using your academy username and password. The homepage has a series of links across the top of the page that include *Projects, Methodology, Resources, Index* and *About.*

- Under the Projects tab you can access many different research areas. Many of the Projects listed do include Guidelines, but *not all projects contain guidelines*! Some projects contain systematic reviews used to support academy position papers. If you click on a project and see "Grade Chart" to the left, the Grade Chart is for the conclusion statements of systematic reviews.

- The Methodology tab includes the Academy Evidence Analysis Manual as well as information on the steps in the evidence analysis process and guideline development process.
- The Resources tab brings you to the EAL tutorials and other helpful resources for navigating and understanding the EAL website and process. The tutorial is made up of four modules and takes less than an hour to complete.

APPLICATION 12.3

Complete the four tutorials on the Evidence Analysis Library. Complete the quiz, print, and hand it in.

ADDITIONAL SYSTEMATIC REVIEWS AND GUIDELINES

In addition to the EAL, other professional review resources may be useful for nutrition professionals. These include the U.S. Department of Agriculture's Nutrition Evidence Library (NEL), Cochrane Database of Systematic Reviews, and the National Guidelines Clearinghouse (Agency for Healthcare Research & Quality). Let's take a closer look at each of these.

NUTRITION EVIDENCE LIBRARY (NEL)

The USDA Nutrition Evidence Library is an online resource of systematic reviews. The NEL works with scientists and stakeholders to complete a wide range of systematic review projects that answer food and nutrition questions and inform users of federal nutrition policy and programs. For example, the NEL supports the Dietary Guidelines Advisory Committee's (DGAC) scientific review process in the ongoing development of the Dietary Guidelines for Americans. In addition to the 2015 Dietary Guidelines Advisory Committee, the NEL has several ongoing projects, which are listed in **Table 12.7**.

Table 12.7 Projects of the Nutrition Evidence Library (of USDA)

NEL project	2015 DGAC	Nutrition education	Dietary patterns 2014	Birth to 24 months
Primary Task	Performed systematic reviews used in Scientific Report of the 2015 DGAC.	Perform systematic reviews to further the understanding of childhood and adolescent nutritional habits and ways to deliver nutrition education to improve this outcome.	12 systematic reviews were done to understand the relationship between dietary patterns and public health outcomes and concerns.	Provide guidance for parents, caregivers, and the medical profession on babies from birth to 24 months based on a variety of systematic reviews.

The NEL website is easy to navigate and provides a list of comprehensive systematic reviews by project (under the "Projects" tab) or topic (under the "Reviews" tab). The topics include the following:

1. Foods and Dietary Patterns
2. Nutrients
3. Energy Balance (Body Weight)
4. Behavior/Environment
5. Health Conditions
6. Special Populations
7. Nutrition Education
8. Food Safety

Each topic is further broken down into subtopics. For example, subtopics for "Food and Dietary Patterns" include Dairy, Vegetables/Fruits, Dietary Patterns, and more. By clicking on a subtopic, you can view a series of systematic reviews related to each category. **Figure 12.6** shows a screenshot of what is revealed if you click on "Dairy." As you can see, further details about each systematic review can then be accessed by clicking on the various links. In addition, each systematic review is rated for overall strength and categorized as Limited, Moderate, or Strong. The NEL staff assigns a rating for each systematic review using a state-of-the-art methodology and review process.

Cochrane Database of Systematic Reviews

Cochrane is an international network of researchers, medical professionals, and patients from 120 different countries who do not accept any commercial funding. Their mission is to provide quality information to help those involved in health care make informed decisions. Established over 20 years ago, Cochrane's work is globally recognized for its quality health-related information. Many of the Cochrane contributors are

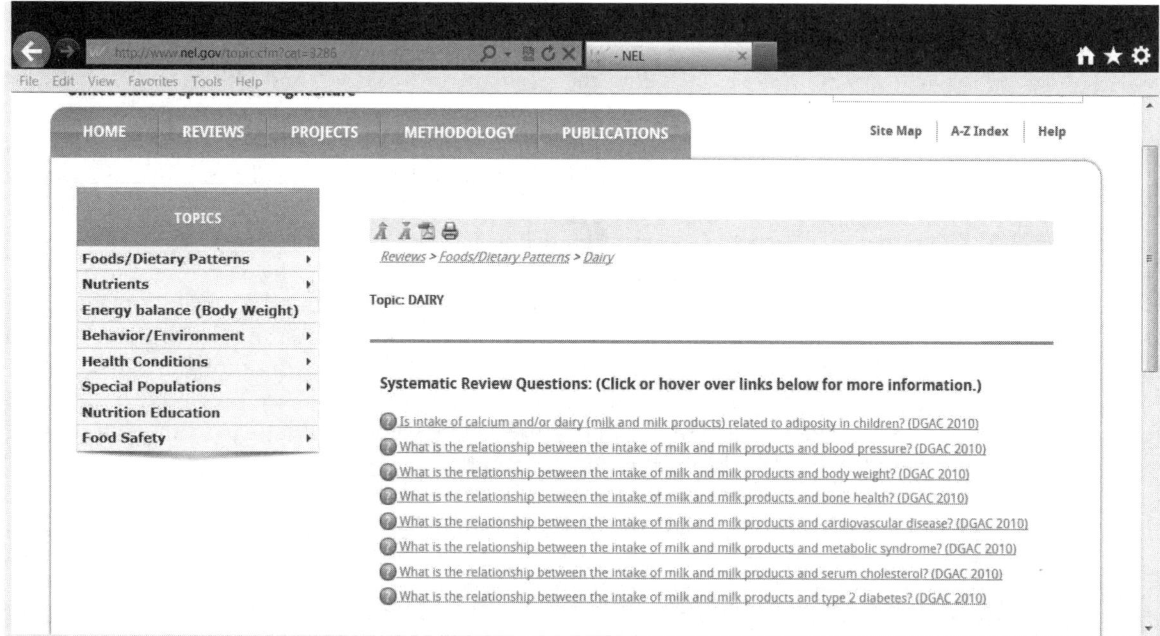

FIGURE 12.6 A Screenshot from the Nutrition Evidence Library of the USDA

Reproduced from U.S. Department of Agriculture. Retrieved from: http://www.nel.gov/topic.cfm?cat=3286

world-renown leaders in various medical fields and have affiliations with top academic and medical institutions.

The Cochrane Database of Systematic Reviews (CDSR) is a comprehensive online tool that houses health care and health policy literature reviews otherwise known as the "Cochrane Reviews." They are found at www.cochranelibrary.com. The CDSR is internationally recognized for providing the highest standard in health care–related systematic reviews. The CDSR comprises 12 monthly issues each year, which are updated regularly to incorporate emerging evidence. This makes the CDSR unique in that the literature reviews are never dated.

The Cochrane reviews are written by authors who must register their reviews with one of the 52 Cochrane Review Groups. Each Cochrane Review Group (CRG) focuses on one topic area and includes an editorial team to provide support and peer review. The Cochrane editorial process ensures consistency by following a strict protocol to monitor the review process from beginning to end. The Cochrane Review Group topics are organized in alphabetical order from Acute Respiratory Infections to Wounds.

As of 2016, 52 categories of CRGs have been established. CRGs are linked to further information about each topic. To find a review on a particular topic, go to the homepage for the Cochrane Library (www.cochranelibrary.com) and click on "Cochrane Reviews." Then you can search by using "Search CDSR," "Browse by Topic," or "Browse by Review Group."

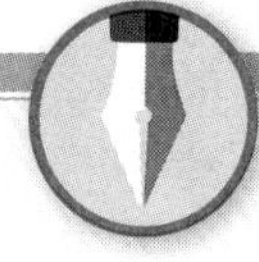

TIP

When you use PubMed to find articles, you can click on "Systematic Reviews" under "Article Types" to include them in your search results.

NATIONAL GUIDELINES CLEARINGHOUSE

The National Guidelines Clearinghouse (NGC) is a public electronic database that compiles evidence-based practice guidelines for health care research and policy from many organizations, including the Academy of Nutrition and Dietetics. The NGC is maintained by the Agency for Healthcare Research and Quality in partnership with the American Medical Association (AMA) and the American Association of Health Plans (AAHP) Foundation. One of the unique features of this site is that it is updated weekly with new content that can easily be accessed by visiting the "New This Week" section on the NGC home page (www.guideline.gov).

On the home page for the NGC, you can search using the Search box or by clicking on "Guideline Summaries" and then browsing by clinical specialty, organization, or MeSH tag. You can also click on "in Progress" and "Archive." Their website also provides (under "Expert Commentaries") insights written by thought leaders in the respective fields who discuss their opinion about the evidence presented and current trends or issues related to the topic at hand. This section is helpful in further interpreting the evidence and relating it to current trends.

In summary, the NGC can be a useful tool when researching a nutrition-related topic, especially if you want a quick glance at the latest evidence.

APPLICATION 12.4

Find one systematic review from each of these sources, if available, on the topic of the effect of potassium on blood pressure.

SUMMARY

1. Systematic reviews and narrative reviews analyze data from primary research studies. Compared to narrative reviews, systematic reviews have more focused research questions, more comprehensive literature searches, more rigor in appraising studies, and more often a meta-analysis. Overall systematic reviews are more transparent and rigorous, and they are used to lay the foundation for evidence-based nutrition practice guidelines. Narrative review articles are considered secondary research, and systematic reviews are tertiary research.
2. Table 12.1 illustrates the steps in a systematic review: formulate the research question, define inclusion and exclusion criteria for studies, develop a search strategy, conduct the literature search, screen the records for eligibility, access the full text of selected studies for abstracting and final eligibility check, critically assess the risk of bias in each study, synthesize the evidence, summarize and discuss the findings, and publish. Figure 12.1 shows a standardized way to display the process of selecting studies.
3. Table 12.2 provides guidelines for assessing the quality of a systematic review.
4. To assess the risk of bias, some researchers use a tool from the Cochrane Collaboration that assesses these domains: random sequence generation, allocation concealment, blinding of participants and personnel, blinding of outcome assessment, incomplete outcome data, and selective outcome reporting.
5. Effect size is at the heart of meta-analysis. Effect size tells you about both the strength and the direction of the effect, and it may be expressed as a correlation, a ratio (relative risk or odds ratio) or a difference between mean values for two groups.
6. The results of a meta-analysis will vary depending on whether the outcomes are continuous or dichotomous (binary data). With continuous data, effect size is measured using either mean difference or standardized mean difference. With binary data, effect size is measured using risk ratios and odds ratios.
7. The method used in meta-analysis to weight studies is called inverse-variance weighting. Another concern in a meta-analysis is heterogeneity. Ideally, the results of the different studies should be similar. Many researchers use the random effects model for meta-analysis because it adjusts for the variability between the studies.
8. Guidelines are given for interpreting forest plots. The vertical line represents the point where there is no intervention effect. If the black diamond, which represents the summary estimate, crosses over the vertical line, the difference between the groups is not statistically significant.
9. The EAL work group teams conduct systematic reviews using these steps: determine the evidence analysis question(s), gather and classify the evidence, critique each study for risk of bias using the Quality Criteria Checklist (Table 12.4), summarize the evidence, write the conclusion statement, and assign a grade: good (I), fair (II), limited (III), expert opinion only (IV), or not assignable (V).
10. The EAL work group teams also develop evidence-based nutrition practice guidelines using their systematic reviews and the nutrition care process. Each guideline may encompass many recommendations. The first statement in a recommendation explains what the dietitian should do (or not do), and the next statement explains why. Each recommendation is rated based on the strength of the evidence: Strong, Fair, Weak, Consensus, Insufficient Evidence. Each rating is also given a label: conditional or imperative. Imperative recommendations have no conditions attached to their use, but conditional recommendations use an "if, then" format so you know in which situations they can be used.
11. The EAL contains guidelines, recommendations, and evidence analysis questions with conclusions. Figure 12.5 describes the components and the relationships between guidelines, recommendations, and evidence analysis review.

12. You can also search for systematic reviews at the U.S. Department of Agriculture's Nutrition Evidence Library (NEL) and the Cochrane Database of Systematic Reviews. The National Guidelines Clearinghouse (Agency for Healthcare Research and Quality) includes guidelines from AND as well as many other health care associations.

REVIEW QUESTIONS

1. When researchers rigorously examine and interpret the findings of research studies using a qualitative method, it is called:
   A. meta-analysis
   B. meta-synthesis
   C. mixed methods systematic review
   D. guidelines
2. A systematic review often includes which of the following?
   A. primary research studies
   B. non-English studies
   C. working papers
   D. unpublished quality research
   E. all of the above
3. Which type of error does *bias* represent?
   A. random error
   B. measurement error
   C. attrition error
   D. systematic error
4. In a randomized clinical trial, a doctor sees that the next person to be admitted will get into the experimental group. So the doctor encourages a patient later that day to enter the trial. This is a problem with:
   A. random sequence generation
   B. allocation concealment
   C. blinding of participants
   D. blinding of assessors
5. At the heart of meta-analysis is:
   A. statistical significance
   B. standard mean difference
   C. effect size
   D. heterogeneity
6. As sample size increases, so does effect size.
   A. true
   B. false
7. A relative risk of 1 means there is a slight difference between groups.
   A. true
   B. false
8. A case control study uses which of the following effect sizes?
   A. mean difference
   B. standardized mean difference
   C. risk ratio
   D. odds ratio
9. In a forest plot, the summary estimate has which shape?
   A. square
   B. octagon
   C. diamond
   D. any of the above
10. The first step in the academy's EAL guidelines for conducting systematic reviews is:
    A. gather the evidence (data)
    B. critique each article for subjectivity/bias
    C. determine the evidence analysis question
    D. present the evidence
11. What is the name of the tool used by the EAL work group to assess the risk of bias in each study?
    A. Data Extraction Tool (DET)
    B. Quality Criteria Checklist (QCC)
    C. Cochrane Database of Systematic Reviews (CDSR)
    D. Evidence Analysis Library (EAL)
12. What is the final step in the evidence analysis process?
    A. write conclusion statements
    B. assign a grade
    C. critique each article
    D. present the evidence
13. Each recommendation on the EAL is given:
    A. a conclusion statement and grade
    B. a rating and label
    C. a Resources tab
    D. all of the above

14. Most evidence analysis questions on the EAL are organized using the Nutrition Care Process categories.
    A. true
    B. false
15. Which of the following is characteristic of the Cochrane Database of Systematic Reviews?
    A. Features 12 monthly issues per year
    B. Literature is continuously updated
    C. Each systematic review is written to address a specific question
    D. All of the above
16. How are a meta-analysis and a meta-synthesis different? Describe at least two ways in which they differ.
17. Find the title of a narrative review and the title of a systematic review. Compare and contrast the two types of reviews.
18. Explain the concepts of publication bias, selection bias, detection bias, attrition bias, and reporting bias.
19. Why is it important to have two reviewers involved in screening studies?
20. In a study looking at stroke in patients with systolic blood pressure either 130 and below or 130 and higher, the relative risk was 2.0. Interpret the meaning of the relative risk.
21. Compare and contrast the steps taken by the EAL work group to do a systematic review versus to develop an evidence-based nutrition practice guideline.
22. Describe the group behind the Cochrane Database of Systematic Reviews. What is a Cochrane Review Group, and what do they do?

CRITICAL THINKING QUESTIONS

1. Answer the following questions for this systematic review: Nissensohn, M. Roman-Vinas, B., Sanchez-Villegas, Al., Piscopo, S., & Serra-Majem, L. (2016). The effect of the Mediterranean diet on hypertension: A systematic review and meta-analysis. *Journal of Nutrition Education and Behavior, 48*, 42–53.
    A. Why was this systematic review done? What is the research question?
    B. Name the inclusion and exclusion criteria.
    C. How many articles did their initial search identify? How many articles were used in the systematic review? Were two reviewers used in the selection of articles?
    D. How did they assess risk of bias and present the results? How many studies overall showed moderate risk? How was moderate risk defined?
    E. How many total participants were in the studies used in the meta-analysis?
    F. Read through the data about the studies included in the systematic review and describe the control groups in this review.
    G. What outcome is measured, and when is it measured?
    H. How was effect size measured in the meta-analysis?
    I. Interpret what you see in the forest plots in Figures 2 and 3, including the level of heterogeneity.
    J. What were the results?
    K. What were the limitations of this systematic review?
2. Answer the following questions for this systematic review: Mumme, K., & Stonehouse, W. (2015). Effects of medium-chain triglycerides on weight loss and body composition: A meta-analysis of randomized controlled trials. *Journal of the Academy of Nutrition and Dietetics, 115*, 249–263.
    A. Why was this systematic review done? What is the research question?
    B. Name the inclusion and exclusion criteria.
    C. How many articles did their initial search identify? How many articles were used in the meta-analysis? Were two reviewers used in the selection of articles?
    D. What were the primary outcome measures?

E. How did they assess risk of bias and present the results?
F. What were the results for the *primary* outcome measures?
G. Interpret what you see in the forest plots in Figures 3 and 5, including the level of heterogeneity. Which outcome(s) used mean difference, and which outcome(s) used standardized mean difference?
H. What were the limitations of this systematic review?
I. What future research do they recommend?

3. Use Table 12.2 to *evaluate* this systematic review: Dall'Oglio, I., Nicolo, R., Di Ciommo, V., Bianchi, N., Cilento, G., Gawronski, O., Pomponi, M., Roberti, M., Tiozzo, E., & Raponi, M. (2015). A systematic review of hospital foodservice patient satisfaction studies. *Journal of the Academy of Nutrition and Dietetics, 115*, 567–584. doi: 10.1016/j.jand.2014.11.013
4. Using the EAL, find any recommendations for sodium restriction for patients with high blood pressure, chronic kidney disease, diabetes, or heart failure. Write down each recommendation and note how each is rated and labeled. For one recommendation, also note one of the evidence analysis questions used to develop it, with its conclusion and grade.
5. Use the Cochrane Database of Systematic Reviews (www.cochranelibrary.org) to find any systematic reviews on the effect of weight loss on blood pressure. Include pertinent information such as the project title, dates, editorial group, and an abstract of results.

SUGGESTED READINGS AND ACTIVITIES

1. Academy of Nutrition and Dietetics. (2012). *Evidence Analysis Manual: Steps in the Academy Evidence Analysis Process.* Available at www.andeal.org/evidence-analysis-manual.
2. Center for Evidence-Based Medicine at the University of Oxford (U.K.). *The Five Stages of Evidence-Based Medicine.* Available at http://www.cebm.net/category/ebm-resources/tools/.
3. Higgins, J., & Green, S. (Eds.). (2011). *Cochrane Handbook for Systematic Reviews of Intervention* (Version 5.1.0). Retrieved from http://handbook.cochrane.org.
4. Orientation tutorials on Evidence Analysis Library website: https://www.andeal.org/tutorials, consisting of four video modules; each only 15 minutes in duration. The modules will further your understanding of the EAL layout and methodology and RDNs can earn 1 hour of continuing education.

REFERENCES

Academy of Nutrition and Dietetics Evidence Analysis Library. (2016). *Criteria for Recommendation Ratings.* Retrieved from http://www.andeal.org/recommendation-ratings

Academy of Nutrition and Dietetics. (2016). *Definition of Terms List.* Retrieved from http://www.eatrightpro.org/~/media/eatrightpro%20files/practice/scope%20standards%20of%20practice/definition%20of%20terms%20list.ashx

Academy of Nutrition and Dietetics. (2012). *Evidence Analysis Manual: Steps in the Academy Evidence Analysis Process.* Retrieved from https://www.andeal.org/vault/2440/web/files/2012_Aug_EA_Manual.pdf

Blumberg-Kason, S., & Lipscomb, R. (2006). Evidence-Based Nutrition Practice Guidelines: A valuable resource in the Evidence Analysis Library. *Journal of the American Dietetic Association, 106*, 1935–1936. doi: 10.1016/j.jada2006.10.025

Cook, D. J., Mulrow, C. D., & Haynes, R. B. (1997). Systematic reviews: Synthesis of best evidence for clinical decisions. *Annals of Internal Medicine, 126*, 376–380. doi:10.7326/0003-4819-126-5-199703010-00006

Eden, J., Levit, L, Berg, A., & Morton, S. (Eds.), for the Institute of Medicine. (2011). *Finding What Works in Health Care: Standards for Systematic Reviews.* Washington, DC: National Academies Press.

Franz, M. J., Boucher, J. L., Green-Pastors, J., & Powers, M. A. (2008). Evidence-based nutrition practice guidelines for diabetes and scope and standards of practice. *Journal of the American Dietetic Association, 108*, S52–S58. doi: 10.1016/j.jada.2008.01.021

Garg, A., Hackam, D., & Tonelli, M. (2008). Systematic review and meta-analysis: When one study is just not enough. *Clinical Journal of the American Society of Nephrology, 3*, 253–260. doi: 10.2215/CNJ.01430307

Graham, L. (2011). Where can I find reliable consumer nutrition information? *Journal of the American Dietetic Association, 111*, 1626. doi: 10.1016/j.jada.2011.08.013

Graham, R., Mancher, M., Miller Wolman, D., Greenfield, S., & Steinberg, E. (Eds.), for the Institute of Medicine. (2011). *Clinical Practice Guidelines We Can Trust*. Washington, DC: National Academies Press.

Handu, D., Moloney, L., Wolfram, T., Ziegler, P., Acosta, A., & Steiber, A. (2016). Methodology for conducting systematic reviews for the Evidence Analysis Library. *Journal of the Academy of Nutrition and Dietetics, 114*, 311–318. doi: 2.1016/j.jand.2016.02.116

Hemingway, P., & Brereton, N. (2009). *What is a systematic review?* (What Is? Series). Retrieved from http://www.medicine.ox.ac.uk/bandolier/painres/download/whatis/syst- review.pdf

Higgins, J., & Green, S. (Eds.). (2011). *Cochrane Handbook for Systematic Reviews of Intervention* (Version 5.1.0). Retrieved from http://handbook.cochrane.org

Higgins, J., Altman, D. G., Gotzsche, P., Juni, P., Moher, D., Oxman, A., . . . Sterne, J. (2011). The Cochrane Collaboration's tool for assessing risk of bias in randomised trials. *BMJ, 343*, d5928. doi: 10.1136/bmj.d5928

Johns, D. J., Hartmann-Boyce, J., Jebb, S. A., & Aveyard, P., for the Behavioural Weight Management Review Group. (2014). Diet or exercise interventions vs combined behavioral weight management programs: A systematic review and meta-analysis of direct comparisons. *Journal of the Academy of Nutrition and Dietetics, 114*, 1557–1568. doi: 10.1016/j.jand.2014.07.005

Lewis, S., & Clarke, M. (2001). Forest plots: Trying to see the wood and the trees. *BMJ, 322*, 1479–1480. doi: 10.1136/bmj.322.7300.1479

Liberati, A., Altman, D. G., Tetzlaff, J., Mulrow, C., Gotzsche, P. C., Ioannidis, J., . . . Moher, D. (2009). The PRISMA statement for reporting systematic reviews and meta-analyses of studies that evaluate health care interventions: Explanation and elaboration. *PLoS Medicine, 6*, e1000100. doi:10.1371/journal.pmed.1000100

Moher, D., Pham, B., Jones, A., Cook, D. J., Jadad, A. R., Moher, M., . . . Klassen, T. P. (1998). Does quality of reports of randomised trials affect estimates of intervention efficacy reported in meta-analyses? *Lancet, 352*, 609–613. doi: 10.1016/S0140-6736(98)01085-X

Moher, D., Liberati, A., Tetzlaff, J., Altman, D. G., & The PRISMA Group. (2009). Preferred reporting items for systematic reviews and meta-analyses: The PRISMA statement. *PLoS Medicine, 6*, e1000097. doi: 10.1371/journal.pmed.1000097

Richardson, W. S., Wilson, M. C., Nishikawa, J., & Hayward, R. (1995). The well-built clinical question: A key to evidence-based decisions. *ACP Journal Club, 123*, A12–A13.

Robinson, E., Thomas, J., Aveyard, P., & Higgs, S. (2014). What everyone else is eating: A systematic review and meta-analysis of the effect of informational eating norms on eating behavior. *Journal of the Academy of Nutrition and Dietetics, 114*, 414–429. doi: 10.1016/j.jand.2013.11.009

Schulz, K. F., Chalmers, I., Hayes, R. J., & Altman, D. G. (1995). Empirical evidence of bias: Dimensions of methodological quality associated with estimates of treatment effects in controlled trials. *Journal of the American Medical Association, 273*, 408–412. doi:10.1001/jama.1995.03520290060030

Schwingshackl, L., & Hoffmann. G. (2015) Diet quality as assessed by the Healthy Eating Index, the Alternate Healthy Eating Index, the Dietary Approaches to Stop Hypertension Score, and health outcomes: A systematic review and meta-analysis of cohort studies. *Journal of the Academy of Nutrition and Dietetics, 115*, 780–800. doi: 10.1016/j.jand.2015.12.009

Spahn, J. M., Lyon, J., Altman, J. M., Blum-Kemelor, D. M., Essery, E. V., Fungwe, T.V., . . . Wong, Y. P. (2011). The systematic review methodology used to support the 2010 Dietary Guidelines Advisory Committee. *Journal of the American Dietetic Association, 111*, 520–523. doi: 10.1016/j.jada.2011.01.005

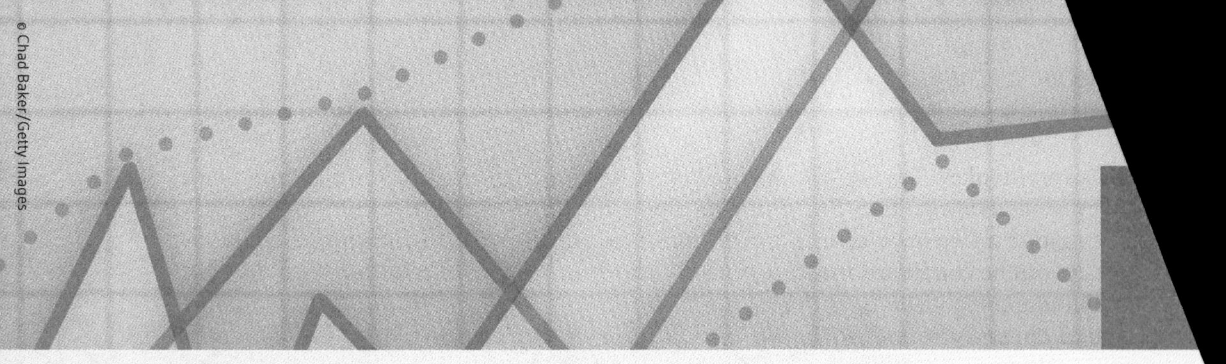

How to Develop and Use Surveys in Research

KAREN EICH DRUMMOND, EDD, RDN, LDN
NATALIE K. COOKE, PHD

CHAPTER OUTLINE

- Introduction
- Survey Basics
- Pick a Sample
- Construct and Refine the Cover Letter and Questionnaire
- Test the Reliability and Validity of a Survey
- Collect and Analyze Survey Data

LEARNING OUTCOMES

- State advantages and disadvantages of paper, email, telephone, and face-to-face surveys.
- Distinguish between cross-sectional, retrospective, and longitudinal surveys, and be able to identify each in a research study.
- Differentiate between probability and nonprobability sampling and give examples of each.
- Explain how sampling size may be determined and identify factors related to sampling that must be considered when evaluating the quality of a study.
- Develop appropriate questions and responses for the questionnaire to answer specific research questions/objectives.
- Explain how to sequence questions, layout the questionnaire, and use cognitive interviews and debriefing to pretest the questionnaire.
- Discuss the different types of reliability and validity for questionnaires/instruments, including how they are tested.
- Explain the basics of collecting and analyzing data including how to increase the response rate, reduce nonsampling errors, and develop a codebook.

INTRODUCTION

You have no doubt taken a survey before; perhaps, it was a marketing survey you responded to on the telephone, a form you completed at the end of the semester when asked to evaluate a college course, or a questionnaire you completed online using

CHAPTER 13

…EVELOP AND USE SURVEYS IN RESEARCH

…eys are questionnaires that are self-administered or administered …re a staple method for asking a question or a series of questions … a specific topic from a representative sample of people. Sur- … many ways: by phone or mail, in person, or on the Internet. …ave to pick the most appropriate answer from a list, the resulting …tered into a statistical program for analysis.

…k of the questionnaire as the "survey," but the questionnaire is simply … the survey process. Surveys involve setting objectives, selecting respon- …mining the most appropriate delivery method, developing and pretesting …onnaire, ensuring validity and reliability, and collecting and analyzing results. … nutrition research, surveys are crucial, for example, to the success of the **…ional Nutrition Monitoring and Related Research Program (NNMRRP)**. …he NNMRRP uses a multidisciplinary approach to provide information about:

- the diet and nutritional status of Americans,
- factors affecting diet and nutritional status, and
- how diet affects the health of Americans.

The National Health and Nutrition Examination Survey (NHANES) is an important component of the NNMRRP. The dietary intake interview part of NHANES obtains two (nonconsecutive) days of dietary intake using 24-hour recalls from a nationally representative sample of individuals of all ages that reside in households. In addition to the 24-hour recall, a Dietary Behavior Questionnaire asks questions such as "Have you heard of MyPlate?" and "In the past 12 months, did you buy food from fast food or pizza places?"

Surveys are used in other research as well, such as in clinical nutrition research, nutrition epidemiological research, program evaluation research, and agricultural research.

- In clinical nutrition research, researchers may use questionnaires to obtain basic demographic and medical information, to determine physical activity levels (using a tool such as the validated International Physical Activity Questionnaire), or 24-hour diet recalls to assess diet quality. Information from a 24-hour recall can be evaluated using a measure of diet quality such as the Healthy Eating Index, which is based on the Dietary Guidelines for Americans.
- The field of nutrition epidemiology (think of the Framingham Heart Study or the Nurses' Health Study as examples) relies a lot on surveys and diet assessment tools such as validated food frequency questionnaires. Researchers may develop and test hypotheses between certain foods or nutrients and their health outcomes, such as a heart-healthy dietary pattern and heart disease in women.
- Surveys are integral to the evaluation of nutrition programs. Evaluation is the "use of scientific methods to judge and improve the planning, monitoring, effectiveness, and efficiency of health, nutrition, and other human service programs" (Boyle & Holben, 2013, p. 115). You have no doubt completed questionnaires to evaluate the courses you have taken and possibly your academic program as well. Feedback such as this is vital to program improvement. Surveys are also used to evaluate the impact of interventions. For example, Hand et al. (2014) used a 10-question survey (Family Nutrition and Physical Activity Screening Tool) with low-income families before and after an intervention. The survey was used to evaluate whether the families had adopted healthy behaviors after the intervention.
- Companies, such as Press Ganey, administer patient satisfaction surveys to inpatients, discharged patients, and outpatients in a healthcare facility or a group

practice. Patients take the survey and provide comments regarding specific aspects of care.
- The U.S. Department of Agriculture is one of the largest collectors of survey data in the federal government. Agricultural research uses surveys to obtain diverse types of data, from the types and amounts of foods being grown on U.S. farms to pest management practices to the economic impact of organic food production.

Surveys are not limited to the types of research just described and are used in many other types of research as well, both descriptive and causal.

This chapter introduces you to the basic principles involved in the survey process. The "Suggested Readings and Activities" list at the end of the chapter will lead you to more in-depth information.

SURVEY BASICS

Surveys can be useful *when*:

- You need information that is *not* readily available from other sources.
- You can clearly identify who you want to take the questionnaire.
- You can access a representative sample of that population.
- You define the research question and variables *before* writing your questionnaire. (This will help you focus your questions.)
- The questions you want to ask are mostly **closed-ended questions**—questions that have specific answers to choose from. Sometimes surveys will include free response questions, which are **open-ended questions** that allow respondents to fill in their own answers and provide more context than choosing from a set of specific responses. Surveys typically limit the number of open-ended questions because they can create a time burden for participants. If you are looking for in-depth responses to your questions, typically individual interviews or focus groups are going to be more appropriate.
- You want anonymous feedback so respondents are more candid. (This is only possible with self-administered questionnaires.)
- You do not have a lot of money to spend.

When questionnaires are completed independently, they can be a cost-effective way to obtain needed data, hearing from a larger number of people more quickly.

SURVEY METHODS

How surveys are delivered or administered to potential respondents, referred to as **survey methods**, vary and include these options:

- *Paper surveys* can be delivered to respondents via the mail. They also can be handed to individuals to complete.
- *Electronic surveys* are delivered to respondents and completed using computers, tablets, and sometimes cell phones.
- *Oral surveys* are completed with the help of an interviewer either on the phone or in person.

The advantages and disadvantages of each method are listed in **Table 13.1**. Keep in mind that more than one mode may be chosen to encourage respondents to answer in the format they find most comfortable.

Table 13.1 Advantages and Disadvantages of Different Survey Methods

Survey method	Advantages	Disadvantages
Paper Survey Sent Via Mail	Less expensive than giving survey directly to respondents or phone/face-to-face interviews. Possible to reach a larger group of respondents in a broad geographic location. No potential for interviewer bias. Respondents seem to be comfortable answering questions on sensitive topics because of anonymity. Easy to include incentives, such as money. May include visuals such as pictures.	Easy for respondents to ignore and throw out. Usually requires incentives and follow-up contacts to improve response. Respondent may wonder about how to fill out survey—the survey has to be self-explanatory and not too long. Open-ended questions often get brief responses. Subject to nonresponse bias, especially among people with low education.
Electronic Surveys	Least expensive to administer of all methods. Short length of data collection. Websites, such as SurveyMonkey, make it easy to collect and analyze data. Easier to make changes to questionnaire than printed version. Possible to reach a larger group of respondents in broad geographic location. No potential for interviewer bias. Questionnaire may include a variety of visual aids such as pictures, drop-down lists, etc.	Respondents must have a computer, Internet access, and the ability to navigate the software. Do not necessarily have a better response rate than mailed surveys. Researcher needs to be familiar with constructing computer questionnaires and using survey software to produce an accessible, understandable instrument. Survey cannot be too long; 10 minutes or less works best. Requires sending reminder messages to improve response. Easy for respondents to ignore. Respondents do not always feel anonymous. Subject to nonresponse bias, especially among people with lower education and minimal computer experience.
Telephone Survey	Interviewer establishes rapport so more questions are answered. Interviewer can answer questions if respondent is unsure about something. Response rate is usually better than mail or email. Length of questionnaire may be a little longer than mail or electronic survey. Can increase the number of completed questionnaires by contacting more people.	Cost is higher than mail or electronic survey, but less costly than face-to-face surveys. Each question and responses must be brief because only the interviewer can see the questionnaire. Interviewers must be thoroughly trained. Interviewer may introduce bias. Many potential respondents resent the request/phone calls and may use screening devices (caller ID) to avoid the call. More people have no landline phone, and cell phone surveys are more expensive and have lower response rates than landline phone surveys (Pew Research Center, 2015).

Table 13.1 Advantages and Disadvantages of Different Survey Methods (continued)		
Survey method	**Advantages**	**Disadvantages**
Face-to-Face Survey	Very good response rate; higher than for telephone interviews. Interviewer establishes rapport so more questions are answered. Interviewer can answer questions if respondent is unsure about something. Length of questionnaire may be longer than mail or electronic survey and can be more complex. Works well for complex questions and for open-ended questions.	Most expensive method. Time-consuming and can take about as long to collect data as a mail survey. Interviewers may introduce bias; therefore, interviewers must be trained to reduce potential for bias. Respondent may not be comfortable answering questions on sensitive topics. Respondent may tell interviewer what he/she thinks the interviewer wants to hear.

Sources: *Designing Surveys, A Guide to Decisions and Procedures* by J. Blair, R. F. Czaja, and E. A. Blair, 2014, Thousand Oaks, CA: Sage; *Survey Research Methods* (5th ed.), by F. J. Fowler, 2014, Thousand Oaks, CA: Sage; "Collecting Survey Data," by Pew Research Center, 2015, retrieved from http://www.pewresearch.org/methodology/u-s-survey-research/collecting-survey-data/.

The survey method you decide to use will depend on many factors, including these:

- Your budget will inform your choice. Certain methods, such as email or mail, are much cheaper to use.
- The characteristics of your respondents, such as do they use email, will they block calls for a phone interview, or will they mind an interview while waiting for a medical appointment? Also consider where they are located, your access to them, their language and literacy level, and their ability and willingness to participate.
- The complexity or length of the questionnaire may favor using interviewers rather than self-administered methods.
- The sensitivity of the information being requested may require more anonymous collection methods, such as mail.

Using one or perhaps two collection methods will ensure that you are collecting data from an appropriate sample.

Cross Sectional, Retrospective, and Longitudinal Surveys

Surveys can vary in terms of how frequently they are administered and to whom.

- A **cross-sectional survey** is administered at only one point in time.
- A **retrospective survey** is also administered at one point in time, but it asks respondents to report *past* behaviors, beliefs, events, and so forth.
- A **longitudinal survey** is administered more than once. There are several types:
  - A **repeated cross-sectional (or trend) survey** asks the same questions at several points in time to a new group of respondents each time. For example, NHANES uses questionnaires to obtain information on the health and nutritional status of Americans using a representative sample of about 5,000 people each year. Their research can show trends in supplement use over the years by asking a simple question, such as "Have you used or taken any vitamins, minerals, herbals or other dietary supplements in the past 30 days?"

- A **panel survey** also asks the same questions at different points in time—but to the *same* respondents. A study that uses a pretest and a posttest questionnaire is considered to be a panel survey. For example, Hand et al. (2014) used a 10-question survey (Family Nutrition and Physical Activity Screening Tool) before and after an intervention for low-income families to encourage healthy behaviors. Scores on the Family Nutrition and Physical Activity Screen Tool improved significantly after the intervention, showing that parents reported behavior changes.
- In a cohort study, the researcher surveys a group of people over time who have experienced a common event or starting point and then observes them for health changes. In some cohort studies, the researchers survey respondents about their lifestyle and health over time, and then analyze the way lifestyle factors correlate with their health. A **cohort survey** is used by the Nurses' Health Study, a cohort study started in 1976 that is the longest-running investigation of women's health issues. The survey for the current cohort, Nurses' Health Study 3, is completely web-based.

Table 13.2 summarizes types of surveys based on frequency of administration.

APPLICATION 13.1

Read the summary of this study and then answer the questions that follow.

Hand and Abram (2016) sent out more than 12,000 invitations via email for Registered Dietitian Nutritionists (RDNs) to participate in a survey during June/July 2014 and then again 6 months later. The survey asked RDNs to self-report their familiarity and use of evidence-based practice guidelines for prediabetes from different organizations including the Academy for Nutrition and Dietetics. During the time between surveys, the Academy announced publication of its Evidence-Based Nutrition Practice Guidelines for the Prevention of Diabetes in the Evidence Analysis Library. The authors wanted to know, in part, if RDNs would report using the new Academy guidelines before they were published. Measuring implementation of guidelines by health professionals in the field is difficult because we tend to offer the "right" answer—yes, we are using the guidelines—when it may not be true.

1. What other methods could researchers use to measure whether RDNs are indeed knowledgeable about and using evidence-based practice guidelines?
2. Why are surveys useful in this type of study?
3. Why was an electronic survey chosen for this study? What were its advantages and disadvantages?
4. What type of survey was this (cross-sectional, etc.)?

Table 13.2 Types of Surveys Based on When Administered

Retrospective Survey	Cross-Sectional Survey	Longitudinal Survey
Administered at one point in time, but it asks respondents to report *past* behaviors, beliefs, events, etc.	Administered at one point in time, useful to compare groups at a single point in time.	Administered more than once. 1. A *repeated cross-sectional (or trend) survey* asks the same questions at several points in time to a new group of respondents each time. 2. A *panel survey* asks the same questions at different points in time, but to the *same* respondents (for example pretest and posttest). 3. A *cohort survey* is completed by the same respondents at numerous points over a period of time. Some questions change from time to time.

Table 13.3 Steps in the Survey Process

1. Use the research questions and literature review to help you.
   A. Define the target population and survey objectives.
   B. Operationalize the research questions as survey items.
   C. Formulate possible hypotheses, and how you will test them.
2. Determine who will be sampled.
   A. Select a method of sample selection (probability or nonprobability-based).
   B. Create a sampling frame (if used).
   C. Determine a sample size.
   D. Select the sample.
3. Create and test the questionnaire (instrument).
   A. Choose the survey method: mail, Internet, telephone, face-to-face, other.
   B. Draft the questions.
   C. Design the questionnaire and cover letter.
   D. Pretest and revise the questionnaire (may include expert panel and cognitive interviews with the sample to assess content validity).
   E. Pilot test the questionnaire for reliability and validity.
4. Contact respondents and collect data.
   A. Prenotify respondents that the questionnaire is coming.
   B. Deliver/administer the cover letter and survey.
   C. Send reminders and follow-ups to reduce nonresponse.
   D. Send thank-you notes, and if applicable, compensation (e.g., raffle ticket) to those who completed the questionnaire.
5. Enter and analyze data.
6. Write up results and present/disseminate results.

Choosing a survey method and determining when, and how frequently, to administer the questionnaire are just parts of the survey process. **Table 13.3** shows the steps in the survey process.

PICK A SAMPLE

Before discussing how to pick a sample, it is important to learn about various errors and biases that can prevent you from obtaining an accurate picture of the population from your sample. First, **sampling error** (also called **sample variance**) happens when a characteristic from your sample does not match the population being sampled. In any sample, even when appropriately chosen, there will be chance variation. The best way to control for sampling error is to make sure you use a large enough sample size. Larger samples have a better chance of producing results closer to the real population.

Sample bias happens when the members of your sample are systematically different from the population in some way. It can occur due to:

- **Coverage bias.** This is when a segment of the population is excluded from the sample. For example, if the survey is online and a segment of your population does not have computers or computer skills, such as older or low-income individuals, you will be missing this segment in your results.
- **Selection bias.** This happens when some groups in the population have a higher or lower chance of being selected than others.
- **Nonresponse bias.** This occurs when the percentage of people who do not respond to the survey varies among the different groups in the sample. In other words, there might be a certain characteristic about individuals that makes them more or less likely to respond to your survey.

Sample bias does not improve if you increase the sample size. Getting the right information from the right people is more important than how many people are in your sample. To get the right people, you need to select a sample that fairly represents the entire population and obtain data from as much of the sample as possible.

Most researchers aim for a sample that is representative of the population of interest to get data that accurately reflects the population. To do so, you need to distinguish between the following terms.

- The **target population** refers to the people who are the focus of the study. For example, a population might be postmenopausal women with breast cancer. The target population is the group to whom you want to apply your results.
- The **accessible (source) population** is a subset of the target population to whom you can get access. It is crucial that the accessible population accurately reflects the target population. For a researcher studying postmenopausal breast cancer, a specific accessible population may be members of several cancer registries. A list of names of women with postmenopausal breast cancer from these registries are then called a **sampling frame**. A sampling frame is a list of members of the accessible population from which the sample is drawn.
- The **sample** includes the people from the accessible population who you have asked to participate. Keep in mind that some members of the sample may be eliminated if they do not completely meet the eligibility criteria for the study/survey.

Figure 13.1 displays these concepts.

Once the accessible population is identified, you can identify potential respondents in one of two ways: probability sampling or nonprobability sampling. In probability sampling, each person in the population has an equal probability or chance of being selected because the method for choosing respondents is random. Using probability sampling allows you to use probability-based statistics, such as hypothesis tests, with your data.

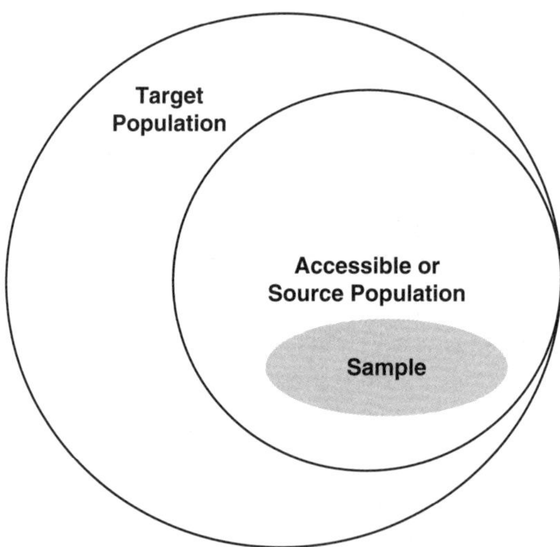

FIGURE 13.1 Target Population, Accessible Population, and the Sample.

PROBABILITY SAMPLING

These random probability methods may be used to pick a sample:

- **Simple random sampling**: randomly selecting individuals on a numbered list using either a table of random numbers or an online random sample generator. Using a table of random numbers can be cumbersome when you are seeking a larger sample.
- **Systematic random sampling**: selecting every *n*th individual from a list after a random start point, such as choosing every 35th person after starting with the 23rd person. The interval (every *n*th person) is determined by dividing the number in the sampling frame by the desired sample size.
- **Stratified random sampling**: dividing the accessible population into groups (based on age or gender, for example) and then using simple random sampling for each group (also called strata). The random sampling is usually, but not always, done proportionally so that more respondents are drawn from the larger strata.
- **Cluster random sampling**: dividing the population into clusters (such as geographic clusters), randomly picking some of the clusters, and then randomly sampling within each of those clusters.

Technologies such as random-digit dialing or random mail/email access make it easier to do random surveys.

Stratified sampling is useful for splitting the accessible population into groups (or strata) based on a factor that could influence the variable being measured—such as age, gender, or urban/rural location. Then you use simple random sampling within each group. It is only possible when you know what proportion of the population belongs to each group. Researchers use stratified sampling to make sure the sample accurately represents the different groups in the population.

In cluster sampling, the population is separated into groups called clusters, such as schools or nursing homes. Clusters are more or less alike, each resembling the overall population. Cluster sampling is useful when the population is widely distributed geographically and occurs in natural clusters. To use cluster sampling, the researcher randomly picks some clusters and then randomly obtains the sample from just those clusters. Cluster sampling is used to make sampling more practical or affordable.

TIP

Keep in mind that cluster sampling differs from stratified sampling in that cluster sampling only draws a sample from the randomly chosen clusters. With stratification, researchers draw a sample from *all* of the groups. See **Figure 13.2** for a graphic displaying this.

Many large national studies use **multistage sampling**. Multistage sampling refers to sampling plans in which the sampling is carried out in stages using smaller and smaller sampling units at each stage. In reality, cluster sampling is an example of multistage sampling because it involves at least two stages. In **multistage (multilevel) cluster sampling**, a large area, such as the United States, is first divided into smaller units, such as states, and some of these smaller units are randomly selected. In the second stage, the selected states are split into smaller units (such as counties), and a random

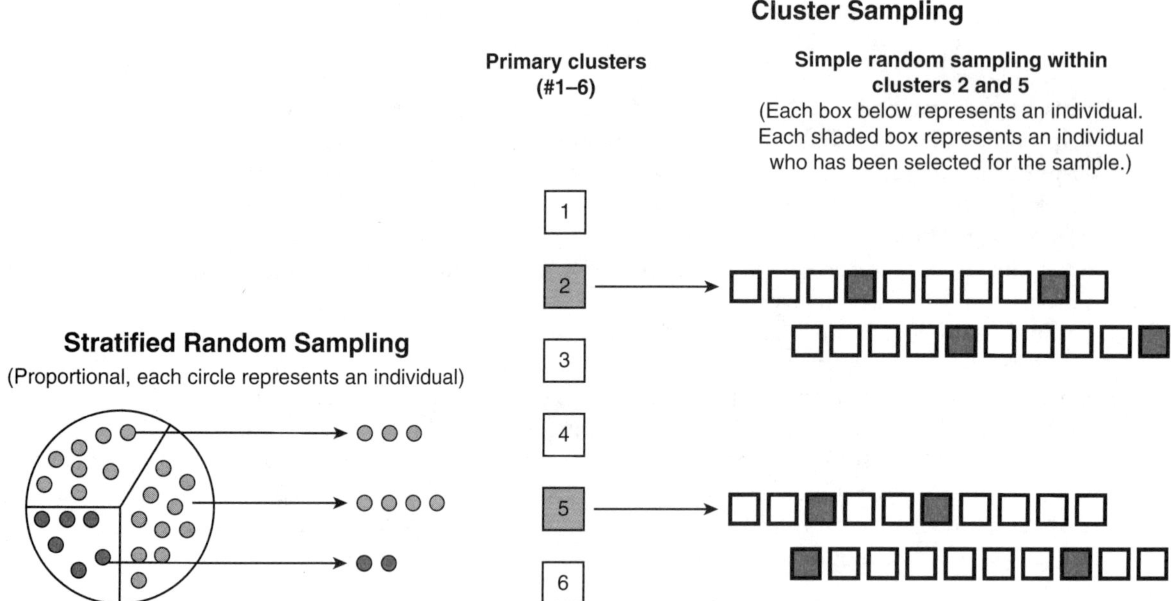

FIGURE 13.2 Stratified Random Sampling and Cluster Sampling

selection is made of counties within each state. In the third stage, a random selection is made of yet smaller areas (such as census tracts) of the counties. Often this yields an area that can be randomly sampled without being too big. **Table 13.4** provides examples of each probability sampling method.

NONPROBABILITY SAMPLING

Nonprobability sampling is based on respondents being selected by convenience or judgment. These methods are much less likely than probability samples to produce representative samples. Here are common nonprobability sampling methods.

- **Convenience sampling** is when members of the population are chosen simply because they are easy to reach and the researcher often has a comfort level asking them to complete a survey. It is the weakest form of sampling, but it is frequently used in research.
- **Quota sampling** is similar to convenience sampling, but quotas (limits) are placed on the number of people in the sample of a particular gender, age, race, or other characteristic. Often the quotas are based on the proportions found within the population: such as 50% male, 50% female. Researchers first identify the groups within the population and figure out how many should be drawn from each group, much like in stratified random sampling, only these respondents are not being drawn randomly.
- **Purposive or judgment sampling** is also a convenience sample, but in this case, the researchers choose respondents specifically based on whether the respondent is a good representative of the population.
- **Network (snowball) sampling** is used when locating respondents with the characteristics you want is difficult. Basically, when you find a few respondents who are appropriate for the study, you ask them to direct you to further potential

Table 13.4 Probability Sampling Methods with Examples

Probability Sampling Method	Examples
Simple random sampling (selecting individuals on a numbered list using either a table of random numbers or an online random sample generator) OR *Systematic random sampling* (selecting every *n*th individual from a list after a random start point)	Leong, Madden, Gray, Waters, and Horwath (2011) used a self-administered mail survey to collect data about the speed of eating and degree of obesity in New Zealand women aged 40 to 50 years old (*target population*). This age bracket was chosen because of the high prevalence of obesity and because women often gained weight at this time. The *accessible population* was female residents who were eligible to vote. A sample of 2,500 New Zealand women was randomly selected from the national electoral rolls (the *sampling frame*) using either simple or systematic random sampling (the study does not say which). The survey's response rate was 65.8%. Results showed that as BMI significantly increased so did self-reported speed of eating.
Stratified random sampling (dividing the accessible population into groups or strata and then using simple random sampling to select from each group)	Ritchie et al. (2015) conducted an online and mail survey of child care sites in California (*target population*) in 2012. The purpose was to determine if policies (one federal and one state) enacted since their prior survey (2008) had improved the quality of the beverages served to children aged 2 to 5 years. State databases of all licensed child care centers and family homes in California served as the *sampling frame*. The researchers randomly picked 1,484 child care sites—equal numbers from each of six categories (or *strata*): Head Start, state preschool, etc. The survey's response rate was 31%. Results showed improvements in the serving of healthy beverages from 2008 to 2012.
Cluster random sampling (dividing the population into clusters, such as geographic clusters, randomly picking some of the clusters, and then randomly sampling within each of those clusters)	A researcher wanted to learn whether Latinos in an urban setting use and understand the Nutrition Facts label. The Latino area of the city was split into 16 clusters of similar population size. Five of the clusters were randomly chosen. Next, 150 households were randomly selected within each cluster. Interviewers asked for the adult most involved in food purchasing and preparation to be surveyed in each household. (This is a simple two-stage cluster sample.)
Multistage cluster sampling (using cluster sampling that is carried out in stages using smaller and smaller sampling units at each stage)	NHANES (2011–2014) used a four-stage sample design. In the first stage, counties were randomly chosen (in some cases counties were combined to keep them big enough). In the second stage, a random selection was made of census blocks (or combinations of blocks) within the selected counties. In the third stage, households (or dwelling units) were selected, and in the fourth stage a person within the household was selected. In each stage, the rates required for sampling individuals were based on sex, age, race, Hispanic origin, and income. Hispanics were oversampled because more reliable information was needed for this population group (Johnson, Dohrmann, Burt, & Mohadjer, 2014).

respondents. So the first few respondents are picked using purposive sampling, then the remaining respondents are picked using network or snowball sampling. This method is more often used in qualitative studies rather than in quantitative studies.

The data from nonprobability sampling may not be representative of the population and is often prone to selection bias and sampling error. **Table 13.5** provides examples of each type of nonprobability sampling.

Table 13.5 Nonprobability Sampling Methods with Examples

Nonprobability Sampling Methods	Example
Convenience sampling (when members of the population are chosen simply because they are easy to reach and the researcher may have a comfort level asking them to complete a survey)	Algert, Baameur, and Renvall (2014) surveyed 83 gardeners using community gardens in San Jose, California, including what vegetables they grew in their gardens. The gardeners were recruited from four community gardens. Ten of the 83 gardeners also weighed the output of their gardens from spring through summer. Results showed that their crop yields were higher than conventional agriculture, and the gardeners saved about $435/plot on vegetable purchases (after expenses for seed, etc.).
Quota sampling (determine the groups within the population and figure out how many should be drawn from each group, which is done using convenience sampling)	Iglesia et al. (2015) conducted a cross-sectional survey in 13 countries to describe total fluid intake in children and adolescents and how it varies by age and sex. In some countries, the sample was selected using quota sampling. The quotas were based on age, sex, region of the country, habitat, and socioeconomic characteristics. Results showed that many children and adolescents are at risk of inadequate fluid intake, especially males and adolescents.
Purposive sampling (when researchers choose respondents based on whether or not the respondent is a good representative of the population)	Patel, Kennedy, Blickem, Reeves, and Chew-Graham (2016) conducted interviews with British South Asian adults with diabetes living in Greater Manchester, U.K. The purpose was to explore their beliefs and practices on managing diabetes when they spent the holidays (often several months) in the Indian subcontinent. Some of the respondents were purposely recruited from mosques, religious classes, and Muslim day centers to obtain a broad sample. Results showed that some respondents did not continue their medication on holiday, which suggests a poor understanding of diabetes.
Network or snowball sampling (when researchers find a few good respondents and then ask them to direct you to other potential respondents)	Doub, Small, and Birch (2015) examined child feeding beliefs and practices, types of recipes, and their associations in food blogs written by mothers of preschoolers. They used an initial sample of 100 blogs to find further blog recommendations—a snowball sample of 168 blogs, of which 8 were included in the study. Results showed that blogs often described involving children in food preparation and preparing foods that children readily accept. (Note: This example shows how snowball sampling was used to find blogs that were evaluated using a survey tool, not to find respondents.)

Here is some advice for picking your sample.

1. Use probability sampling as much as possible. It is not unusual to use both probability and nonprobability sampling together. For example, if you are doing a face-to-face survey involving nursing homes and know you are limited geographically, consider developing a sampling frame, a list of nursing homes in the area. Then use a random number table to help you randomly pick nursing homes from your list. Make sure you have variety and diversity in your sample.
2. Work hard to get responses from as many people in your sample as possible; this will minimize nonresponse bias.
3. Include all groups to minimize coverage bias.
4. Know the limitations of your sample, and be sure to include these limitations, along with a thorough description of how the sample was picked, in your research paper.

Even without a perfect sample, your data is probably quite usable.

Sample Size and Power Analysis

Before you choose a sample, you need to know how many respondents you will need—in other words, your **sample size**. Determining an appropriate sample size can be complicated, and you should consult a statistician, but here are some basics you need to know.

In a descriptive study, you may want to estimate a population parameter (such as a Healthy Eating Index score for adolescents with type I diabetes) using survey data. Sample size is based on confidence level, confidence intervals, and the size of the target population.

- The **confidence level** is a percent and is usually set at 95%, sometimes at 99%.
- **Confidence intervals** are constructed at a confidence level, such as 95%. You will need to know the width of the expected confidence interval.

You also need to have an estimate of the mean outcome.

Sample size calculators are available online, and several are listed at the end of the chapter under "Suggested Readings and Activities." Another factor that can affect sample size is response distribution, or the percentage of participants who pick each answer. Normally you should use the worst case percentage (50%) as this will require a higher sample size.

If your survey data is from two or more groups or subgroups, and is being used in a correlational, quasi-experimental, or experimental study, the deciding factor for sample size is power. **Power** refers to the ability of a study to detect statistically significant differences or relationships in the groups when they really do exist. In other words, the power of a hypothesis test is the probability of rejecting the null hypothesis when you should reject it. To have enough power in a study, you need to do a **power analysis** to calculate the minimum sample size needed to detect the difference you are looking for. In general, *increasing sample size increases power*. A power analysis is used for experimental, quasi-experimental, and correlational studies.

First, let's review a few key statistical concepts.

- Alpha (α) is the probability of a type I error.
- Beta (β) is the probability of a type II error.
- The quantity $1 - \beta$ is the power of a test (the probability of *avoiding* a type II error).

In a power analysis, power is normally set at 80%, which means there is a 20% chance of *failing to observe a difference when there is one* (a type II error).

Power analysis uses the relationships among the following factors to determine sample size (Grove, Burns, & Gray, 2013):

- *The level of significance being used—the alpha level.* Often the alpha level is set at 0.05 or lower—meaning that the chance making a Type I error is 1 in 20 or lower. If you want to use a level of 0.01, you need a much larger sample size.
- *The power level* is usually set at 0.80, so there is a 20% chance of a type II error. You may wonder why the type I error is set a lot lower than the type II error. This is because *making a type I error is more serious than making a type II error.* You don't want to disseminate results that say a treatment or intervention was successful when it really was not.
- *The expected effect size* is the magnitude or size of the difference between the groups. For example, if a study showed that the Healthy Eating Index of the experimental group was 65/100 and the control group was 54/100, the difference between the groups is 11. The effect size is often estimated by taking the

difference between the two groups and dividing it by the standard deviation of the participants. If the result is between 0.3 and 0.5, the effect size would be considered moderate (although it varies depending on the context and other factors). For a power analysis, you need to look at previous studies (if available) to see what the difference might be between the groups. The smaller the effect size, the larger the necessary sample size because it will be harder to detect. If the effect size is fairly large, you do not need as large a sample. Researchers often use a value of 0.5 for effect size because it indicates a moderate to large difference.

- *The sample size.*

When working with a statistician or using a power or sample size program, you will be expected to provide information on the effect size as well as the level of type I and type II error that you are willing to accept. Other factors to consider are the type of study, number of variables, expected standard deviation, method of data analysis, and sample design.

Doing a power analysis enables you to determine whether the available sample is adequate to answer your research questions and to detect important effects or associations. When sample size is too small, you run the risk of concluding that the groups were not different when in fact they were (type II error). If you need a sample of, let's say, 1,100 people, you will need to include more than that in your initial sample to account for attrition. For more information on calculating sample size, consult Boushey (2008) and Hulley, Cummings, Browner, and Grady (2013). Sample size calculators are available online, and some are noted at the end of the chapter under "Suggested Readings and Activities."

TIP

When reading survey data from two or more groups in a correlational, quasi-experimental, or experimental study, look in the Methods section for information on whether and how a power analysis was performed. For example, Kullen, Iredale, Prvan, and O'Connor (2015) used a survey to evaluate the general nutrition knowledge of members of the Australian Regular Army (a convenience sample, split up by occupation within the Army) and Australian civilians. Because there were no previous studies in this area, the authors did a pilot study to gain some knowledge about the effect size. They describe how they calculated sample size: "It was determined that to observe a difference of 10% in total GNKQ (General Nutrition Knowledge Questionnaire) score between groups at $\alpha = .05$ and power of 80%, a minimum of 68 respondents was required in each group" (Kullen et al., 2015, p. 253).

APPLICATION 13.2

Identify the type of sampling used in each of these studies and explain why you chose your answer.

Study 1: Garza, Ding, Owensby, and Zizza (2016) used a survey to examine "the association between impulsivity and consumption of fast food among middle-aged employed adults in a region with high rates of obesity and diabetes" (p. 62). They also asked why they chose to eat at fast food restaurants. Respondents were recruited via email to all employees of a large university in the southeastern United States.

Study 2: The target population for the Minnesota Heart Study is the Minneapolis–St. Paul metropolitan area. For the study, this area was separated into geographic regions that have approximately equal number of households. A certain number of regions were randomly selected. Then within each region, 5% of households were randomly selected. An interviewer called each household.

CONSTRUCT AND REFINE THE COVER LETTER AND QUESTIONNAIRE

WRITE A COVER LETTER

For both written and emailed questionnaires, you need a cover letter to encourage respondents to take your survey. When the survey is introduced properly, the response rate is better, so you can really think of the cover letter as a marketing tool. Dillman, Smyth, and Christian (2014) and Blair, Czaja, and Blair (2014) recommend the following items be included in the cover letter.

1. What the study is about and why it is important (especially if there are any benefits to the respondent).
2. Why the respondent is important to the study and how he or she was selected.
3. The voluntary nature of respondent participation and promise of confidentiality (meaning the respondent is not associated with his or her answers).
4. The incentive you may be providing for participation.
5. An estimate of the time to complete the questionnaire with directions to complete and return the survey.
6. A phone number and person's name for the respondent to call with questions.

Printed cover letters should be on official letterhead and signed. To make the cover letter quick and easy to read, keep it to one page and use bullet points where appropriate.

The cover letter is *separate* from an informed consent document. Studies using surveys must be approved beforehand by the appropriate Institutional Review Board, and appropriate consent forms must be used.

WRITE QUESTIONS

Initially you want to develop a pool of questions. Because some questions will be eliminated during this process, it is a good idea to start with a large pool. Before writing questions, check your literature review to see whether other researchers have measured any of the concepts you want to measure. There is no point is reinventing the wheel, especially if someone else has tested the questions for validity and reliability (although you will likely test them again because they were modified or it had been a long time since they were last validated). Of course, you still have to consider whether these questions are appropriate for your research goals as well ask for permission.

Questions can measure many concepts, including knowledge, attitudes, opinions, personal attributes, or behaviors (such as eating behaviors). Questions can be asked in one of two ways: open-ended or closed-ended. Open-ended questions allow respondents to respond to questions in their own words. If the respondent is being interviewed, the interviewer writes down the entire answer. Closed-ended (fixed-alternative) questions give respondents specific answers from which to choose.

Questions are most often closed-ended, in large part because they require less time for respondents to complete. For the researcher, closed-ended questions are easy to quantify, enter into statistical analysis software, and analyze. Close-ended questions are also subject to less interviewer bias. However, closed-ended questions are harder to write than open-ended questions. As a researcher, you have to construct quality close-ended questions and test them many times before using them in a survey.

Because open-ended questions are not restrictive, they can yield more and richer information, especially when respondents express themselves well. Answering open-ended questions does require more time than close-ended questions, so too many open-ended or free responses questions will make a survey too long. For the researcher, answers to open-ended questions need to be read, interpreted, and coded (put into categories) before the results can be analyzed, so the process is more time-consuming. Another disadvantage is that there can be errors/bias in how open-ended answers are interpreted and coded.

When writing the questions, it is important to carefully consider the possible respondents so the questionnaire is understandable and easy to use. Here are some questions to help you determine whether your questions need some work.

1. Does the question measure something directly related to one of the research questions?
2. Will most respondents understand the question as it is intended?
3. Is the question brief, free of bias, and free of double negatives?
4. Is only one question posed? (Avoid double-barreled questions such as "Do you know how to find and interpret scientific studies?" Trying to measure two things at once will not yield accurate answers.)
5. Will most respondents be willing to answer the question?
6. Are specific time references included for questions that require recall?
7. Will most respondents have the information to answer the question?
8. Do all respondents need to answer this question?
9. Does the question provide a list of acceptable responses?
10. Are the response categories both comprehensive and mutually exclusive (the response options do not overlap or conflict)?

Sometimes it may be appropriate to check the readability level of the questions, which can often be done using word processing software.

WRITE RESPONSES

The choice of response format depends on the question and the information you want to collect. **Table 13.6** shows some possible closed-ended response formats with examples. The type of response format you use can affect how respondents answer the question, so you need to give it a lot of thought. Also, your answer choices should anticipate all possibilities.

A number of response formats use **scales**, a set of possible answers representing ordered points on a continuum. You are probably familiar with the Likert scale, which asks respondents to indicate their level of agreement with a number of statements using an ordinal (ranked) scale from Strongly Agree (1), Agree (2), Neither Agree nor Disagree (3), Disagree (4) to Strongly Disagree (5). Notice how the scale is balanced, with two "agree" types of statements and two "Disagree" types of statements. The **Likert scale** (or Likert-type scales) is useful for measuring opinions, attitudes, and feelings—constructs that are not observable. To be a true Likert scale, a question would have these features (Uebersax, 2006):

1. Several target statements are given (see Table 13.6 for an example).
2. Response choices (from Strongly Disagree to Strongly Agree) are arranged horizontally and anchored with numbers (usually 1 through 5).
3. The middle choice is "Neither Agree nor Disagree," which is neutral.

Table 13.6 Types of Response Formats for Close-Ended Questions

Types of close-ended response formats	Examples
Dichotomous (Respondent must choose one response from two choices.)	Do you currently take multivitamins? • Yes • No
Checklist (Respondent may choose more than one response.)	Which of the following beverages are available at lunch in the cafeteria? • Sugar sweetened beverages (soda, sweetened iced tea, etc.) • Diet beverages (diet sodas, diet iced teas, etc.) • Water • Whole or reduced-fat milk • Chocolate milk • Low-fat or nonfat milk • Milkshakes • Other (please specify)__________________
Likert Scale (Respondent chooses a level of agreement with a list of statements using the ordinal scale shown.)	1 Strongly Agree 2 Agree 3 Neither Agree Nor Disagree 4 Disagree 5 Strongly Disagree 1. I am confident about my nutritional knowledge. 2. I know where to get nutrition information. 3. I am comfortable that I have the nutritional information needed to care for my children.
Traditional Ordinal Rating Scale (The respondent evaluates an attribute by choosing one of several ordered choices.)	How would you judge the availability of healthy foods in the school cafeteria? Excellent ☐ Good ☐ Fair ☐ Poor ☐ Very Poor ☐
Verbal Frequency Scale (The respondent chooses how often he or she has undertaken an action.)	How many multivitamins do you take per week? ☐ 2 or less ☐ 3 – 5 ☐ 6 – 9 ☐ 10 or more
Rank Order Scale (The respondent ranks items in a list, usually starting with 1 being the first choice, 2 being the second choice, and so on.)	Rank each physical activity in the order of your preferences. (1 = most preferred, 5 = least preferred) A. Walking ____ B. Biking ____ C. Swimming _____ D. Organized Sport _____ E. Going to the Gym _____
Semantic Differential Scale (Respondent checks a space on a line scale that has polar opposite statements at the two ends of the scale. A 7-point scale is commonly used, and numbers (1–7) could be used as anchors.	Depressed ___:___:___:___:___:___:___: Cheerful 1 2 3 4 5 6 7

(*continues*)

Table 13.6 Types of Response Formats for Close-Ended Questions (continued)

Types of close-ended response formats	Examples
Visual Analog Scales (VAS) (Respondent makes a mark along a line anchored by terms describing opposite values of a subjective dimension. The line used should measure 100 mm in length (so researchers can score it from 0 to 100.)	Depressed ________________X___Cheerful
Hedonic Scale (A sensory evaluation scale rating food characteristics such as flavor or texture, from "like extremely" to "dislike extremely.")	Sample 76 Sample 90 Cake Color ________ ________ Cake Tenderness ________ ________ Cake Flavor ________ ________ Scale: 9 = Like extremely 8 = Like very much 7 = Like moderately 6 = Like slightly 5 = Neither like nor dislike 4 = Dislike slightly 3 = Dislike moderately 2 = Dislike very much 1 = Dislike extremely
Nonverbal Hedonic Scale for Children (A sensory evaluation scale using smiley faces that children can use to communicate how much they like a food.)	Source: "Evaluation of a Pictorial Method to Assess Liking of Familiar Fruits and Vegetables Among Preschool Children," by V. Carraway-Stage, H. Spangler, M. Borgres, and L. S. Goodell, 2014, *Appetite, 75*, p. 16. Copyright 2014 by Elsevier. Reprinted with permission.

When using a scale, a midpoint such as "Neutral" or "Neither Agree Nor Disagree" is sometimes used. When a midpoint is available, survey research shows that quite a few respondents choose it. Blair, Czaja, and Blair (2014) recommend using a midpoint if you think a sizable number of respondents do not feel strongly about the statement. If you use the midpoint in a question, Bradburn, Sudman, and Wansink (2004) have found that "it does not usually change the ratio of support to opposition" (p. 142). In addition to a neutral point, some researchers like to add "Not sure" to some questions to discourage random guessing. To discourage skipped questions, you may want to use "Prefer to not answer" as a response. The length of a questionnaire can affect your response rate. The shorter the questionnaire, the more likely it will be completed, so make every question count.

Sequence the Questions

How you sequence the questions in the questionnaire can affect whether a respondent gets frustrated and completes the questionnaire, or whether his or her answers have been influenced by earlier questions. Here are some guidelines:

- The first few questions should be easy to answer, engaging, and connected to the survey purpose. You want to build interest and rapport with the respondent. The first question is most important because it has the power to get people to complete, or toss, the questionnaire.
- The questionnaire needs to be well organized with appropriate section headings and similar questions grouped together—this makes it easier for the respondents to focus on one area at a time.
- When testing knowledge or ability, arrange items from easy to difficult to build confidence.
- Go from general questions to more specific ones.
- Ensure that earlier questions do not affect how respondents answer later questions. For example, if respondents see two questions as related, they may answer both questions similarly.
- Any questions dealing with sensitive issues should be toward the end of the questionnaire and placed after neutral questions.
- Some researchers put demographic questions at the end so respondents do not get bored and not finish the questionnaire.

Lay Out the Questionnaire

When laying out your questionnaire, remember to start with an introduction that includes instructions and a brief thanks and as well as how to hand it in at the end.

1. Headings and subheadings act as road signs. Use color with your headings and subheadings to help respondents navigate easily through the questionnaire.
2. Number all questions and number all pages. For online surveys, use a progress bar to indicate the number of questions or sections remaining.
3. Use a larger size font (such as 14 points) and an easy-to-read font.
4. Avoid words in all capital letters. When all capitals are used, words take a similar rectangular form and become more difficult to read.
5. Use contrast between question stems and responses by making the questions a little larger in size (or bolded) and having the responses a little smaller.
6. The right-hand margin should not be justified as this leaves unexplained spaces between words that make text harder to read.
7. The use of white space is important to reduce clutter and increase user-friendliness. Where margins are set determines in part the amount of white space.
8. For a paper questionnaire, make sure the color of the paper provides high contrast with the ink and that the paper is low-gloss or no-gloss to decrease glare.
9. Be consistent in your layout and design elements.
10. Any pictures and illustrations should be simple, clear, realistic, and be placed in the right spot to reinforce the content.

The Online Survey Design Guide is an excellent resource for designing Web-based survey instruments (www.lap.umd.edu/survey_design/).

PRETEST THE QUESTIONNAIRE

Pretesting your questionnaire on individuals similar to your respondent population (preferably) as well as other students or faculty is a *must*! You need to get feedback on the clarity of the questions, usefulness of the response options, and how user-friendly the whole questionnaire is. Keep in mind that **pretesting** the questionnaire is not the same as pilot testing. Pretesting is always preliminary to pilot testing. Pilot testing is a full-dress-rehearsal of the survey in actual field conditions.

Some researchers use **cognitive interviews** to get feedback and to assess face validity. Carbone, Campbell, and Honess-Morreale (2002) describe cognitive interviews as "asking the target population to describe all the thoughts, feelings, and ideas that come to mind when examining specific questions or messages and to provide suggestions to clarify wording as needed" (p. 690). There are two main types of cognitive interviews: think-aloud and probing. Using the think-aloud method, each respondent is asked to think out loud about what comes to mind when answering questions—from understanding the question, recalling the information to answer the question, deciding if the information is relevant to the question, picking the best answer for a closed-ended question, to explaining a written answer for an open-ended question. The interviewer asks questions as appropriate, such as "Can you tell me more about what you meant when you said that the question_____?"

When using the probing method, the interviewer probes the respondent after answering a question or at natural breaks to allow the respondent to maintain a train of thought while decreasing interruptions. The interviewer can either record the session or make notes during it. Cognitive interviews are always completed individually.

Cognitive interviewing is useful for reducing response error, which can happen when respondents interpret the question in different ways. Cognitive interviewing has

APPLICATION 13.3

Each of these survey questions and/or responses has faults. Identify the problems and then rewrite the question and/or responses.

1. Did you eat breakfast yesterday? ___ Yes ___ No
2. Please rate the instructor from 1 (most negative) to 4 (most positive). ______
3. Do you work full-time or part-time? ________
4. Do most of your meals include vegetables? ___ Yes ____ No
5. From which source do you get most of your nutrition information?
   __ radio
   __ television
   __ magazines
   __ while at home
6. How concerned are you that you will get breast cancer?
   __ Very concerned
   __ Somewhat concerned
   __ Slightly concerned
   __ Not at all concerned
7. Trying to diet and exercise to lose weight is hard.
   Strongly Agree Agree Disagree Always Disagree
8. How often do you eat spinach?
   Daily Weekly Monthly

Table 13.7 Pretesting Checklist

1. How long does the survey take to complete?
2. Did the time to complete the survey vary widely among the test respondents?
3. Are the instructions for each section clear and unambiguous?
4. Do the different sections flow reasonably from one to the next?
5. Are the questions within each section logically ordered?
6. Are all questions necessary to meet your survey objectives?
7. Are the questions and response options easy to understand and concise?
8. Are the questions measuring what they are intended to measure?
9. Are examples and foods relevant for individuals of other cultures?
10. Are there questions that made respondents feel uncomfortable, annoyed, or confused?

been used to refine many surveys, including food frequency questionnaires and diet recalls used in national surveys.

Additional methods for pretesting surveys are individual debriefing and group debriefing. In **individual debriefing**, a respondent takes the survey in its entirety. Once completed, the researcher goes through each question with the respondent and asks open-ended questions to get feedback on what was helpful, what was confusing, and so on. In **group debriefing**, a group of respondents complete the questionnaire and then sit together for a focus group discussion of the instrument. The researcher can see which issues may be larger or smaller by observing how many respondents chime in on them.

Table 13.7 is a checklist that can be used to make sure you are getting the most out of the pretesting process.

Pretesting is useful to ascertain face validity. You also need a panel of experts to look at a questionnaire's content validity to ensure that it contains everything it should and is not missing anything. These are both discussed in the next section. **Figure 13.3** is a summary of this section.

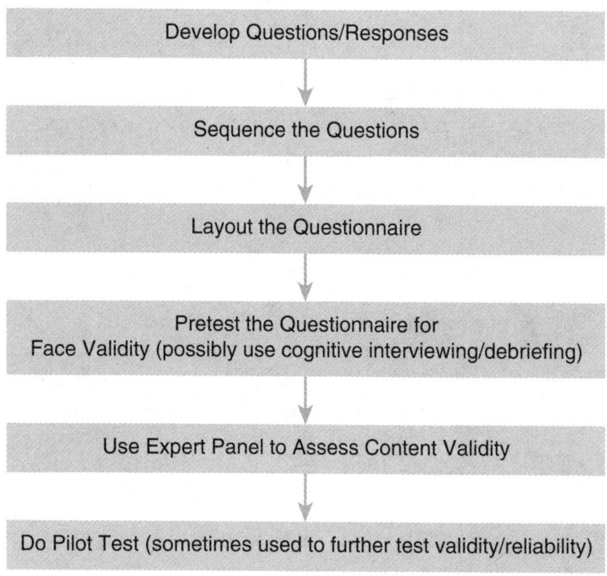

FIGURE 13.3 Steps in Developing and Testing the Questionnaire

TEST THE RELIABILITY AND VALIDITY OF A SURVEY

Reliability and **validity** are important because they tell you about the quality and believability of your questionnaire (or any instrument you are using to measure something). A questionnaire is reliable if it obtains consistent results on repeated trials. When you see "reliability" in research, think "repeatability." A reliable instrument gives consistent results. Consider the SAT, for example; it is reliable because a student who takes it twice within a year will have a similar score (as long as the student did not change how he or she prepared for it). Validity is important too. Your questionnaire is only valid if it accurately measures the constructs it is supposed to measure. In other words, a valid questionnaire improves the likelihood that your results accurately represent what is being studied. For example, the SAT is considered a valid test because the higher score you get, the higher your GPA during the first year of college.

RELIABILITY

These are some ways to test whether a survey is reliable or consistent over time.

1. **Test-retest reliability** (also known as stability reliability) is measured by having the same respondents take the *same survey at two different times* to see how consistent or stable their answers are (**Figure 13.4**). If the respondents take the questionnaire just a few days apart, they often just repeat the same answers. If they take the questionnaire again after a long period of time, some things may have changed for them and they may answer some questions differently. The optimal time period between measurements may depend on characteristics of the participants, variability of the variables being measured, or other relevant factors.

   For questions with interval or ratio answers, such as the number of teaspoons of salt used in cooking, Pearson's correlation coefficient is used to assess test-retest reliability. For ordinal answers, such as ranking something, the Spearman nonparametric rank correlation coefficient could be used. A correlation coefficient of at least 0.70 to 0.80 is generally considered good (r value can range from 0.00 to 1.00). You can also assess the test-retest reliability of a continuous variable by using a paired t-test. For categorical variables, you could simply calculate the percentage of times the test-retest scores are in agreement.

   Many researchers prefer to use the intraclass correlation coefficient (ICC) instead of Pearson's correlation coefficient. Pearson's correlation coefficient measures linear trends between two measures, but it does not measure agreement.

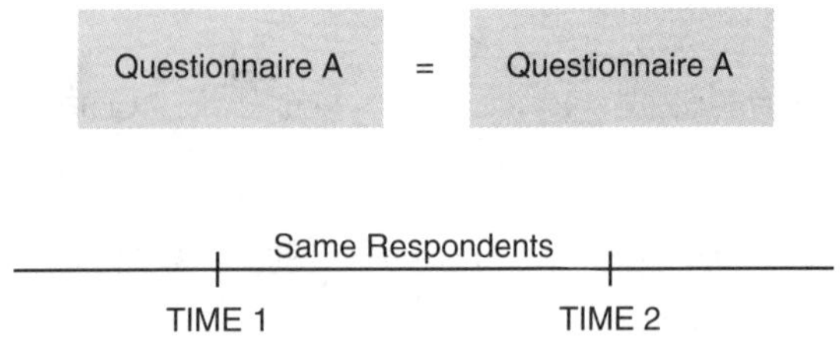

FIGURE 13.4 Test-retest reliability. The same respondents take the same test at two separate points in time.

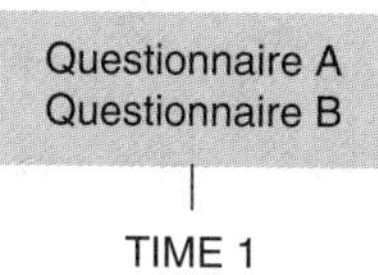

FIGURE 13.5 Parallel forms reliability. One set of respondents take different questionnaires at the same time.

The ICC (there are several types) assesses the *agreement* between the results of the two questionnaires, so it is a better indicator for test-retest reliability. Similar to the Pearson's correlation coefficient, if the ICC is 0.70 or higher, the measure is considered reliable.

2. **Equivalence reliability** looks at whether measurements from two versions of a test *or* from two observers observing the same event are consistent. When researchers develop *two tests with different questions that address the same constructs*, this is called **parallel forms reliability**. When repeated measurements are collected from the same subjects in a study, two tests can improve the study design. Parallel forms reliability can be tested by administering the two tests/surveys at the same time to one group of people (**Figure 13.5**). The scores between the tests are then correlated to evaluate the consistency of results across alternate versions. A coefficient of 0.80 or higher is desirable.

   Inter-rater reliability measures the *consistency of two or more raters (not the people taking the survey)* who have to, for example, categorize answers to open-ended questions or observe and record an event (as in a qualitative study). Inter-rater reliability is used to test how similarly raters (or observers) categorize, score, or simply measure something. You can use the same statistical tools to measure inter-rater reliability that were used in measuring test-retest reliability, including the ICC. A rating closer to 0.90 (or 90%) is desirable for inter-rater reliability.

3. **Internal consistency reliability** (or inter-item reliability) looks at *how well different questions measuring the same construct produce similar results*. Testing internal consistency requires less money and time than test-retest or parallel forms reliability, and it may be used by some researchers to estimate reliability. To use it, you administer the questions to a group of people on one occasion. Each question measuring the same construct should be highly correlated to show internal consistency. Cronbach's alpha coefficient is the most common internal consistency reliability coefficient, and it is used for interval and ratio level data. It ranges from 0.00 (no internal consistency) to 1.00 (perfect internal consistency). The higher the coefficient, the more internally consistent the questions. If Cronbach's alpha coefficient is 0.80, it indicates the test is 80% reliable with 20% random error (DeVon et al., 2007). A coefficient of 0.80 or higher is desirable, and a reliability coefficient less than 0.60 is considered low.

See **Table 13.8** for examples of each form of reliability. Reliability is necessary for validity—the next topic.

VALIDITY

Validity looks at whether the survey accurately measures what it is intended to measure. There are various types of validity (**Table 13.9**). Face and content validity are the assessments used most often—in part because they are easier to accomplish—and they

Table 13.8 Forms of Reliability: Definitions and Examples

Forms of reliability	Examples
Test-Retest Reliability "Extent to which repeated measurements of the same concept for a given individual will be similar to one another" (Gleason, Harris, Sheean, Boushey, & Bruemmer, 2010, p. 410).	Francis and Stevenson (2012) assessed the reliability and validity of a short dietary questionnaire designed to assess dietary intake of saturated fat and free sugars. Participants included students at an Australian college. Twenty-nine students took the questionnaire at two different times approximately 158 days apart. The intraclass correlation coefficient between scores at first and second administration was 0.83, which indicates good reliability.
Parallel Forms Reliability The extent to which two versions of the same tests are equivalent.	Boeckner, Pullen, Walker, Abbott, and Block (2002) tested parallel forms reliability of the 1998 Block Health Habits and History Questionnaire. In this study, the two forms used had the same content; however one was administered as a paper form and the other as an online form (with different presentation). Each participant took both forms, and Pearson correlations were used to assess agreement between the two forms on an individual level. When comparing the two forms, the researchers concluded there was adequate reliability.
Inter-Rater Reliability "Extent to which different raters or observers of a given measure come up with the same value of the measure for a given case; also known as inter-observer reliability" (Gleason et al., 2010, p. 410).	Falbe, Kenney, Henderson, and Schwartz (2011) developed and tested the Wellness Child Care Assessment Tool (WCCAT) for validity and reliability. Trained raters used the WCCAT to score the comprehensiveness and strength of written nutrition and physical activity polices at 94 child care centers in Connecticut (all participated in the Child and Adult Care Food Program). A random sample of 18 policies coded by the same two raters were used to determine inter-rater reliability. The scores each rater assigned for the comprehensiveness and strength scores (overall and also for each of five subscales) were used to calculate correlation coefficients. Interrater reliability for all scores was high (intraclass correlation coefficients of 0.84 to 0.99).
Internal Consistency Reliability The extent to which different questions measuring the same construct produce similar results.	Takeuchi, Edlefsen, McCurdy, and Hillers (2006) developed a survey to assess consumers' readiness to use a food thermometer when cooking small cuts of meat. Two of the questions were designed to do the same thing: categorize participants into stages of change regarding thermometer use. One question used a simple format, and the other was more detailed and complex. The researchers kept both questions in the questionnaire when it was pilot tested to determine which question more accurately classified participants into the appropriate stage. Results showed that the detailed question more accurately classified participants ($\alpha = 0.73$).

are useful for reducing the chances of bias. However, criterion and construct validity are also critical.

1. **Face validity**. Establishing a questionnaire's credibility often starts with face validity. The survey questions are reviewed by untrained judges, such as people similar to your potential respondents (although sometimes researchers ask content experts to look at face validity). They are asked to judge (subjectively) whether the format, questions, and procedures are clear and easy to use, and whether the survey measures what it is supposed to measure.

Table 13.9 Forms of Validity: Definitions and Examples

Forms of validity	Example
Face Validity "Extent to which a measure appears to most observers to capture the concept it is intended to reflect" (Gleason et al., 2010, p. 410).	Anderson, Must, Curtin, and Bandini (2012) developed a questionnaire to assess family mealtime environments and child mealtime behaviors. The questionnaire was designed to be completed by the parent/guardian of a children between 3 and 11.9 years old. It was initially pretested with 10 parents to identify design or wording issues. After revision, the interdisciplinary research team also reviewed it for face validity.
Content Validity "Extent to which a measure covers all dimensions present in the concept it is intended to reflect" (Gleason et al., 2010, p. 410).	Whelan et al. (2013) developed a survey to measure research involvement among Registered Dietitians in the United Kingdom. Six experts rated each survey item in terms of its relevance. A content validity index was developed by coming up with a proportion of the number of reviewers who rated the item as *quite relevant* or *very relevant* to the total number of reviewers. The content validity index for the entire survey was 0.92 (recommended minimum is 0.90).
Criterion Validity "Any type of validity based on a comparison of a test measure to a criterion intended to reflect the exact value of the concept the measure is intended to reflect" (Gleason et al., 2010, p. 410).	Boucher et al. (2006) asked respondents to take an adaptation of Block's food frequency questionnaire (FFQ), and also asked the same respondents to take two 24-hour diet recalls via telephone. The researchers evaluated the agreement of 32 nutrient intakes between the adapted FFQ and the diet recalls for each respondent. Correlation coefficients showed moderate to high validity.
Construct Validity An experimental demonstration that a test measure is measuring the construct that it is intended to measure.	Cooke, Nietfeld, and Goodell (2015) developed the Childhood Obesity Prevention Self-Efficacy Survey (COP-SE) which measures medical students' self-efficacy in skills needed to prevent and treat childhood obesity. The pilot survey of 43 items was administered to 444 medical students. The exploratory factor analysis revealed a two-factor structure: Factor 1 (10 items) assesses self-efficacy in nutrition counseling and Factor 2 (8 items) measures self-efficacy to assess readiness to change and initiate nutrition lifestyle changes. The final, validated survey contains 18 items (**Figure 13.6**).

2. **Content validity**. Before developing any survey questions, we assume the researchers identified exactly *what needed to be measured*, and then selected appropriate questions for each domain. A panel of experts (and sometimes a statistician) is used to look at a survey's content validity. They usually perform an organized review of the survey's content to ensure that it contains everything it should and is not missing anything. The panel may *rate the content relevance of each item using a rating scale* such as a 4-point scale from 1 (irrelevant) to 4 (extremely relevant) (Lynn, 1986). The ratings can then be used to calculate a Content Validity Index for each question and also for the whole instrument (Lynn, 1986). Content validity establishes a survey's relevance and the breadth of what it is measuring.
3. **Criterion validity**. This is a measure of *how well your survey/instrument stacks up against another survey/instrument or predicts something*. Criterion validity can be subdivided into concurrent and predictive validity. **Concurrent validity** refers to the degree to which your survey correlates with another previously established and valid instrument, perhaps a gold standard. For example, a tool to assess nutrition status in the elderly may be tested against the Mini-Nutritional Assessment, a validated nutrition assessment tool used to identify patients age 65 and above

For each question, indicate your level of agreement by clicking one of the 5 options in the column, ranging from Strongly Disagree to Strongly Agree. **For the purpose of this survey, "child" is defined as being between the ages of 5 and 10.**

	I am confident that I can . . .				
	Strongly Disagree	Disagree	Neutral	Agree	Strongly Agree
1. Describe to an obese child's family members what a healthy diet should include.					
2. Use motivational interviewing to guide an obese child's family members to make lifestyle changes.					
3. Describe to an obese child how to increase fruit and vegetable consumption.					
4. Discuss with an obese child's family members the benefits of making lifestyle changes.					
5. Determine if an obese child is ready to make lifestyle changes.					
6. Counsel an obese child in a way that helps them overcome barriers to change.					
7. Describe to an obese child how to choose healthy foods to consume.					
8. Determine if an obese child recognizes they need to make lifestyle changes.					
9. Use motivational interviewing to guide an obese child to make lifestyle changes.					
10. Describe to an obese child what a healthy diet should include.					
11. Counsel an obese child's family members in a way that helps them overcome barriers to change.					
12. Describe to an obese child's family members how to choose healthy foods to consume.					
13. Describe to an obese child how to choose healthy snack alternatives.					
14. Describe to an obese child's family members how to increase fruit and vegetable consumption.					
15. Determine if an obese child's family members recognize they need to make lifestyle changes.					
16. Describe to an obese child's family members how to choose healthy snack alternatives.					
17. Discuss the health impacts of obesity with an obese child's family members.					
18. Determine if an obese child's family members are ready to make lifestyle changes.					

FIGURE 13.6 Childhood Obesity Prevention Self-Efficacy Survey

Reproduced from "The Development and Validation of the Childhood Obesity Prevention Self-Efficacy (COP-SE) Survey," by N. K. Cooke, J. L. Nietfeld, & L. S. Goodell, 2015, *Childhood Obesity, 11*, p. 4. Copyright by Mary Ann Liebert, Inc. Reprinted with permission.

who are malnourished or at risk of malnutrition (Marshall, Young, Bauer, & Isenring, 2015). **Predictive validity** evaluates how well your survey/instrument predicts a specific outcome: a survey asking adults about their attitudes toward healthy eating may predict the quality of their diets.

4. **Construct validity**. This measure of validity can be difficult to assess but is very valuable. Construct validity *experimentally tests the quality of an instrument to determine if it is really measuring what it is supposed to measure.* In other words, it is the extent to which the instrument measures the theoretical concept being measured. An example using factor analysis is provided in Table 13.9.

   In addition, **factor analysis** can be used to determine an instrument's construct validity. To use factor analysis, the survey must first be administered to a large, representative group. Factor analysis is a statistical technique that looks at interrelationships among many variables to identify clusters of variables that are most closely linked together. In **exploratory factor analysis**, each factor or cluster is identified. For example, if a 20-item questionnaire is really a valid measure of the construct "nutrition literacy," a factor analysis on the scores of the questionnaire should result in one factor that can explain most of the variances in these 20 items. If an item is not included in a factor, in other words it does not correlate well with other items, the item may be removed. Then the researcher can develop models and use **confirmatory factor analysis** for statistical hypothesis testing on these proposed models.

Keep in mind that validity is somewhat of an imprecise science.

APPLICATION 13.4

Jones et al. (2015) went through a number of steps to assess the reliability and validity of a nutrition knowledge questionnaire to be used for adults in California. Which form of reliability or validity has been assessed in each of these examples?

1. University students took the nutrition knowledge questionnaire. Some of the students had taken a college nutrition course, some had not. The researchers compared knowledge scores of the two groups.
2. A group of Californian adults participated in cognitive interviews.
3. A group of university students completed the questionnaire twice, about 2 weeks apart.
4. A committee including nutrition college faculty, postdoctoral scholars, and registered dietitians reviewed the questionnaire to make sure it included everything it needed to have.
5. In a pretest of the survey, questions in each domain were tested to see if they measured consistently.

COLLECT AND ANALYZE SURVEY DATA

Once you have the questionnaire ready to use, you will need approval from the Institutional Review Board (IRB). Surveys do involve human subjects and must therefore get approval from the IRB before implementation.

Before sending out any questionnaires, you also need to assign an anonymous unique identifier (usually a random number) to each person in the sample. This unique identifier is also put on the survey so you can track whether you get the survey back.

Researchers often maintain a spreadsheet with basic information for each respondent, which is used to track and audit when the advance letter is sent, the questionnaire is sent, reminders are sent, questionnaire is received, and so on.

Steps in collecting data for mail and email questionnaires usually include the following:

- Send out a letter or email in advance of the questionnaire, explaining that a questionnaire will be coming, a little about the survey, and why it is important for the respondent to complete the survey. Advance letters help to increase response. Having a pamphlet or Web page where potential respondents can learn more about the project increases their confidence in the legitimacy of the study.
- Send the questionnaire out (if by mail, include stamped addressed envelope for return) with the cover letter.
- If the questionnaire is not returned within a certain period of time, send a reminder. If the questionnaire is received, send a thank-you.
- Send out the second questionnaire to nonresponders.

The number of times reminders and questionnaires are sent out, and how they are spaced out, needs to be determined in advance. You need to log these events for each person in your sample.

Increasing **response rate** (the percentage of your sample who complete the questionnaire) increases the usefulness of your results. One way to increase the response rate is to offer an incentive for participation, which can be anything from cash to gift cards to simply a summary of the survey results. Additional ways to increase response rate include the following (Dillman et al., 2014):

1. Briefly explain why the survey results will be useful.
2. Do not make the survey too long, too dull, or too complex to complete. Fill the questionnaire with interesting questions in an attractive visual design, and make it easy and convenient to complete and return.
3. Show that the survey is being done by a legitimate, trustworthy organization such as a university by using appropriate letterhead, enclosing/attaching a pamphlet about the study, or setting up a website about the study.
4. Ask for your respondents' help.
5. Do not ask for too much sensitive information.
6. Assure confidentiality to respondents and that the data is protected.

It is important to always act professionally throughout the survey process.

As you collect data, consider the errors that can occur during this time, which we call **nonsampling errors**. Examples of nonsampling errors include interviewer errors, response errors, and coding errors.

1. **Interviewer errors** occur any time the interviewer does not administer the survey the way it was intended. Perhaps the interviewer skipped a question, misread a question, or does not probe an answer when required. Interviewers need to be trained properly and observed occasionally. Researchers also need to verify that interviews took place.
2. **Response errors** occur when the respondent does not understand a question, the respondent answers a question that he does not really have an answer for, or the respondent does not provide accurate answers on sensitive questions.
3. **Coding errors** can occur at any point when the respondent or the interviewer checks the wrong box on the survey, uses the wrong code, or enters an answer incorrectly.

Appropriate interviewer training, pretesting of questions, and double-checking data entry (along with data cleaning) can help prevent these errors.

After the questionnaires have been collected, the researcher needs to enter the data into a database or spreadsheet. You can then upload the data into your statistical software. In some cases, students enter data directly into the statistical software. When using computer-assisted interviewing software, data entry takes place during the interview. To enter data, make sure you are familiar with these terms.

- *Case*. A case is one row in a spreadsheet; it represents the scores/values for every variable (question) for one respondent.
- *Variables*. Each column in a spreadsheet represents a variable. At the top of each column is the variable name.
- *Data file*. A set of cases makes up a data file.

Many researchers use a codebook to help manage their data. Some statistical software will help you create a codebook. A **codebook** is a technical description of the data that was collected for a study or survey. A codebook for a questionnaire should include this information:

- Variable name and label. The variable name is at the top of each column. The variable name should be short enough to put at the top of the column and long enough to have some meaning when you look at it. For each column, you can also assign a variable label, which can be much longer and is often the survey question. In SPSS you can hover over the variable name and see the variable label, which is very helpful.
- Where each variable is located in the data files.
- How the variable was measured (whether the responses were nominal, ordinal, or scale—includes interval and ratio).
- How the variable was recorded in the raw data (numeric or string—may contain numbers and/or letters) and how many characters wide it is.
- Codes used for each response (such as "M" or "1" for male). In the case of open-ended questions, you have to develop coding categories so you can group each response into a category (this is often done by two coders so you can assess the reliability of the codes). Each code for an open-ended question should be defined and a couple of examples given.
- How missing data was coded.

A more complete codebook would include an overall description of the survey process including sampling design and data collection. **Figure 13.7** shows part of a codebook.

Some guidelines for managing data include the following:

- Using the original records, spot check that data was entered correctly.
- Check for entries that really stick out from the norm (such as "5" when the only possible responses were lower than that).
- Be careful when assigning variable names so they do not cause confusion.
- Check for duplicate entries.
- Decide how to handle missing data, and code missing values according to the guidelines given by the statistical software you are using.
- Make sure your data is backed up and properly secured according to policy and the IRB.

You also need to know basic characteristics of your sample such as the range and distribution of each variable, whether there are outliers, and the normality of continuous

Question Number	Variable Name	Question	Variable Type	Variable Length	Codes
1	INTDATE	{Date of interview}	date	8	- Enter as DD-MM-YYYY
2	AGE	What is your age in years?	numeric	3	- Enter number - Missing = {leave blank}
3	SEX	What is your sex?	text	1	- Male = M - Female = F - Missing = {leave blank}
4	WORK	Which of the following categories best describes your work status?	text	10	- Working full time = FULLTIME - Working part time = PARTTIME - Unemployed but want to work = UNEMP - Retired = RETIRED - Student = STUDENT - Homemaker = HOME - Other = OTHER → If OTHER go to 4b, otherwise skip to 5
4b	WORK_ OTHER	Other occupational description	text	50	-{Enter text as reported by respondent}
5	STUDENT	Are you currently enrolled in school?	text	1	- Yes = Y - No = N - Don't know/Missing/ Refused = D
6	ALC	How often do you drink alcohol?	numeric	1	- Never = 0 - Less than 1x/month = 1 - About 1x/month = 2 - About 2x/month = 3 - About 1x a week = 4 - About 2-3x/week = 5 - About 4-5x/week = 6 - Every day or almost every day = 7 - Don't know = 8 - Refused/missing = 9
7	DIA	Do you have diabetes?	numeric	1	- Yes = 1 - No = 2 - Don't know = 7 - Refused to answer = 8 - Missing = 9

FIGURE 13.7 Example of codebook entries.

variables. Some researchers will go through a more thorough process, known as **data cleaning**, to detect, diagnose, and edit faulty data.

In the early stages of survey development, researchers write up the hypotheses they want to test and consider how each variable is to be defined, measured, and statistically analyzed. The dependent (also called outcome) variable, such as blood pressure, is typically proposed to change as a result of the independent variable, which could be sodium intake. The statistical tests you can use on a variable depend on whether the variable is categorical or continuous. See Chapter 6 for statistical tests you can use when testing one independent and one dependent variable.

APPLICATION 13.5

You are doing a survey of students at your university, and you are ready to send your sample an advance email about the study. Your study examines student perceptions of the availability of healthy foods on campus. Write an email that will help keep your response rate high.

SUMMARY

1. Surveys are used in nutrition monitoring programs such as NHANES, clinical nutrition research, nutrition epidemiological research, program evaluation research, and other research.
2. Survey methods include paper surveys delivered by mail for the respondent to fill out, electronic surveys, and oral surveys that are completed with an interviewer either on the phone or in person. Table 13.1 discusses advantages and disadvantages of each method. Surveys sent by mail or email are cheaper, but using interviewers can increase the response rate.
3. Most surveys are cross-sectional (administered at one time). Retrospective surveys are also administered at one time, but they ask respondents to discuss past behaviors, etc. Longitudinal surveys are administered more than once and include repeated cross-sectional (or trend) surveys, panel surveys, and cohort surveys (see Table 13.2).
4. The major steps in the survey process include using the research question and literature review to guide your survey objectives; determine who will be sampled; create and test the questionnaire; contact respondents; collect, enter, and analyze data; and write up and disseminate results.
5. The best way to control for sampling error is to use a large enough sample size. Sample bias occurs when the members of your sample are different from the population in some way (such as coverage bias, selection bias, or nonresponse bias). Increasing sample size does not improve sample bias.
6. Figure 13.1 shows how a sample is part of the accessible population, which is a subset of your target population. A sampling frame is a list of members of the accessible population from which the sample is drawn.
7. Using probability sampling, each person in the population has an equal probability or chance of being selected. Examples include simple random sampling, systematic random sampling, stratified random sampling, and cluster random sampling (see Figure 13.2 and Table 13.4).
8. Nonprobability sampling is based on respondents being selected by convenience or judgment and is less likely to produce representative samples. Examples include convenience sampling, quota sampling, purposive or judgment sampling, and network (snowball) sampling (see Table 13.5).
9. In a descriptive study, sample size is based on confidence intervals, confidence level, the size of the target population, and

response distribution. In correlational, quasi-experimental, or experimental studies, a power analysis is used to determine sample size. Power analysis uses the relationships among the alpha level (level of significance), power level, effect size, and sample size to calculate sample size. Additional factors may be used as well.

10. Figure 13.3 lists the steps in developing and testing the questionnaire.
11. Guidelines are given for developing a cover letter, questions, and responses. There are many close-ended response formats such as dichotomous, checklist, Likert scale, traditional ordinal rating scale, verbal frequency scale, rank order scale, semantic differential scale, visual analog scale, hedonic scale, and nonverbal hedonic scale for children (see Table 13.6).
12. Using a midpoint in a scale, such as "Neutral," does not usually change the results. To discourage random guessing, you may add "Not sure." To discourage skipped questions, you may use "Prefer to not answer" as a response.
13. Guidelines are given for sequencing the questions and laying out the questionnaire so it is easy for respondents to use.
14. Pretesting the questionnaire, often through cognitive interviews or debriefing, is important to get feedback on the clarity of the questions, usefulness of response options, and user-friendliness of the questionnaire.
15. Ways to test whether a questionnaire (instrument) has reliability (repeatability) include test-retest reliability, parallel forms reliability, inter-rater reliability, and internal consistency reliability (see Table 13.8).
16. Validity looks at whether the survey accurately measures what it is intended to measure. The survey can be tested for face validity, content validity, criterion validity, and construct validity (see Table 13.9).
17. Ways to increase response rate include offering an incentive, explaining why the survey results will be useful, making sure the survey is easy and convenient to complete, showing the survey is being done by a trustworthy organization, asking for your respondents' help, assuring confidentiality, and not asking for too much sensitive information.
18. As data is collected, you need to watch for nonsampling errors such as interview errors, response errors, or coding errors.
19. A codebook is a technical description of the data that was collected for a study (see Figure 13.7).
20. Guidelines are given for managing data.

REVIEW QUESTIONS

1. Surveys can be useful when:
   A. you need information that is not readily available from other sources
   B. your questions are mostly closed-ended
   C. you can access a representative sample
   D. all of the above
2. Which of these survey methods is the least expensive to administer?
   A. mail survey
   B. electronic survey
   C. telephone survey
   D. face-to-face survey
3. Which of these survey methods is the most expensive and has an excellent response rate?
   A. mail survey
   B. electronic survey
   C. telephone survey
   D. face-to-face survey
4. A survey that asks the same questions at several points in time to a new group of respondents each time is a:
   A. cross-sectional survey
   B. trend survey
   C. panel survey
   D. cohort survey

5. Larger samples have a better chance of preventing:
   A. sample bias
   B. nonresponse bias
   C. sampling error
   D. all of the above
6. Which of the following is the group to whom you want to apply your results?
   A. target population
   B. accessible population
   C. sampling frame
   D. source population
7. Which type of sampling involves dividing the accessible population into groups and then using simple random sampling for each group?
   A. systematic random sampling
   B. stratified random sampling
   C. cluster random sampling
   D. multistage sampling
8. Sampling plans where the sampling is carried out in stages using smaller and smaller sampling units is called:
   A. systematic random sampling
   B. stratified random sampling
   C. cluster random sampling
   D. multistage sampling
9. ____________ sampling is when members of a population are chosen because they are easy to reach.
   A. purposive
   B. network
   C. convenience
   D. quota
10. Which of the following is *not* needed to do a power analysis?
    A. level of significance
    B. margin of error
    C. effect size
    D. power level
11. Getting feedback on the design of your questionnaire and the clarity of the questions and responses is called:
    A. pretesting
    B. pilot testing
    C. content validity
    D. construct validity
12. A measure that looks at how well different questions measuring the same construct produce similar results is called:
    A. test-retest reliability
    B. internal consistency reliability
    C. inter-rater reliability
    D. content reliability
13. When you compare the results of your dietary intake questionnaire against a proven food frequency questionnaire, that would be testing its:
    A. face validity
    B. content validity
    C. criterion validity
    D. construct validity
14. Describe the six steps in the survey process.
15. Explain three ways sample bias can occur.
16. How is simple random sampling different from systematic random sampling?
17. How is stratified random sampling different from cluster random sampling?
18. Why is a probability sampling technique more desirable than a nonprobability sampling technique in a survey?
19. List five guidelines for sequencing the questions in a questionnaire, and also list five guidelines for laying out a questionnaire.
20. Compare and contrast cognitive interviews and debriefing (individual and group).
21. List five ways to increase response rate.
22. Live five guidelines for managing data and describe what a codebook is.
23. As part of your job in a small Women, Infants, and Children program (WIC) office, you have been asked to develop a brief survey (no more than 10 questions) asking your clients about their satisfaction with your services. The survey will be handed to clients to fill out before they leave. Before developing your questionnaire, learn about WIC and what clients could be asked to evaluate. Carefully put together your questions and response categories. Finally, lay out your questionnaire on one page, being sure to include instructions.

CRITICAL THINKING QUESTIONS

1. Read this article and answer the following questions.
   Wilson, M. M., Reedy, J., & Krebs-Smith, S. M. (2016). American diet quality: Where it is, where it is heading, and what it could be. *Journal of the Academy of Nutrition and Dietetics, 116*, 302–310.
   A. How will diet quality be measured in this study?
   B. Describe basic information about the NHANES survey (type of survey, who is picked, who conducts the survey, how survey is conducted, etc.).
   C. Who was excluded from this study?
   D. What is the objective of this study, and how will the researchers reach the objective (in other words, explain the methods)? Be concise, but do not leave out any major details.
   E. Has diet quality improved from 1999–2000 to 2011–2012? If so, by how much?
   F. Will the American diet in 2020 meet the *Healthy People 2020* objectives or the 2010 Dietary Guidelines for Americans? Describe.
   G. Which part(s) of the American diet has not shown improvement over time?
2. Read this open-access article and answer the following questions.
   Lakerveld, J., Mackenbach, J., Horvath, E., Rutters, F., Compernolle, S., Bardos, H., … Brug, J. (2016). The relation between sleep duration and sedentary behaviours in European adults. *Obesity Reviews, 17*, 62–67.
   A. Describe the objectives of this study.
   B. The study took place in five urban areas in Europe. How was the sampling accomplished? Was it random or nonrandom?
   C. What topics were covered in the survey, and how was the survey administered?
   D. What was the response rate?
   E. Briefly describe the survey results.
3. Read this article and answer the following questions.

   Yaroch, A., Tooze, J., Thompson, F., Blanck, H., Thompson, O., Colon-Ramos, U., … Nebeling, L. (2012). Evaluation of three short dietary instruments to assess fruit and vegetable intake: The National Cancer Institute's Food Attitudes and Behaviors Survey. *Journal of the American Dietetic Association, 112*, 1570–1577.
   A. Explain the objective of the study.
   B. Who did the sampling frame include, and how were respondents chosen?
   C. What is it called when the researchers compared estimates from each of the screeners to estimates from the 24-hour recalls?
   D. Describe the Automated Multiple Pass Method.
   E. How was test-retest reliability tested for the screeners?
   F. What were the conclusions of the researchers?

SUGGESTED READINGS AND ACTIVITIES

1. Blair, J., Czaja., R., & Blair, E. (2014). *Designing surveys: A guide to decisions and procedures.* Thousand Oaks, CA: Sage Publications Inc.
2. Boushey, C. J. (2008). Estimating sample size. In E. R. Monsen & L. Van Horn (Eds.), *Research: Successful approaches* (pp. 373–381). Chicago, IL: American Dietetic Association.
3. Dillman, D., Smyth, J., & Christian, L. (2014). *Internet, phone, mail and mixed-mode surveys: The tailored design method.* Hoboken, NJ: John Wiley & Sons, Inc.
4. Dilorio. C. K. (2005). *Measurement in health behavior: Methods for research and evaluation.* San Francisco, CA: Jossey-Bass.
5. Fink, A. (2002). *The survey kit.* Thousand Oaks, CA: Sage Publications Inc.
6. Fowler, F. J. (2014). *Survey research methods.* Thousand Oaks, CA: Sage Publications Inc.

7. Gleason, P., Harris, J., Sheean, P., Boushey, C., & Bruemmer, B. (2010). Publishing nutrition research: Validity, reliability and diagnostic test assessment in nutrition-related research. *Journal of the American Dietetic Association, 110*, 409–419. doi: 10.1016/j.jada,2009.11.022.05.012
8. Online Sample Size Calculators. For surveys: http://www.raosoft.com/samplesize.html; for clinical trials, crossover studies, and studies to find an association: http://hedwig.mgh.harvard.edu/sample_size/size.html
9. Online Survey Design Guide. www.lap.umd.edu/survey_design
10. Ruel, E., Wagner, W., & Gillespie, B. (2016). *The practice of survey research: Theory and applications*. Thousand Oaks, CA: Sage Publications Inc.
11. Schaeffer, N., & Presser, S. (2003). The science of asking questions. *Annual Review of Sociology, 29*, 65–88. doi: 10.1146/annurev.soc.29.110702.110112

REFERENCES

Algert, S., Baameur, A., & Renvall, M. (2014). Vegetable output and cost saving of community gardens in San Jose, California. *Journal of the Academy of Nutrition and Dietetics, 114*, 1072–1076. doi: 10.1016/j.jand.2014.02.030

Anderson, S., Must, A., Curtin, C., & Bandini, L. (2012). Meals in our household: Reliability and initial validation of a questionnaire to assess child mealtime behaviors and family mealtime environments. *Journal of the Academy of Nutrition and Dietetics, 112*, 276–284. doi: 10.1016/j.jada.2011.08.035

Blair, J., Czaja., R., & Blair, E. (2014). *Designing surveys: A guide to decisions and procedures*. Thousand Oaks, CA: Sage Publications Inc.

Boeckner, L. S., Pullen, C. H., Walker, S. N., Abbott, G. W., & Block, T. (2002). Use and reliability of the World Wide Web version of the Block Health Habits and History Questionnaire with older rural women. *Journal of Nutrition Education and Behavior*, 34, S20-S24.

Boucher, B., Cotterchio, M., Kreiger, N., Nadalin, V., Block, T., & Block, G. (2006). Validity and reliability of the Block food-frequency questionnaire in a sample of Canadian women. *Public Health Nutrition, 9*, 84–93. doi: http://dx.doi.org/10.1079/PHN2005763

Boushey, C. J. (2008). Estimating sample size. In E. R. Monsen & L. Van Horn (Eds.), *Research: Successful approaches* (pp. 373–381). Chicago, IL: American Dietetic Association.

Boyle, M. A., & Holben, D. H. (2013). *Community nutrition in action: An entrepreneurial approach*. Belmont, CA: Wadsworth/Cengage.

Bradburn., N., Sudman, S., & Wansink, B. (2004). *Asking questions: The definitive guide to questionnaire design for market research, political polls, and social and health questionnaires*. New York: John Wiley & Sons, Inc.

Carbone, E., Campbell, M., & Honess-Morreale, L. (2002). Use of cognitive interview techniques in the development of nutrition surveys and interactive nutrition messages for low-income populations. *Journal of the American Dietetic Association, 102*, 690–696. doi: 10.1016/S0002-8223(02)90156-2

Cooke, N. K., Nietfeld, J. L., & Goodell, L. S. (2015). The development and validation of the Childhood Obesity Prevention Self-Efficacy (COP-SE) Survey. *Childhood Obesity, 11*, 114–121. doi:10.1089/chi.2014.0103

DeVon, H. A., Block, M. E., Moyle-Wright, P., Ernst, D. M., Hayden, S. J., Lazzara, D. J., . . . Kostas-Polston, E. (2007). A psychometric toolbox for testing validity and reliability. *Journal of Nursing Scholarship, 39*, 155–164. doi: 10.1111/j.1547-5069.2007.00161.x

Dillman, D., Smyth, J., & Christian, L. (2014). *Internet, phone, mail and mixed-mode surveys: The tailored design method*. Hoboken, NJ: John Wiley & Sons, Inc.

Doub, A., Small, M., & Birch. L. (2015). An exploratory analysis of child feeding beliefs and behaviors included in food blogs written by mothers of preschool-aged children. *Journal of Nutrition Education and Behavior.* Advance online publication. doi: 10.1016.j.jneb.2015.09.001

Falbe, J., Kenney, E., Henderson. K., & Schwartz, M. (2011). The Wellness Child Care Assessment Tool: A measure to assess the quality of written nutrition and physical activity policies. *Journal of the American Dietetic Association, 111*, 1852–1860. doi: 10.1016/j.jada,2011.11.022.09.006

Fowler, F. J. (2014). *Survey research methods*. Thousand Oaks, CA: Sage Publications Inc.

Francis, H., & Stevenson, R. (2012). Validity and test-retest reliability of a short dietary questionnaire to assess intake of saturated fat and free sugars: A preliminary study. *Journal of Human Nutrition and Dietetics, 26*, 234–242. doi: 10.111/jhn.12008

Garza, K., Ding, M., Owensby, K., & Zizza, C. (2016). Impulsivity and fast-food consumption: A cross-sectional study among working adults. *Journal of the Academy of Nutrition and Dietetics, 116*, 61–68. doi: 10.1016/j.jand.2015.05.003

Gleason, P., Harris, J., Sheean, P., Boushey, C., & Bruemmer, B. (2010). Publishing nutrition research: Validity, reliability and diagnostic test assessment in nutrition-related research. *Journal of the American Dietetic Association, 110*, 409–419. doi: 10.1016/j.jada,2009.11.022.05.012

Grove, S. K., Burns, N., & Gray, J. R. (2013). *The practice of nursing research: Appraisal, synthesis, and generation of evidence*. St. Louis, MO: Elsevier Saunders.

Hand, R., & Abram, J. (2016). Sense of competence impedes uptake of new Academy Evidence-Based Practice Guidelines: Results of a survey. *Journal of the Academy of Nutrition and Dietetics*. Advance online publication. doi: 10.1016.j.jand.2015.12.020

Hand, R., Birnbaum, A., Carter, B., Medrow, L., Stern, E., & Brown, K. (2014). The RD Parent Empowerment Program creates measurable change in the behaviors of low-income families and children: An intervention description and evaluation. *Journal of the Academy of Nutrition and Dietetics*, *114*, 1923–1931. doi: 10.1016/j.jand.2014.08.014

Hulley, S. B., Cummings, S. R., Browner, W. S., & Grady, D. G. (2013). *Designing clinical research* (4th ed.). Philadelphia, PA: Lippincott, Williams & Wilkins.

Iglesia, I., Guelinckx, I., De Miguel-Etayo, P., Gonzalez-Gil, E., Salas-Salvado, J., Kavouras, S., … Moreno, L. (2015). Total fluid intake of children and adolescents: Cross-sectional surveys in 13 countries worldwide. *European Journal of Nutrition*, *54*, S57–S67. doi: 10.1007/s00394-015-0946-6

Johnson. C. L., Dohrmann, S. M., Burt, V. L., & Mohadjer, L. K. (2014). *National Health and Nutrition Examination Survey: Sample design, 2011–2014* (Vital and Health Statistics Report No. 162). Atlanta, GA: National Center for Health Statistics.

Jones, A. M., Lamp. C., Neelon, M., Nicholson, Y., Schneider, C., Wooten Swanson, P., & Zidenberg-Cherr, S. (2015). *Journal of Nutrition Education and Behavior*, *47*, 69–74. doi: 10.1016/j.jneb.2014.08.003

Kullen, C., Iredale, L., Prvan, T., & O'Connor, H. (2015). Evaluation of general nutrition knowledge in Australian military personnel. *Journal of the Academy of Nutrition and Dietetics*, *116*, 251–258. doi: 10.1016/j.jand.2015.08.014

Leong, S. L., Madden, C., Gray, A., Waters, D., & Horwath. C. (2011). Faster self-reported speed of eating is related to higher body mass index in a nationwide survey of middle-aged women. *Journal of the American Dietetic Association*, *111*, 1192–1197. doi: 10.1016/j.jada.2011.05.012

Lynn, M. R. (1986). Determination and quantification of content validity. *Nursing Research*, *35*, 3820–3850. doi: 10.1097/00006199-198611000-00017

Marshall, S., Young, A., Bauer., J., & Isenring, E. (2015). Malnutrition in geriatric rehabilitation: Prevalence, patient outcomes, and criterion validity of the Scored Patient-Generated Subjective Global Assessment and the Mini Nutritional Assessment. *Journal of the Academy of Nutrition and Dietetics*. Advance online publication. doi: 10.1016/j.jand.2015.06.013

Parmenter, K., & Wardle, J. (1999). Development of a general nutrition knowledge questionnaire for adults. *European Journal of Clinical Nutrition*, *53*, 298–308.

Patel, N., Kennedy, A., Blickem, C., Reeves, D., & Chew-Graham, C. (2016). "I'm managing my diabetes between two worlds": Beliefs and experiences of diabetes management in British South Asians on holiday in the East—A qualitative study. *Journal of Diabetes Research*, *2016*, 1–8. doi: 10.1155/2016/5436174

Pew Research Center. (2015a). *Cell phone surveys*. Retrieved from http://www.people-press.org/methodology/collecting-survey-data/cell-phone-surveys/

Pew Research Center. (2015b). *Collecting survey data*. Retrieved from http://www.pewresearch.org/methodology/u-s-survey-research/collecting-survey-data/

Ruel, E., Wagner, W., & Gillespie, B. (2016). *The practice of survey research: Theory and applications*. Thousand Oaks, CA: Sage Publications Inc.

Ritchie, L.D., Boyle, M., Chandran, K., Spector, P., Whaley, S.E., James, P., . . . Crawford, P. (2012). Participation in the Child and Adult Care Food Program is associated with more nutritious foods and beverages in childcare. *Childhood Obesity*, *8*, 236–241. doi: 10.1089/chi.2011.0061

Ritchie, L., Sharma, S., Gildengorin, G., Yoshida, S., Braff-Guajardo, E., & Crawford, P. (2015). Policy improves what beverages are served to young children in child care. *Journal of the Academy of Nutrition and Dietetics*, *115*, 724–730. doi: 10.1016/j.jand.2014.07.019

Shafer, K., & Lohse, B. (2005). How to conduct a cognitive interview: A nutrition education example. Washington, DC: National Institute of Food and Agriculture, USDA.

Takeuchi, M. T., Edlefsen, M., McCurdy, S. M., & Hillers, V. N. (2006). Development and validation of Stages-of-Change questions to assess consumers' readiness to use a food thermometer when cooking small cuts of meat. *Journal of the American Dietetic Association*, *106*, 262–266.

Uebersax, J. S. (2006). *Likert scales: Dispelling the confusion*. Retrieved from http://john-uebersax.com/stat/likert.htm

Whelan, K., Copeland, E., Oladitan, L., Dip, P., Murrells, T., & Gandy, J. (2013). Development and validation of a questionnaire to measure research involvement among Registered Dietitians. *Journal of the Academy of Nutrition and Dietetics*, *113*, 563–568. doi: 10.1016/j.jand.2012.08.027

CHAPTER 14

Writing and Disseminating a Research Proposal and Paper

CHAPTER OUTLINE

- Introduction
- Identify a Topic and Research Question/Objective
- Search the Literature and Write the Literature Review
- Write the Introduction
- Write the Methods
- Use a Style Manual to Format Your Paper
- Write the Results, Discussion, and Conclusion
- Write a Title and Abstract
- The 3 P's of Dissemination: Posters, Presentations, and Publications

LEARNING OUTCOMES

- List elements in a research proposal and research paper.
- Identify and develop a researchable problem.
- Explain the purposes of a Literature Review.
- Write a research proposal including an Introduction, Literature Review, and Methods.
- Use a style manual consistently throughout a written project.
- After completing a research proposal, complete the study and write a research paper to include an Introduction, Literature Review, Methods, Results, Discussion, Conclusion, and Abstract.
- Discuss the importance and channels of dissemination of research findings.
- Develop a poster and explain how to conduct a poster session.

INTRODUCTION

This chapter will take you through the steps involved in a research study, from formulating a problem to writing a proposal and full paper to presenting your work. As you consider a research project, it is important to know the state of the research in the area that interests you. This will help you determine whether the proposed problem has already been answered. Whether you are conducting research for work or as part of your studies, a good research project must always address a problem. Nutrition evidence is ever changing, and RDNs and other nutrition professionals will continue to have numerous opportunities to participate in research.

Following are the typical sections of a research study or thesis that a student will complete as part of an undergraduate or graduate program. Note that a research proposal only includes the first three chapters (but you may be asked to add more to the proposal such as possible results, etc.), whereas a full research paper or thesis includes all chapters. Also note that the Literature Review is in its own section or chapter, although a number of studies from the Literature Review will be mentioned in the Introduction.

Chapter 1 – Introduction
Chapter 2 – Literature Review
Chapter 3 – Methods
Chapter 4 – Results
Chapter 5 – Discussion/Conclusions
References
Appendices

Be sure to use the guidelines provided by your department and your professor. Read the guidelines carefully; they will undoubtedly include other important things such as length and the style manual to use. **Table 14.1** shows an example of a table of contents for a thesis that examined the effectiveness of an educational program (with a theoretical background) for older adults to take steps to prevent osteoporosis.

From time to time you will run across a research proposal in a journal that is called a study protocol. Researchers will have the protocol published before or while conducting the study. You can tell that it is a protocol because the abstract only includes up to the Methods. In the Suggested Readings and Activities at the end of this chapter, you will find a study protocol for the Baptist Employee Healthy Heart Study and another study protocol for the Live Well, Viva Bien randomized trial (both are open access). They are excellent examples of research proposals/protocols that you can refer to as you read the chapter.

IDENTIFY A TOPIC AND RESEARCH QUESTION/OBJECTIVE

The best research starts with a question that interests you. To come up with possible topics, you may want to use the PICO framework, which is used to do a literature search:

P—Participants, population (Is there a particular group you want to look at?)
I—Intervention/Observation (Is there a particular intervention or exposure/observation of interest to you?)
C—Comparison (What do you want to compare?)
O—Outcome (What outcomes do you want to examine?)

Another way to brainstorm ideas is to browse the table of contents of journals in your area of interest. For example, if you are interested in a diabetes topic, look at diabetes-specific journals (such as *Diabetes Care* and *Diabetes*) as well as general medical journals (such as *New England Journal of Medicine* and *Lancet*).

Be aware that you will probably need to narrow your focus. This is quite common and a normal part of the research process. **Table 14.2** gives examples of topics that were narrowed down to research questions that describe the variables and population.

Table 14.1 Example of a Table of Contents for a Thesis

- Abstract
- Chapter 1. Introduction
  - Overview
  - Problem Statement
  - Aim
  - Research Question and Hypothesis
  - Limitations
  - Definitions
- Chapter 2. Literature Review
  - Osteoporosis and Its Health Effects
  - Role of Calcium and Vitamin D in Reducing Hip Fractures in Older Adults
  - Osteoporosis Prevention Education Programs
  - Conceptual Framework: Revised Health Belief Model
  - Summary
- Chapter 3. Methods
  - Research Design
  - Participants
  - Intervention
  - Instruments
  - Procedures
  - Statistical Analyses
  - Summary
- Chapter 4. Results
  - Participant Characteristics
  - Baseline Comparability and Attrition
  - Effect of Intervention on Knowledge, Self-Efficacy, and Health Beliefs
  - Effects of Intervention on Calcium and Vitamin D Intake
  - Summary
- Chapter 5. Discussion
  - Relationship of Results to Other Research
  - Limitations and Strengths
  - Implications and Recommendations
  - Summary (Conclusion)

Table 14.2 Narrowing Down from a Broad Topic

Broad topic	Narrowed topic	Focused topic	Research question
Children's Health	Children and Food Allergies	Children with food allergies and food allergy status of siblings.	In a family with one child who has food allergies, how often are siblings sensitized or clinically reactive to the same food(s)?
Men's Health	Men and Prostate Health	Men with prostate cancer and lycopene intake.	Is there a decreased risk of prostate cancer in men who consume a diet high in lycopene?

Once you have come up with some ideas, *examine the literature to see what is known up to this point in your area(s) of interest* as you consider possible research questions. You do not want to research something that has already been thoroughly examined or pick an idea that has little or no published research. Too little research could be a sign that the idea is not very relevant or significant or that it is a very new area of research.

TIP

Do not forget that your research question is based on a problem statement. The problem statement (discussed in both the Introduction and the Literature Review) identifies the specific gap or problem into which the researchers want to gain further insight.

When examining the literature, here are some valuable tips to help you find a suitable research question:

- Locate recent articles in your area of interest and *read the Introduction carefully*. The Introduction provides the *problem statement* and a *brief Literature Review* of the topic. The problem statement describes the problem addressed in the study, and why it is important. The Literature Review may provide references for other articles that you should include in your Literature Review.
- Also *look at the Methods section for "how" the research question was answered*. If you are just writing a research proposal, you have more freedom to pick a research design because you do not have to carry out or implement the study. If you are writing a proposal *and* carrying out the study, you need to think realistically about a research design you can carry out, and whether that design is appropriate to answer the research question.
- Then read the Results and especially *focus on any ideas for future research* given in the Discussion section.
- *Use recent narrative reviews and systematic reviews* to give you a picture of the research already completed in a specific area. To find these types of articles on PubMed, select "Reviews" and "Systematic Reviews" and limit the publication date to less than 5 years.

Once you have a research question, state it as a research objective with clearly identified variables and the population of interest.

Use the following checklist before you move on to the Literature Review. You may also need to get approval from your professor at this point; be sure to check on that.

1. Does your research question address some aspect of a significant problem?
2. Is your research question relevant and important?
3. Does your research question identify the variables being studied and indicate the type of relationship being examined?
4. Is your topic neither too broad nor too narrow in scope?
5. Have you chosen an appropriate and feasible research method to answer the research question?
6. Is the research study ethical?

If you can answer "yes" to these questions, you will be less likely to encounter problems as you move forward.

SEARCH THE LITERATURE AND WRITE THE LITERATURE REVIEW

The next step is either to write the Introduction or the Literature Review. If you write the Literature Review first, writing the Introduction will be easier. That is because the Literature Review gives you the information you need for the problem statement and the brief literature review used in the Introduction.

Writing an effective Literature Review requires a great deal of time, thought, and attention. Besides showing your reader that you have a good grasp of the research in an area, the Literature Review has several other purposes (Caulley, 1992).

1. Define and describe the problem/gaps in research.
2. Compare and contrast studies (methods, results, etc.).
3. Critique studies.
4. Highlight the best studies.
5. Summarize the state of the literature and how your study fits in.

Doing a Literature Review will also help you understand your topic better.

Before diving into the Literature Review, let's look at a couple of things *you should not do*:

- *Do not write a summary of the articles you read.* A Literature Review is not a summary of the articles you read on your topic; it is a *synthesis* of the literature. In a synthesis you compare and contrast the recent literature, as well as find common ideas and themes. In a Literature Review you may provide a summary of two studies, but then you must explain how they had slightly different methods but similar results, for example.
- *Do not include every article ever published about the research topic.* You must decide which articles to include and which to exclude. Researchers tend to include both recent (within the last 5 years) and seminal articles. Why focus on the recent literature? Nutrition knowledge and understanding is constantly changing, and it is important that researchers present the most up-to-date understanding of their research topic. There is an important exception to this general rule: seminal articles. Seminal articles are those ground-breaking articles that presented an idea of great importance or influence within a discipline, generally for the first time. You can identify them because they are frequently mentioned by researchers. For example, if you are researching the dietary practices of immigrants who have come to the United States, you will probably see a number of references to an article on dietary acculturation by Satia-Abouta, Patterson, Neuhouser, and Elder (2002) published in the *Journal of the American Dietetic Association.*

TIP

Choose articles for the Literature Review that meet the requirements set by your professor. Normally you will be required to use mostly, if not all, original research articles (primary research). You may also have a minimum number of articles or date requirements, so be sure you are meeting all requirements.

As you search for articles to include in your Literature Review, *keep track of the search terms you use for each database* and define some exclusion criteria so you consistently remove irrelevant articles from the search. Also, use a **citation management tool**, which can help you:

- Import citations from both databases and websites
- Build and organize bibliographies
- Format references for your research paper
- Take and save notes on articles
- Save PDFs and other files for your research (MIT Libraries, 2016).

The three most popular citation tools are EndNote, Zotero, and Mendeley. EndNote is a popular choice for students and researchers in the health sciences because it has the longest history and is great for large collections of articles. Zotero is popular for researchers who want to gather citation records for PDF and non-PDF content. Mendeley is the newest of the three citation tools and is best when your research content is mostly in PDF files. Zotero and Mendeley are free tools, as is a basic version of EndNote. You can purchase a more powerful version of EndNote.

While selecting studies, *keep in mind that a Literature Review needs a clear line of argument, which helps justify why the study should be done.* **Figure 14.1** is an example of a very brief Literature Review completed for a study on garden-based nutrition education for children. It begins with a *broad focus* on the importance of early eating patterns on health, then *narrows* to how school-based programs, and then gardening programs in schools, can improve eating habits. Each statement is backed up by research studies, and the review ends by showing conflicting results from gardening studies, which helps to justify this study.

Once you have completed a comprehensive literature search and found articles relevant to your topic, *critically read and highlight each article.* As you read, *it is a good idea to use*

Studies have shown that eating patterns (specifically of food choices regarding fruits and vegetables) are developed at an early age and can be traced into and through adulthood (5,6). Proper adolescent nutrition can reduce overweight and obesity and can reduce risk factors for diet-related diseases later in life (6-8). As a result, experts suggest developing interventions and effective nutrition programming early in a child's life as a tool for increasing healthful dietary patterns and reducing the risk of chronic disease later in life (5,9).

School-based programs represent an important venue for nutrition behavior change. There is great potential for affecting behaviors and health risks that persist into adulthood, such as food choices and obesity (10-13). Schoolyard gardens are emerging as health education tools in academic settings (14-16). A study of California teachers found that school gardens were perceived as an effective tool for promoting healthful eating habits (15). Morris and Zidenberg-Cherr (17) found that garden-enhanced nutrition education was effective in improving nutrition knowledge and vegetable preferences of fourth-grade students. In a related study, third-grade and fifth-grade students' attitudes toward vegetables became more positive after gardening, but fruit and vegetable consumption did not improve significantly (18).

FIGURE 14.1 A Brief Literature Review for a Garden-Based Nutrition Education Study

Reproduced from "Garden-based Nutrition Education Affects Fruit and Vegetable Consumption in Sixth-Grade Adolescents." by J. D. McAleese & L. L. Rankin, 2007, *Journal of the American Dietetic Association, 107*, p. 662. Reprinted with permission.

Article Title/ Date	Objective/ Hypothesis	Methods	Results/ Discussion	Study Limitations	Additional Notes
1.					
2.					
3.					
4.					
5.					
6.					
7.					
8.					
9.					
10.					

FIGURE 14.2 Literature Review Matrix

a table or matrix (**Figure 14.2**) and list key parts of each article there along with notes such as comparisons, critical comments, or themes you might see emerging between a group of articles. The matrix will make it easier for you to pinpoint similarities and differences between studies and to find themes or common threads. Look for findings that appear most frequently, the consistency of the evidence, gaps in the evidence, what methods worked or did not work, and whether the results varied based on setting or population. Writing up the matrix will also help you see where your proposed study fits in. The matrix involves work, but it will make it *easier to organize and write a good Literature Review*.

Depending on the situation, it may be helpful to enter the studies in the matrix in chronological order or to customize a column heading to better meet your needs. The studies you are reading are likely to be either mostly experimental/quasi-experimental or nonexperimental. Therefore, you may want to change a column heading to focus your matrix a little differently.

Now, it's time to organize your thoughts logically *into an outline for the Literature Review* (if you have not already done this). The Literature Review often starts with a broad focus and then narrows down. For example, let's say your proposed study is to explore the effectiveness of an online behavioral weight management program for college students. You know you need to justify your study idea and give an in-depth review of the existing literature, so you write up this outline:

- You discuss the studies showing how many college students are obese/overweight and the consequences (broad statement of the problem). You include the topic of weight gain among college students and what is known about who gains weight and why.
- Next, you discuss studies of behavioral weight management programs used with college students, including comparing methods and results and critically examining pertinent studies. Your Literature Review revealed some research on weight management programs for college students, but the bulk of this research is on adults who are a bit older.

- Finally, you justify why you want to study an online program. Your Literature Review showed that an online program has never been studied with college students before, so you can show the gap (narrowed statement of the problem). You then discuss studies that showed how this technique worked for adults, describing overall results, explaining any inconsistencies among the studies, and showing how this may be a good technique to try with busy, tech-savvy college students.

That is a good, logical outline for the Literature Review; it justifies your study as well as informs the reader of the current literature so the reader knows where your study will fit in. Now you can write a rough draft of your Literature Review.

APPLICATION 14.1

A researcher has been looking at the problem of iron deficiency during pregnancy. She wonders whether pregnant women who are food insecure are more likely to have an iron deficiency than pregnant women who are food secure, and she finds only one study in this area. Develop a tentative outline for a Literature Review.

Following are guidelines for writing the Literature Review.

1. Start with a clear introduction explaining how the review is organized and the purpose of the proposed research. (You may want to write the introductory paragraph after you have written some or all of the Literature Review.)
2. Use headings to organize the Literature Review in a logical manner to guide the reader.
3. Start each paragraph with a strong topic sentence that clearly states the main idea of the paragraph. Use active rather than passive tense.
4. Use transition words and phrases to connect ideas between sentences and paragraphs (see **Table 14.3**).
5. Always acknowledge and be respectful of results and opinions that do not agree with your thesis. It is okay to indicate when results are conflicting or inconclusive and why you think so, just use a professional tone.

Table 14.3 Transition Words and Phrases to Connect Ideas in a Literature Review

To propose an opinion or idea	states, claims, argues, discusses, contends, suggests, asserts, proposes, according to
To add to an idea	furthermore, in addition, also, moreover
To give an example	for example, for instance, such as, as an illustration, to illustrate
To link similar ideas/opinions	in addition, also, similarly, likewise, similar to, in a like manner
To contrast	however, on the other hand, on the contrary, although, in contrast, though, conversely, but
To emphasize	indeed, especially, importantly, undoubtedly, in fact, particularly, clearly
To show cause	because of, due to, in view of
To argue a point	although, even though, despite, on the other hand, admittedly, in spite of
To dismiss	in any case, in any event, either way, whatever happens
To clarify	to put it another way, in other words

6. When necessary, use quotations, but do so sparingly. A Literature Review with too many quotations is difficult to read.
7. Write in an academic style (see Chapter 2).
8. Consistently reference the literature in your discussion.
9. Be careful not to plagiarize.
10. Write a summary at the end.

WRITE THE INTRODUCTION

Following are common sections found in the Introduction. The sections you will include in your Introduction depend on the requirements of your course or program.

- Background of the Problem
- Statement of the Problem
- Purpose (Aim) of the Study
- Research Objectives
- Hypothesis (if applicable)
- Limitations of the Study
- Operational Definitions

The Introduction goes from a broad focus and continually narrows down, like a funnel (**Figure 14.3**). The Introduction of a journal article would end at the hypothesis, but you may be asked to include study limitations and operational definitions in your Introduction.

If you have already written your Literature Review, you can easily write up the background of the problem and the statement of the problem. *Be brief here and convey the most important points.* For example, if you are studying the effectiveness of an online behavioral weight management program for college students, the background of the problem would include how many college students are obese/overweight, risk factors for gaining weight in college, and the consequences of being overweight or obese. The statement of the problem would explain that there are few weight management studies using college students, and none using online behavioral management techniques, yet these techniques have worked in the general adult population.

The purpose of the study describes what you want to achieve from carrying out this research. Generally speaking, the purpose is broader in scope than the research objectives, which are more specific. When you write up the purpose, think about the big picture.

Now you are leading up to what everyone wants to see—the research objective, the formal stated goal of the study or desired outcome. Be sure the research objective identifies the variables being studied and indicates the type of relationship being examined.

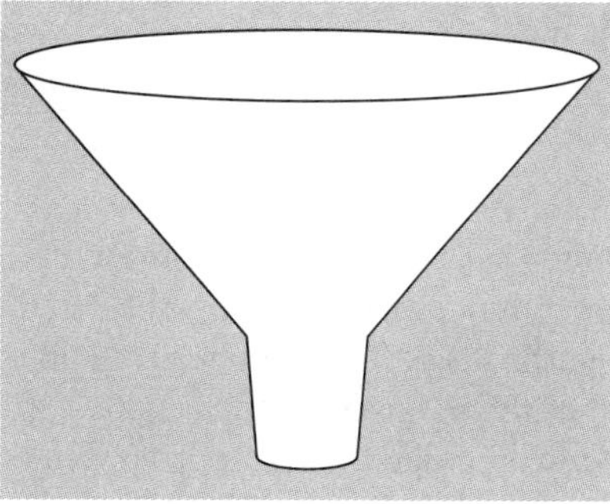

FIGURE 14.3 Use a Funnel Approach When Writing Your Introduction.

A research objective should be relevant, important, and ethical. In the college weight loss study, the research objective was to see how effective an online behavioral weight management program was for overweight and obese college students compared to overweight/obese college students taking part in a Weight Watchers program with weekly classes. There may be more than one research objective.

A hypothesis may also be included in the Introduction, usually after the objective, especially if the study has an intervention. The hypothesis describes the predicted relationship between the variables, the population being studied, and sometimes other information such as the time frame. For the college weight loss study, the hypothesis was that the overweight/obese college students using the online behavioral weight management program would lose significantly more weight than those students attending weekly classes by the end of the program.

In the Introduction of a proposal or thesis, you may have to address topics you would not see in the Introduction of a research article, such as limitations of the study (usually put into the Discussion) and operational definitions of variables. Limitations could include using a convenience sample, having the participants self-report their body weight or dietary intake, having a small sample size, or using measurement tools that have not been tested for reliability and validity. Operational definitions are needed so that readers know exactly how you will measure the variables.

APPLICATION 14.2

Give an example of an operational definition for body fat.

WRITE THE METHODS

In the Methods section, avoid these problems:

- Lack of a well-thought-out rationale for the research design and methods
- Insufficient details
- Lack of details about research instruments
- Limited discussion of data analysis that will be done
- No attention to ethical procedures

As usual, this section requires a lot of thought.

The Methods section has a number of subsections. How you set them up will vary depending on your course requirements and on the type of study you are conducting. Here are some typical subsections:

- Research design
- Participants and setting
- Tools and instruments
- Procedures
- Statistical analysis

If your study has an intervention, you may want an Intervention subsection.

If you are writing a research proposal, write the Methods section in the future tense. If you have conducted the research and are writing up the research study, then the Methods section should be in the past tense.

When you discuss the research design, be sure to provide plenty of detail, including the variables, and include a rationale for your choice. If the design is a little complex, you may want to include a diagram to help explain it (see **Figure 14.4**).

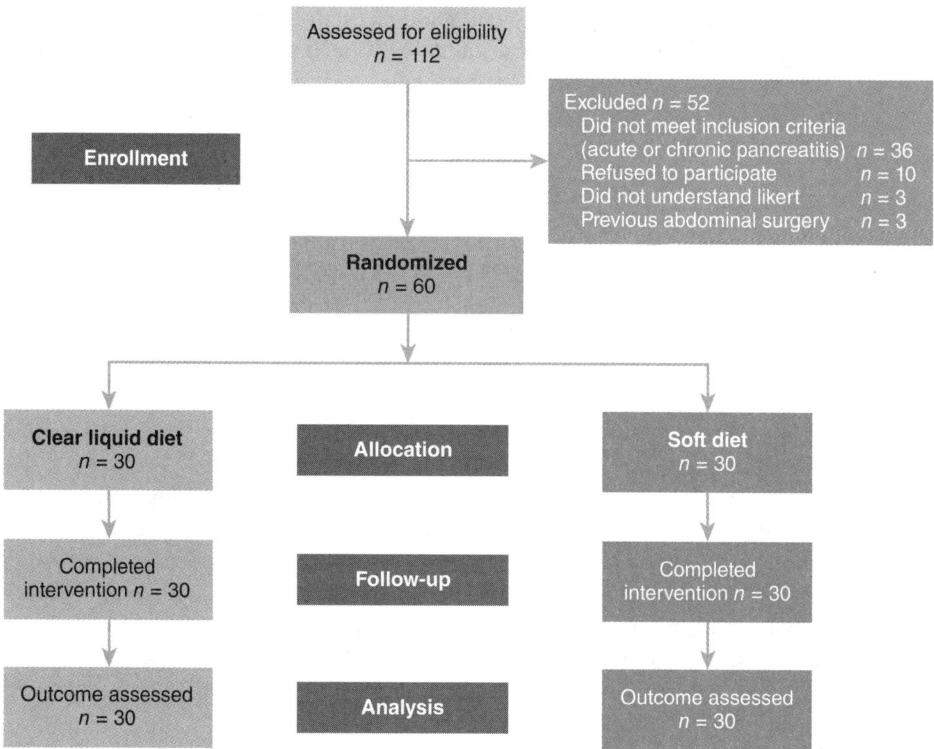

FIGURE 14.4 Flow Diagram of the Participants Through a Study

Reproduced from "Clear Liquid Diet vs Soft Diet as the Initial Meal in Patients with Mild Acute Pancreatitis: A Randomized Interventional Trial," by N. Rajkumar, V. S. Karthikeyan, S. M. Ali, S. C. Sistla, and V. Kate, 2012, *Nutrition in Clinical Practice, 28,* p. 367. Reprinted by Permission of SAGE Publications, Inc.

When you discuss participants, be sure to answer these questions.

1. Who will the participants be (geographic location, gender, age, socioeconomic status, etc.)? Include any inclusion or exclusion criteria.
2. How will they be chosen (sampling method)? How will they be recruited?
3. Will participants be paid or receive some other type of remuneration?
4. How many participants will there be? How are you going to determine the sample size?
5. How are you going to measure participant characteristics that you want to assess?
6. How will participants be assigned to a group?

You also need to describe the type of setting where the study will take place, such as an outpatient clinic in an urban hospital or the office of a primary care physician, and any important features of the setting.

Before discussing the tools and instruments you will use, operationalize your variables (in other words, determine how you will measure each variable). Nutrition research uses a variety of methods and instruments to measure variables, from self-reported dietary recalls and food frequency questionnaires to anthropometric, laboratory, and clinical measurements. Once you know exactly what you want to measure in a study, you can assess which instruments to use and how they are to be used, taking into account factors such as each instrument's advantages and disadvantages, the budget, time frame, and number of participants. In evaluating the quality of an instrument, consider both its reliability (consistency in measuring under similar circumstances) and its validity (the instrument is measuring what it is supposed to measure).

Provide the background and important features of all instruments that you use. If you use the Healthy Eating Index, for example, you need to explain how the grading works. If you have participants being weighed, you need to provide information about the make and model of the scale and how each person will be weighed, such as shoes and jackets will be removed and the nurse will do the weighing.

If you are using a survey, you need to include a copy of the survey (as a Table or Appendix) and explain how each section of the survey works and the rationale for the questions. You also need to explain how you tested for reliability and validity, and the results of any tests that were done (listed here):

- Tests for reliability: test-retest reliability, parallel forms reliability, inter-rater reliability, internal consistency reliability
- Tests for validity: face validity, content validity, criterion validity, construct validity

You should also describe any pretesting and pilot testing that was done. Chapter 12 explains these concepts.

The procedures subsection includes everything about *how* the study will be conducted, from beginning to end, that has not already been discussed in another subsection of Methods. Some procedures, such as how groups are determined, may appear in the Participants subsection. The procedures should include how you will obtain Institutional Review Board approval, how you will get informed consent, when and how data will be obtained, all instructions to participants, who will have contact with the participants, and so on. If you are using raters or observers, you need to explain how they will be chosen and trained, and the statistic used to calculate agreement.

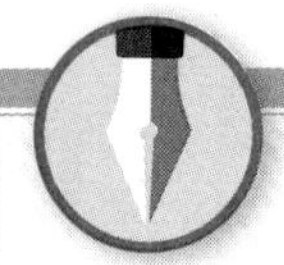

TIP

When writing up the procedures, think of yourself as a participant and describe the steps you will go through during the study so you do not forget anything.

If you have a subsection in Methods for the intervention, use it to describe exactly how the intervention was administered to all groups. If your intervention involves the use of education materials, be sure to describe these materials and, as appropriate, include them in the Appendices.

The last Methods subsection identifies the statistical analysis that will be done. Identify the questions in your study that you wish to use statistics to answer. Usually this begins with using statistics to examine your groups/participants. Then you will be using statistics to answer your research questions or to test hypotheses. **Table 14.4** can help you find appropriate statistical tests to use.

APPLICATION 14.3

Name two statistical tests often used to compare groups to see how equivalent they are (usually discussed at the start of the Results section).

USE A STYLE MANUAL TO FORMAT YOUR PAPER

When writing a research article, various documentation styles can be used. A documentation style is a standard approach to writing, formatting, and citing references within

Table 14.4 Finding Appropriate Statistical Tests

Statistics That Look at Differences

Name	Test statistic	Purpose	Number of groups	Measurement level of dependent variable
Independent samples *t*-test	t	To test the difference between the means of two independent groups.	2	Interval/ratio
Paired samples *t*-test (or dependent *t*-test)	t	To test the difference between the means from two paired groups (such as before-and-after observations on the same subject).	2	Interval/ratio
One-way analysis of variance (ANOVA)	F	To test the difference among means of more than two independent groups for one independent variable (with more than one level).	More than 2 groups	Interval/ratio
Two-way analysis of variance (ANOVA)	F	To test the difference among means for 2 independent variables, of which each may have multiple levels.	More than 2 groups	Interval/ratio
Repeated measures ANOVA (one-way within-subjects)	F	To test the difference among 3+ means in the same group over time. (Extended design of dependent samples *t*-test).	1 group	Interval/ratio
Chi square	χ^2	To analyze nominal and ordinal data to find differences between groups.	2 or more groups	Nominal/Ordinal

Statistics That Look at Association

Name	Test statistic	Purpose	Measurement level of dependent variable
Pearson product-moment correlation	r	To measure the strength and direction of the relationship between two variables.	Interval/ratio
Spearman rank-order correlation	ρ	To measure the strength and direction of the relationship between two variables. (Nonparametric version of Pearson product-moment correlation)	Ordinal, interval, or ratio
Linear regression		To predict the value of a dependent variable, and measure the size of the effect of the independent variable on a dependent variable while controlling for covariates.	Interval/ratio
Logistic regression		Same as linear regression; used when dependent variable is binary.	Binary/dichotomous

the text and at the end of the paper. If you are writing a paper for a college course, your instructor will require a specific documentation style, so it is important to understand the requirements before getting started. Once you are clear on the preferred documentation style, it is imperative that you apply the rules consistently. The primary writing styles used by medical or scientific authors are the American Medical Association (AMA) or American Psychological Association (APA) formats. Each journal specifies the writing/formatting style that authors should follow. For example, the *Journal of the Academy of Nutrition and Dietetics* uses AMA style.

AMA STYLE

The AMA style dates back to 1962 when the first edition of the editorial manual for scientific journals was published. The latest edition includes electronic guidelines and an increased emphasis and explanation on ethical and legal considerations.

General Guidelines for Documenting Using AMA Style

- Double spaced with 1 inch margins on all sides.
- Times New Roman or Courier Font 12 is preferred for the body content.
- Arial or Tahoma Font is preferred for table and figures.
- Left justify the text.
- The first line should be indented 0.5 in.
- Pages should be numbered and number placed in the upper right corner in the header.
- A running head or title header should be included at the top page aligned to the left. The page header is a shortened version of your manuscript title that does not exceed 50 characters.

General Guidelines for Documenting In-Text Citations Using AMA Style

- Use superscript Arabic numerals for citations (e.g., [1, 2, 3]).
- The superscript number [1] is inserted in the document immediately next to the material, idea, or fact being cited (e.g., *Glutathione is a powerful antioxidant found in every cell in the body.*[1]).
- The superscript number is inserted after periods and commas (e.g., *Glutathione is a powerful antioxidant found in every cell in the body.*[1]).
- The superscript number is inserted on the inside before colons and semicolons (e.g., *Glutathione is a powerful antioxidant found in every cell in the body*[2]*; vitamin C is also very important for neutralizing free radicals.*).
- If citing more than one reference at one location in the text, the numbers are separated with commas and no spaces between (e.g., [1,2,3]).
- When citing more than two references at the same location in the manuscript, use commas to separate the numbers and hyphens to join the numbers together (e.g., *As previously studied,*[1,6-1,14,18] *glutathione is a powerful antioxidant found in every cell in the body.*[2]).

General Guidelines for Documenting References Using AMA Style

- References are numbered in order as they appear in the text and are listed in the reference list in numerical order.
- When citing authors' names, last name is stated first followed by only initials for the first and middle names. No periods are used between initials. Use a comma between authors.
- Capitalize only the first word and proper nouns and abbreviations in article titles.

- Use only journal abbreviations that are used by the National Library of Medicine Catalog. Enter in the title of the journal at this website (http://www.ncbi.nlm.nih.gov/nlmcatalog/journals) and you will get the abbreviation.
- When citing a journal, the issue number is stated in parentheses after the volume number. If there is no issue number, state the month before the year.

American Psychological Association (APA) Style

The APA writing style dates back to 1929, when a group of psychologists, anthropologists, and business managers convened to establish a simplified method of scientific writing. Today, the APA style is the most commonly used documentation style in the social sciences. In 2016, the American Psychological Association announced that they will transition away from the APA format by the year 2020 and cease use of the APA style. In addition, they will no longer publish the sixth edition of the American Psychological Association. The American Psychological Association plans to transition to the AMA style for scientific writing to be more consistent with physician research documentation.

General Guidelines for Documenting Using APA Style

- Document is double spaced with 1 inch margins on all sides.
- Times New Roman Font 12 is preferred.
- A page header, also known as a running head or title header, should be included at the top of the page aligned to the left. The page header is a shortened version of your manuscript title that does not exceed 50 characters (all capitals).
- Document sections include Title Page, Abstract, Main Body, and References.

General Guidelines for Documenting In-Text Citations Using APA Style

- References are cited in the sentence using the author's last name and year date: *A cross-sectional online survey was conducted with participants recruited using a mass electronic mailing (Williams, 2016).*
- When stating titles of sources within your paper, capitalize the first letter of all words with four or more letters.
- Books, movies, and other titles are set italic or underlined.

General Guidelines for Documenting References Using APA Style

- References are listed in alphabetical order by last name of the first author in the manuscript.
- List authors' names beginning with last name first, followed by the initial of the first name and middle initial if applicable. If the manuscript has several authors, list only the first six authors and then use an ellipsis followed by last author. (An ellipsis is a set of three periods [...] that indicates an omission has occurred.)
- With more than one article by the same author, list in chronological order from the earliest to the most recent publications.
- The first letter of all major words in journal titles are capitalized.
- Use italics for titles of journals and books.

Table 14.5 summarizes the basics of both AMA and APA styles.

APPLICATION 14.4

Take a quiz on AMA style references at the AMA website: http://www.amamanualofstyle.com/page/style-quizzes#Practice_Editing_Tables. Take a quiz on APA style at citationgame.org.

Table 14.5 Basics of AMA and APA Styles

	Basic set-up	In-text citation	Reference examples
AMA	Spacing: double spaced Margins: 1 inch all sides Fon: Times New Roman, Courier 12 Headings: Aligned to the left with a shortened version of title (not to exceed 50 characters)	Superscript Arabic numbers within text, inserted *after* a period or comma and *before* a colon or semicolon. Separate superscript Arabic numbers with a comma if citing more than one reference at one location. In-text citation example: This evidence was refuted in another study.[1]	**Journal:** Garza KB, Owensby JK. Impulsivity and fast food consumption: a cross-sectional study among working adults. *J Acad Nutr Diet.* 2016;116(3):61–68. doi: 10.1016.6661 **Book:** Riegelman RK, Kirkwood B. *Public Health 101: Healthy People—Healthy Populations.* 2nd ed. Burlington, MA: Jones & Bartlett Learning; 2015. **Website:** Nutrient Data Laboratory. Nutrition. Gov website. https://www.nutrition.gov/whats-food, Updated November 30, 2015.
APA	Spacing: double spaced Margins: 1 inch all sides Font: Times New Roman 12 Headings: aligned to the left with a shortened version of title (not to exceed 50 characters)	Use author's last name and year date; use semicolons between multiple entries. Use p. or pp. (for more than one page) when quoting. In-text citation example: This evidence was refuted in another study (Cole & Jones, 2011).	**Journal:** Jacoby, W. G. (1994). A cross-sectional study among working adults. *Journal of the Academy of Nutrition and Dietetics, 116,* 61–68. doi: 10.1016.6661 **Book:** Riegelman, R. K., & Kirkwood, B. (2015). *Public health 101:Healthy people-healthy populations.* Burlington, MA: Jones & Bartlett Learning. **Website:** Nutrient Data Laboratory. (2016). *Foods high in vitamin A.* Retrieved from https://ndb.nal.usda.gov/

Sources: *AMA Manual of Style: A Guide for Authors and Editors* (10th ed.), by AMA Manual of Style Committee, 2007, Oxford (U.K.): Oxford University Press; *Publication Manual of the American Psychological Association* (6th ed.), by the American Psychological Association, 2010, Washington, DC: American Psychological Association.

WRITE THE RESULTS, DISCUSSION, AND CONCLUSION

RESULTS

The Results section is limited to the data generated by your study; put any interpretation of the data in the Discussion section. Strive for maximum organization and clarity in this section. Start the Results section with the basic demographics and other pertinent characteristics of the participants, including any pretest data (such as weight or blood pressure). If you have one group, show the number and percentage of total participants with various characteristics, such as ethnicity and age. For other characteristics, such as body mass index and fruit intake, show the mean and standard deviation.

If you have two or more groups, here is where you will show the results of the statistical tests performed to see how similar the groups are (see **Table 14.6**). Note that *t*-tests were used for continuous variables and χ^2 tests for categorical variables. If there are differences between the groups, the differences observed on the dependent variable may be due to the nonequivalence of the groups, which can threaten the internal validity of the study. If the groups are nonequivalent, this should be noted in the limitations section in the Discussion.

Before you start writing this section, look at your results and organize them into a logical order of appearance. The results most directly related to the research objectives

Table 14.6 Example of Comparison of Demographic and Baseline Characteristics in Study with Two Groups

Variable	Intervention group (n = 105)	Control group (n = 110)	*P*-value*
Age, mean (SD), y	46.9 (11.4)	45.3 (10.9)	.91
Weight, mean, (SD), lb	225.6 (39.2)	220.3 (38.4)	.39
Body mass index, mean, (SD)	36.2 (6.7)	36.0 (6.5)	.87
Female sex, No. (%)	69 (66)	72 (65)	.19
Race/ethnicity, No. (%)			.42
White	84 (80.0)	88 (80.0)	
Hispanic	5 (4.8)	8 (7.3)	
Black	10 (9.5)	10 (9.1)	
Other	6 (5.7)	4 (3.6)	
Medical Conditions, No. (%)			
Hypertension	61 (58.1)	66 (60.0)	.64
Diabetes	14 (13.3)	22 (20.0)	.39

* *t*-tests were used for continuous variables and χ^2 tests for categorical variables.

normally appear first. Next, put your results into tables and other displays. If some of your results are not lengthy and can be stated concisely, you may not need a table and can simply provide the results in the text. Do not use a table to display just two or three numbers. Once you have the tables and figures ready, write your narrative, being sure to reference the appropriate table or figure in the text.

Tables and figures are not the same thing. **Tables** present lists of numbers with text in well-organized columns and formats. **Figure 14.5** shows the components of a table. **Figures** usually contain some data but also some artwork to illustrate concepts. For example, a flow diagram (such as Figure 14.4 earlier in this chapter), a bar chart, a line graph, or a photograph are all considered figures (see **Figure 14.6** for examples).

When you make a table, format it for easy reading and keep it as small as possible. Other tips include the following:

1. Have an informative title.
2. Use appropriate column headings.
3. Note the population size.
4. Give dates for data points if applicable.
5. If data are presented as percentages, the numbers used to calculate the percentages should also be provided.
6. Note the name of the statistic used.

Do not try to make the table smaller (or bigger) by using a different font. Use the appropriate font called for in your style manual.

When you create a figure, make sure it is drawn professionally, such as by using Excel to draw a graph. Also do the following:

1. Make sure the display is clear and free of unnecessary detail. You want the figure to be readable and simple.

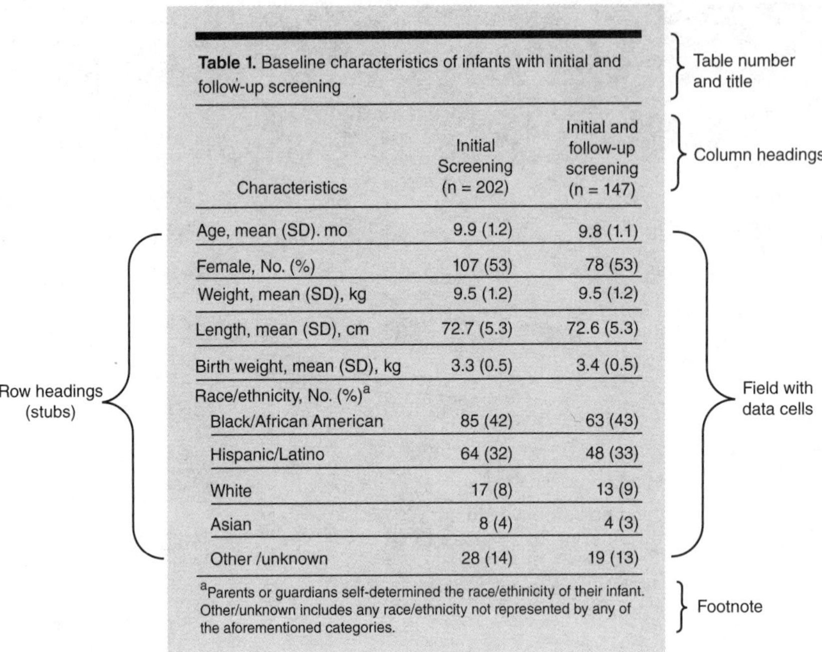

Table 1. Baseline characteristics of infants with initial and follow-up screening

Characteristics	Initial Screening (n = 202)	Initial and follow-up screening (n = 147)
Age, mean (SD). mo	9.9 (1.2)	9.8 (1.1)
Female, No. (%)	107 (53)	78 (53)
Weight, mean (SD), kg	9.5 (1.2)	9.5 (1.2)
Length, mean (SD), cm	72.7 (5.3)	72.6 (5.3)
Birth weight, mean (SD), kg	3.3 (0.5)	3.4 (0.5)
Race/ethnicity, No. (%)[a]		
Black/African American	85 (42)	63 (43)
Hispanic/Latino	64 (32)	48 (33)
White	17 (8)	13 (9)
Asian	8 (4)	4 (3)
Other /unknown	28 (14)	19 (13)

[a]Parents or guardians self-determined the race/ethnicity of their infant. Other/unknown includes any race/ethnicity not represented by any of the aforementioned categories.

FIGURE 14.5 Components of a Table

Reproduced from *AMA Manual of Style: A Guide for Authors and Editors* (10th ed.), p. 83, by AMA Manual of Style Committee, 2007, Oxford (U.K.): Oxford University Press.

2. Use an appropriate chart or graph format for your data. For example, line charts often work best for time series data.
3. Label all axes appropriately.
4. Use a key to identify any symbols, shading, color, etc.
5. Pay attention to size and scale.
6. Be sure the figure communicates what you want to say.
7. Keep figures visually honest.

Both the APA and AMA style manuals give in-depth guidance and examples on setting up many different kinds of tables and figures. *Use the manuals to help you develop clear and concise tables and figures.* Check with your professor for where to place tables and figures in the paper.

DISCUSSION AND CONCLUSION

In the Discussion section, explain and interpret your results in light of what is already known about the topic. The major goal of this section is to show how the study results fit into the bigger picture of research in this area. The Introduction goes from a broad to a narrow focus, whereas the Discussion does the opposite as you compare the relationship of your results to previous literature and also look at prospects for future research. The Discussion section generally includes this information and may follow this sequence:

1. Summarize your results. If a hypothesis was stated, summarize how the results either supported or did not support your hypothesis.
2. Compare your results to other studies mentioned in the Literature Review and Introduction. Try to explain any agreements and differences.

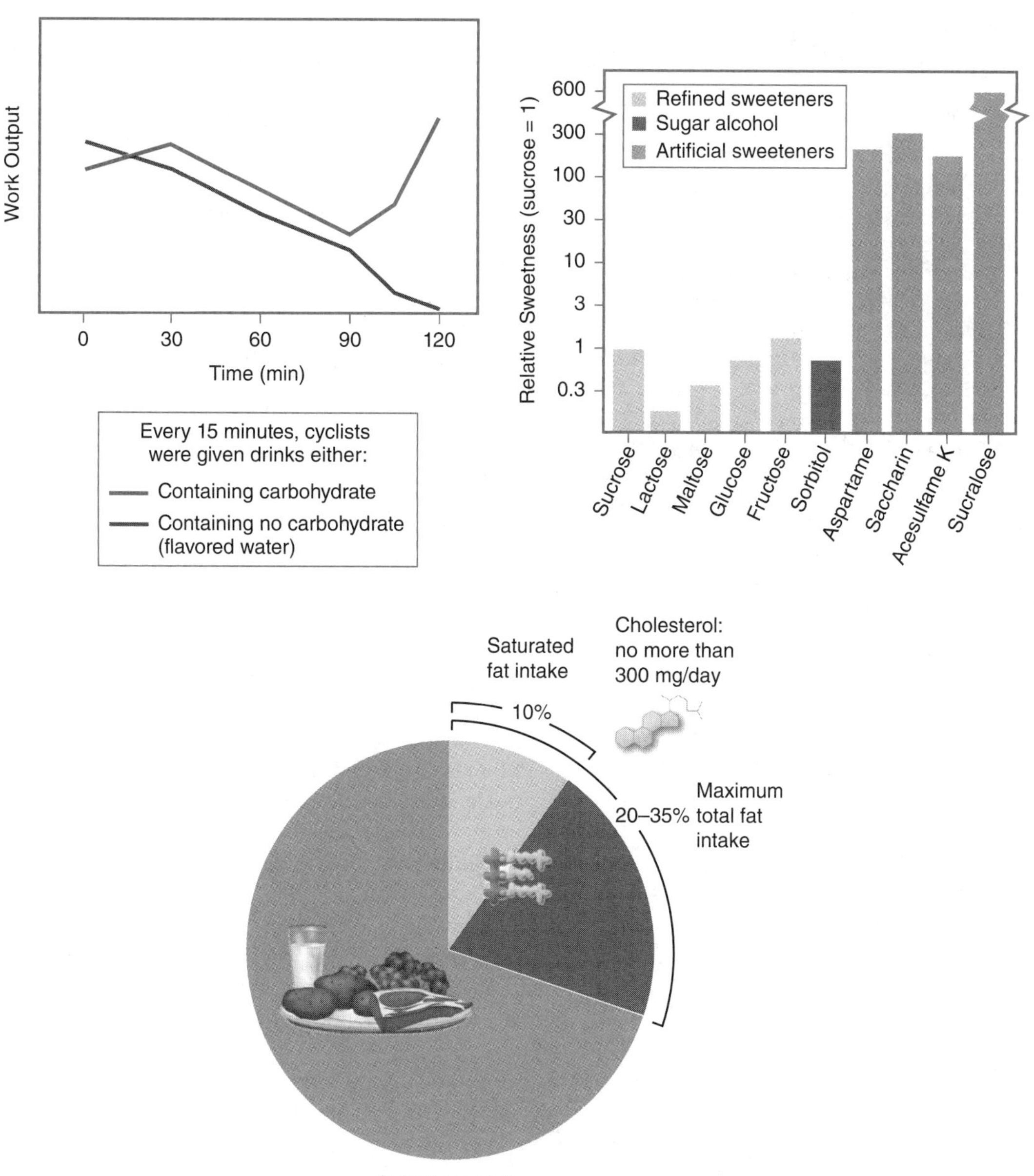

FIGURE 14.6 Examples of an Effective Line Chart, Bar Graph, and Pie Chart

3. After considering the results of other studies, do you have a new understanding of the problem or the solution? If so, explain.
4. Mention any limitations of the study. You may also mention strengths if there are any that stand out.
5. Do you have any ideas for future research? If so, explain.

Because each research article has its own unique findings, the Discussion section can differ a lot in terms of length and structure.

APPLICATION 14.5

Critique these article titles for clarity, length, and interest. Rewrite a title if you can improve it. In your opinion, which is the best title and why?

1. Frequent Consumption of Sugar- and Artificially Sweetened Beverages and Natural and Bottled Fruit Juices Is Associated with an Increased Risk of Metabolic Syndrome in a Mediterranean Population at High Cardiovascular Disease Risk
2. Greater Healthful Dietary Variety Is Associated with Greater 2-Year Changes in Weight and Adiposity in the Preventing Overweight Using Novel Dietary Strategies (POUNDS Lost) Trial
3. Development and Validation of an Empirical Dietary Inflammatory Index
4. Consuming Iron-Fortified Beans Increases Iron Status in Kenyan Women after 180 Days in a Randomized Controlled Feeding Trial
5. Proximity to Fast-Food Outlets and Supermarkets as Predictors of Fast-Food Dining Frequency
6. Adding a Social Marketing Campaign to a School-Based Nutrition Education Program Improves Children's Dietary Intake: A Quasi-Experimental Study*

**Note the use of a subtitle in the last title. A subtitle is often provided to describe the research method used.*

Avoid these common problems with the Discussion section (Cone & Foster, 1993):

1. First, this is the Discussion section; it is not a repeat of the Results section. You are done stating and summarizing the results. It is time to analyze, interpret, compare, and synthesize a new understanding of the topic.
2. It is not all about statistical significance. *P*-values do not tell you anything about the size or the practical significance of the differences between groups. Consider effect size information too.
3. If findings approached statistical significance, do not discuss them as though they are significant. They are not.
4. You cannot conclude that a relationship is causal simply based on correlation because no attempt is made to manipulate an independent variable in correlational designs. Also, be careful about causation in general. Keep in mind that no matter how powerful the findings of a quantitative study are, nothing is ever 100% proven.
5. When data is self-reported, it does not mean the reported data is what actually happened. So make sure you say something such as this, "Older adults *reported* that they exercised on average 20 minutes a day."

The conclusion is a general statement of the answer to the original research question along with any scientific implications. Be sure to show the reader the logic behind your conclusion, and stay on the conservative side. Your conclusion may also include some practical advice.

WRITE A TITLE AND ABSTRACT

You have written a research proposal or a full research paper, and now you need a good title. Make your title as brief as possible, yet still informative and clear. If you can, choose a title that sounds more interesting than "Self-Perceived Eating Habits of Australians." That title is clear and informative, but it certainly is not exciting. Brainstorm and write down different ideas for your title, and ask for feedback from others before you make a final choice.

The abstract is a short summary of the paper and should include the background, research objective, research design and methods, major results, and conclusions. The length and what to include in the abstract are normally stipulated by each journal or professional association in the case of submitting an abstract for a poster or presentation (our next topic). Be as detailed as possible within the word count limit you have. Limit your description of each section of the study, such as methods or results, to two or three sentences, if possible.

Your abstract is like an advertisement for your article, so make sure it is interesting as well as understandable and accurate. The abstract helps readers decide whether they want to read the rest of the paper, so enough key information must be included. **Figure 14.7** shows a well-done abstract with 270 words.

To write your abstract, first determine the sections you will use, unless they are given to you. Next write a summary for each section of the abstract. Count up the number of words and see if you are over or under the requirement. Most times you will be over, but at least now you can consider where you can condense without losing meaning. As you continue to refine the abstract and get to a final version, be sure to get someone's feedback on it.

Habitual intake of anthocyanins and flavanones and risk of cardiovascular disease in men.

A. Cassidy, M., Bertoia, S. Chiuve, A. Flint, J. Forman, & E.B. Rimm.

Abstract

Background: Although increased fruit intake reduces cardiovascular disease (CVD) risk, which fruits are most beneficial and what key constituents are responsible are unclear. Habitual intakes of flavonoids, specifically anthocyanins and flavanones, in which >90% of habitual intake is derived from fruit, are associated with decreased CVD risk in women, but associations in men are largely unknown.

Objective: We examined the relation between habitual anthocyanin and flavanone intake and coronary artery disease and stroke in the Health Professionals Follow-Up Study.

Design: We followed 43,880 healthy men who had no prior diagnosed CVD or cancer. Flavonoid intake was calculated with the use of validated food-frequency questionnaires.

Results: During 24 y of follow-up, 4046 myocardial infarction (MI) and 1572 stroke cases were confirmed by medical records. Although higher anthocyanin intake was not associated with total or fatal MI risk, after multivariate adjustment an inverse association with nonfatal MI was observed (HR: 0.87; 95% CI: 0.75, 1.00; $P = 0.04$; P-trend = 0.098); this association was stronger in normotensive participants (HR: 0.81; 95% CI: 0.69, 0.96; P-interaction = 0.03). Anthocyanin intake was not associated with stroke risk. Although flavanone intake was not associated with MI or total stroke risk, higher intake was associated with a lower risk of ischemic stroke (HR: 0.78; 95% CI: 0.62, 0.97; $P = 0.03$, P-trend = 0.059), with the greatest magnitude in participants aged ≥65 y (P-interaction = 0.04).

Conclusions: Higher intakes of fruit-based flavonoids were associated with a lower risk of nonfatal MI and ischemic stroke in men. Mechanistic studies and clinical trials are needed to unravel the differential benefits of anthocyanin- and flavanone-rich foods on cardiovascular health.

FIGURE 14.7 Example of an Abstract

From "Habitual Intake of Anthocyanins and Flavanones and Risk of Cardiovascular Disease in Men," by A. Cassidy, M., Bertoia, S. Chiuve, A. Flint, J. Forman, and E.B. Rimm, 2016, *American Journal of Clinical Nutrition*, *104*, p. 587. doi:10.3945/ajcn.116.133132. Reprinted with permission.

THE 3 P'S OF DISSEMINATION: POSTERS, PRESENTATIONS, AND PUBLICATIONS

According to Schmidt and Brown (2015), **dissemination** is the "communication of clinical, research, and theoretical findings for the purpose of transitioning new knowledge to the point of care" (p. 505). The key aim of dissemination is to transmit useful knowledge and practices to appropriate target audiences. Effective dissemination relies on the use of varied channels: posters and presentations at professional conferences and meetings; publications, reports, blogs and podcasts; and, of course, person-to-person communication. The most common dissemination methods in nutrition are posters, presentations, and publications.

Publication usually involves getting a research study published in a journal, but also includes publishing in professional periodicals such as newsletters as well as lay and trade publications. Getting published in a scholarly journal requires a high-quality study and manuscript on a timely topic. The publications you choose to submit to will depend on questions such as these: What type of articles does the journal publish? What type of audience does it reach? You also need to understand the status of the journal. A scientific journal has an impact factor, which is one way to learn about the importance that journal has within the field. If you have never published before, it would be wise to look at lower-tier journals. If you are interested in publishing in a journal, go to the "For Authors" section on the journal's website and read the detailed information about the different types of articles they publish, requirements for manuscript preparation, author responsibilities, author queries, and more.

Oral presentations are also an effective way to disseminate new knowledge. Presentations are commonly given at professional and other meetings from the local to the national and global levels. If you want to do an oral presentation, do some research on the groups who would be interested in your topic, and examine their websites as well as contact them to see what type of opportunities are available. **Table 14.7** provides some tips for oral presentations.

Table 14.7 Speaker's Checklist

Do You . . .	Action
_______	Check room, equipment, podium, and lighting prior to speech?
_______	Focus on communications objectives?
_______	Project a strong, positive image?
_______	Maintain direct eye contact with audience?
_______	Use gestures effectively for emphasis and to convey feeling?
_______	Eliminate nervous habits (clearing throat, clutching podium, etc.)?
_______	Remain calm and relaxed?
_______	Exhibit enthusiasm?
_______	Project voice adequately?
_______	Smile and use humor?
_______	Vary tone, pitch, volume, and pace?
_______	Avoid undue dependence on notes?
_______	Enunciate clearly?
_______	Maintain sincerity, credibility?
_______	Use visual aids and technology appropriately and effectively?
_______	Anticipate questions?
_______	Listen carefully to questions?

Many professional associations put out a call for abstracts and sessions for their annual conferences quite some time before the conference. The call for programs includes *detailed* submission guidelines and a deadline date. An abstract is often required to present a poster or a brief oral presentation of your study, although some organizations will just have posters. Abstracts are usually blind reviewed (meaning the reviewers do not have your name) and evaluated to determine who will do a poster presentation, or possibly a brief oral presentation, depending on the sponsoring group.

To submit an abstract for either type of presentation, carefully read the guidelines provided. The guidelines will tell you what to include in the abstract and also the maximum number of words. The guidelines may also explain that there are categories for the abstracts (such as a research abstract or program report) and list areas/topics that are likely to be chosen. Pay attention to all of these details because they can help you be successful. If you are selected, you will be expected to attend the conference, usually at your own expense.

TIP

Once you have an abstract ready to submit, check that you have followed all directions. Also check for any spelling and grammar mistakes, and ask someone to read it and give you feedback. Then do a final check before submission.

MAKING A POSTER

A poster combines text and graphics to present your research/program in a visually interesting manner to others. Each poster presenter is normally given a table and board in a room where students and professionals can walk through and speak with presenters whose topics interest them. The size of your poster is normally specified, probably somewhere between 24 × 36 inches and 48 × 72 inches. You can create large posters in PowerPoint, and your college may provide you with a template for it. Large posters have to be specially printed usually using plotter printing, but many commercial printers have that capability. The poster should be printed on non-glossy white paper for maximum legibility.

The content of a poster for a research study normally includes the title, authors, purpose, methods, results, discussion, summary, and any acknowledgments. **Figure 14.8** shows the layout for an evidence-based practice poster.

An effective poster is well organized, attractive, and easy to read. The title is very important as it is at the top of your poster. According to Erren and Bourne (2007), "the title is your equivalent of a newspaper headline—short, sharp, and compelling" (p. e102). Your poster title does not need to be the same as the study title. A poster title in the form of a question is easy for someone to read and may attract more people to your poster.

Once you have a good title, work on each section one at a time before you start laying out the poster. According to Purrington (2015), the number one poster problem is that they are jam packed with way too many words and sentences, so aim for fewer than 800 words total. Each section should contain no more than 10 sentences, and you should really think about how to replace some text with bullet lists or appropriate graphics to make it more appealing and readable.

When designing your poster, keep in mind the 10–10 rule, which is that the average person will scan your poster for 10 seconds while standing about 10 feet away (Boullata & Mancuso, 2007). Make sure your poster draws attention with graphics and text that is readable from a distance. **Table 14.8** provides some tips for creating a quality poster.

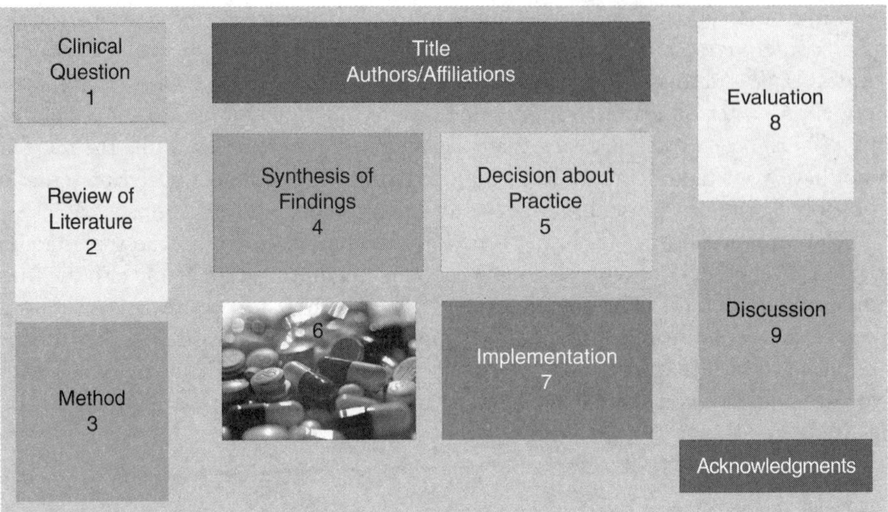

Image © Photos.com

FIGURE 14.8 Logical Layout for an Evidence-Based Practice Poster

Reproduced from *Evidence-Based Practice for Nurses: Appraisal and Application of Research* (3rd ed.), p. 512, by N. A. Schmidt & J. M. Brown, 2015, Burlington (MA): Jones & Bartlett Learning. Reprinted with permission.

APPLICATION 14.6

Search the Internet for scientific poster examples. Use this website to find nutrition posters presented at the Society for Nutrition Edcation and Behavior Annual Conference: http://www.jneb.org/content/usda_poster_abstracts. Find and print a poster that you think meets many of the criteria listed here and explain why.

PRESENTING A POSTER

Normally, poster presenters are together in one or more rooms for a specific time slot. Your job is to arrive at your table at the proper time and get set up. To make it easy for a conference attendee to take home information from your poster, have copies of your poster on standard size paper and include your contact information. Have a sheet available for attendees to put down their contact information if you want to follow up with them.

Once the session starts, you can ask and answer questions from attendees and encourage discussion. Here are more tips for presenting a poster:

- Let attendees read the poster and ask questions. As you answer questions, other people will be listening, and this will attract more people.
- Do not give all your attention to just one or a few people. Keep your eyes scanning around to make eye contact with everyone in your area. This encourages people to ask questions or make comments.
- Encourage attendees to take a copy of your handout.

Table 14.8 Tips for Creating a Quality Poster

1. Layout and Color
• The viewer's eye is drawn to the upper center part of the poster, so place your title and most important information there, which could include a graphic. Notice how the poster in Figure 14.8 has the findings and practice implications in this upper central area.
• White space is important. White space is the space surrounding and between the content/graphics of a poster. Adequate white space creates a balanced, professional poster that is easy for viewers to navigate and understand.
• White space also can be used to provide focus and emphasis. Your poster should have a focal point that draws in viewers.
• Do not overdo color. Stick to two to three complementary colors. Too much color is distracting and makes your poster harder to read.
2. Text
• Use a sans serif font such as Arial or Helvetica because they are easier to read. Sans serif letters do not have the little flourishes or lines.
• Use a font size of at least 24 points.
• All text should be concise and clear.
• Avoid blocks of text 10 sentences or longer.
• Avoid words/sentences spelled in all capital letters; they are harder to read.
• Use bullets and numbering when possible to make text easier and quicker to read.
3. Graphics (Diagrams, Photos, Flowcharts, etc.)
• When possible, consider using graphics such as flowcharts, graphs, bar charts, or photographs to illustrate an idea or a concept. An appropriate graphic in the right place can act as a focal point to draw people in.
• A good balance of graphics to text is about 50/50.
• Avoid three-dimensional graphics (and text); they are hard to read.
• Graphics should be between 150 to 300 dpi. Web images are usually less than 150 dpi, so they will not look good when printed.
• Use a credit line for any graphic you did not create.

SUMMARY

Follow these steps when writing a research paper:

1. Before doing any writing, make sure you have a good research topic and question by answering "yes" to each of these questions. Use the literature to help you find a suitable research question.
   - **A.** Does your research question address some aspect of a significant problem?
   - **B.** Is your research question relevant and important?
   - **C.** Does your research question identify the variables being studied and indicate the type of relationship being examined?
   - **D.** Have you found enough pertinent research articles to write a Literature Review?

   E. Have you chosen an appropriate and feasible research method to answer the research question?
   F. Is the research study ethical?
2. Search the literature and write the Literature Review.
   A. As you search for articles to include in your Literature Review, keep track of the search terms you use for each database, and define some exclusion criteria so you consistently remove irrelevant articles from the search. Also, use a citation management tool.
   B. Keep in mind that a Literature Review needs a clear line of argument, which helps justify why the study should be done.
   C. Critically read each article you are considering for the Literature Review, and enter key points into a table/matrix along with notes such as comparisons, critical comments, or themes you might see emerging between a group of articles.
   D. Also use the matrix to look for findings that appear most frequently, the consistency of the evidence, gaps in the evidence, what methods worked or did not work, or whether the results varied based on setting or population.
   E. Organize your thoughts logically into an outline for the Literature Review, starting with the broad statement of the problem and narrowing it down. By the end you should have justified the reason for your study and also shown the reader where your study fits into the literature.
   F. Use headings to organize the Literature Review, include an introductory and summary paragraph, and use strong topic sentences along with transition words and phrases.
3. Write the Introduction using a funnel approach.
   A. The Introduction begins with a broad focus and continually narrows down as you move from the background to the statement of the problem and the overall purpose of the study.
   B. Now you are leading up to what everyone wants to see—the research objective, or if it is stated as question, the research question. Be sure the research objective identifies the variables being studied and indicates the type of relationship being examined.
   C. A hypothesis may also be included in the Introduction, usually after the objective, especially if the study has an intervention. The hypothesis describes the predicted relationship between the variables, the population being studied, and sometimes other information such as the time frame.
   D. You may have to include other information, such as study limitations and definitions, in the Introduction.
4. Organize and write your Methods section with details including rationale.
   A. Typical subsections include research design, participants and setting, instruments, procedures, and statistical analysis.
   B. If you are writing a research proposal, write the Methods section in the future tense. If you have conducted the research and are writing up the research study, he Methods section should be in the past tense.
5. Report your Results.
   A. Start the Results section with the basic demographics and other pertinent characteristics of the participants, including any pretest data (such as weight or blood pressure), and any statistical analysis.
   B. Organize Results into the same order of appearance that was stated in the Methods section. Normally the results most directly related to the research objectives appear first. Next, put your results into tables and other displays. Make sure each table and figure can stand alone and be interpreted.
   C. Once you have the tables and figures ready, write your narrative, being sure to reference the appropriate table or figure in the text.
   D. Both the APA and AMA style manuals give in-depth guidance and examples on setting up many different kinds of tables and figures. Use the manuals to help you develop clear and concise tables and figures. Check with your professor for where to place tables and figures in the paper.

6. Write your Discussion and Conclusion.
   A. Compare your results to other studies mentioned in the Literature Review and Introduction. Try to explain any agreements and differences.
   B. After considering the results of other studies, do you have a new understanding of the problem or the solution? If so, explain.
   C. Mention any limitations of the study. You may also mention strengths if there are any that stand out.
   D. Do you have any ideas for future research? If so, explain.
   E. Be sure to show the reader the logic behind your conclusion, and stay on the conservative side.
7. Now write a brief, informative, and clear title and abstract. Your abstract is like an advertisement for your article, so make sure it is interesting as well as understandable and accurate.
8. Use the guidelines provided by your professor.
9. Consistently use the style manual to format and type your paper.
10. Write in a scholarly and professional manner.

REVIEW QUESTIONS

1. A thesis is divided into:
   A. sections
   B. chapters
   C. books
   D. references
2. A research proposal does *not* include which of the following?
   A. Introduction
   B. Literature review
   C. Methods
   D. Results
3. What is the PICO framework and what does PICO stand for?
4. Give three reasons it is important to look at the literature on a topic before deciding to do a research study in the area.
5. Name three purposes of a Literature Review.
6. Give five tips on how to write a Literature Review.
7. Explain how and why the Introduction uses a funnel approach.
8. Name the major subsections of the Methods section.
9. For the following journal article and book, write the reference in APA and AMA styles. Also show how to use an in-text citation for the journal article and book, using APA and AMA styles.

   Journal Article: "Evaluating the Influence of the Revised Special Supplemental Nutrition Program for Women, Infants, and Children (WIC) Food Allocation Package on Healthy Food Availability, Accessibility, and Affordability in Texas" by Wenhua Lu, Lisako J. McKyer, Diane Dowdy, Alexandra Evans, Marcia Ory, Deanne M. Hoelscher, Suojin Wang, and Jingang Miao. Journal of the Academy of Nutrition and Dietetics, Volume 116 , Issue 2, pages 292–301

   Book: Designing Clinical Research, 4th edition, by Stephen B. Hulley, Steven R. Cummings, Warren S. Browner, Deborah G. Grady, and Thomas B. Newman, published 2013 by Lippincott Williams & Wilkins in Philadelphia.
10. Compare when to use a table versus when to use a figure.
11. Compare writing the Results section to writing the Discussion.
12. Define dissemination and describe the 3 Ps of dissemination.
13. Give five tips for creating a poster.

CRITICAL THINKING QUESTIONS

1. Two research proposals (both open access) are listed under Suggested Readings and Activities. Pick one of them and discuss what was done well in each major section of the proposal. Next, discuss something from the proposal that could have been improved.
2. You are working on a new research project that is looking at the impact of a diabetes prevention intervention on a group of adults who have prediabetes. The intervention will be delivered at the worksite. Develop an outline of what you would want to include in the Literature Review and the order in which you would discuss each topic.
3. You are working on a new research project, a cohort study looking at the duration of adulthood overweight and obesity and its possible effect on cancer risk in women. Develop an outline of what you would want to include in the Literature Review and the order in which you would discuss each topic.
4. Critique this title for a study that was published as a protocol, giving the positives and negatives. Rewrite the title to make it shorter.

   Rationale and design of the Baptist Employee Healthy Heart Study: A randomized trial assessing the efficacy of the addition of an interactive, personalized, web-based lifestyle intervention tool to an existing health information web platform in a high-risk employee population.
5. For the following study, write your own abstract. Your abstract is limited to 250 words. Use these headings: Background, Objectives, Methods, Results, Conclusions.

   "Evaluating the Influence of the Revised Special Supplemental Nutrition Program for Women, Infants, and Children (WIC) Food Allocation Package on Healthy Food Availability, Accessibility, and Affordability in Texas" by Wenhua Lu, Lisako J. McKyer, Diane Dowdy, Alexandra Evans, Marcia Ory, Deanne M. Hoelscher, Suojin Wang, and Jingang Miao. *Journal of the Academy of Nutrition and Dietetics, Volume 116*, Issue 2, pages 292–301
6. Use the abstract from Figure 14.7 to develop a poster. If your college has a template, go ahead and use that. If not, you will find a number of poster templates at http://colinpurrington.com/tips/poster-design.

SUGGESTED READINGS AND ACTIVITIES

1. Gans, K. M., Gorham, G., Risica, P. M., Dulin-Keita, A., Dionne, L., Gao, T., Peters, S., & Principato, L. (2016). A multi-level intervention in subsidized housing sites to increase fruit and vegetable access and intake: Rationale, design, and methods of the 'Live Well, Viva Bien' cluster randomized trial. *BMC Public Health, 16*(521), 1–14. doi: 10.1186/s12889-016-3141-7
2. Post, J. M., Ali, S. S., Robertson, L. L., Aneni, E. C., Shaharyar, S., Younus, A., ... Nasir, K. (2016). Rationale and design of the Baptist Employee Healthy Heart Study: A randomized trial assessing the efficacy of the addition of an interactive, personalized, web-based lifestyle intervention tool to an existing health information web platform in a high-risk employee population. *Trials, 17*(308), 1–9. doi: 10.1186/s13063-016-1424-z
3. Take a quiz on AMA style at http://www.amamanualofstyle.com/page/style-quizzes.
4. Do a tutorial on APA style at http://www.apastyle.org/learn/index.aspx,
5. Review this excellent website on poster design, which includes poster templates: http://colinpurrington.com/tips/poster-design.

REFERENCES

AMA Manual of Style Committee. (2007). *AMA manual of style: A guide for authors and editors* (10th ed.). Oxford, UK: Oxford University Press.

American Psychological Association. (2010). *Publication manual of the American Psychological Association* (6th ed.). Washington, DC: American Psychological Association.

Boullata, J. I., & Mancuso, C. E. (2007). A "How-To" guide in preparing abstracts and poster presentations. *Nutrition in Clinical Practice, 22*, 641–646. doi: 10.1177/0115426507022006641

Caulley, D. N. (1992). *Writing a critical review of the literature.* Bundoora, Australia: La Trobe University.

Cone, J. D., & Foster, S. L. (1993). *Dissertations and theses from start to finish: Psychology and related fields.* Washington, DC: American Psychological Association.

Denicolo, P., & Becker, L. (2012). *Developing research proposals.* London, UK: Sage Publications.

Erren, T. C., & Bourne, P. E. (2007). Ten simple rules for a good poster presentation. *PLOS Computational Biology, 3*, e102.

Garrard, J. (2014). *Health sciences literature review made easy: The matrix method* (4th ed.). Burlington, MA: Jones & Bartlett Learning.

Heard, S. B. (2016). *The scientist's guide to writing: How to write more easy and effectively throughout your scientific career.* Princeton, NJ: Princeton University Press.

Jha, K. N. (2014). How to write articles that get published. *Journal of Clinical & Diagnostic Research, 8*, XG01–XF03. doi: 10.7860/JCDR/2014/8107.4855

Locke, L. F., Wyrick Spirduso, W., & Silverman, S. J. (2014). *Proposals that work: A guide for planning dissertations and grant proposals.* Los Angeles, CA: Sage.

Matthews, J. R., & Matthews, R. W. (2014). *Successful scientific writing: A step-by-step guide for the biological and medical sciences* (4th ed.). Cambridge, UK: Cambridge University Press.

McAleese, J. D., & Rankin, L. L. (2007). Garden-based nutrition education affects fruit and vegetable consumption in sixth-grade adolescents. *Journal of the American Dietetic Association, 107*, 662–665. doi: 10.1016/j.jada.2007.01.015

MIT Libraries. (2016). *Overview of citation software at MIT: Managing your references.* Retrieved from http://libguides.mit.edu/references

Pautasso, M. (2013). Ten simple rules for writing a Literature Review. *PLOS Computational Biology, 9*, e1003149. doi: 10.1371/journal.pcbi.1003149

Purrington, C. B. (2015). Designing conference posters. Retrieved from http://colinpurrington.com/tips/poster-design

Satia-Abouta, J., Patterson, R.E., Neuhouser, M.L., & Elder, J. (2002). Dietary acculturation: Application to nutrition research and dietetics. *Journal of the American Dietetic Association, 102*, 1105–1118. doi: 10.1016/S0002-8223(02)90247-6

Turabian, K. L. (2013). *A manual for writers of research papers, theses, and dissertations: Chicago style for students & researchers.* Chicago, IL: University of Chicago Press.

CHAPTER

15

Securing Grants for Nutrition Research

CHAPTER OUTLINE

- Introduction
- Government Funding
- Nongovernment Funding
- Plan Your Application
- Develop and Write Your Grant Proposal

LEARNING OUTCOMES

- Identify where to find grant funding using government and nongovernment sources.
- Distinguish between government and nongovernment funding.
- Given an idea for a grant, locate appropriate funders.
- Plan, develop and write a simple grant proposal.

INTRODUCTION

Standard Four of the Standards of Professional Performance for Registered Dietitians states that "The registered dietitian applies, participates in, or generates research to enhance practice" (Academy Quality Management Committee and Scope of Practice Subcommittee, 2013, p. S40). Without adequate funding, it is difficult to move forward with your research ideas. To secure a grant, you need a good understanding of how to find funding sources that support your research questions and hypotheses, and how to put forth a strong research proposal. A grant is the way a federal or nonfederal organization provides funding for your ideas, projects, or services. If this is your first time seeking a grant or funding for your research, the process can seem daunting. Fortunately, there are resources available to help you get started. Conducting research as a student can be very rewarding, and it will look great on your resume. Opportunities for funding are often underutilized by students because students do not know where to start looking. Research will allow you to take your classroom knowledge and apply it to a real world setting.

The following steps will help you get started on your first research proposal:

1. *Establish the need for your research and demonstrate a clear and thorough understanding of your topic and your research strategy*. If you are trying to secure funding for a topic or an idea, you better know your facts. Insufficient knowledge and incorrect details about the current state of research in your field will surely lead to a rejected proposal. Demonstrating knowledge of the current state of research in your field is essential for getting approval. Familiarize yourself with the current literature and be able to identify the gap you want to investigate and why it is important. Also, remember that research is not necessary, nor will it be monetarily supported, if it does not answer new questions. A good solid research proposal should consist of a thought-provoking question and plenty of details to support your idea. Your proposal should give the reviewers a concise and solid understanding of what you will do when you are spending their money. Building a strong relationship with funders will also help you find funding.
2. *Familiarize yourself with the types of funding available, locate the funders whose priorities match your topic/idea, and thoroughly research each possible funding source.* The two primary categories for funding nutrition research include government (federal) and nongovernment grants (nonfederal). Under each of these umbrellas are a variety of funding sources and programs that may be willing to support your endeavor. Your job is to learn as much you can about possible funders and the requirements for each proposal. Especially consider how well you meet a funder's requirements. That will be a major factor in whether you are successful.
3. *Show each potential funder that you have the ability to accomplish what you propose*. Even if you have located the appropriate funders for your project and written a solid proposal, if the funders are at all shaky about whether you can pull this off, they will likely pick someone else. Make sure your credentials and those of anyone else on your team are appropriately highlighted in the application/proposal.

This chapter will help you navigate the funding environment and provide you with the tools necessary to secure grant money for your research. First, we discuss funding sources, and then how to write a proposal.

GOVERNMENT FUNDING

The federal government funds much of the research in the United States. Some of the funding agencies include the National Institutes of Health, Centers for Disease Control and Prevention, National Institute for Food & Agriculture, Agency for Healthcare Research and Quality, and the National Science Foundation. Grants.gov is the federal government's centralized site for grant seekers to access information about federal grants. The site is useful in many, many ways, from searching for grants to accessing federal forms and getting information on grants already handed out. To apply for a grant, your organization must be registered on Grants.gov.

Keep in mind that some grant money is also available from state governments. States can apply for a **pass-through grant** from the federal government and then pass the federal money on to applicants. One advantage of applying for a state pass-through grant is that you compete only against other applicants in your state, but the awards tend to be smaller than at the federal level.

National Institutes of Health (NIH)

The NIH is the main source of government grants supporting nutrition research and clinical trials. Past NIH research has paved the way for breakthroughs in new treatments and disease prevention.

The NIH comprises 27 Institutes and Centers (ICs), many of which support nutrition research. Examples include the following:

- National Cancer Institute (NCI)
- National Heart, Lung and Blood Institute (NHLBI)
- National Institute on Aging (NIA)
- National Institute for Diabetes, Digestive and Kidney Disorders (NIDDK)
- National Center for Complementary and Alternative Medicine (NCCAM)

Of the 27 ICs, 24 provide funding for research. Approximately 80% of the NIH budget each year supports research in colleges, universities, medical schools, and other research organizations globally. An additional 10% of the NIH budget goes to NIH researchers who work in the laboratories at the headquarters in Bethesda, Maryland.

Intramural NIH research is conducted by scientists employed by the federal government. Many of them work on the NIH campus in Bethesda, Maryland. **Extramural NIH research** is done across the United States and in some foreign countries by investigators who have been awarded grants through the NIH grant program.

Congress provides funding to each of the ICs, and they then decide how these funds will be distributed to the proposed grants. The amount of funds distributed to a grant application is based on scientific peer review, public health necessity, and scientific need. Generally speaking, research that has been awarded funding has received a high merit rating in the peer review process.

As a researcher seeking funding, it is important to do your homework and understand the unique mission and focus of each IC. For example, if you conduct research on factors contributing to health and disease in older people, you would seek funding from the Division of Geriatrics and Clinical Gerontology of the National Institute on Aging (NIA). The ICs are interested in supporting research and in turn providing funding to studies that support their unique mission.

Some research may be appropriate for submission to more than one IC. In that case, scientific program officials who are employed at the NIH can assist you in determining the best IC choice for your research. The NIH also has a matchmaker tool, the **NIH RePorter**, that can assist you in finding the most compatible IC for your research as well as contact information for program officials. The NIH RePorter is a repository of information about NIH-funded research projects, and you can look at current projects and consider how your research might be a little different or unique, which can be an advantage when you submit your proposal.

The NIH categorizes most of its grant funding available into the types shown in **Table 15.1**. The Research Grants (R Series) are the most commonly utilized for basic research and comprise the largest category of funding and support by the NIH. The R Series grants are often awarded to colleges, universities, medical schools, hospitals, research institutes, and other government institutions that conduct research in the biomedical sciences. The funding is used for researcher salaries, equipment, supplies, travel, and any additional expenses needed to carry out the study. The NIH has defined activity codes (e.g., R01, R02, etc.) to categorize research-related programs where funding is available through the ICs. **Table 15.2** provides a description of the various R Series Activity codes and the type of research they support.

Table 15.1 Types of NIH Grants

Type of NIH grant	Highlights
Research Grants (R Series)	Most commonly used grant program.
Career Development Awards (K Series)	Funds research training opportunities for college bound individuals including those in undergraduate, graduate, and postdoctoral programs.
Research & Training Fellowships (R & T Series)	Funds research training opportunities for college bound individuals including those in undergraduate, graduate, and postdoctoral programs.
Program Project/Center Grants (P Series)	Provides support for project-based research that involves multiple independent investigators who share the same resources and are contributing to a common research theme.
Resource Grants (Various Series)	Provides funding and support for resources used to execute research projects. Funds education projects to generate and promote interest in biomedical research by providing training and communicating advances in science via community applications.
Trans-NIH Programs	A program that supports new initiatives in biomedical research that requires efforts from more than one NIH institute to gain new scientific knowledge and interpret it for public health benefits.

Modified from "Types of Grant Programs," by the National Institutes of Health, 2016b. Retrieved from https://grants.nih.gov/grants/funding/funding_program.htm

Table 15.2 Frequently Used R Series Research Grants

Activity code	Title	Description
R01	NIH Research Project Grant Program	• Used to support a discrete, specified, research project. • NIH's most commonly used grant program. • No specific dollar limit unless specified in Funding Opportunity Announcement (FOA). • Generally awarded for 3 to 5 years. • Utilized by all ICs.
R03	NIH Small Grant Program	• Provides limited funding for a short period of time to support a variety of types of projects, including pilot or feasibility studies, collection of preliminary data, secondary analysis of existing data, etc. • Limited to 2 years of funding. • Not renewable. • Utilized by more than half of the NIH ICs.
R13	NIH Support for Conferences and Scientific Meetings	• Support for high-quality conferences/scientific meetings that are relevant to NIH's scientific mission and to public health. • Requires advance permission from the funding IC. • Support for up to 5 years may be possible.
R15	NIH Academic Research Enhancement Award (AREA)	• Supports small-scale research projects in the biomedical and behavioral sciences conducted by undergraduate or graduate students and faculty in institutions of higher education that have not been major recipients of NIH research grant funds. • Eligibility limited. • Project period limited to up to 3 years. • Utilized by most NIH ICs.

Table 15.2 Frequently Used R Series Research Grants (continued)

Activity code	Title	Description
R21	NIH Exploratory/ Developmental Research Grant Award	• Encourages new, exploratory, and developmental research projects by providing support for the early stages of project development. Sometimes used for pilot and feasibility studies. • Limited to up to 2 years of funding. • No preliminary data is generally required. • Utilized by most NIH ICs.
R34	NIH Clinical Trial Planning Grant Program	• Designed to permit early peer review of the rationale for the proposed clinical trial and support development of essential elements of a clinical trial. • Usual project period of 1 year, sometimes up to 3 years. • Used only by select ICs.

Modified from "Types of Grant Programs," by the National Institutes of Health, 2016b. Retrieved from https://grants.nih.gov/grants/funding/funding_program.htm

The **Funding Opportunity Announcements (FOAs)** include specific eligibility criteria for the research grants and which ICs participate. All federal grant-making agencies publish FOAs at Grants.gov to notify potential applicants of the requirements, forms to apply for grant funding, and the number of grants to be given. For any application you submit to NIH, you will apply through an FOA.

Panels of expert scientists review all grant applications submitted to the NIH in a process known as **peer review**. Although a number of factors contribute to whether your application will be funded, great emphasis is placed on how the reviewers rate the scientific merit of your proposal. Section V of every FOA details the review criteria that will be used to assess your application.

Centers for Disease Control and Prevention (CDC)

The CDC provides funding mostly related to disease prevention programs targeted to improve public health. The CDC also supports nutrition-related research, mostly clinical trials that also target disease prevention. Under the CDC umbrella, the centers that support nutrition-related research include the National Center for Birth Defects and Developmental Disabilities, National Center for Chronic Disease Prevention and Health Promotion, and the National Center for HIV/AIDS, Viral Hepatitis, STD and TB Prevention.

National Institute for Food and Agriculture (NIFA)

NIFA, formerly known as CSREES, is the USDA's primary source of funding for individuals, institutions and various profit and nonprofit organizations. NIFA supports nutrition-related research mostly to advance agriculture-related sciences and address agricultural problems that affect consumers and communities. NIFA also provides a comprehensive list on their website of all funded research projects.

AGENCY FOR HEALTHCARE RESEARCH AND QUALITY (AHRQ)

AHRQ is an operating division of the U.S. Department of Health and Human Services. The division focuses on research in these areas: making health care safer and improving quality and improving healthcare affordability, accessibility, and efficiency.

NATIONAL SCIENCE FOUNDATION (NSF)

NSF provides funding for research mostly in the areas of science and engineering. A large portion of their funding is awarded as federal support to over 2,000 K–12 school systems, colleges and universities (graduate and postgraduate research), and businesses /science organizations that are involved in basic research. To apply for a grant with NSF, you must register and use FastLane, an online portal.

APPLICATION 15.1

Compare the number and type of nutrition grants available at NIH versus the National Science Foundation.

NONGOVERNMENT FUNDING

When discussing nongovernment sources of grants, you will frequently hear the term **foundations**. In the nonprofit sector, foundations are not precisely defined but generally refer to an organization that makes grants to institutions, organizations, or individuals for scientific, educational, or other reasons. In addition to funding grants, many foundations engage in their own programs and charitable activities. Private foundations are usually established with funds from an individual, a family, or a company. Examples include the Allen Foundation, the Bill and Melinda Gates Foundation, and the Sodexo Foundation. Corporate foundations, such as the Nestle Foundation, are usually set up as private foundations.

Various foundations can be excellent sources of nutrition-related research funding; however, there may be some risk. These organizations may cease funding with little notice, property from the study may not belong to the researcher, and it may be more difficult to adhere to ethical practices. Written agreements can counter some of these potential issues.

PRIVATE FOUNDATIONS AND DISEASE-SPECIFIC ORGANIZATIONS

Table 15.3 highlights organizations that provide funding for research related to health, wellness, nutrition, and food insecurity. A comprehensive list of foundations, some of which support nutrition-related research, can be found at http://foundationcenter.org This site compiles a listing of more than 2,000 organizations and specifies the funding interests, grant allotments, processes for applying, and contact information. The site requires a subscription, but many public and university libraries offer free access.

Table 15.3 Private Foundations and Disease-Specific Funding Organizations

Organization	Disease focus	Funding focus	Website
American Heart Association (AHA)	Heart disease	Diet, Lifestyle, CV Research	http://www.heart.org Click on "Research"
American Cancer Society (ACS)	Cancer	Diet, Lifestyle, Cancer Research	http://www.cancer.org/ Click on "Explore Research"
American Institute for Cancer Research	Cancer	Diet, Lifestyle, Cancer Research	http://www.aicr.org/
Susan G. Komen Foundation	Cancer	Diet, Lifestyle, Cancer Research	http://ww5.komen.org/ Click on "Grants Central"
American Diabetes Association Research Foundation	Diabetes	Diet, Lifestyle, Diabetes Research	www.diabetes.org Click on "Research and Practice"
Celiac Disease Foundation	Celiac disease	Celiac Disease Research and Awareness	https://celiac.org/ Click on "Celiac Disease" and "For Researchers"
Food Allergy Research and Education (FARE)	Food allergies	Food Allergy Research and Awareness	http://www.foodallergy.org/research/apply-for-a-grant
Robert Wood Johnson Foundation	Health promotion	Health, Wellness, and Nutrition	www.rwjf.org
Allen Foundation	Health promotion	Health, Wellness, and Nutrition	https://www.allenfoundation.org
Bill & Melinda Gates Foundation	Food insecurity	Women and Children in Developing Countries	http://www.gatesfoundation.org/What-We-Do/Global-Development/Nutrition
International Nutrition Foundation	Food insecurity	Nutrition and Health Issues in Developing Countries	http://www.inffoundation.org/
No Kid Hungry—Share Our Strength	Food insecurity	Access to Healthy Food	https://bestpractices.nokidhungry.org/

Academy of Nutrition and Dietetics Foundation and Dietetic Practice Groups

Several professional organizations set aside funding for nutrition-related research. The Academy of Nutrition and Dietetics Foundation (ANDF) was established in 1966 to promote nutrition and dietetics research conducted by Registered Dietitian Nutritionists (RDNs). The foundation seeks donations and focuses on investing in nutrition research to promote RDNs and to move the profession forward. ANDF has expanded efforts to make funding available on an annual basis for academy members. This funding supports the ongoing need and desire of academy members to conduct research in an effort to keep abreast of the emerging areas of our profession. This, in turn, will help the profession provide the most up-to-date and accurate nutrition information to consumers, and it highlights the role of the RDN as the nutrition expert. ANDF has a comprehensive list of available grants and past grant recipients on its website.

In addition, various dietetic practice groups support nutrition-related research. Many of the practice groups do not have active grants; however, some are working to raise funds to support practice-specific research.

INDUSTRY SOURCES

Industry funding for nutrition-related research is another viable option. Some examples of industries that might support your research include pharmaceutical companies, food companies, nutrition supplement manufacturers, cooperative extensions, and health equipment companies. **Table 15.4** summarizes some corporate foundations that support nutrition-related research.

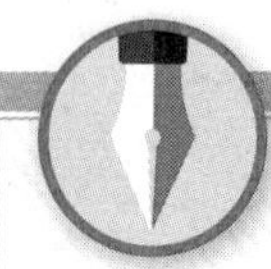

TIP

In general, foundations offer smaller grants than many of the government programs. Also, their grants tend to be in more focused areas.

Table 15.4 Corporate Foundations

Industry	Funding interest	Website
Aetna Foundation	Health, Wellness, and Nutrition	https://www.aetna-foundation.org/
Atkins Foundation	Weight Management, Cardiovascular Disease, Diabetes	http://www.atkinsfoundation.org/
Bristol Myer-Squibb Foundation	Cancer, Cardiovascular Disease, Infectious Disease, Metabolic Disorders	http://www.bms.com/foundation/Pages/home.aspx
Campbell's Soup Foundation	Health, Wellness, and Nutrition, with an emphasis on Youth Programs	http://www.campbellsoupcompany.com/Foundation.aspx
ConAgra Foods Foundation	Access to Healthy Food	http://www.conagrafoods.com/our-commitment/child-hunger
General Mills Foundation	Food Insecurity, Sustainability, and Agriculture	https://www.generalmills.com/Responsibility/general-mills-foundation
Gerber Foundation	Nutrition for Infants and Children up to age 3.	http://www.gerberfoundation.org/pd-research/research/pediatric-nutrition/8-research-general
H. J. Heinz Company Foundation	Nutrition	http://www.heinz.com/sustainability/communities/heinz-foundation.aspx
W. K. Kellogg Foundation	Wellness, Public Health	http://www.wkkf.org/grants
Nestle Foundation	Wellness, Public Health, Maternal and Childhood Nutrition	http://www.nestle.com/csv/nutrition/nutriton-health-research
Newman's Own Foundation	Nutrition Awareness, Education, and Fresh Food Access	http://newmansownfoundation.org
Nutritional Research Foundation	Diabetes, Cardiovascular Disease, Cancer, Autoimmune Diseases	https://www.nutritionalresearch.org/
Sodexo Foundation	Hunger	http://ysa.org/grants/sodexoyouth/

APPLICATION 15.2

Compare and contrast the opportunities for nutrition-related grants from Robert Wood Johnson Foundation, ANDF, and the Gerber Foundation.

PLAN YOUR APPLICATION

First you need to spend time identifying funders who would be a good fit for your proposed project. The best place to start learning more about funders is through their websites, where you can start becoming familiar with their priority areas, grant guidelines, and special funding initiatives. Lists of current and previously funded programs also can be found on these websites. Familiarizing yourself with previously funded programs is a great way to gain a better understanding on what the organizations are looking for, and it will help you think about how your project will be original and exert a powerful influence in the field.

Another way to learn about funders is to contact them. A brief email inquiry can plant the seed as you briefly explain your intent and inquire about the appropriateness of the project for the funder. Another approach is to place a call directly to the foundation or federal agency. Although you may think that a huge funder, such as NIH, really does not have time to talk to you, NIH recommends you contact them prior to submitting an application. This will start the conversation and build a relationship, and you may also get feedback on your proposed idea. Whether emailing or calling, be prepared to answer questions about your project and be knowledgeable about the funder.

If you plan to ask a private sector funder for money, check to see if you first need to send an initial **letter of inquiry**. Many private foundations want to review a letter of inquiry first to determine whether they have an interest in your project before accepting a full application/proposal. The foundation may have specific guidelines on length, or may ask you to submit your inquiry using an online form. An inquiry letter should include the following information in three pages or less:

- *Introduction.* Introduce your organization and then present an abstract of what is written in the rest of the letter.
- *Statement of need.* Describe the problem and the need for the project, as well as the solution.
- *Project description.* State the methodology, timetable, amount of funding to be requested, and expected outcomes. Include names, titles, and key qualifications of researchers.
- *Connection to funder's purpose.* Show how your organization and project meets the funder's interests and priorities.
- *Closing.* Restate how the project fits their organization. Request a follow-up conversation to answer further questions, say thank-you for their consideration, and provide contact information.

When targeting private foundations, you may want to invite the funder or grant maker to tour your organization. Building good relationships with foundations requires many conversations. Funders want to know you will put their money to good use and that you have a reliable team to execute the study and communicate progress on an ongoing basis.

When planning your application, there are many possible facets to consider at this early stage.

- *Carefully read each application's guidelines several times.* Are you/your organization eligible? Is the deadline too soon? Is the range of the grant award appropriate for your project? What will the application require? Will the application be peer reviewed, and if so, what are the criteria? Can you deliver what the grantor is looking for?
- *Will you need collaborators?* Most likely you will. Who will they be? Qualified collaborators can fill in any gaps in credentials or expertise, so spend some time finding appropriate collaborators. For NIH applications, you will need letters of commitment, Memoranda of Understanding, or Memoranda of Agreement from anyone who will be working with you. These documents are working agreements that spell out the services of each party.
- *Evaluate the resources and support you have available where you work, and what you will need to put into the proposed budget.* If you are requesting funding from a particular funder for the first time, keep in mind that you are less likely to get the maximum amount of funding until you have had some experience working successfully with them.
- *You will need assurances from your Institutional Review Board* that this study will receive approval.

Develop a time line to complete all parts of the application, including getting feedback and review, so that the application is handed in (often electronically, which can require additional time) on time.

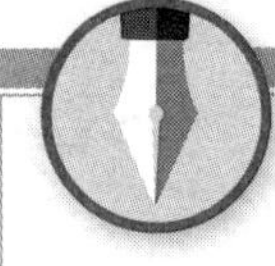

TIP

Many researchers have to hand in a grant application to their own internal Research Office well before the deadline to allow for review. So you need to work extra time into your time line.

DEVELOP AND WRITE YOUR GRANT PROPOSAL

Once you have established the need for your research, determined eligibility, and know where to go to secure funding, you are ready to start writing your proposal. The length and format of your proposal will vary depending on the funder, but in general you will be writing a narrative in these areas.

1. Cover letter
2. Abstract (executive summary)
3. Statement of need/problem statement
4. Research design/methodology
5. Evaluation
6. Background of organization
7. Budget

If the funder is the federal government, you will prepare a grant application. If the funder is a private foundation or corporate grant, it is still called a grant application but is also frequently called a **proposal**. Some private foundations may ask you to use the Common

Grant Application format (much like you may have used the Common Application to apply to college), which is available online.

You can find examples of completed NIH grant applications online. Just use Google or go to this website: https://www.niaid.nih.gov/researchfunding/grant/pages/appsamples.aspx#r21r33

Table 15.5 lists some reasons grant applications may be rejected. Applications may be rejected if the applicant did not follow all the details specified by the grantor—even something as simple as using a certain size font. When you submit a federal grant application, it may first be reviewed to see whether you have submitted all the required forms and to verify that the document is formatted properly and not longer than specified. Only if you have paid attention to these details will your application continue to the next step to be fully reviewed.

Write a Compelling Need/Problem Statement

This section explains the reason for the application. The statement of need shows that the project will address an unmet need, an important gap, or a community problem. If you have done your homework, you have already picked possible grantors whose mission and initiatives align with your statement of need.

Suggestions for writing the statement of need include these points:

- *Do not use generalities*. Use well-documented data that is clearly cited, and make sure the information is accurate and current.
- *Demonstrate a thorough understanding of the problem and/or gaps* addressing the problem, including social and economic costs.
- *Do not present only quantitative data*. If you can, use qualitative data to help persuade funders of the importance of your project. For example, use real stories or documentaries of people who are affected by the problem.
- *Use attention-grabbing visuals* such as comparison charts, bar graphs, and so forth to communicate key points.
- *Be clear and compelling.*
- *Toward the end, give some brief information on how this problem might be solved.*

Cite all the sources that you use in this section.

Define Clear Goals and Objectives

Once you have constructed a compelling problem statement, the next step is to write your goals and objectives. **Goals** are broad-based statements of what your project will accomplish. **Objectives** are measurable steps that are taken to achieve each

Table 15.5 Why Grant Proposals Are Rejected
1. The proposal was not a "good fit" for the funder.
2. The proposal was not complete; one or more elements were missing.
3. One or more elements of the proposal were not completely clear or described in sufficient detail.
4. The problem was not sufficiently important.
5. The research design was not suited to the objective or likely to produce new or useful information.
6. The quality of the writing was poor, or the proposal showed lack of attention to details.
7. The proposed study appeared to be beyond the capacity of the authors in terms of their experience, training, and available resources.
8. The cost of the proposed study was high/unrealistic.

goal. Measurable objectives are necessary to determine the success of your program once the study has been completed. Objectives should be specific, measurable, achievable, relevant, and time-bound (SMART). **Table 15.6** provides an example of a well-constructed goal with SMART objectives.

It is important that your goals and objectives be aligned with the purpose of the funding you are requesting. It is also important that your goals aim to produce information that is new or useful. If your application is going to be successful, you cannot test something that has already been done a number of times. There has to be a novel element, and it should be reflected in your goals and objectives.

DEVELOP THE RESEARCH DESIGN/METHODOLOGY

This section helps funders understand how you will accomplish the goals and objectives. The research design includes all the details of how your project will be carried out and evaluated, and generally includes the overall research design, sampling methods, instrumentation, and procedures. Because this section tends to be long, it is crucial to have good organization (such as a time line for implementation) and transparency to make sure reviewers do not miss an item of critical importance. Reviewers look especially hard at whether your research design is:

- suited to the objectives,
- explicit, detailed, and well thought out,
- rigorous, and
- likely to yield unbiased results.

Whichever methodology you choose, be prepared to answer these questions clearly in the application:

- How was the methodology determined to be the best one to solve the problem presented?
- Does it build on models already in existence, or is it a different approach?
- If it is different, why is it different?

In any case, the methodology must be rigorous.

Funders also want to know details about staffing the study and the qualifications of those involved. If you will be hiring personnel once you get the grant, you still need to provide information on the qualifications for those positions. For many of the personnel in the study, a paragraph highlighting the relevant qualifications and designating the percentage of the position that will be charged to the grant budget is sufficient. However,

Table 15.6 Example of Goal and Objectives

Goal	Objectives
All children in Boston public schools will have access to healthy fresh produce.	1. Boston public schools will offer two or more fresh fruit choices as part of the school breakfast program by the end of the school year. 2. Boston public schools will offer at least two fresh fruit and two fresh vegetable choices with the school lunch program by the end of the school year. 3. Boston public schools will offer two or more fresh fruit or vegetable choices with the after school snack program by the end of the school year. 4. Children in Boston public schools will consume at least two or more fruits or vegetables daily while attending school by the end of the school year.

more information is required for the lead researcher, called the **principal investigator** (PI), for a grant in the sciences. Federal grants usually ask for a biographical sketch (with page limits) of the PI, including education/training, personal statement, positions and honors, peer-reviewed publications, and other ongoing or completed research grants.

The PI is responsible for managing the project and ensuring that it is successful. The PI plans and controls the project, communicates with others, oversees evaluation, and monitors the use of all resources, including money. The PI also periodically reports project progress to the grantor. Reviewers want to know that the PI and other personnel have the necessary qualifications to carry out the project successfully.

Keep in mind that the Methods section should be written to ensure that all components are realistic and attainable using the proposed resources. In addition, make sure the resources and each activity are tied to your program budget.

Prepare the Evaluation

Evaluating a program focuses on process evaluation and outcome evaluation.

- **Process evaluation** looks at measurements taken during the project itself to assure or improve its quality. Process evaluation answers the question, "Was the project implemented successfully?"
- **Outcome evaluation** focuses on measuring the end results to see if the goals and objectives have been met. Outcome evaluation answers the question, "Did the project achieve its goals?"

In addition, a program may use formative evaluation. **Formative evaluation** is usually conducted when a new program or activity is being developed or when an existing one is being adapted or modified. It ensures that a program or activity is appropriate, reasonable, and acceptable (to the stakeholders) before it is fully implemented.

When writing this section, use the following questions as a guide:

- What data (quantitative and qualitative) should be collected (based on goals and objectives)?
- What is the specific evaluation design?
  - When will data be collected?
  - Using what strategies or instruments?
  - Using what comparison group or baseline, if any?
- Who will collect the data? Have they been trained to collect data?
- Who will receive the results?
- Who will analyze the data and report the results?
- What procedures will be used to determine whether the program was implemented as planned?
- When will corrective actions be taken if the data shows problems with implementation or outcomes?
- Have you addressed the grantor's guidelines on evaluation?
- Does your evaluation plan align with your goals and objectives?

Writing this section will help you see the strengths and weaknesses of your proposal and provide you with the opportunity to make adjustments as needed to strengthen your project.

Writing the evaluation requires critical thinking and the ability to see the big picture. Also, remember that you need to visualize the end but also take into consideration how the findings will be used and how the program will improve the lives of a specific community or population served.

DEVELOP THE PROJECT BUDGET

Another component of your written proposal is to establish a written program budget. A detailed budget is critical to your grant proposal because it will show specifics on how the funding will be allocated. For this section of the application, make sure that:

- your costs are reasonable,
- your costs are justified by the results of the project, and
- each cost is directly related to an activity to meet a goal and objective.

When developing a program budget, begin by reviewing the grant application instructions to determine the budget requirements. Funders may require a standard budget template with specific instructions and financial data that should be recorded. The instructions also may address what *not* to include in your budget. Once you understand the instructions, you can begin to organize and create your budget. This step will require some time and research to determine how much it will cost for various supplies, services, and personnel. Once you have a handle on the budget instructions and approximate costs, you can begin to write your budget. The budget section of the application usually requires you to complete a budget summary, a table that shows expenses for all line items, and also a budget narrative.

Budgets are typically written for a calendar year, a fiscal year, or for the duration of the grant. Expenses are usually broken down into direct and indirect costs. **Direct costs** are expenses directly related to your project. **Indirect costs**, also called **overhead costs**, cover things such as rent, utilities, and telephone. **Table 15.7** lists some examples of both. Indirect costs may be calculated in some way by the grantor and be reimbursed (especially if you have a federal grant). In other cases, indirect costs will not be reimbursed.

After you have completed your spreadsheet and recorded all of the projected expenses, summarize your budget in a narrative format known as a **budget narrative** or **budget justification**. This section explains your budget and provides further clarification to the funder. The budget justification should accompany your budget summary, and it should be written in a format that is clear and concise.

If you are writing a grant to obtain funding for a new or an ongoing program, you will probably have to address how you will continue your program once the grant money and other funding sources are exhausted (known as sustainability). Because funds are limited to the terms of the grant, funders like to know how you will continue to support the program after the grant period. This section is often overlooked in the proposal, but it may be essential to the success of winning a grant. Funders want to know that your efforts and their money will not go to waste and that the program will continue after the grant comes to a close. In some cases, this section may not be listed as a requirement in

Table 15.7 Direct and Indirect Costs

Direct costs	Indirect costs
Salaries	Utilities
Benefits	Office space
Grant-related travel	Grants management
Equipment	IT support
Supplies and materials	Equipment rental

the grant guidelines; however, it is advisable to include this information to show funders that you are thinking about your program beyond the life of the initial grant. This will instill confidence in the funder's decision to support you. Future funding can be sought from a variety of sources:

Continuation Grants from Grantors. Although funders typically like to support new programs, they may fund your ongoing efforts. This is one reason it is important to build strong relationships with the funders.

Fees for Service. In some cases, clients may be asked to pay a fee for an ongoing service. If this is your approach to ongoing funding, be sure to write this into your proposal.

Sales of Items or Activities. In some cases, a nonprofit organization can generate revenue from various sources such as an onsite gift shop, publications, or educational symposiums. This approach should also be written into your proposal.

A detailed sustainability plan will instill confidence in your funder and result in you winning the grant and beginning to build a great relationship for future projects.

Tips for Writing Grants

Wisdom, Riley, and Myers (2015) reviewed more than 1,000 abstracts of articles about writing successful grant proposals for faculty in the health science field. They narrowed down the number of articles to 53 (using inclusion criteria). The 53 articles gave 445 separate recommendations, which were then condensed into the following 10 recommendations for writing successful grant proposals (p. 1721):

1. Research and identify appropriate funding opportunities.
2. Use key components of the proposal to persuade reviewers of the project's significance and feasibility.
3. Describe proposed activities and their significance persuasively, clearly, and concisely.
4. Seek advice from colleagues to help develop, clarify, and review the proposal.
5. Keep the study design simple, logical, feasible, and appropriate for the research questions.
6. Develop a time line that includes time for possible resubmission to guide the grant proposal process.
7. Choose a novel, high-impact project with long-term potential.
8. Conduct an exhaustive literature review to clarify the present state of knowledge about the topic.
9. Ensure budgets request only essential items and reflect an honest portrayal of the funding that the team needs to successfully carry out the work.
10. Consider interdisciplinary collaborations.

Table 15.8 provides some additional tips from NIH for writing grants.

APPLICATION 15.3

Where does this list of tips from NIH overlap with the list from Wisdom, Riley, and Myers (2015)?

Table 15.8 Tips for Writing Grants

TIP 1. Make Your Project's Goals Realistic

Do not propose more work than can be reasonably done during the proposed project period.

- Before you start writing the application, think about the budget and how it is related to your research plan. Remember that everything in the budget must be justified by the work you have proposed to do.
- Be realistic. Do not propose more work than can be reasonably done during the proposed project period. Make sure that the personnel have appropriate scientific expertise and training. Make sure that the budget is reasonable and well-justified.

TIP 2. Be Organized and Logical

Why? Reviewers are accustomed to finding information in specific sections of the application. This creates an efficient evaluation process and saves reviewers from hunting for required information.

Start with an outline, following the suggested organization of the application. The thought process of the application should be easy to follow.

- Write clear headings.
- Use subheadings, short paragraphs, and other techniques to make the application as easy to navigate as possible. Be specific and informative, and avoid redundancies.
- Bookmark major sections.
- Use diagrams, figures and tables, and include appropriate legends, to assist the reviewers to understand complex information. These should complement the text and be appropriately inserted. Make sure the figures and labels are readable in the size they will appear in the application.
- Use bullets and numbered lists for effective organization. Indents and bold print add readability. Bolding highlights key concepts and allows reviewers to scan the pages and retrieve information quickly.
- Utilize white space effectively.

TIP 3. Write in Clear Concise Language

Why? A reviewer must often read 10 to 15 applications in great detail, so your application has a better chance of being successful if it is easy to read and well written.

- Write a clear topic sentence for each paragraph with one main point or idea. This is key for readability.
- Make your points as direct as possible. Avoid jargon or excessive language.
- Write simple and clear sentences, keeping to about 20 words or less in each.
- Be consistent with terms, references, and writing style.
- Use the active, rather than passive, voice. For example, write "We will develop an experiment, " not "An experiment will be developed."
- Spell out all acronyms on first reference.
- If writing is not your forte, seek help!

TIP 4. Sell Your Idea on Paper

Capture the reviewers' attention by making the case for why the funder should fund your research!

- Include enough background information to enable an intelligent reader to understand your proposed work.
- Support your idea with collaborators who have expertise that benefits the project.

TIP 5. Edit Yourself, but also Enlist Help

You have most likely been looking at the same words, sentences, and paragraphs repeatedly! Allow someone with fresh eyes to read your content, check your punctuation, and give you feedback on whether the content flows.

- Have zero tolerance for typographical errors, misspellings, grammatical mistakes, or sloppy formatting. A sloppy or disorganized application may lead the reviewers to conclude that your research may be conducted in the same manner.
- **Remember the Details!** There are format requirements, such as font size, margins, and spacing. Make sure you are familiar with them before submitting your application and label sections as directed. You do not want your application delayed because any of these details are not incorporated.
- If more than one investigator is contributing to the writing, it would be helpful to have one editor not only review for punctuation errors, but ensure that the application has a consistent writing style.

Table 15.8 Tips for Writing Grants (continued)

TIP 6. Share for Comments

You have most likely been looking at the same words over and over! Allow someone with fresh eyes to read your content, check your punctuation, and give you feedback on whether the content flows.

- Request your colleagues or mentors to review a first draft of your specific aims early in the process. This step can save lots of valuable time.
- Allow time for an internal review by collaborators, colleagues, and mentors and make revisions/edits from that review. If possible, have both experts in your field and those who are less familiar with your science provide feedback.
- Ask those who are providing a review to use a critical eye and evaluate the application using the peer-review criteria.
- Allow sufficient time to put the completed application aside, and then read it from a fresh vantage point yourself. Also, try proofreading by reading the application aloud.
- Conduct your own review based on the peer review criteria. How would you rate your own application?

Modified from "Write Your Application" by the National Institutes of Health, 2016c. Retrieved from https://grants.nih.gov/grants/how-to-apply-application-guide/format-and-write/write-your-application.htm

SUMMARY

1. Numerous opportunities exist for securing grants to conduct nutrition-related research. When seeking grants as part of an organization or as an individual, remain diligent in your efforts to secure funding. There is plenty of money to be found. The grant-seeking process takes patience and time.
2. Conducting nutrition-related research can be very rewarding, looks great on your resume, and will allow you the opportunity to apply your classroom knowledge to the real world. The opportunities for funding are often underutilized because students do not know where to look.
3. When seeking a grant, familiarize yourself with the current research on your topic, the types of funding available, and demonstrate to funders that you can accomplish what you propose.
4. Government funding is awarded from federal, state, and local agencies. The NIH comprises 27 Institutes and Centers (ICs) and is the main source of government funding with 24/27 ICs supporting research. Approximately 80% of the NIH budget goes toward research in academic institutions, medical schools, and other global research organizations.
5. Nongovernment funding, through nonprofit and private foundations, disease-specific and professional organizations, industries, and academic institutions, also are excellent sources of nutrition-related research funding. In general, nonprofit funding tends to support more focused areas and to award smaller grants when compared to government funding.
6. When planning your grant application, it is important to identify funders who are compatible with your proposed project. Familiarize yourself with their websites, initiatives, and previously funded programs. Make sure you and your organization are a good match for the grant you are pursuing.
7. Writing a strong grant proposal can lead to a substantial amount of income if written strategically. Make sure to evaluate the readiness of your organization to receive the funding before submitting your proposal.
8. Establishing a positive rapport with funders is key to securing funds. Funders want to know that you will put their money to good use and that you have a reliable team to execute the study and communicate the research results. Having a good understanding as to why grant proposals are rejected is helpful.

9. The length and format of your proposal will vary depending on the funder, but in general you will want to include all of the following areas: problem statement, research design/methodology, evaluation, budget, and background of the organization.

REVIEW QUESTIONS

1. The main source of grant funding, which comprises 27 Institutes and Centers (ICs), is the:
   A. NIH
   B. CDC
   C. NIFA
   D. AHRQ
2. Which of the following is an example of a private foundation (family founded)?
   A. ANDF
   B. Allen Foundation
   C. Kellogg Foundation
   D. Nestle Foundation
3. When developing a proposal idea, it is good to:
   A. do your research on the funders so you have clarity on their mission
   B. involve everyone involved in the potential research in planning
   C. make sure you can successfully implement the research study if granted funding
   D. all of the above
4. The most important aspect of the Evaluation section in a proposal is to:
   A. explain the procedures that will be used to see that the program is implemented as planned
   B. show compelling evidence of a problem or gap
   C. set goals and objectives
   D. all of the above
5. The section of your proposal that shows funders that you are thinking about your program beyond the life of the initial grant is called the:
   A. Evaluation section
   B. Budget section
   C. Sustainability section
   D. all of the above
6. Compare and contrast government and nongovernment funding. Are there any advantages in applying for a government or a nongovernment grant?
7. List the common components of a grant application/proposal and briefly describe each component.
8. Give 10 grant writing tips.

CRITICAL THINKING QUESTIONS

1. You are seriously considering doing an experimental study on the role of resistance training in overweight people trying to lose weight. You want to compare results of a traditional behavioral weight loss program with walking to the same program but also with resistance training 3 times a week.
   A. Find at least one government grant that might be a good match for your study. Explain why it could be a good match.
   B. Find at least one nongovernment grant that might be a good match, and explain why.
   C. Write a compelling statement of need for your project.
   D. Develop the goals and objectives for the project.
   E. What research design would you use? Write down the steps involved in implementing the research, and show them in a time line.

F. How would you evaluate whether the weight loss program with resistance training was more successful than the traditional program?
G. How would you evaluate whether the goals and objectives have been met?
H. What are some examples of direct costs that a grant would cover?

2. Not all grants are used to pay for research studies. Many nutrition grants are used to provide nutrition programs to a variety of audiences—from children in a preschool program to older adults in a community center. Think of a nutrition program you would like to be able to provide. Then answer these questions.

A. Find at least two grants that might be a good match for your study. Explain why either could be a good match.
B. Write a compelling statement of need for your project.
C. Develop the goals and objectives for the project.
D. Describe the steps involved in implementing the program, and show these steps in a time line.
E. How would you evaluate whether the goals and objectives have been met?
F. List the expenses you would want the grant to pay, including salaries.

SUGGESTED READINGS AND ACTIVITIES

1. View a video (1 hour 13 minutes) on "Fundamentals of Effective Grant Writing" found in the Video Library at the University of Wisconsin School of Medicine and Public Health. http://videos.med.wisc.edu/videos/4447
2. View a video (22 minutes) on "What Happens to Your NIH Grant Application: An Overview of Peer Review." https://www.nih.gov/about-nih/nih-research-planning
3. View a video (15 minutes) on "NIH Grants Process: The Big Picture." https://www.youtube.com/watch?v=rNwsg_PR90w
4. National Science Foundation. (2002). *The 2002 User-Friendly Handbook for Project Evaluation*. Arlington, VA: The National Science Foundation.

REFERENCES

Academy Quality Management Committee and Scope of Practice Subcommittee of the Quality Management Committee. (2013). Academy of Nutrition and Dietetics: Revised 2012 Standards of Practice in Nutrition Care and Standards of Professional Performance for Registered Dietitians. *Journal of the Academy of Nutrition and Dietetics*, *113*, S29–S45. doi: 10.1016/j.jand.2012.12.007

Locke, L. F., Spirduso, W. W., & Silverman, S. J. (2014). *Proposals that work: A guide for planning dissertations and grant proposals*. Los Angeles, CA: Sage.

National Institutes of Health. (2016a). *Plan your application*. Retrieved from https://grants.nih.gov/grants/planning_application.htm#idea

National Institutes of Health. (2016b). *Types of grant programs*. Retrieved from https://grants.nih.gov/grants/funding/funding_program.htm

National Institutes of Health. (2016c). *Write your application*. Retrieved from https://grants.nih.gov/grants/how-to-apply-application-guide/format-and-write/write-your-application.htm

National Science Foundation. (2002). *The 2002 User-Friendly Handbook for Project Evaluation*. Arlington, VA: The National Science Foundation.

O'Neal-McElrath, T., & Carlson, M. (2013). Winning grants step by step: The complete workbook for planning, developing, and writing successful proposals (4th ed.) Hoboken, NJ: John Wiley & Sons, Inc.

Thompson, C. A. (2007). Funding nutrition research: Where's the money? *Nutrition in Clinical Practice*, *22*, 609–617. doi: 10.1177/0115426507022006609

Wisdom, J. P., Riley, H., & Myers, N. (2015). Recommendations for writing successful grant proposals: An information synthesis. *Academic Medicine*, *90*, 1720–1725. doi: 10.1097/ACM.0000000000000811

APPENDIX A

FULL LENGTH QUASI-EXPERIMENTAL RESEARCH ARTICLE: GARDEN-BASED NUTRITION EDUCATION AFFECTS FRUIT AND VEGETABLE CONSUMPTION IN SIXTH-GRADE ADOLESCENTS

Jessica D. McAleese, MPH
Linda L. Rankin, PhD, RD, FADA

ABSTRACT

Schoolyard gardens are emerging as a nutrition education tool in academic settings. The purpose of this study was to investigate the effects of garden-based nutrition education on adolescents' fruit and vegetable consumption using a nonequivalent control group design. Sixth-grade students (n = 99) at three different elementary schools made up a control and two treatment groups. Students in the treatment groups participated in a 12-week nutrition education program, and one treatment group also participated in garden-based activities. Students in all three groups completed three 24-hour food-recall workbooks before and after the intervention. A repeated-measures analysis of variance showed that adolescents who participated in the garden-based nutrition intervention increased their servings of fruits and vegetables more than students in the two other groups. Significant increases were also found in vitamin A, vitamin C, and fiber intake. Although further research is needed, the results of this study seem to indicate the efficacy of using garden-based nutrition education to increase adolescents' consumption of fruits and vegetables.

J Am Diet Assoc. 2007;107:662-665.

Research supports the role of fruit and vegetable consumption in cancer and heart disease prevention (1-3). Increasing scientific evidence also suggests a protective role for fruits and vegetables in strokes and possibly cataract formation, chronic obstructive pulmonary disease, diverticulosis, and hypertension (1). Despite this evidence, poor dietary patterns, combined with other unhealthful behaviors, such as sedentary lifestyles, have contributed to the epidemic of overweight and obesity affecting not only adults, but also children and adolescents in the United States (4).

Reproduced from "Garden-Based Nutrition Education Affects Fruit and Vegetable Consumption in Sixth-Grade Adolescents," by J.D. McAleese and L.L. Rankin, 2007, *Journal of the American Dietetic Association*, 107, p. 662-665. Reprinted with permission.

J. D. McAleese is patient advocate, Portneuf Medical Center, Pocatello, ID; at the time of the study, she was a graduate student in the Department of Health and Nutrition Sciences, Idaho State University, Pocatello. L. L. Rankin is an associate professor, Department of Health and Nutrition Sciences, Idaho State University, Pocatello.
Address correspondence to Linda L. Rankin, PhD, RD, FADA, Idaho State University, Department of Health and Nutrition Sciences, Box 8109, Pocatello, ID 83209. E-mail: ranklind@isu.edu

0002-8223/07/10704-0015$32.00/0
doi: 10.1016/j.jada.2007.01.015

Studies have shown that eating patterns (specifically of food choices regarding fruits and vegetables) are developed at an early age and can be traced into and through adulthood (5,6). Proper adolescent nutrition can reduce overweight and obesity and can reduce risk factors for diet-related diseases later in life (6-8). As a result, experts suggest developing interventions and effective nutrition programming early in a child's life as a tool for increasing healthful dietary patterns and reducing the risk of chronic disease later in life (5,9). School-based programs represent an important venue for nutrition behavior change. There is great potential for affecting behaviors and health risks that persist into adulthood, such as food choices and obesity (10-13). Schoolyard gardens are emerging as health education tools in academic settings (14-16). A study of California teachers found that school gardens were perceived as an effective tool for promoting healthful eating habits (15). Morris and Zidenberg-Cherr (17) found that garden-enhanced nutrition education was effective in improving nutrition knowledge and vegetable preferences of fourth-grade students. In a related study, third-grade and fifth-grade students' attitudes toward vegetables became more positive after gardening, but fruit and vegetable consumption did not improve significantly (18).

The current study was designed to measure the effects of garden-based education on fruit and vegetable consumption. The primary study hypothesis was to determine whether adolescents who participated in a garden-based nutrition intervention would increase their fruit and vegetable consumption more than those participating in a nutrition education intervention without any garden activities. A control school was included for comparison.

METHODS

Subjects included 122 sixth-grade students at three similar elementary schools in southeast Idaho. The ages ranged from 10 to 13 years, with a mean age of 11.11 years. The sample populations at each school contained a similar representation of ethnic, cultural, and socioeconomic traits. Selected schools were convenience samples. A nonequivalent control group design was used. A control school and one experimental school (experimental school 1) were randomly assigned, and a second experimental school (experimental school 2) was assigned based on garden availability. Approval for the study was received from the Human Subjects Committee at Idaho State University. Participants in the study were required to be in grade six attending Public School District 25 in Bannock County, Pocatello, ID. In addition, subjects were only eligible if they had turned in signed parental consent and child assent forms.

After confirmation of student eligibility, participants completed three consecutive 24-hour food-recall work-books before as well as after the 12-week intervention. The workbook was developed and validated by Barbara Jendrysik (19). Food-recall workbooks were administered in assigned classrooms by the sixth-grade teachers. Teachers received training before the study and were encouraged to respond to student questions without guiding student answers. Before the first food-recall workbook administration, subjects received instructions from the principal investigator on how to report food intake accurately. Food-recall workbooks also included age-appropriate instructions, portion size illustrations, and other explanations that assisted in completion of the workbooks. After the workbooks were completed, students placed them in a manila envelope, which was then sealed and given to the principal investigator at the end of the day. Food recalls were checked for completeness by the principal investigator, ensuring confidentiality as required by the Institutional Review Board.

Subjects at the control school completed three food-recall workbooks before and three after the intervention. No further intervention was carried out at the control school. In addition to the food-recall workbooks, the subjects at one experimental school also participated in a 12-week nutrition education program. The nutrition curriculum guide, *Nutrition in the Garden*, developed by Lineberger and Zajicek (20), was used. The curriculum provided lessons and activities that combined nutrition and horticulture. At a second experimental school, the subjects completed three food-recall workbooks before and three after the intervention, and participated in the 12-week nutrition education program. In addition, at the experimental school 2 subjects participated in hands-on, garden-based activities designed to correspond with the nutrition curriculum.

The school garden was within walking distance of experimental school 2. It was approximately 25×25 feet with two raised strawberry beds, a large herb garden, and a variety of fall crops including potatoes, corn, peppers, peas, beans, squash, cantaloupe, cucumbers, broccoli, tomatoes, spinach, lettuce, and kohlrabi. Subjects participated in maintaining the garden over the 12-week period through weeding, watering, and harvesting. They also engaged in other garden activities that included but were not limited to a salsa making workshop, class cookbook, "add a veggie to lunch day," planting and harvesting, herb drying, and food experiences with fruits and vegetables harvested from the garden.

Participants who did not complete at least two food-recall workbooks before and two food-recall workbooks after the intervention were dropped from the behavioral analysis. As a result, a total of 99 subjects were included in the statistical analyses. Food consumption and nutrient intake were determined using the Diet Analysis Plus software program (version 6.1, 2004, Thomson Wadsworth, Atlanta, GA). A repeated-measures one-way factorial analysis of variance (ANOVA) was conducted using the number of fruit and vegetable servings consumed and the daily intake of vitamin A, vitamin C, and fiber before and immediately after the 12-week intervention. Data were analyzed using the Statistical Package for the Social Sciences (version 13.0, 2004, SPSS Inc, Chicago, IL). A P value of 0.05 was selected to indicate statistical significance.

The ANOVA was conducted using the daily number of servings of fruits and vegetables, vitamin A intake (μg retinol activity equivalents [RAE]/day), vitamin C intake (mg/day), and fiber intake (g/day) as the dependent variables. The ANOVA compared fruit and vegetable consumption and selected nutrient intake at two different times for subjects at three different elementary schools. The within-subjects factor was the time of measurement (before vs after), and the between-subjects factor was the school (control, experimental school 1, and experimental school 2). The ANOVA showed a significant interaction effect between fruit and vegetable consumption, vitamin A intake, vitamin C intake, and fiber intake and school before and after the intervention. The ANOVA was followed up with a post hoc analysis using a Bonferroni adjustment to determine where the interaction occurred.

RESULTS AND DISCUSSION

Schoolyard gardening programs are springing up across the country. There are currently 1,100 projects in the registry for school garden projects at www.kidsgardening.com (21). There are also numerous Web sites devoted to encouraging and helping schools implement schoolyard gardening programs. French and Wechsler (22) examined various school-based interventions to promote fruit and vegetable consumption. They suggest that school gardens are a new direction in the school-based promotion of fruit and vegetable consumption, but point to the lack of research examining the effectiveness of such programs. Our study's findings show that garden-based nutrition education did have a significant effect on adolescents' consumption of fruits and vegetables and selected nutrient intake.

Forty-four percent of the subjects were male, and 56% were female. The ages ranged from 10 to 13 years, with 88% of all participants being 11 years old. There were no significant differences in fruit servings, vegetable servings, vitamin A, vitamin C, or fiber intake based on sex or age.

When comparing fruit servings, vegetable servings, vitamin A intake, vitamin C intake, and fiber intake before and after the intervention, all values increased significantly for the students at experimental school 2 (Table 1). Students participating in the nutrition education curriculum along with garden-based activities increased their numbers of fruit servings, vegetable servings, vitamin A intake, vitamin C intake, and fiber intake more than those students attending the control school and more than those students who participated in the nutrition education curriculum without garden activities.

Fruit consumption significantly increased (before to after) by 1.13 servings ($P < 0.001$) for students at experimental school 2, and vegetable consumption significantly increased by 1.44 servings ($P < 0.001$). Combined, the number of servings of fruits and vegetables more than doubled, from 1.93 to 4.50 servings per day. This is slightly below the recommended intake of five servings per day.

The mean vitamin A intake increased significantly at experimental school 2 by 181.99 μg RAE to 612.35 ± 359.60 μg RAE/day ($P = 0.004$). The dietary reference intake (DRI) of 600 μg RAE per day for 9-year-old to 13-year-old children was met (23). Vitamin C mean consumption also increased significantly at experimental school 2 by 85.27 mg/day ($P = 0.016$) and exceeded the DRI of 45 mg (24). The mean fiber intake of students at experimental school 2 significantly increased by 4.24 g to 16.90 ± 7.40 g/day ($P = 0.001$). This amount is still lower than the DRI of 31 g for 9-year-old to 13-year-old boys and 26 g for girls ages 9 to 13 years (25).

Table 1. Intakes of fruits, vegetables, fiber, and vitamins A and C of sixth-grade adolescents at three schools in southeast Idaho, before and after study interventions, using repeated-measures analysis of variance and Bonferroni post hoc analysis (n = 99)

	CS[a] (n = 25)		ES1[b] (n = 25)		ES2[c] (n = 45)			
	Before	After	Before	After	Before	After	F[d]	*P* Value
	← mean ± SD[e] →							
Fruits (servings)	0.7 ± 0.6	0.6 ± 0.7	0.3 ± 0.5	0.5 ± 0.7	0.8 ± 0.8	1.9 ± 1.4	10.98	<0.001
Vegetables (servings)	1.7 ± 0.7	1.4 ± 0.7	1.8 ± 1.1	1.7 ± 1.0	1.2 ± 0.6	2.6 ± 1.7	15.00	<0.001
Vitamin A (µg RAE[f])	621.4 ± 294.1	549.5 ± 248.9	428.5 ± 247.9	358.8 ± 273.3	430.4 ± 244.1	612.4 ± 359.6	5.86	0.004
Vitamin C (mg)	83.1 ± 115.6	76.2 ± 129.5	47.5 ± 48.5	60.8 ± 126.6	58.2 ± 62.2	143.4 ± 144.5	4.31	0.016
Fiber (g)	15.3 ± 6.0	12.6 ± 8.0	10.7 ± 5.2	9.9 ± 5.0	12.7 ± 4.6	16.9 ± 7.4	8.21	0.001

[a]CS=control school, children did not participate in nutrition education curriculum or gardening activities.

[b]ES1=experimental school 1, children participated in nutrition education curriculum only, no gardening activities.

[c]ES2=experimental school 2, children participated in nutrition education curriculum and corresponding gardening activities.

[d]F statistic for interaction of school and before-and-after test results from repeated-measures analysis of variance.

[e]SD=standard deviation.

[f]RAE=retinol activity equivalents.

No significant changes occurred in fruit, vegetable, vitamin A, vitamin C, or fiber intakes at the control school or at experimental school 1.

To ensure that home gardens and access to garden activities outside the school did not impact the results, participants were asked whether they had a fruit and/or vegetable garden at home. Using the χ^2 test of independence, it was found that the "garden effect" was not significant and that there was no school that had proportionally more individuals with home gardens than the other schools.

In our subjects, the garden-based activities along with nutrition education resulted in significant increases in fruit and vegetable consumption. In addition, vitamin A, vitamin C, and fiber intakes showed significant increases. These results help to show the importance of hands-on activities when attempting to change nutrition-related behavior such as fruit and vegetable consumption. Similar studies have shown the importance of exposure to fruits and vegetables, building self-efficacy regarding the preparation of fruits/vegetables, increasing nutrition knowledge and awareness, and creating experiential opportunities with fruits and vegetables (9,18,26,27). The results from this study hopefully will aid future researchers in their development of effective nutrition education programs.

This study is not without limitations. Although the sixth-grade participants at experimental school 2 significantly increased their intakes of fruits and vegetables during this study, it is important to note that prolonged behavior change cannot be implied because of the nature of the study time (12 weeks). Complete behavior change is difficult to evaluate after only 12 weeks. Thus, to accurately measure prolonged behavior change regarding the increased consumption of fruits and vegetables, future studies should be conducted. Because this was a nonrandomized trial, the scope of inference is limited to the specific study population. In addition, these results should be approached cautiously because of the nature of self-reported data as well as other influences on the students' fruit and vegetable intake. Factors such as eating at home, parental influences, and additional classroom activities could have affected the results.

CONCLUSIONS

The results from this study illustrate the efficacy of using garden-based nutrition education when attempting to increase adolescents' consumption of fruits and vegetables. The persistent annual increase in adolescent overweight/ obesity must be addressed to meet the goals and objectives of Healthy People 2010 (2), as well as many other governmental initiatives, including the *Dietary Guidelines for Americans* (28), and to decrease the risk factors for many chronic diseases. It is heartening to speculate that garden-based nutrition education, when implemented during adolescence, may be one small tool with tremendous impact.

REFERENCES

1. Van Duyn MA, Pivonka E. Overview of the health benefits of fruit and vegetable consumption for the dietetics professional: Selected literature. *J Am Diet Assoc*. 2000;*100*:1511-1521.
2. US Department of Health and Human Services. *Healthy People 2010: Conference Edition*, Vol I. Washington, DC: US Government Printing Office; 2000.
3. Hyson D. The health benefits of fruits and vegetables: A scientific overview for health professionals. Produce for Better Health Foundation, 2002. Retrieved January 30, 2005, from http://www.5aday.com/pdfs/research/health_benefits.pdf.
4. Hedley AA, Ogden CL, Johnson CL, Carroll MD, Curtin LR, Flegal KM. Prevalence

of overweight and obesity among US children, adolescents, and adults, 1999-2002. *JAMA*. 2004;*291*:2847-2850.

5. Sandeno C, Wolf G, Drake T, Reicks M. Behavioral strategies to increase fruit and vegetable intake by fourth-through sixth-grade students. *J Am Diet Assoc*. 2000;*100*:828-830.
6. O'Dea J. Children and adolescents' eating habits and attitudes: Preliminary findings from the national nutrition and physical activity study. *NutriDate*. 2004; *15*:1-4.
7. Deckelbaum RJ, Williams CL. Childhood obesity: The health issue. *Obes Res*. 2001;*9*(suppl 4):239S-243S.
8. Odea J. Prevention of child obesity: "First, do no harm." *Health Educ Res*. 2005;*20*:259-265.
9. Domel SB, Baranowski T, Davis H, Thompson WO, Leonard SB, Riley P, Baranowski J, Dudovitz B, Smyth M. Development and evaluation of a school intervention to increase fruit and vegetable consumption among 4th and 5th grade students. *J Nutr Educ*. 1993;*25*:345-349.
10. Dietz WH, Bellizzi MC. Introduction: The use of BMI to assess obesity in children. *Am J Clin Nutr*. 1999; *70*(suppl 1):123S-125S.
11. Lytle LA, Kelder SH, Perry CL, Klepp KI. Covariance of adolescent health behaviors: The class of 1989 study. *Health Educ Res*. 1995;*10*:133-146.
12. Story M, Neumark-Sztainer D. School-based nutrition education programs and services for adolescents. *Adolescent Medicine: State of the Art Reviews*. 1996; 7:287-302.
13. Stokes MM. Adolescent nutrition: Needs and recommendations for practice. *The Clearinghouse*. 2002;*75*: 286-291.
14. Graham H, Lane Beall D, Lussier M, McLaughlin P, Zidenberg-Cherr S. Use of school gardens in academic instruction. *J Nutr Educ Behav*. 2005;*37*:147-151.
15. Graham H, Zidenberg-Cherr S. California teachers perceive school gardens as an effective nutritional tool to promote healthful eating habits. *J Am Diet Assoc*. 2005;*105*:1797-1800.
16. Graham H, Feenstra G, Evans AM, Zidenberg-Cherr S. Davis school program supports life-long healthy eating habits in children. *Calif Agric*. 2004;*58*:200-205.
17. Morris JL, Zidenberg-Cherr S. Garden-enhanced curriculum improves fourth-grade school children's knowledge of nutrition and preferences for some vegetables. *J Am Diet Assoc*. 2002;*102*:91-93.
18. Lineberger SE, Zajicek JM. School gardens: Can a hands-on teaching tool affect students' attitudes and behaviors regarding fruit and vegetables. *Horticulture Technology*. 2000;*10*:593-597.
19. Jendrysik B. A comparison of children's dietary information using a workbook recall method to reported intake and observation [thesis]. Blacksburg, VA: Department of Human Nutrition and Foods, Virginia Polytechnic Institute and State University; 1991.
20. Lineberger SE, Zajicek JM. Nutrition in the garden: A curriculum guide. College Station, TX: Texas Agricultural Extension Service; 1998.
21. National Gardening Association. School Garden Registry. Available at: http://www.kidsgardening.com. Accessed March 24, 2006.
22. French SA, Wechsler H. School-based research and initiatives: Fruit and vegetable environment, policy, and pricing workshop. *Prev Med*. 2004;*39*(suppl 2): S101-S107.
23. Institute of Medicine. *Dietary Reference Intakes for Vitamin A, Vitamin K, Arsenic, Boron, Chromium, Copper, Iodine, Iron, Molybdenum, Nickel, Silicon, Vanadium and Zinc*. Food and Nutrition Board. Washington, DC: National Academies Press; 2001.
24. Institute of Medicine. *Dietary Reference Intakes for Vitamin C, Vitamin E, Selenium, and Carotenoids*. Food and Nutrition Board. Washington, DC: National Academies Press; 2000.
25. Institute of Medicine. *Dietary Reference Intakes for Energy, Carbohydrate, Fiber, Fat, Fatty Acids, Cholesterol, Protein and Amino Acids*. Food and Nutrition Board. Washington, DC: National Academies Press; 2002.
26. Quinn LJ, Horacek TM, Castle J. The impact of cook-shop on the dietary habits and attitudes of fifth graders. *Topics in Clinical Nutrition*. 2003;*18*:42-48.
27. Dundas M, Cook K. Impact of the Special Supplemental Nutrition Program for Women, Infants and Children on the healthy eating behaviors of preschool children in eastern Idaho. *Topics in Clinical Nutrition*. 2004;*19*:273-279.
28. US Department of Health and Human Services, US Department of Agriculture. *Dietary Guidelines for Americans 2005*. 6th ed. Washington, DC: US Government Printing Office; 2005.

APPENDIX B

FULL LENGTH EXPERIMENTAL RESEARCH ARTICLE—CLEAR LIQUID DIET VS SOFT DIET AS THE INITIAL MEAL IN PATIENTS WITH MILD ACUTE PANCREATITIS: A RANDOMIZED INTERVENTIONAL TRIAL

Nagarajan Rajkumar, MS[1]
Vilvapathy Senguttuvan Karthikeyan, MS[2]
Sheik Manwar Ali, MS[1]
Sarath Chandra Sistla, MS[1]
Vikram Kate, MS, FRCS(Eng), FRCS(Ed), FRCS(Glasg), PhD, MNAMS, FIMSA, FACS, FACG[1]

ABSTRACT

Background: Patients recovering from mild acute pancreatitis are usually started on a liquid diet and advanced to a solid diet. Evidence suggests a soft diet as the initial meal is tolerated well by such patients. However, the results are controversial. *Objectives*: To assess the safety of starting an early soft diet compared with a liquid diet in patients with mild acute pancreatitis as the initial meal. *Methods*: We randomized 60 patients with mild acute pancreatitis into 2 groups to receive either a clear liquid diet (CLD) or a soft diet (SD) as the initial meal, and parameters such as tolerance to diet, recurrence of pain, length of hospitalization (LOH), need to stop feeding, post-refeeding length of hospitalization (PRLOH), and postdischarge readmission rate within 30 days were analyzed. *Results*: The demographic and baseline parameters (amylase, total leucocyte count, Balthazar score) in the 2 groups were comparable. Patients in both groups tolerated the diet well except 1 patient in the SD group, who developed vomiting

Reproduced from N. Rajkumar, V.S. Karthikeyan, S.M. Ali, S.C. Sistla, and V. Kate, *Nutrition in Clinical Practice*, 28(3), "Clear Liquid Diet vs Soft Diet as the Initial Meal in Patients with Mild Acute Pancreatitis: A Randomized Interventional Trial," p. 365-370, copyright © 2012. Reprinted by Permission of SAGE Publications, Inc.

From the [1]Department of Surgery and [2]Department of Urology, Jawaharlal Institute of Postgraduate Medical Education and Research, Puducherry, India.

Financial disclosure: None declared.

This article originally appeared online on December 13, 2012.

Corresponding Author:
Vikram Kate, MS, FRCS(Eng), FRCS(Ed), FRCS(Glasg), PhD, MNAMS, FIMSA, FACS, FACG, Professor, Department of Surgery, Jawaharlal Institute of Postgraduate Medical Education and Research, Puducherry 605006, India.
Email: drvikramkate@gmail.com.

and diarrhea, not severe enough to stop feeding. LOH and PRLOH were significantly lower in the SD group (4.23 ± 2.08 and 1.96 ± 1.63 days, $P < .0001$) compared with the CLD group (6.91 ± 2.43 and 4.10 ± 1.64 days, $P < .0001$). PRLOH in the SD group was 2.14 days less when compared with the CLD group. *Conclusion*: In patients with mild acute pancreatitis, a soft diet as the initial meal is well tolerated and leads to a shorter total length of hospitalization. (*Nutr Clin Pract.* 2013;28:365-370)

KEYWORDS

pancreatitis; nutrition therapy; diet

Acute pancreatitis (AP) is a common condition presenting with acute abdominal pain in emergency medical services worldwide.[1] Most of these cases are classified as mild AP, and 70%–90% of them usually resolve spontaneously in 5–10 days with conservative management.[1,2] The management of mild AP conventionally involves avoidance of oral feeding, intravenous (IV) hydration, and adequate analgesia until pain improves. Patients recovering from mild AP traditionally receive a clear liquid diet (CLD) initially and are gradually advanced to a soft diet (SD). Hospital discharge is planned based on tolerance to a solid diet. It is not clear whether resumption of feeding with CLD is actually essential as the timing and method of resumption of oral feeding after mild AP are based on anecdotal experience rather than scientific study.[3] The conventional sequence of progressing oral feeds from CLD to solid diet may pointlessly prolong the patient's hospitalization, causing inconvenience and incurring needless expenditure. Some studies in the literature have reported favorable outcomes with solid diet as the initial meal in patients with mild AP.[4,5] However, reports are controversial.[6] Hence, this study was conducted with the aim to analyze the safety of starting an early SD compared with a liquid diet in patients with mild acute pancreatitis as the initial meal.

METHODS

PATIENTS

This was a hospital-based, randomized interventional trial done in 60 patients with mild AP admitted to the Department of Surgery in a tertiary care referral center, catering to around 200 cases of pancreatitis a year, mostly from South India, pre-dominantly men, working as daily wage laborers and addicted to alcohol intake. After obtaining clearance from the institute research council and institute ethics committee, the study was conducted between September 2008 and June 2010.

All consecutive patients diagnosed with mild AP based on the inclusion criteria were eligible for the study. Written informed consent was obtained from all the patients. The inclusion criteria were patients presenting within 48 hours after the onset of abdominal pain with elevated serum or peritoneal fluid amylase or ultrasound features suggestive of AP, leukocyte count <16,000/mm^3, temperature <101.6°F at admission, oxygen saturation >90%, systolic blood pressure >90 mm Hg, serum creatinine <2 mg/dL (or >2 mg/dL with preexisting renal insufficiency), and Balthazar score[7] ≤D. Patients with previous abdominal surgery, trauma, cancer, ischemic bowel disease, short bowel syndrome, or pregnancy and patients receiving enteral nutrition (EN) or parenteral narcotics for abdominal pain on the day of refeeding and cases of acute on chronic pancreatitis were excluded from the study.

Assignment

Patients were randomized into 2 groups to receive CLD or SD by computer-generated randomization.

Allocation Concealment and Randomization

Block randomization was done with a block size of 10 using Microsoft Excel 2007 (Microsoft Corp, Redmond, WA). Allocation concealment was performed using a serially numbered opaque-sealed envelope technique. Randomization and sealed envelopes were prepared by a person independent of the investigators. Envelopes were opened and group allocation was done by a person not involved in the research once the patients were ready to be started on the diet.

Study Protocol

After randomization, a brief history was taken and the patients were kept on conservative management with IV fluids, adequate analgesia, and nil orally until symptomatic improvement ensued, that is, complete absence of pain. Patients were started on CLD or SD based on the group allocation. The standard CLD comprised plain water and tender coconut water. The standard SD included prescribed local food items (patients had to choose from South Indian food items in the form of *idli* or *idiyappam*—made by steaming fermented rice batter; fermentation breaks down starches so that they are more readily metabolized). They were advised and supervised to adhere strictly to the standard CLD or SD. The intake of fluid was recorded. After starting oral feeds, the patients were evaluated for recurrence of pain and intolerance to diet in the form of vomiting and diarrhea, if any. Tolerance to diet and pain was determined by using a 5-point Likert scale.[8] After initiation of diet (CLD or SD), the patients were instructed to stop oral feeding when they developed pain of moderate or severe intensity (Likert score ≥3/5) or more than 2 episodes of vomiting or an episode of diarrhea. Decisions about diet advancement and hospital discharge were done without input from the study members. Hospital discharge was based on the patient's tolerance to SD. Patients were discharged on a uniform basis when they had tolerated the SD for more than 24 hours without recurrence of pain and at the discretion of the treating surgeons.

Outcome

The primary outcome of our study was total length of hospitalization (LOH). The secondary outcomes were recurrence of pain, need to stop feeding, post-refeeding length of hospitalization (PRLOH), and postdischarge readmission rate within 30 days. The sample size of 60 was calculated based on the requirement to detect a reduction in LOH of 2 days with 95% power.

Statistical Analysis

Statistical analysis was done using GraphPad version 3.6 (GraphPad Software, La Jolla, CA) and SPSS version 16 for Windows (SPSS, Inc, an IBM Company, Chicago, IL). Continuous variables were summarized as mean with standard deviation. Median with interquartile range was used for continuous variables with nonnormal distribution. Analysis was performed using an unpaired *t* test. Categorical variables were summarized in numbers and percentages and analyzed using the χ^2 test. A P value <.05 was considered statistically significant.

RESULTS

PARTICIPANT FLOW

The flow diagram (**Figure 1**) shows the number of patients assessed for participation in the study. It also shows the number of patients excluded for various reasons and the number of patients finally eligible for randomization into 2 groups who completed the study protocol. In all, 52 patients were not included because of the reasons shown in the flowchart (Figure 1).

BASELINE CHARACTERISTICS

The baseline clinical and laboratory parameters and Balthazar score have been summarized in **Table 1**. Most patients in both groups were men between 21 and 40 years of age. The etiology of pancreatitis was similar in both groups (P = .54), and the commonest cause was alcohol intake (Table 1).

TIME TO FIRST MEAL AND TOLERANCE TO DIET

The mean time interval between admission and the first meal was comparable between the 2 groups (2.97 ± 2.08 days in the CLD group and 2.30 ± 1.12 days in the SD group; P = .13).

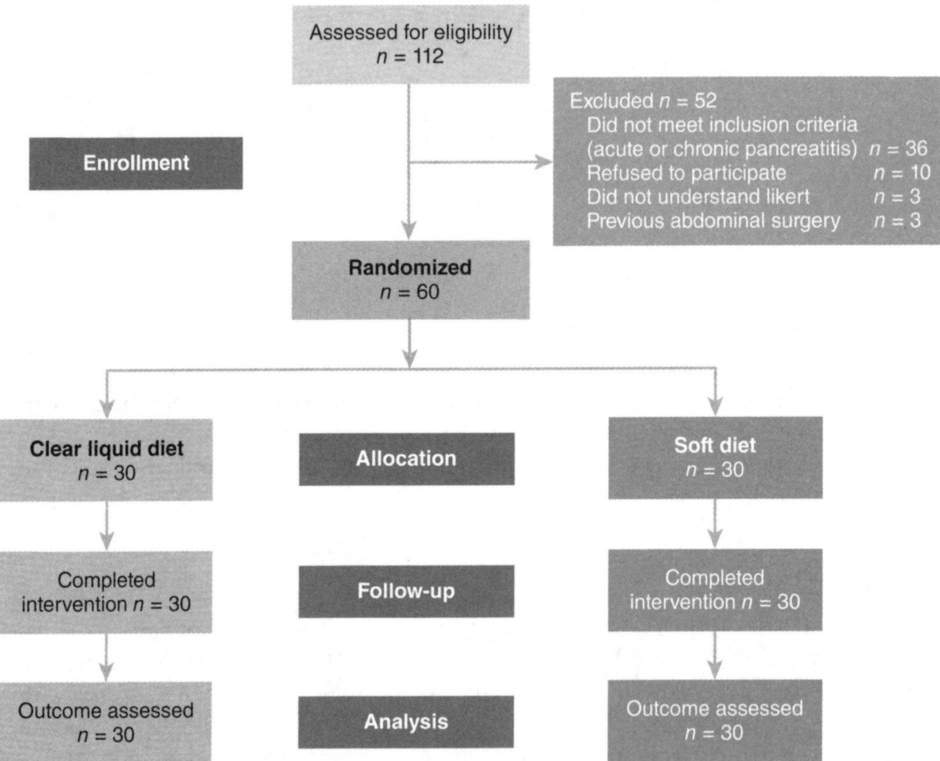

FIGURE 1. Flow diagram of the participants through the study.

Table 1. Patient Characteristics in the Study Groups.

Patient Characteristics	Clear Liquid Diet, n = 30	Soft Diet, n = 30
Age, y, mean ± SD	36.33 ± 7.69	37.90 ± 10.42
Sex, No. (%)		
Male	28 (93.3)	27 (90.0)
Female	2 (6.7)	3 (10.0)
Etiology, No.		
Alcohol	27	27
Gallstones	2	3
Pancreatic divisum	1	0
Amylase, IU/L, median ± IQR	535.5 ± 723.75	486 ± 876.50
Total leukocyte count, per mm^3, median ± IQR	7500 ± 2550	7050 ± 2725
Temperature, °F, mean ± SD	98.4 ± 0.1	98.5 ± 0.1
Oxygen saturation, %, mean ± SD	97.2 ± 1.4	96.8 ± 1.6
Systolic blood pressure, mm Hg, mean ± SD	119 ± 11.2	118.4 ± 13.4
Serum creatinine, mg/dL, mean ± SD	0.9 ± 0.4	0.9 ± 0.3
Balthazar class, No.		
B	7	10
C	14	14
D	6	5

IQR, interquartile range; SD, standard deviation.

All 30 (100%) patients in the CLD group tolerated the diet well. Only 1 of the 30 patients (3.33%) in the SD group had vomiting and diarrhea, which was not severe enough to stop oral refeeding. The differences with regard to tolerance to diet and vomiting were not statistically significant in both groups ($P = 1.00$) (**Table 2**).

Table 2. Comparison of Tolerance to Diet in the Study Groups.

Parameters	Clear Liquid Diet, n = 30	Soft Diet, n = 30	*P* Value[a]
Time interval from admission to starting orals, d, mean ± SD	2.97 ± 2.08	2.30 ± 1.12	.13
Tolerance to diet, No. (%)	30 (100.0)	29 (96.7)	1.00
Recurrence of pain, No. (%)	6 (20.0)	6 (20.0)	1.00
Length of hospitalization, d, mean ± SD	6.91 ± 2.43	4.23 ± 2.08	**<.0001**
Post-refeeding length of hospitalization, d, mean ± SD	4.10 ± 1.64	1.96 ± 1.63	**<.0001**

SD, standard deviation.

[a]Bold *P* values represent the significant *P* values ($P < 0.05$).

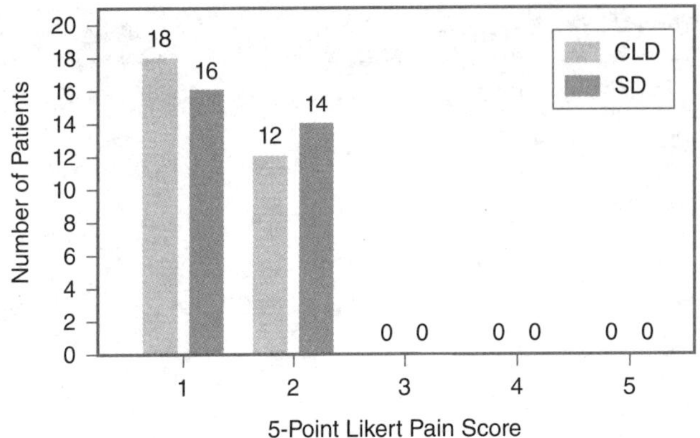

FIGURE 2. Distribution of Likert scores in the study groups.

LOH

The total LOH was significantly lower in the patients initiated on SD than those initiated on CLD ($P < .0001$). The mean LOH in the CLD and SD groups was 6.91 ± 2.43 days and 4.23 ± 2.08 days, respectively (Table 2).

PRLOH

The PRLOH was significantly lower in patients initiated on SD than those initiated on CLD ($P < .0001$). The mean PRLOH was 4.10 ± 1.64 days in the CLD group and 1.97 ± 1.63 days in the SD group (Table 2).

Recurrence of Pain

Recurrence of pain was observed in 6 patients in each group, although the pain was not severe enough (Likert score <3) to stop feeding ($P = 1.00$) (**Figure 2**). Patients were continued on their respective diet, and they tolerated it well. Twenty-nine patients (96.7%) in the SD group tolerated the diet well, whereas all 30 patients in the CLD group tolerated the diet well ($P = 1.00$) (Table 2).

DISCUSSION

Practice management guidelines regarding time of refeeding and the form of nutrition in AP are still evolving concepts. Despite sufficient evidence to support oral feeding in AP, questions regarding the role of nutrition support, the mode of delivery, and the form of diet in these patients remain unanswered.[9] In mild AP, which constitutes a majority of cases, dietary management is not yet optimized.[10] Many clinicians start CLD when there is symptomatic improvement in the form of absence of pain, vomiting, and abdominal tenderness.[5,11] This diet is then gradually progressed from a soft diet to a normal diet, and then the patients are discharged based on their tolerance to the solid diet. However, the time to resume oral feeding and the choice of the diet are based on anecdotal experience rather than scientific study.[5] Many authors in the past believed that starting patients on an early solid diet would stimulate the pancreatic secretion, thereby aggravating pain,[12] but these concepts are no longer valid.

Etiology

In the West, gallstone disease is the commonest cause of mild AP, and hence it is almost equally distributed among men and women (1:1).[5] In our study population, alcohol consumption was the commonest cause (54/60; 90%) for AP, which also reiterates the Indian statistics, and hence the disease was more prevalent in males (male/female ratio: 11:1).

Grading of Pancreatitis

Jacobson et al[5] (**Table 3**) used the Acute Physiology and Chronic Health Evaluation II (APACHE II) scoring system to grade pancreatitis. We used the Balthazar scoring system[13] to grade pancreatitis because it was more feasible in our institute. Moreover, there is a wide variation in the relationship of prognostic indicator systems such as APACHE II, Ranson, and Glasgow criteria and early computed tomography (CT) findings in AP.[13] Excellent correlation has been documented between CT findings in AP and LOH, complications, and death in a series by Balthazar et al[14] in 1990. Also, we studied the effect of diet only in cases of mild AP, and to classify AP based on Ranson criteria, there was a need to wait for 48 hours, by which time many of our patients had resolution of symptoms and were ready for oral feeds. On the other hand, using CT criteria as proposed by Balthazar et al was sensitive and specific for classifying patients based on severity and was objective, as the overall sensitivity and specificity of the numeric systems ranged between 57%–85% and 68%–85%, respectively.[13]

Table 3. Comparison With Similar Studies.

Study	Groups and Population Characteristics	No. of Patients	Parameters	Results
Present study	CLD and SD; daily wage laborers of South India	CLD, 30 SD, 30	Total LOH, recurrence of pain, need to stop feeding, PRLOH, postdischarge readmission rate within 30 days	SD was safe, feasible and LOH and PRLOH were significantly lower in SD ($P < .0001$)
Sathiaraj et al[4]	CLD and SD; not mentioned	CLD, 52 SD, 49	Frequency of pain, total LOH and PRLOH, dietary intake	Decreased LOH and PRLOH ($P < .001$) in SD; more calories consumed in SD group ($P < .001$)
Jacobson et al[5]	CLD and LFSD; not mentioned (review of electronic medical records system)	CLD, 66 LFSD, 55	LOH, PRLOH, readmission rate within 28 days	LFSD was safe but did not result in shorter LOH
Cshebli et al[6]	Single group; not mentioned	130	Post-refeeding pain, LOH	Pain relapse maximum on days 1 and 2 of refeeding and increased LOH ($P < .01$)
Moraes et al[15]	CLD, SD, solid diet; not mentioned	CLD, 70 SD, 70 Solid, 70	LOH, PRLOH within 7 days, pain relapse, dietary intake	Solid diet was well tolerated ($P = .000$) and shorter LOH ($P < .001$)

CLD, clear liquid diet; LFSD, low-fat solid diet; LOH, length of hospitalization; PRLOH, post-refeeding LOH; SD, soft diet.

LOH and PRLOH

The main advantage of starting SD in patients with mild AP lies in the reduction of LOH and PRLOH. In our study, both groups were comparable with respect to the time of starting orals ($P = .13$). It was found that the total LOH ($P < .0001$) and the PRLOH ($P < .0001$) were significantly lower in patients initiated on SD than in patients initiated on CLD. This clearly shows that there was an average difference of 2 days in LOH and PRLOH between the groups. This could be explained by the delay in graduating to SD in patients initiated on CLD. Patients in the CLD group were kept on a tolerated amount of standard fluids the first day, supplemented with IV fluids and a full fluid diet (plain water, tender coconut water, clear filtered juices, buttermilk) on the next day before they could be started on SD, whereas patients in the SD group were started on SD right away, when they were ready to receive oral feeding. This ensued in a shorter hospital stay as the time interval from admission to the starting of orals was comparable between both groups ($P = .13$). Thus, bypassing a step in the resumption of oral feeding resulted in a decreased LOH in the SD group. This finding was rather consistent with an earlier study done by Sathiaraj et al[4] (Table 3). A similar finding was also noted by Moraes et al[15] (Table 3) that a shorter hospital stay ensued when patients received a full solid diet as the initial meal compared with CLD and SD.

Recurrence of Pain

In our study, 6 (20%) patients in each group had recurrence of pain but was not severe enough to interfere with oral refeeding ($P = 1.00$). Recurrence of pain was seen in both the groups, and it had no association with the type of diet initiated. The respective diets were tolerated well by patients in both groups, with a very low incidence of vomiting and diarrhea, which again reinforces that initiating a soft diet in mild AP was tolerated well by these patients.

Jacobson et al[5] found that there was no difference in the LOH and PRLOH between patients started on CLD or a low-fat solid diet (LFSD). This could have been due to 2 reasons. A prolonged delay before refeeding might have diminished the chance of achieving a shortened LOH. They also explained that physicians made discharge decisions based not only on a patient's diet tolerance but also on other factors independent of diet, which affected the discharge and thereby the LOH.

In our study, there was no need to stop feeding during the entire study period, and none of the patients in the SD group were readmitted within 30 days of discharge for recurrence of pain. Sathiaraj et al[4] in their study observed recurrence of pain severe enough to cause cessation of feeding in 3 (5.76%) patients in the CLD group and 4 (8.16%) patients in the SD group ($P = .85$). Vomiting led to cessation of feeding in 4 (7.69%) patients in the CLD group; however, none of the patients in the SD group had to stop oral refeeding due to vomiting ($P = .12$). Neither of the diets was associated with significantly increased rates of feeding cessation.

Thus, initiating soft diet in mild AP does not lead to recurrence of pain or vomiting severe enough to cause cessation of feeding. On the contrary, Jacobson et al[5] reported failure to tolerate initial feeding in mild AP as a significant problem affecting 8% of their study population, attributable to reasons aforementioned. They also found increased abdominal pain scores on the day of refeeding and failure to tolerate an oral diet. Our patients, however, were asymptomatic on the day of refeeding in both groups.

Chebli et al[6] in their study offered a similar diet to all 130 patients and found that pain relapse was 25%, especially on the first or the second day, and this relapse of pain prolonged LOH ($P < .01$) and the overall costs of disease treatment (Table 3).

CONCLUSION

Resumption of oral feeding with an SD as the initial meal in patients with mild AP is well tolerated, feasible, and a viable option as it shortens the hospital stay without the need to stop refeeding or recurrence of symptoms.

ACKNOWLEDGMENT

The authors sincerely acknowledge the efforts of Dr T. Mahalakshmy, Assistant Professor, Community Medicine, Indira Gandhi Medical College and Research Institute, Pondicherry, India, in study design and statistical analysis.

REFERENCES

1. Steer M. Acute pancreatitis. In: Wolfe M, Davis G, Farraye F, Giannella R, Malagelada, eds. *Therapy of Digestive Disorders*. Philadelphia, PA: Elsevier; 2006:417-426.
2. Mitchell R, Byrne M, Baillie J. Pancreatitis. *Lancet*. 2003;*361*:1447-1455.
3. Lankisch PG, Banks PA. *Pancreatitis*. Berlin, Germany: Springer-Verlag;1998.
4. Sathiaraj E, Murthy S, Mansard MJ, Rao GV, Mahukar S, Reddy DN. Clinical trial: oral feeding with a soft diet compared with clear liquid diet as initial meal in mild acute pancreatitis. *Aliment Pharmacol Ther*. 2008;*28*:777-781.
5. Jacobson BC, Vander Vliet MB, Hughes MD, Maurer R, McManus K, Banks PA. A prospective, randomized trial of clear liquids versus low-fat solid diet as the initial meal in mild acute pancreatitis. *Clin Gastroenterol Hepatol*. 2007;*5*:946-951.
6. Chebli JM, Gaburri PD, De Souza AF, et al. Oral refeeding in patients with mild acute pancreatitis: prevalence and risk factors of relapsing abdominal pain. *J Gastroenterol Hepatol*. 2005;*9*:1385-1389.
7. Balthazar EJ. CT diagnosis and staging of acute pancreatitis. *Radiol Clin North Am*. 1989;27:19-37.
8. Likert R. A technique for the measurement of attitudes. *Arch Psychol*. 1932;*22*:55.
9. Dervenis C. Enteral nutrition in severe acute pancreatitis: future development. *JOP*. 2004;*5*:60-63.
10. Eckerwall GE, Tingstedt BB, Bergenzaun PE, Andersson RG. Immediate oral feeding in patients with mild acute pancreatitis is safe and may accelerate recovery: a randomized clinical study. *Clin Nutr*. 2007;*26*:758-763.
11. Whitcomb DC. Acute pancreatitis. *N Engl J Med*. 2006;*354*:2142-2150.
12. Abou-Assi S, O'Keefe SJD. Nutritional support during acute pancreatitis. *Nutrition*. 2002;*18*:938-943.
13. Balthazar EJ. Acute pancreatitis: assessment of severity with clinical and CT evaluation. *Radiology*. 2002;*223*:603-613.
14. Balthazar EJ, Robinson DL, Megibow AJ, Ranson JH. Acute pancreatitis: value of CT in establishing prognosis. *Radiology*. 1990;*174*:331-336.
15. Moraes JM, Felga GE, Chebli LA, et al. A full solid diet as the initial meal in mild acute pancreatitis is safe and result in a shorter length of hospital-ization: results from a prospective, randomized, controlled, double-blind clinical trial. *J Clin Gastroenterol*. 2010;*44*:517-522.

APPENDIX C

CONSORT 2010 CHECKLIST OF INFORMATION TO INCLUDE WHEN REPORTING A RANDOMIZED TRIAL*

Section/Topic	Item No.	Checklist Item	Reported on Page No.
Title and Abstract			
	1a	Identification as a randomized trial in the title	
	1b	Structured summary of trial design, methods, results, and conclusions (for specific guidance see CONSORT for abstracts)	
Introduction			
Background and objectives	2a	Scientific background and explanation of rationale	
	2b	Specific objectives or hypotheses	
Methods			
Trial design	3a	Description of trial design (such as parallel, factorial) including allocation ratio	
	3b	Important changes to methods after trial commencement (such as eligibility criteria), with reasons	
Participants	4a	Eligibility criteria for participants	
	4b	Settings and locations where the data were collected	
Interventions	5	The interventions for each group with sufficient details to allow replication, including how and when they were actually administered	
Outcomes	6a	Completely defined prespecified primary and secondary outcome measures, including how and when they were assessed	
	6b	Any changes to trial outcomes after the trial commenced, with reasons	
Sample size	7a	How sample size was determined	
	7b	When applicable, explanation of any interim analyses and stopping guidelines	

Section/Topic	Item No.	Checklist Item	Reported on Page No.
Randomization			
Sequence	8a	Method used to generate the random allocation sequence	
Generation	8b	Type of randomization; details of any restriction (such as blocking and block size)	
Allocation concealment mechanism	9	Mechanism used to implement the random allocation sequence (such as sequentially numbered containers), describing any steps taken to conceal the sequence until interventions were assigned	
Implementation	10	Who generated the random allocation sequence, who enrolled participants, and who assigned participants to interventions	
Blinding	11a	If done, who was blinded after assignment to interventions (for example, participants, care providers, those assessing outcomes) and how	
	11b	If relevant, description of the similarity of interventions	
Statistical methods	12a	Statistical methods used to compare groups for primary and secondary outcomes	
	12b	Methods for additional analyses, such as subgroup analyses and adjusted analyses	
Results			
Participant flow (a diagram is strongly recommended)	13a	For each group, the numbers of participants who were randomly assigned, received intended treatment, and were analyzzed for the primary outcome	
	13b	For each group, losses and exclusions after randomization, together with reasons	
Recruitment	14a	Dates defining the periods of recruitment and follow-up	
	14b	Why the trial ended or was stopped	
Baseline data	15	A table showing baseline demographic and clinical characteristics for each group	
Numbers analyzed	16	For each group, number of participants (denominator) included in each analysis and whether the analysis was by original assigned groups	
Outcomes and estimation	17a	For each primary and secondary outcome, results for each group, and the estimated effect size and its precision (such as 95% confidence interval)	
	17b	For binary outcomes, presentation of both absolute and relative effect sizes is recommended	

Section/Topic	Item No.	Checklist Item	Reported on Page No.
Ancillary analyses	18	Results of any other analyses performed, including subgroup analyses and adjusted analyses, distinguishing prespecified from exploratory	
Harms	19	All important harms or unintended effects in each group (for specific guidance see CONSORT for harms)	
Discussion			
Limitations	20	Trial limitations, addressing sources of potential bias, imprecision, and, if relevant, multiplicity of analyses	
Generalizability	21	Generalizability (external validity, applicability) of the trial findings	
Interpretation	22	Interpretation consistent with results, balancing benefits and harms, and considering other relevant evidence	
Other Information			
Registration	23	Registration number and name of trial registry	
Protocol	24	Where the full trial protocol can be accessed, if available	
Funding	25	Sources of funding and other support (such as supply of drugs), role of funders	

*We strongly recommend reading this statement in conjunction with the CONSORT 2010 Explanation and Elaboration for important clarifications on all the items. If relevant, we also recommend reading CONSORT extensions for cluster randomized trials, noninferiority and equivalence trials, nonpharmacological treatments, herbal interventions, and pragmatic trials. Additional extensions are forthcoming: for those and for up-to-date references relevant to this checklist, see www.consort-statement.org.

APPENDIX D

STROBE STATEMENT—CHECKLIST OF ITEMS THAT SHOULD BE INCLUDED IN REPORTS OF OBSERVATIONAL STUDIES

	Item No.	Recommendation
Title and Abstract	1	(*a*) Indicate the study's design with a commonly used term in the title or the abstract
		(*b*) Provide in the abstract an informative and balanced summary of what was done and what was found
Introduction		
Background/rationale	2	Explain the scientific background and rationale for the investigation being reported
Objectives	3	State specific objectives, including any prespecified hypotheses
Methods		
Study design	4	Present key elements of study design early in the paper
Setting	5	Describe the setting, locations, and relevant dates, including periods of recruitment, exposure, follow-up, and data collection
Participants	6	(*a*) *Cohort study*—Give the eligibility criteria, and the sources and methods of selection of participants. Describe methods of follow-up *Case-control study*—Give the eligibility criteria, and the sources and methods of case ascertainment and control selection. Give the rationale for the choice of cases and controls *Cross-sectional study*—Give the eligibility criteria, and the sources and methods of selection of participants
		(*b*) *Cohort study*—For matched studies, give matching criteria and number of exposed and unexposed *Case-control study*—For matched studies, give matching criteria and the number of controls per case
Variables	7	Clearly define all outcomes, exposures, predictors, potential confounders, and effect modifiers. Give diagnostic criteria, if applicable

	Item No.	Recommendation
Data sources/ measurement	8*	For each variable of interest, give sources of data and details of methods of assessment (measurement). Describe comparability of assessment methods if there is more than one group
Bias	9	Describe any efforts to address potential sources of bias
Study size	10	Explain how the study size was arrived at
Quantitative variables	11	Explain how quantitative variables were handled in the analyses. If applicable, describe which groupings were chosen and why
Statistical methods	12	(*a*) Describe all statistical methods, including those used to control for confounding
		(*b*) Describe any methods used to examine subgroups and interactions
		(*c*) Explain how missing data were addressed
		(*d*) *Cohort study*—If applicable, explain how loss to follow-up was addressed *Case-control study*—If applicable, explain how matching of cases and controls was addressed *Cross-sectional study*—If applicable, describe analytical methods taking account of sampling strategy
		(*e*) Describe any sensitivity analyses
Results		
Participants	13*	(a) Report numbers of individuals at each stage of study—e.g., numbers potentially eligible, examined for eligibility, confirmed eligible, included in the study, completing follow-up, and analyzed
		(b) Give reasons for nonparticipation at each stage
		(c) Consider use of a flow diagram
Descriptive data	14*	(a) Give characteristics of study participants (e.g., demographic, clinical, social) and information on exposures and potential confounders
		(b) Indicate number of participants with missing data for each variable of interest
		(c) *Cohort study*—Summarize follow-up time (e.g., average and total amount)
Outcome data	15*	*Cohort study*—Report numbers of outcome events or summary measures over time
		Case-control study—Report numbers in each exposure category, or summary measures of exposure
		Cross-sectional study—Report numbers of outcome events or summary measures

	Item No.	Recommendation
Main results	16	(*a*) Give unadjusted estimates and, if applicable, confounder-adjusted estimates and their precision (e.g., 95% confidence interval). Make clear which confounders were adjusted for and why they were included
		(*b*) Report category boundaries when continuous variables were categorized
		(*c*) If relevant, consider translating estimates of relative risk into absolute risk for a meaningful time period
Other analyses	17	Report other analyses done—e.g., analyses of subgroups and interactions, and sensitivity analyses
Discussion		
Key results	18	Summarize key results with reference to study objectives
Limitations	19	Discuss limitations of the study, taking into account sources of potential bias or imprecision. Discuss both direction and magnitude of any potential bias
Interpretation	20	Give a cautious overall interpretation of results considering objectives, limitations, multiplicity of analyses, results from similar studies, and other relevant evidence
Generalizability	21	Discuss the generalizability (external validity) of the study results
Other Information		
Funding	22	Give the source of funding and the role of the funders for the present study and, if applicable, for the original study on which the present article is based

*Give information separately for cases and controls in case-control studies and, if applicable, for exposed and unexposed groups in cohort and cross-sectional studies.

Note: An Explanation and Elaboration article discusses each checklist item and gives methodological background and published examples of transparent reporting. The STROBE checklist is best used in conjunction with this article (freely available on the websites of PLoS Medicine at http://www.plosmedicine.org/, Annals of Internal Medicine at http://www.annals.org/, and Epidemiology at http://www.epidem.com/). Information on the STROBE Initiative is available at www.strobe-statement.org.

APPENDIX E

PRISMA 2009 CHECKLIST

Section/Topic	#	Checklist Item	Reported on Page #
Title			
Title	1	Identify the report as a systematic review, meta-analysis, or both.	
Abstract			
Structured summary	2	Provide a structured summary including, as applicable: background; objectives; data sources; study eligibility criteria, participants, and interventions; study appraisal and synthesis methods; results; limitations; conclusions and implications of key findings; systematic review registration number.	
Introduction			
Rationale	3	Describe the rationale for the review in the context of what is already known.	
Objectives	4	Provide an explicit statement of questions being addressed with reference to participants, interventions, comparisons, outcomes, and study design (PICOS).	
Methods			
Protocol and registration	5	Indicate if a review protocol exists, if and where it can be accessed (e.g., Web address), and, if available, provide registration information including registration number.	
Eligibility criteria	6	Specify study characteristics (e.g., PICOS, length of follow-up) and report characteristics (e.g., years considered, language, publication status) used as criteria for eligibility, giving rationale.	
Information sources	7	Describe all information sources (e.g., databases with dates of coverage, contact with study authors to identify additional studies) in the search and date last searched.	
Search	8	Present full electronic search strategy for at least one database, including any limits used, such that it could be repeated.	
Study selection	9	State the process for selecting studies (i.e., screening, eligibility, included in systematic review, and, if applicable, included in the meta-analysis).	
Data collection process	10	Describe method of data extraction from reports (e.g., piloted forms, independently, in duplicate) and any processes for obtaining and confirming data from investigators.	

Section/Topic	#	Checklist Item	Reported on Page #
Data items	11	List and define all variables for which data were sought (e.g., PICOS, funding sources) and any assumptions and simplifications made.	
Risk of bias in individual studies	12	Describe methods used for assessing risk of bias of individual studies (including specification of whether this was done at the study or outcome level), and how this information is to be used in any data synthesis.	
Summary measures	13	State the principal summary measures (e.g., risk ratio, difference in means).	
Synthesis of results	14	Describe the methods of handling data and combining results of studies, if done, including measures of consistency (e.g., I^2) for each meta-analysis.	
Risk of bias across studies	15	Specify any assessment of risk of bias that may affect the cumulative evidence (e.g., publication bias, selective reporting within studies).	
Additional analyses	16	Describe methods of additional analyses (e.g., sensitivity or subgroup analyses, meta-regression), if done, indicating which were specified.	
Results			
Study selection	17	Give numbers of studies screened, assessed for eligibility, and included in the review, with reasons for exclusions at each stage, ideally with a flow diagram.	
Study characteristics	18	For each study, present characteristics for which data were extracted (e.g., study size, PICOS, follow-up period) and provide the citations.	
Risk of bias within studies	19	Present data on risk of bias of each study and, if available, any outcome level assessment (see item 12).	
Results of individual studies	20	For all outcomes considered (benefits or harms), present, for each study: (a) simple summary data for each intervention group (b) effect estimates and confidence intervals, ideally with a forest plot.	
Synthesis of results	21	Present results of each meta-analysis done, including confidence intervals and measures of consistency.	
Risk of bias across studies	22	Present results of any assessment of risk of bias across studies (see Item 15).	
Additional analysis	23	Give results of additional analyses, if done (e.g., sensitivity or subgroup analyses, meta-regression [see Item 16]).	
Discussion			
Summary of evidence	24	Summarize the main findings including the strength of evidence for each main outcome; consider their relevance to key groups (e.g., healthcare providers, users, and policy makers).	
Limitations	25	Discuss limitations at study and outcome level (e.g., risk of bias), and at review-level (e.g., incomplete retrieval of identified research, reporting bias).	
Conclusions	26	Provide a general interpretation of the results in the context of other evidence, and implications for future research.	
Funding			
Funding	27	Describe sources of funding for the systematic review and other support (e.g., supply of data); role of funders for the systematic review.	

For more information, visit www.prisma-statement.org

GLOSSARY

A

abstract: A summary of a research article.

Academy of Nutrition and Dietetics Health Informatics Infrastructure (ANDHII): A Web platform for Registered Dietitian Nutritionists to report and track outcomes for individual patients and promote evidence-based nutrition practice research.

accessible (source) population: The subset of the target population to which the researcher has access for sampling.

accuracy: The degree to which a measurement approximates the true value.

acquiescence bias: A form of response bias in which respondents are more likely to answer questions positively, such as agreeing with a list of statements rather than disagreeing.

adjusted odds ratio: An odds ratio that controls for confounding variables.

adjustment (controlling): The isolating or controlling of confounding variables so that any change in the dependent variable can be attributed to the independent variable.

allegiance bias: When a researcher's results risk being biased, or a study not published, because of allegiances to a funder or an employer, for example.

alpha level: Probability of making a type I error; typically designated as 0.05 or 0.01 at the end of the tail in a distribution.

amodal: A data set that does not have a mode.

analysis of variance (ANOVA): Inferential statistical test used to compare and analyze the means of more than two groups or the variable is measured more than two times; data must be interval or ratio.

analytic epidemiology: The study of the relationship and strength of association between exposures and outcomes.

analytic research: Research that analyzes the relationship between an intervention or exposure on an outcome.

applied epidemiology: The application of epidemiological concepts and methods to control and prevent disease in the community.

applied research: Research completed to gain knowledge to solve problems and improve practice.

articulation: When qualitative researchers apply a theory or model to explain how parts of the research topic fit together.

assent forms: Forms used to obtain a child's affirmative agreement to participate in research.

associative hypothesis: A hypothesis about two variables in which when one variable changes, the other changes too; does not indicate cause and effect.

associative relationship: A relationship between variables, such that when one changes, the other variable changes too.

attrition: The loss of study participants over time.

auxiliary documents: Documents that are relevant, but not central, to the research question.

axial coding: Second phase of analysis in grounded theory research in which researchers reread transcripts and compare preliminary codes, themes, and subthemes that have been identified, trying to make connection between the open codes.

B

baby theory: A young theory being developed.

basic research: Research completed to produce knowledge alone or build a theory, but not to solve an immediate problem.

Belmont Report: Ethical principles for research including respect for persons, beneficence, and justice; drafted by U.S. commission in 1979.

between-groups design: A study design in which participants are assigned to only one group (usually the experimental group or the control group); also called between-subjects design.

bias: Systematic errors not due to chance; any influence in a study that causes the results to deviate from the true value.

biased selectivity: Any bias in selecting and recording data as part of document analysis in qualitative research.

bimodal: A data set with two modes.

bivariate analysis: The use of statistics to describe the relationship between two variables.

blinding: In a research study, concealing the group to which a participant is assigned from the participant or from study personnel.

bracketing: A method used in qualitative research in which the researcher puts aside all personal biases and opinions in order to be objective; often achieved through writing.

budget narrative or justification: A summary of a budget in a narrative format.

C

carryover effects: The effect that one treatment in an experiment can have on the response to subsequent treatments.

case-control design: A type of retrospective nonexperimental study involving a group of individuals with a disease or condition who are matched and compared to others without the disease, especially in regard to the proportion of people in each group exposed to certain risk factors.

cases: Participants in a case-control study who have the disease or health-related condition; in qualitative research, an individual, group of people, organization, or institution in a case study.

case studies: A qualitative research design that seeks to understand the complexity of a case (such as an individual, group, or organization) in a thorough manner using multiple sources of data; the researchers identify the case and the boundaries of the case.

categorical data: Data that consists of counts or observations in specific categories; nominal data.

categorical variable: Variables that have discrete values (such as male/female).

causal hypothesis: A hypothesis that proposes a cause and effect interaction between variables.

Chi square: A common statistic used to analyze nominal and ordinal data to find differences between groups.

citation management tool: Software used to import article citations, save articles, and build and format reference lists.

clinical practice guidelines: Systematically developed guidelines to assist practitioners in making healthcare decisions that enhance patient care.

clinical studies: Studies using human subjects to help researchers add to medical knowledge.

clinical trial: Studies in which participants receive new treatments, drugs, or medical devices to determine their efficacy and safety; usually a randomized controlled trial.

closed-ended questions: Questions that have specific answers for the respondent to choose from.

cluster random sampling: A type of sampling that first divides the population into clusters, randomly picking some of the clusters, and then randomly sampling within each cluster.

code: A label used to describe a segment of data (image, group of sentences).

codebook: A document that provides a detailed list of all codes and code definitions created for a single database in qualitative research; a document of the variables used in a study/survey, such as their names, how they were defined, and how response options were coded.

coding: The process of reading qualitative data and finding patterns, and giving a label (code) to that part of the text.

coding error: In surveys, errors due to the interviewer or respondent not entering information correctly.

cognitive interview: A method to pretest a questionnaire by having respondents (individually) think aloud while working their way through a questionnaire with the interviewer asking probing questions to get additional information as appropriate; reduces response error.

cohort: A group of individuals who share a common characteristic (such as gender or geographical location) and, in research, are observed over time to gather information.

cohort design: An epidemiologic research design in which a group of individuals with a common characteristic are observed over a period of time so researchers can gather data about exposures (risk factors) and outcomes.

cohort survey: A survey used in a cohort study that surveys people over time observing for health changes.

Common Rule: A short name for "The Federal Policy for the Protection of Human Subjects" and was adopted by a number of federal agencies in 1991.

complex hypothesis: A hypothesis that predicts the relationship between three or more variables.

concept: Words or phrases that abstractly describe a phenomenon, idea, or object.

concurrent validity: Extent to which a measure correlates with another previously established and valid measure/instrument.

confidence interval: The range of values in which the population parameter is estimated to lie based on a sample and specified probability; a narrower interval indicates higher precision.

confidence level: The frequency with which a given confidence interval will contain the true value of the parameter being estimated; usually set at 95%.

confirmation bias: The bias that results when a researcher selectively interprets information to confirm his or her beliefs.

confirmatory factor analysis: A statistical method used to test whether new data fit a hypothesized factor model.

confounding variable: A type of extraneous variable that cannot be controlled or is not recognized until the study starts.

consensus coding: When coders discuss why they coded the same data differently, and try to come to an agreement (consensus) on one appropriate code.

construct: Concepts that are quite complex and at high levels of abstraction.

constructivist paradigm: A worldview in which reality is mentally constructed by individuals in different ways so studies should focus on the individual; associated with qualitative research.

construct validity: Extent to which the researchers are actually measuring the theoretical concepts or constructs in the study.

content validity: Extent to which a measure covers all the dimensions it is supposed to; often used to develop tests and questionnaires.

continuous data: Interval- or ratio-level data that use a continuum of numeric values with equal intervals.

continuous variable: Variables that can take on an infinite range of values on a continuum with equal intervals (such as weight).

control: The use of rules and procedures that regulate conditions and variables in an experiment so the study outcomes accurately reflect reality.

control group: In experimental research, the group that is not exposed to the experimental treatment or procedures.

controlled clinical trials: Intervention studies with a control group, but may not assign participants in a strictly random manner.

convenience sample: A sample based on ready availability of participants.

convenience sampling: A nonprobability sampling method based on ready availability of members.

correlated *t*-test: A variation of the *t*-test used when there is only one group or when groups are related; paired *t*-test.

correlation: A statistical procedure used to measure the strength of a linear relationship between two variables.

correlation coefficients: An estimate, ranging from 0.00 to +1.00, that indicates the reliability of an instrument; statistic used to describe the relationship among two variables.

cost-effectiveness: A comparison of the costs and outcomes/benefits of a treatments.

covariates (covariables): Variables that affect the dependent variable but are not the independent variable.

coverage bias: A bias in which a segment of the population is improperly excluded from consideration in the sample.

covered entities: According to the Health Insurance Portability and Accountability Act, the health care providers, insurance companies, and other agencies that must comply with specific rules to protect the privacy and security of health information and to provide individuals with certain rights with respect to their health information.

Cox's proportional hazards model (Cox regression): A statistical technique used to build models that analyze the effect of one or more independent variables on the time before an event takes place (survival time); results in a hazard ratio.

criterion validity: Extent to which a measure stacks up against another measure or predicts something.
cross-sectional study: A study in which data is collected at one point in time.
cross-sectional survey: A survey administered at one point in time.

D

data cleaning: After data collection, a process to detect, diagnose, and edit or remove faulty data.
Declaration of Helsinki: Ethical principles for medical research with human subjects, amended periodically and used by physicians and institutions around the world.
degrees of freedom: A statistical concept used to refer to the number of sample values that are free to vary; $n - 1$.
de-identified health data: Health data that does not contain certain elements that could be used to identify the person, their relatives, or employer.
dependent variable (outcome measure): The variable/outcome measured in research that is assumed to be influenced by the independent variable. The variable that captures the outcome of an intervention.
descriptive cross-sectional study: A research design that collects information about variables at one point in time without changing the environment, manipulating any variables, or seeking to establish cause and effect; often used to obtain information on prevalence and distribution.
descriptive design: A variety of research designs that collect information about variables without changing the environment, manipulating any variables, or seeking to establish cause and effect; nonexperimental research.
descriptive epidemiology: Describes the distribution of disease by person, place, and time.
descriptive research: A category of research that describes or categorizes a wide variety of phenomena such as a person's or group's characteristics or how often something occurs.
descriptive statistics: Collection and presentation of data that explain characteristics of variables found in the sample.
dichotomous: Nominal measurement when only two possible fixed responses exist such as yes or no.
Dietetics Outcomes Registry (DOR): Part of ANDHII, this database makes anonymous data available for nutrition research and quality improvement projects.
digital object identifier (DOI): A unique persistent identifier for a published article that provides a link to its location on the Internet.
direct costs: Any costs that can be specifically identified with a particular project, such as salaries, equipment, and supplies.
direction: The way two variables covary.
directional hypothesis: A hypothesis that gives the expected direction of the relationship between variables.
dissemination: The act of spreading information to many people; in science, the communication of study findings through posters, presentations, publications, and other ways.
document analysis: A method of systematically collecting, authenticating, and analyzing documents.

double-blind study: A study in which both the participants and the researchers/data collectors who interact with the participants do not know the group assignment for each individual.

E

effectiveness: Ability of a treatment to provide a beneficial effect under usual circumstances.

effect size: A statistic showing the magnitude (or size) of the relationship between two variables or the magnitude of the difference between groups on a variable.

efficacy: Ability of a treatment to provide a beneficial effect under ideal, controlled conditions.

epidemiologic design: Study designs used in epidemiology.

epidemiology: A branch of medical science that investigates factors that determine the presence or absence of diseases and disorders in groups of people, and the application of this work to control health problems.

equivalence reliability: Extent to which measurements from two versions of a test or from two observers observing the same event are consistent.

evidence analysis: Appraising and synthesizing research results in a specific area.

Evidence Analysis Library Reviews: Systematic reviews undertaken by the work group teams of the Evidence Analysis Library of the Academy of Nutrition and Dietetics.

evidence-based dietetics practice: Practice in nutrition and dietetics that is based on using the best available research evidence along with professional know-how and the client's needs and values.

evidence-based nutrition practice guidelines: Systematically developed guidelines and treatment algorithms to assist Registered Dietitian Nutritionists when making nutrition care decisions to enhance quality patient care.

evidence-based practice: Practice based on using the best available research evidence along with professional know-how and the client's needs and values.

Evidence Summary: In the Evidence Analysis Library of the Academy of Nutrition and Dietetics, a narrative synthesis of studies reviewed as part of the systematic review process, which will include a statistical analysis when appropriate.

evidence synthesis: Integrating studies' findings in a specific area; studies can be integrated descriptively (such as finding themes) or quantitatively (such as using meta-analysis).

exclusion criteria: Requirements identified by the researcher that would prevent someone or something from taking part in a study. Can also be applied to the qualitative process (data analysis) when researchers develop a set of "rules" for excluding a specific portion of data from being coded.

exempt review: A procedure the Institutional Review Board uses to review studies that involve no or minimal risk.

expectation bias: When researchers' expectations of what they believe the study results should be get in the way of accurately taking measurements and reporting results.

expedited review: A procedure the Institutional Review Board uses to review studies that do not present more than minimal risk.

experimental design: Research designs that involve manipulation of the independent variable, control of extraneous variables, and random assignment to groups to provide the control necessary to examine possible cause-and-effect relationships.

exploratory factor analysis: A statistical method for identifying underlying dimensions (factors) from a large set of variables; used to reduce data and build scales.

exposure: Any factor that may be associated with an increased occurrence of disease or other health-related outcome or condition; risk factor.

external validity: Extent to which a study's findings can be generalized to other individuals, settings, and time periods.

extramural NIH research: NIH-funded research conducted in colleges, universities, and medical schools in the United States and in some foreign countries.

extraneous variables: A variable that interferes in the relationship between the independent and dependent variables that researchers try to control through research design.

extreme response set bias: A bias in which participants pick the most extreme answers, even when they are not accurate.

F

fabrication: Reporting results/data that was made up.

face validity: Extent to which a measure appears to measure the desired content; often used to develop tests and questionnaires.

factor: The independent variables in a factorial design.

factor analysis: A family of mathematical procedures used to remove duplication from a large set of correlated variables in order to cluster variables into homogenous sets and identify underlying factors; a data reduction tool often used in developing scales.

factorial design: An experimental design in which two or more independent variables (must be categorical) are manipulated to see their joint effect and separate effects on a dependent variable.

falsification: Manipulating data, equipment, or processes resulting in an inaccurate research report.

field notes: Notes written when a researcher observes something, such as a focus group interview, and records the behaviors, activities, and so forth that were observed.

figure: Visual presentations, often in a book or journal, that may include graphs, diagrams, photos, drawings, maps, as well as some text to illustrate concepts.

fishing: Searching unsystematically through a data set and doing statistical tests to find significant differences or relationships to report.

focus groups: A qualitative data collection method in which a group leader uses a semi-structured group interview process to capture information such as values, beliefs, or motivations from a small group of people with characteristics relevant to the research question.

forest plot: In meta-analysis, a graph listing the study titles on the left side, and the corresponding effect size for each study (represented by a square) on the right side; diamond shape at the bottom represents the overall effect size.

formative evaluation: Evaluation done before a program is fully implemented to make sure the program is appropriate and feasible.

foundations: In the nonprofit sector, generally refers to organizations that engage in their own programs and charitable activity; also make grants to institutions, organizations, or individuals for scientific, educational, or other reasons; private foundations usually are established with funds from an individual, a family, or a company.

full board review: A procedure the Institutional Review Board uses to review studies that involve more than minimal risk.

Funding Opportunity Announcements (FOAs): A notice at Grants.gov of a federal grant opportunity; FOAs from the National Institutes of Health are either program announcements (PAs) or requests for applications (RFAs).

G

goals: Broad-based statements of what a project will accomplish.

grounded theory: A qualitative research design that aims to better understand a process among the participants and often results in the development of a theoretical model.

group debriefing: A method to pretest a questionnaire in which a group of respondents complete the questionnaire and then take part in a focus group discussion on it.

guide: A protocol used by qualitative researchers when doing individual interviews or focus groups.

H

Hawthorne effect: The effect on the behaviors of individuals when they are being observed or taking part in research; a type of measurement bias.

hazard ratio: Comparing the risk of an event in the treated/exposed group to the risk of an event in the control or comparison group; gives instantaneous risk at a point in time.

hazard: In hazard analysis, the probability that an individual at any given time has an event at that time.

hedonic scale: A sensory evaluation scale rating food characteristics such as flavor or texture as well as overall acceptability.

heterogeneity: In meta-analysis, the quality of having very different study outcomes.

heterogeneous: The degree to which elements are diverse or not alike.

history: In research, the influence of events outside of a study on the study results; a threat to internal validity.

homogenous: Elements that share many common characteristics.

hypothesis: A statement that predicts the relationship between the variables in a population.

I

Impact Factor: For a journal, the frequency with which articles in the journal are cited during a specific time frame.

incidence: The number of new cases of a disease in a specific population during a given time period.

inclusion criteria: Requirements identified by the researcher that must be present for someone or something to participate in the study. Can also be applied to the qualitative coding process (data analysis) when researchers develop a set of "rules" for applying a specific code to a portion of data.

independent *t*-test: A variation of the *t*-test used when data values vary independently from one another.

independent variable: The variable that is assumed to affect the dependent variable or outcome. In experimental research, the intervention or treatment that is varied by the researcher to affect the dependent variable.

indirect (overhead) costs: Facilities and administrative costs such as rent and utilities (for office space) and administrative staff such as Human Resources.

individual debriefing: A method to pretest a questionnaire in which a respondent takes the entire survey, and then the researcher goes through it with the respondent and asks open-ended questions to get feedback.

individually identifiable health information (IIHI): Health information, as well as additional information such as demographic data and payments for health care, that identify the individual patient.

inductive: Moving from a form of detailed data to more broad, general ideas, conclusions, and sometimes theory.

inferential statistics: Analysis of data as the basis for prediction related to the phenomenon of interest.

Institutional Review Board (IRB): An independent committee named by an institution or agency that consists of physicians, statisticians, and members of the community (such as a university or hospital) who ensure that research proposals are ethical and that the rights and welfare of participants are protected.

instruments: Measurement devices, such as surveys and scales, used to gather research data.

instrument bias: A bias that occurs when a measuring instrument is not properly calibrated.

intention-to-treat analysis: A technique used to prevent bias due to subject attrition in which all participants are used in the statistical analysis regardless of whether they complete the treatment/study; used in randomized controlled trials.

internal consistency reliability: Extent to which different questions measuring the same construct produce similar results.

internal validity: Extent to which the independent variable produced changes in the dependent variable.

inter-rater reliability: Extent to which two or more raters or observers are consistent in measuring or categorizing something.

interrupted time series design with control group: An interrupted time series design that includes a nonequivalent control group; also called a multiple time series design.

interval level of measurement: A continuum of numeric values with equal intervals but the zero point is not meaningful.

intervention group: In experimental research, the treatment or procedures the experimental group undergoes to determine the outcomes.

intervention research: Research in which an intervention is designed, implemented, and tested to see how well it achieves the desired outcomes under controlled conditions.

interviewer error: Errors by the interviewer related to the administration of the survey, such as skipping questions.

intramural NIH research: The internal research program of the National Institutes of Health.

J

jottings: Brief notes written in the field that will be used to write field notes.

K

Kaplan-Meier survival plot: A survival curve used in research to compare groups' time to event (such as heart attack or cancer remission) without adjusting for variables.

keywords: Words used by a search engine or database to find relevant documents.

kurtosis: The peakedness or flatness of a distribution of data.

L

letter of inquiry: A letter written to a funder that allows the funder to determine if they have an interest in the project described in the letter before accepting a full proposal.

level of significance: The criterion used for rejecting the null hypothesis; the alpha level; often set at either 0.05 or 0.01.

levels of measurement: A system of classifying measurements according to a hierarchy of measurement and the type of statistical test that is appropriate.

Likert scale: A type of scale useful to measure opinions, attitudes, and feelings; response choices vary from Strongly Disagree to Strongly Agree, and the middle choice is neutral.

linear mixed models: A range of statistical models useful to analyze longitudinal data.

linear regression: A form of regression analysis that models the relationship between one or more independent variables on one continuous dependent variable by fitting a linear equation to observed data; requires a linear relationship between the variables and normal distributions of the variables; results include a regression coefficient and R-squared.

literature review: Reading, analyzing, and synthesizing research to summarize what is known and not known in a specific topic area.

logistic regression: A form of regression analysis similar to linear regression except that the outcome is dichotomous; used to analyze data in which one or more independent variables affects a dichotomous dependent variable; results show the impact of each independent variable on the odds ratio of the event of interest (dependent variable).

longitudinal study: A study used to collect data at many points over an extended period, often on the same individuals.

longitudinal survey: A survey that is administered more than once.

M

magnitude: The strength of the relationship existing between two variables.

manipulate: In research, adjusting the independent variable to determine its effect on the dependent variable.

MANOVA: Multivariate analysis of variance; an ANOVA with two or more continuous dependent variables (rather than one dependent variable as in ANOVA).

maturation: Naturally occurring time-related changes in a study participant that can pose a threat to internal validity of a study.

maximum variation: A method of selecting participants for a study sample that will provide the possibility that researchers will hear as many different ideas and experiences as possible.

mean: The mathematical average calculated by adding all values and then dividing by the total number of values.

mean difference: Statistic that measures the absolute difference between the mean value in two groups.

measures of central tendency: Measures (e.g., mean, median, mode) that provide information about the typical case found in the data.

measures of variability: Measures providing information about differences among data within a set; measures of dispersion.

median: The point at the center of a data set.

memo: In qualitative research, recording insights, ideas, or even "hunches" that a researcher thinks of when engaging in data analysis.

MeSH Headings (Medical Subject Headings): U.S. National Library of Medicine's controlled medical vocabulary thesaurus that uses a hierarchical structure to allow searching at various levels.

meta-analysis: A statistical technique in which results from many studies addressing the same research question are pooled into a single estimate of the effect of the intervention.

meta-synthesis: In qualitative research, an attempt to examine, integrate, and interpret related qualitative studies; may be used to build or explain a new theory, or other purpose.

mixed methods research: Research that includes quantitative and qualitative methods, data collection, and data in a single study to more fully understand a specific phenomenon.

mixed methods study: Study that includes quantitative and qualitative methods, data collection, and data in a single study to more fully understand a specific phenomenon.

mixed methods systematic review: Synthesis of findings from both quantitative and qualitative studies.

modality: The number of modes found in a data distribution.

mode: The most frequently occurring value in a data set.

model: A graphical or other representation of concepts/constructs and their interrelationships to help us better understand a real world situation.

moderator: Someone who uses a set of open-ended questions to guide a focus group toward an open and spontaneous discussion to create a web of dialogue.

multicollinarity: In multiple regression, a problem that occurs when the independent variables you are testing are highly correlated with each other, making it hard to determine separate effects on the dependent variable.

multi-method qualitative study: A qualitative study that combines multiple qualitative data collection methods.

multiple linear regression: Linear regression to predict the value of a continuous dependent variable from two or more independent variables (continuous or categorical).

multiple logistic regression: Logistic regression used to explore associations between two or more independent variables and one dichotomous dependent variable.

multiple regression: Inferential statistical test that describes the relationship of three or more variables.
multistage sampling: Sampling plans where the sampling is carried out in stages.
multistage (multilevel) cluster sampling: A type of sampling using cluster sampling that is carried out in stages using smaller and smaller sampling units at each stage.
multivariate analysis: The use of statistics to describe the relationships among three or more variables.

N

narrative reviews: Mainly descriptive reviews in which authors organize, interpret, and summarize evidence from primary studies for a specific topic.
National Nutrition Monitoring and Related Research Program (NNMRRP): Research activities regularly conducted by federal agencies that provide information about the dietary, nutritional, and related health status of Americans, and how diet affects health.
negatively skewed: A distribution when the mean is less than the median and the mode; the longer tail is pointing to the left.
network (snowball) sampling: A nonprobability sampling method where the researcher asks members of the sample for assistance to locate others with similar characteristics.
NIH RePorter: A service of the National Institutes of Health that provides access to reports, data, and analyses of NIH research activities and the results of NIH-supported research.
nominal level of measurement: The lowest level of measurement whereby data are categorized simply into groups.
nondirectional hypothesis: A hypothesis that does not give the expected direction of the relationship between variables.
nonequivalent control group design: A quasi-experimental design that includes an intervention and does not randomly assign subjects to groups, so groups are not likely to be equivalent.
nonparametric: Inferential statistics involving nominal- or ordinal-level data to make inferences about the population.
nonprobability sampling: Nonrandom selection of members; often done using judgment or convenience.
nonresponse bias: In survey sampling, a bias in which the percentage of people who do not respond to the survey varies among the different groups in the sample.
nonsampling error: All sources of error in surveys that are not related to the sampling of respondents.
nonsignificant: When results of the study could have occurred by chance; findings that support the null hypothesis.
normal distribution: Data representation with a distinctive bell-shaped curve, symmetric about the mean.
null (or statistical) hypothesis: A hypothesis that the study will find no relationship between the variables, and that any variation is due to chance; a statistical hypothesis used for statistical testing.
Nuremberg Code: Set of 10 principles for ethical human subjects study developed after World War II; important document in the history of medical research ethics.

O

objective: In research, the aim or purpose of the study; in grants, measurable steps to achieve a goal.

observer's comments: Personal comments of the researcher found in field notes; may include the researcher's feelings, reactions, and so forth.

odds ratio: In logistic regression, a ratio of the odds of an outcome occurring for two groups, of which one group has a characteristic not found in the other group. In case-control studies, the odds of having the exposure among those with the disease (the cases) compared to the odds of having the exposure among those without the disease (the controls). Often interpreted like a relative risk.

open-access journals: Journals that provide unrestricted access to journal articles online; often peer reviewed.

open coding: The process of first reading data and noting themes that are evident.

open-ended questions: Questions that ask the respondent to answer in their own words and usually require more thought than close-ended questions.

open-ended research question: An interrogatory statement that directs a study and may change during the course of the study.

operational definition: A definition of a concept that translates the verbal meaning into a measurement.

ordinal level of measurement: A continuum of numeric values where the intervals are not meant to be equal; used in rank ordering an attribute.

original (primary) research study: Narrative of a single study designed and conducted by the researchers.

outcome evaluation: Taking and analyzing measurements at the end of a project to see if goals and objectives have been met.

outcomes: Changes in a client's health or quality of life that result from health/nutrition care or a research intervention.

outcomes research: Research to test the effectiveness of an intervention under ordinary/usual circumstances.

outcome variable: The outcome or visible result of interest that is measured in research; also called the dependent variable.

P

panel survey: A survey that asks the same questions at several points in time to the same respondents.

parallel forms reliability: Extent to which two tests with different questions that address the same constructs are consistent.

parametric: Inferential statistical tests involving interval- or ratio-level data to make inferences about the population.

pass-through grant: A state applies to the federal government for a grant, and if successful, the state passes the federal money on to applicants who have been chosen for the grant.

Pearson's *r*: An inferential statistic used when two variables are measured at the interval or ratio level; Pearson product–moment correlation.

peer review: When editors, researchers, and experts review and critique a manuscript submitted to a journal for publication to determine whether the manuscript should be published, and if so, any changes that should be made.

percentage distributions: Descriptive statistics used to group data to make results more comprehensible; calculated by dividing the frequency of an event by the total number of events.

percentile: A measure of rank representing the percentage of cases that a given value exceeds.

phenomenology: A qualitative research design used to better understand the common experiences of a group of individuals.

phenomena: Experiences that make up the lives of humans.

pilot test: To test the use of a new tool or instrument to see how it works in the real world and get feedback for possible revisions.

placebo: Any intervention or treatment that is believed to have no effect.

plagiarism: Using someone's words or ideas without giving credit appropriately and obtaining permission when necessary.

population parameters: Characteristics of a population that are inferred from characteristics of a sample.

position of the median: Calculated by using the formula $(n + 1)/2$, where n is the number of data values in the set.

positively skewed: Distribution when the mean is greater than the median and the mode; the longer tail is pointing to the right.

positivist paradigm: A worldview in which there is an orderly reality that can be objectively studied; associated with quantitative research.

power: The ability of a study to detect statistically significant differences or relationships in the groups when they really do exist.

power analysis: A procedure to estimate the minimum sample size needed to detect the difference you are looking for as well as the likelihood of committing a type II error.

practice-based research networks (PBRNs): Groups of primary healthcare clinicians and practices that facilitate collaborative research among clinicians and researchers.

precision: A measure of accuracy.

predictive correlational design: Research designs using regression analysis that use predictor/independent variables to predict an outcome and can also estimate the contributions of the predictor variables on the outcome variable.

predictive validity: Extent to which a measure can predict a specific outcome.

predictor variable: In regression analysis and other models, the variable investigated to assess the strength and direction of its association with the dependent or outcome variable; also called the independent variable.

pretesting: In survey methodology, trying out a new survey under conditions similar to real conditions to get feedback on questions, procedures, and the entire questionnaire; completed before pilot testing.

prevalence: The number of cases of a disease or condition in a given population.

prevalence ratio: An estimate of the magnitude of the association between the exposure and the disease.

primary documents: Documents that are the main focus of the study; original documents that may include audio recordings or photos.

principal investigator: Lead researcher for a grant in the sciences; manages the project including monitoring the use of all resources, including the money.

Privacy Rule Authorization: An individual's signed permission to allow a covered entity to use or disclose the patient's protected health information for research purposes as described in the authorization.

probability: Likelihood or chance that an event will occur in a situation.

problem statement: A description of the gap in the knowledge base or dilemma into which researchers want to gain further insight.

process evaluation: Taking and analyzing measurements during the project to assure/improve its quality.

proposal: Another term used for grant application in the field of grants.

prospective: Looking forward in time.

prospective cohort study: An epidemiologic research design in which a group of individuals with a common characteristic are observed over a period of time so researchers can gather data about exposures (risk factors) and outcomes.

protected health information: Personal health information held by covered entities (such as healthcare providers) that is personally identifiable to the patient; protected by the Health Insurance Portability and Accountability Act.

protocol: A thorough written plan for a research study from background and rationale to methodology and a timetable.

publication bias: The bias that results when researchers seek publication of studies only if they contain statistically significant findings.

purposive or judgment sampling: A nonprobability sampling method in which the researcher picks members based on certain characteristics desired in the sample.

***P*-value:** In statistical significance testing, the probability that the results were due to chance alone.

Q

qualitative research: Research that produces descriptive results without using a hypothesis, statistics, or numbers; although some studies may use some numbers.

Quality Criteria Checklist: A tool used by analysts to critically appraise a study's design and methodological quality as part of the systematic review process used by the Evidence Analysis Library of the Academy of Nutrition and Dietetics; a risk of bias tool.

quality improvement: Identifying problems and testing solutions to improve a process, system, or outcome to improve services within a department/facility.

Quality Rating Summary: A compilation of the Quality Criteria Checklists for each article reviewed as part of the systematic review process used by the Evidence Analysis Library of the Academy of Nutrition and Dietetics.

quantitative studies: Studies that use the scientific method, measure variables using a numerical system, and examine associations and relationships among the variables.

quasi-experimental design: A research design for testing an intervention but lacking randomization into groups.

quota sampling: The same as convenience sampling except a certain number of people are picked from different groups with specific background characteristics (such as male/female).

R

random error: Random variation or imprecision due to chance alone.

randomization: The random assignment of people or elements to treatment conditions in a research study; also called random assignment.

randomized block design: A method to assign participants in which individuals are first divided into blocks or subsets and then randomly placed from those blocks into treatment or control groups.

randomized controlled trials (RCT): A rigorous quantitative design that involves an intervention or treatment, randomization into experimental and control groups, and control of extraneous variables.

random sampling: A technique for selecting people or elements where each has an equal probability of being selected.

range: The difference between the maximum and minimum values in a data set.

ratio level of measurement: The highest level of measurement that involves numeric values with equal intervals between them and a meaningful zero point.

recall bias: A bias in which the ability to recall past events accurately differs between the groups.

regression: Statistical techniques used to predict an outcome variable based on one or more independent variables, and to examine the effect of independent variables on an outcome variable after adjusting for other variables.

regression analysis: Statistical techniques used to investigate and/or predict relationships between independent and dependent variables.

regression coefficient: In regression analysis, how a change in the independent (predictor) variables affects the dependent (outcome) variable; if not standardized, it is expressed in the units of the outcome variable; if standardized, it is called a beta coefficient.

regression to the mean: The tendency for very high or very low scores to become closer to the mean when retesting occurs; a threat to internal validity.

reliability: Obtaining consistent measurements over time.

repeated cross-sectional (trend) survey: A survey that ask the same questions at several points in time to a new group of respondents each time.

repeated-measures ANOVA (one-way): Analysis of variance that compares how a within-subjects group performs at repeated points in time; compares three or more means based on a continuous dependent variable.

repeated-measures design: A design in which multiple or repeated measurements are made on the same participant or experimental unit.

research: A systematic investigation involving collection, analysis, and interpretation of information/data to answer questions to extend knowledge.

research design: A detailed plan that states precisely how a study will be conducted including how controls may be used to increase the validity of the findings.

research editorial: An editorial usually on a specific research article in a journal that discusses the topic within a broad context and offers an opinion.

research framework: The theoretical structure that guides a study; not always highly developed or tested.

research (or alternative) hypothesis: A statement of the expected relationships between variables in a study; alternative hypothesis to the null hypothesis.

research methods: Different tools, techniques, and processes used in research to gather data.

research misconduct: Fabrication, falsification, or plagiarism in research activities.

research objective: In research, the aim or purpose of the study.

research problem: A description of the gap in the knowledge base or dilemma into which researchers want to gain further insight.

research question: An interrogatory statement that directs a study and poses a relationship among variables.

researcher bias: Any bias or judgments that the researcher brings to the research topic.
response bias: A bias in which an error in measurement is due to the study participant.
response error: In surveys, errors due to inaccurate answers because respondents do not understand a question, do not know how to answer a question, or do not give an accurate answer.
response rate: The percentage of a sample that complete a questionnaire or interview.
Responsible Conduct of Research (RCR): The practice of research in an ethical and professional manner.
retrospective: Looking backward in time.
retrospective survey: A survey administered at one point in time that asks respondents to report past behaviors, beliefs, and so forth.
review article: Article that summarizes the existing knowledge on a specific topic.
rigor: In a quantitative study, the strict application of the scientific method in every phase to ensure unbiased results. In a qualitative study, the use of strategies, such as triangulation, to ensure the authenticity and truthfulness of findings (trustworthiness).
risk ratio (relative risk): Comparing the probability of one group (exposed to a risk factor or intervention) of experiencing an outcome to another group's probability of experiencing the same outcome; expresses how much more (or less) likely it is for the exposed person to develop an outcome relative to an unexposed person.
R-squared: A statistical measure of how close data are to the regression line; the percentage of variation in the dependent variable that is accounted for by the independent variable(s); also called the coefficient of determination.
Rule of 68–95–99.7: Rule stating that for every sample 68% of the data will fall within one standard deviation of the mean; 95% will fall within two standard deviations; 99.7% of the data will fall within three standard deviations.

S

sample: A subset of the population selected for a study.
sample bias: A bias in which the members of your sample are systematically different from the population in some way.
sample size: The number of participants or units included in the sample to be studied.
sample statistics: Numerical data describing characteristics of the sample.
sampling distribution: A theoretical distribution representing an infinite number of samples that can be drawn from a population.
sampling error: When the data obtained from a sample differ from the true population parameters; also called sample variance.
sampling frame: The specific source of individuals; usually a list of members of the accessible population.
sampling variance (sampling error): When the data obtained from a sample differ from the true population parameters.
saturation: In qualitative research, when no new information is being obtained and repetition of information is consistently heard.

scale: A self-completed form with questions that are thought to measure a certain construct, such as attitudes; questions usually have a set of possible answers representing ordered points on a continuum.
scatterplot: A graph in which data pairs (x,y) are plotted as individual points to examine the linear relationship (correlation) of the points.
scientific method: Procedures used for investigating questions to pursue knowledge.
secondary data analysis: Analyzing existing data previously collected to answer new research questions.
secondary documents: Documents that interpret and analyze primary documents.
secondary research: Research that summarizes content from primary research studies, such as narrative reviews.
selection bias: A bias in which some groups in the population have a higher or lower chance of being selected than others.
selective coding: Third phase of analysis in grounded theory research in which the researcher identifies, compares, contrasts, and describes the key themes found in the data; key themes are used to develop a visual theoretical model.
seminal article: Classic articles that report a new idea, insight, or major breakthrough in a research area that are cited often by others.
semiquartile range: The range of the middle 50% of the data.
sensitivity: The probability that a test can screen or diagnose a condition accurately.
semi-structured interview: A qualitative research method that involves a set of open-ended questions and the opportunity for the participant to share relevant information.
significant financial interest: When total income/assets that a researcher receives go above a certain level, the researcher may be asked to disclose, manage, or eliminate such financial interests.
simple hypothesis: A hypothesis that predicts the relationship between one independent variable and one dependent variable.
simple interrupted time-series design: A quasi-experimental design in which changes in the dependent variable are observed multiple times before and after an intervention.
simple linear regression: Linear regression to predict the value of a continuous dependent variable from one independent variable (continuous or categorical).
simple logistic regression: Logistic regression used to explore associations between one independent variable and one dichotomous dependent variable.
simple randomization: Randomizing participants based on a single sequence of random assignments, such as flipping a coin or using computer-generated random numbers.
simple random sampling: Basic probability sampling from a population using a fair process such as random digits.
single-blind study: A study in which the participants do not know to which group they are assigned.
skewed: An asymmetrical distribution of data.
snowball sampling: A nonprobability sampling method in which the researcher asks members of the sample for assistance in locating others with similar characteristics; also called purposive sampling.
social desirability bias: A bias in which respondents choose responses to questions that they believe will be viewed favorably by others.

Solomon four-group design: A rigorous experimental design that combines a pretest-posttest design with a posttest-only design; allows researcher to see if the pretest influenced the results.

specificity: The probability that a test yields a negative diagnosis accurately.

standard deviation: A measure of variability used to determine the number of data values falling within a specific interval in a normal distribution.

standardized mean difference: Mean difference (measures absolute difference between the means in two groups) that has been standardized to a uniform scale to allow comparison between studies; used in meta-analysis.

statement of the problem: A description of the gap in the knowledge base or dilemma into which researchers want to gain further insight.

statistical conclusion validity: Extent to which inferences about relationships among variables from the statistical analysis of the data are reasonable and accurate.

statistically significant: When critical values fall in the tails of normal distributions; when findings did not happen by chance alone.

Statistics: The branch of mathematics that collects, analyzes, interprets, and presents numerical data in terms of samples and populations.

statistics: The numerical outcomes and probabilities derived from calculations on raw data.

stratified random sampling: A type of sampling that first involves dividing the accessible population into groups and then randomly sampling each group.

structured interview: A research method in which each person being interviewed is presented with the same series of questions in the same order.

study protocol: A document that describes in detail the purpose of a study as well as the specific steps to carry out the study including ethical considerations/approvals and a timetable.

summary estimate: Pooled intervention effect estimate in a meta-analysis.

survey methods: The way a survey is delivered or administered to potential respondents.

survival analysis: A number of statistical methods that are used to model time-related outcomes, such as estimating the amount of time until the occurrence of a specific event, such as diagnosis of high blood pressure.

survival time: In survival analysis, the time from a defined point to the occurrence of a given event.

systematic random sampling: A type of sampling in which sample members are listed and randomly chosen using an objective procedure such as every 10th person after a random starting point.

systematic reviews: Use of a systematic process to identify, appraise, and synthesize all relevant studies on a topic, often using meta-analysis to synthesize the data.

T

table: A chart that presents lists of numbers/text in a well-organized format such as columns.

tailedness: The degree to which a tail in a distribution is pulled to the left or to the right.

target population: The population that a study is focused on and to which generalizations are to be made.

tertiary research: Research that collects and distills information from both primary and secondary sources.

test-retest reliability: The extent to which repeated measurements for a given person will be similar.

thematic analysis (content analysis): A qualitative research design focused on organizing key ideas that emerge from single or multiple forms of data.

theme: In qualitative research, the patterns researchers discover after reviewing the dataset multiple times.

theoretical definition: The verbal meaning attached to a concept.

theoretical sampling: The process of collecting and analyzing data simultaneously, and deciding during this process which data should still be collected to help develop and refine a theory/model; often used in grounded theory research.

theoretical saturation: In qualitative research, the point at which analyzing data no longer brings addition insights to the research questions and theory development.

theory: A set of relationships among constructs that, when taken together, attempt to explain or predict related phenomena.

tool: Data collection documents used by qualitative researchers when doing observations or document analysis.

translational research: A systematic process of transforming findings from basic science or clinical studies into practical applications and evidence-based practice to improve the health of individuals and populations; research that goes from the researcher's bench to the patient bedside and then to the community.

transcript: A written document of everything spoken in an audio recording.

transcription: The process of making a full written copy of what was spoken and recorded.

treatment fidelity: Implementing the intervention as planned and delivering it in a comparable manner to all participants.

triangulation: Using multiple data sources or methods to investigate and provide additional evidence for understanding the problem under study.

trustworthiness: A determination that a qualitative study is of high quality and credible.

***t* statistic:** Inferential statistical test to determine whether a statistically significant difference exists between groups.

type I error (alpha α error): When the researcher rejects the null hypothesis when it should have been accepted.

type II error (beta β error): When the researcher inaccurately concludes that there is no relationship among the independent and dependent variables when an actual relationship does exist; when the researcher accepts the null hypothesis when it should have been rejected.

U

unimodal: A data set with one mode, such as a normal distribution.

univariate analysis: The use of statistical tests to provide information about one variable.

unstructured interview: A qualitative research method in which the interviewer uses open-ended questions and allows the participant to guide the conversation.

V

validity: Degree to which conclusions are accurate and supported; accuracy of instruments and measurements.

variable: Any quality of a person, group, thing, or situation that varies and can take on different values; any quality that is measured, manipulated, or controlled in research.

visual analog scale: Psychometric response scale used to measure an attitude or characteristic that ranges across a continuum, such as level of pain.

W

washout period: A period of time in a study during which participants receive no treatment and the effects of a previous treatment are washed out of the individual's system.

within-groups design: A study design in which each participant goes through all treatment and control conditions such as in a crossover design; also called within-subjects design.

X, Y, Z

***z* scores:** Standardized units used to compare data gathered using different measurement scales.

INDEX

Note: Page numbers followed by *f* or *t* indicate figures and tables, respectively.

A

abbreviations, 42
abstract, 102, 407, 407*f*
academic journals, 32, 32*t*. *See also* journals
Academy of Nutrition and Dietetics, 338
  Standards of Professional Performance, 31–32
Academy of Nutrition and Dietetics Foundation (ANDF), 423
Academy of Nutrition and Dietetics Health Informatics Infrastructure (ANDHII), 17
accessible (source) population, 358, 358*f*
  defined, 92, 93*f*
accuracy, defined, 91
Achenwall, Gottfried, 116
acquiescence bias, 99
ADA/CDR Code of Ethics, 59*t*, 61, 62*t*
adjusted odds ratio (AOR), 147, 194, 195*t*
adjustment process, 200
Agency for Healthcare Research and Quality (AHRQ), 344, 422
AGRICOLA (Agricultural Online Access), 43
Agricultural Online Access (AGRICOLA), 43
AHA. *See* American Heart Association (AHA)
allegiance bias, 91
allocation concealment, 326
alpha level, 134
α error (type I error). *See* type I error (α error)
alternative hypothesis, 84
American Association of Health Plans (AAHP), 344
American Heart Association (AHA), 98
American Journal of Clinical Nutrition, 32*t*, 34–35
American Medical Association (AMA), 344
  documentation style, 400–401, 402*t*
American Psychological Association (APA)
  documentation style, 401, 402*t*
amodal data, 121
analysis of covariance (ANCOVA), 141
analysis of variance (ANOVA), 139–141, 141*t*, 158*t*, 165, 169, 191, 227
  one-way, 140
  two-way, 140
analytic epidemiology, 18, 186
analytic research, 8
ANDHII. *See* Academy of Nutrition and Dietetics Health Informatics Infrastructure (ANDHII)
Annals of Family Medicine, 220
ANOVA. *See* analysis of variance (ANOVA)
AOR (adjusted odds ratio), 194, 195*t*
applied epidemiology, 18
applied research, 13–14
articles. *See* research article(s)
articulation, 275
assent forms, 67
associative hypothesis, 83, 83*f*
associative relationship, in variables, 79, 79*f*
asymmetric/skewed distributions, 127–128, 127–128*f*
  negatively skewed, 127–128, 127*f*
  positively skewed, 128, 128*f*
attrition, 88
  RCTs, 161
attrition bias, 326
authors, 220–221, 221*t*
auxiliary documents, 250–251

B

baby theory, 289
bar graph, 403, 405*f*
baseline data, 161
basic research, 13–14
Belmont Report (1979), 55
beneficence, 55
β error (type II error). *See* type II error (β error)
between-groups design, 165
biased selectivity, 257
bias(es), 90–92, 256, 324–325
  allegiance, 91
  confirmation, 91
  described, 90–91
  expectation, 90, 156
  instrument, 99

bias(es) (*cont.*)
  nonresponse, 91
  publication, 91
  reducing, 92
  in research (examples), 91, 91*t*
  response, 99
  risk of, assessment of, 324–326, 334, 335*t*-336*t*
  sample, 97
bimodal data, 121
bioactive compounds in fruits and vegetables, researcher interview, 46–47
bivariate analysis, 116
blinding
  defined, 161
  RCTs, 163
Block's food frequency questionnaire (FFQ), 178
blueprint, 6, 244
books, 32, 37
Boolean operators, 42
bracket, 288
budget justification, 430
budget narrative, 430

C

carryover effects, 165
case, 292
case-control design, epidemiological studies, 192–196, 192*f*, 195*t*
case study(ies), 286, 292, 302
  qualitative research designs, 286, 292–293
  strengths and limitations, 293
categorical data, 117
  in ungrouped format, 118*t*
categorical variables, 5, 80, 117
causal hypothesis, 83, 83*f*
causality, in epidemiological designs, 196, 197*t*
CCT. *See* controlled clinical trials (CCT)
CDC. *See* Centers for Disease Control and Prevention (CDC)
CDSR (Cochrane Database of Systematic Reviews), 43
Centers for Disease Control and Prevention (CDC), 421
  data sources for secondary data analysis, 177*t*
central tendency, measures of. *See* measures of central tendency
checklist. *See also specific entries*
  for articles selection, 44–45
Chi-Square tests, 138–139, 140*t*, 141*t*, 227
Childhood obesity prevention self-efficacy survey, 376*f*
CINAHL (Cumulative Index of Nursing and Allied Health), 43
citation management tool, 392
clinical outcomes, 16
clinical practice guidelines, 320
clinical studies, 15
clinical trials, 15
  controlled (CCT), 162
  in experimental designs, 160–165
ClinicalTrials.gov, 162
closed-ended questions, 256, 353, 365
cluster random sampling, 93, 95*t*, 359, 360*f*, 361*t*
cluster sampling, 95*f*
  multistage (multilevel), 94, 95*t*
Cochrane, 325
Cochrane Collaboration, 232
Cochrane Collaboration tool, 325
Cochrane Database of Systematic Reviews (CDSR), 43, 343–344
Cochrane Handbook, The, 161
Cochrane Review Group (CRG), 344
code, defined, 262
"Code of Ethics for the Profession of Dietetics," principles, 59*t*, 62*t*
Code of Federal Regulations Title 21, Parts 50, 55
Code of Federal Regulations Title 45, Part 46, 55
codebook, 263, 265, 266*f*, 379, 380*f*
coding errors, 378
coding process, qualitative research, 262–268
  final stages, 263
  initial stages, 263
  inter-rater reliability *vs.* consensus coding, 267–268
  key concepts, 263
  sample codebook page, 266*f*
  sample codes, 264–265, 266*f*
  visual model, 263, 263*f*
coefficient of variation, 126
cognitive interviews, 370
  probing method, 370
  think-aloud method, 370
cohort, defined, 188
cohort study design, 156, 188–192
  defined, 188
  epidemiological studies, 188–192, 188*f*
  prospective, 188, 188*f*
  retrospective, 188, 188*f*
cohort survey, 356
Collaborative Institutional Training Initiative (CITI), 57
commentaries, 37
commentary articles, 34

Common Rule, 56, 64
comparative design, descriptive quantitative, 172–174
comparison group, 159–160
completed observation tool (qualitative and quantitative), example, 258–259*f*
complex hypothesis, 83–84
concepts, quantitative research, 78–80
conclusion grading table, 337*t*–338*t*
Conclusion section, research article
  qualitative research, 278
    evaluating, 312–313
  quantitative research, 105–106, 107*t*
    evaluating, 230–232, 231*t*
conclusions statements, 334
concurrent validity, 100, 375
conference proceedings, 37
confidence intervals (CIs), 106, 131, 363
confidence level, 363
confirmation bias, 91
confirmatory factor analysis, 377
conflict of commitment, 58–59
conflict of interest, 57–59
  "Code of ethics for the Profession of Dietetics," principles, 59*t*
conflicts
  financial, 57–58, 58*f*
  intellectual, 59
  personal, 59
confounder, exposures, and outcome, relationship among, 200, 200*f*
confounding variables, 79, 200
consensus coding, 268
  described, 268
  vs. inter-rater reliability, 267–268
Consolidated Criteria for Reporting Qualitative Research (COREQ) checklist, 302, 304*f*
CONSORT 2010 checklist, 165, 233, 453–456
construct validity, 87, 90, 377
  defined, 90
  instruments, 100
  threats to, 90
constructivist paradigm, 10
constructs
  qualitative research, 275–276
  quantitative research, 78–80, 87
content analysis. *See* thematic analysis
content validity, 100, 375, 375*t*
contingency table, 187, 187*t*
continuous data, 117
continuous variables, 5, 80
control
  concept of, 10
  for extraneous variables, 157
control group, 6
  experimental designs, 157, 159–160
  interrupted time series design with, 169*t*, 170
  nonequivalent designs, 168–169, 168*t*
controlled clinical trials (CCT), 162. *See also* randomized controlled trials (RCTs)
controlling process, 200
convenience sample, 254
convenience sampling, 94, 96*t*, 360, 362*t*
Cooke, Natalie K., 294–296
Cooking Light, 32
COREQ (Consolidated Criteria for Reporting Qualitative Research) checklist, 302, 304*f*
corporate foundations, 424, 424*t*
correlated *t* test, 139
correlation coefficients, 142, 142*f*, 174
correlational design, 174–176
correlations, 142–143, 145, 174
  scatterplot (positive and negative), 175–176, 175*f*
cost-benefit analysis, 17
cost-effectiveness, 16
cost-effectiveness analysis, 16–17
cost outcomes, 16
covariates/covariables, 80, 200
cover letter, 365
  items be included in, 365
  printed, 365
coverage bias, 97, 357
covered entities, 65, 65*t*
Cox's proportional hazards model (Cox regression), 207–211
criterion validity, 100, 375, 375*t*, 377
cross-sectional study, 6, 105, 156
  advantages, 172
  descriptive, 171–172, 173*t*
  epidemiological research, 187–188, 187*t*
  repeated, 171–172, 173*t*
cross-sectional survey, 355, 356*t*
crossover designs, 165–166, 166*f*
Cumulative Index of Nursing and Allied Health (CINAHL), 43
Cunningham-Sabo, Leslie, 178–179

D

data analysis, qualitative research, 262–273
  coding process, 262–268

data analysis, qualitative research (*cont.*)
  data organization, 262
  evaluating, 310
  memoing, 268–270
  theming, 270–271
  theory development, 271–272
  trustworthiness, 272–273
data cleaning, 381
data collection, qualitative research, 260–262
  document analysis, 261–262
  evaluating, 309–310
  focus groups and interviews, 260–261
  observations, 261
data collection methods, qualitative research, 248–251
  document analysis, 248, 250–251, 251*f*
  focus groups, 248–249
  individual interviews, 249
  observations, 249–250
  strengths and limitations, 252*t*
data collection tools, 255–257
  interview and focus group guides, 255–256
  observation and document analysis tools, 257
data organization, 262
databases. *See also specific entries*
  examples, 37
  Google Scholar, using, 43
  mapping, 39
  MEDLINE/PubMed, using, 39–43, 41*f*
  other, using, 43–44
  searching, using keywords or subject headings, 38–39, 38*t*, 39*t*
  using, to find articles, 37–44
de-identified health data, 65, 66*t*
debriefing, 273
Declaration of Helsinki (1964), 55
decreased risk, 146, 190
degrees of freedom, 137
Department of Health and Human Services (HHS), 14, 55, 56, 65
dependent variables, 5–6, 78–79, 198*t*, 221
descriptive cross-sectional study, 171–172, 173*t*
descriptive designs, 104
descriptive epidemiology, 18, 186
descriptive quantitative designs, 157, 171–176, 220
  comparative design, 172–174
  correlational design, 174–176
  descriptive cross-sectional study, 171–172, 173*t*
  repeated cross-sectional study, 171–172, 173*t*
descriptive research, 8, 157, 171–176
descriptive statistics, 116, 130
  statistical symbols for, 117*t*
detailed (thick) descriptions, 272
detection bias, 326
dichotomous variable, 78, 117
diet quality, 78
Dietary Guidelines for Americans, 78
dietetic practice groups, 423
Dietetics Outcomes Registry (DOR), 17
Dietetics Practice-Based Research Network (DPBRN), 21
digital object identifier (DOI), 35–36
direct costs, 430, 430*t*
direct nutrition care outcomes, 16
direction, 142
directional hypothesis, 83
Discussion section, research article
  qualitative research, 278
    evaluating, 311–312
  quantitative research, 105–106
    evaluating, 230–232, 231*t*
disease detectives, 18
disease-specific funding organizations, 422, 423*t*
dissemination, 408
  aim of, 408
  in nutrition, 408
    posters, 408, 409–411
    presentations, 408–409, 408*f*
    publications, 408
dissertations, 36
distribution patterns, 127–130
  asymmetric/skewed distributions, 127–128, 127–128*f*
  normal distributions (symmetrical shapes), 127, 127*f*
  tailedness, 128–130, 129–130*f*
document analysis
  for data collection, 261–262
  as data collection tool, 257
  qualitative research, 248, 250–251, 251*f*
documentation styles, 398, 400
DOI. *See* digital object identifier (DOI)
DOR. *See* Dietetics Outcomes Registry (DOR)
double-blind study, 161

E

EAL. *See* Evidence Analysis Library (EAL)
EBP. *See* evidence-based practice (EBP)
editorials, 34
effect size, 144–145, 326–330. *See also* meta-analysis
  defined, 86, 144
  expected, 98

effectiveness, interventions, 16
efficacy, 15
  demonstration in RCT, 15–16
electronic surveys, 353, 354*t*
EndNote, 392
enhanced (tailored) intervention (EI), 223
Enhanced Intervention group, 227
epidemiologic designs, 104
epidemiological research, 17–18
  defined, 17, 20*t*
  examples, 20*t*
epidemiological research designs, 185–212
  case-control design, 192–196, 192*f*, 195*t*
  causality in, 196, 197*t*
  cohort design, 188–192, 188*f*
  cross-sectional, 187–188, 187*t*
  overview, 185–186
  predictive correlational designs, 197–211
epidemiologists, 18
epidemiology, 104, 156, 185
  analytic, 18, 186
  applied, 18
  defined, 17–18
  descriptive, 18, 186
  researcher interview, 211–212
equivalence reliability, 373
ERIC, 43
Error Score, 87*f*
error(s)
  categories, 90
  defined, 90
  in measurement, 99
  random, 90, 91
  reduction of, in hypothesis, 132–136
    level of significance, 134–136, 135*f*
    type I error, 133–134, 134*t*
    type II error, 133–134, 134*t*
  sampling, 96–97, 131–132
  systematic (*See* bias(es))
  type I (α error), 85, 85*t*, 97, 133–136, 134*t*
  type II (β error), 85, 85*t*, 97, 133–136, 134*t*
ethics, 53–71
  ADA/CDR Code of Ethics, 61, 62*t*
  code of, 53–54
  defined, 53
  guidelines, 54
  human subjects research and, 60–66
  IRB and, 66–70
  overview, 53–54
  principles, 55
  research, history of, 54–56
  Responsible Conduct of Research (RCR), 56–60
  standards/norms for research, 54
evaluation
  qualitative research, 301–313
    conclusions, 312–313
    data analysis, 310
    data collection, 309–310
    design, 308
    discussion, 311–312
    literature review, 306–307, 306*f*
    overview, 301–302
    results, 311
    review criteria, 302
    statement of problem, 302–305, 305*t*
    subject selection, 309
    trustworthiness, 313
  quantitative research, 219–235
    additional tools, 232–233
    discussion and conclusion, 230–232, 231*t*
    introduction of article, 222–224, 222*t*
    methods, 224–228, 226*t*
    overview, 219–220
    research title and authors, 220–221, 221*t*
    results, 228–230, 229*t*
evidence analysis, 9, 319
Evidence Analysis Library (EAL)
  of Academy of Nutrition and Dietetics, 332–342
  analysts, 232–233
  navigating, 341–342
  reviews, 34
  systematic review process for, 332–338
evidence-based dietetics practice, 320
evidence-based nutrition practice guidelines, 338
  definition of, 338
  development of, 339–341, 339*t*
evidence-based practice (EBP), 131, 147–148, 321
  defined, 7
  RDNs, 31–32
Evidence Summary, 333, 334
exclusion criteria, 92, 253
exempt reviews, 68
expectation bias, 90, 156
expedited review, 68
experimental designs, 8, 104, 157–168, 220–221
  clinical trials, 160–165
  comparison group, 159–160
  control for extraneous variables, 157
  control group, 157, 159–160
  crossover designs, 165–166, 166*f*
  factorial designs, 166–167, 167*f*
  intervention or treatment, 157

experimental designs (*cont.*)
placebo, 160
randomization, 157, 159
randomized controlled trials (RCTs), 160–165
Solomon four-group design, 167–168, 167*t*
exploratory factor analysis, 377
exposures, 18, 104, 145–146, 185–186, 189–190
outcome, and confounder, relationship between, 200, 200*f*
external validity, 87, 88–89
defined, 90
extramural NIH research, 419
extraneous variables, 6, 79, 156
control for, 157
design strategies to control, 80*t*
extreme response set bias, 99

F

fabrication, 60
face-to-face survey, 355*t*
face validity, 100
factor analysis, 100, 377
factorial designs, 166–167, 167*f*
factors, 166
fair subject selection, for human subjects research, 61, 62*t*
falsification, 60
Family Nutrition and Physical Activity Screening Tool, 352
favorable risk-benefit ratio, human subjects research and, 61, 62*t*
FDA. *See* Food and Drug Administration (FDA)
field notes, 260
figures, use of, 403–404
filters, using, 43
financial conflicts, 57–58, 58*f*
Fischer, Joan G., 46–47
fishing, 89
focus groups, 10, 248–249, 255–256, 260–261
Food and Drug Administration (FDA), 15, 55, 56
Food Management, 32, 32*t*
Food Science and Technology Abstracts (FSTA), 44
food science/sensory evaluation, researcher interview, 233–235
FoodService Director, 32*t*
forest plot, 330–332, 332*f*, 333*f*
formative evaluation, 429
foundations, 422
framework, quantitative research, 82
Framingham Heart Study, 189, 191
frequency(ies)
examples, 119*t*
and percentage distributions of ages, 119–120, 119*t*, 120*f*
samples description using, 118–120, 118*t*, 119*t*
frequent peer review, 273
fruits, bioactive compounds in (researcher interview), 46–47
FSTA (Food Science and Technology Abstracts), 44
full board review, 68
Funding Opportunity Announcements (FOAs), 421

G

goals, in grant proposals, 427, 428*t*
Goodell, L. Suzanne, 294–296
Google Scholar, 36, 38
using, 43
grants, for nutrition research, 417–433
government funding, 418
Agency for Healthcare Research and Quality, 422
Centers for Disease Control and Prevention, 421
federal government, 418
National Institute for Food & Agriculture, 421
National Institutes of Health, 419–421
National Science Foundation, 422
state governments, 418
nongovernment funding, 422–424
ANDF and dietetic practice groups, 423
corporate foundations, 424, 424*t*
disease-specific organizations, 422, 423*t*
private foundations, 422, 423*t*
planning application for, 425–426
proposal, developing and writing of, 426–433
evaluation, 429
goals and objectives, 427–428, 428*t*
project budget, 430–431, 430*t*
research design/methodology, 428–429
statement of need, 427
rejection of grant applications, 427*t*
writing of, tips for, 431, 432*t*–433*t*
Grants.gov, 418
"gray literature," 36
Greene, Geoffrey, 107–108
grounded theory, 286, 289–292, 302
example, 290–292, 291*f*
features, 290
goals, 289–290
strengths and limitations, 292
group debriefing, 371

groups, testing for differences between, 137–142, 138*t*
  analysis of variance (ANOVA), 139–141, 141*t*
  Chi-square statistic, 138–139, 140*t*, 141*t*
  t-statistic, 139, 140*t*, 141*t*
Guide for Effective Nutrition Interventions and Education, 21
guides. *See also* data collection tools
  for data collection, 256
  defined, 255

H

hashtag, 262
Hawthorne effect, 91, 165
hazard, defined, 147, 207–208
hazard ratio (HR), 147, 207–208
health belief model, 81*t*
Health Insurance Portability and Accountability Act (HIPAA), 65
Healthy Eating Index, 38, 78, 86
Hedonic scale, 368*t*
heterogeneity, in meta-analysis, 330
heterogeneous data, 124
HHS. *See* Department of Health and Human Services (HHS)
Hill's criteria for causation, 197*t*
HIPAA. *See* Health Insurance Portability and Accountability Act (HIPAA)
history, 88
homogenous data, 124
Hottenstein, Annette, 233–235
HR. *See* hazard ratio (HR)
human subjects research
  defined, 60
  ethics and, 60–66
  informed consent, 63–64, 64*t*
  privacy, 65–66, 65–66*t*
  requirements for, 60–61
  vulnerable populations, 63*t*
hypothesis, 5–6, 222, 224
  alternative, 84
  associative, 83, 83*f*
  causal, 83, 83*f*
  complex, 83–84
  directional, 83
  error, reduction of, 132–136
    level of significance, 134–136, 135*f*
    type I error, 133–134, 134*t*
    type II error, 133–134, 134*t*
  examples, 103*t*
  level of significance, 84
  nondirectional, 83
  null hypothesis, 84
  quantitative research, 83–85
  simple, 83
  statistical, 84
hypothesis testing, 84–85, 86

I

IIHI (individually identifiable health information), 65
Impact Factor, 35–36
incidence, defined, 186
inclusion criteria, 253
increased risk, 146, 190
independent review, for human subjects research, 61, 62*t*
independent *t* test, 139
independent variables, 5, 6, 78–79, 198*t*, 221
indirect costs, 430, 430*t*
individual debriefing, 371
individual interviews, 249
individually identifiable health information (IIHI), 65
inductive qualitative study, 244
industry funding, for nutrition-related research, 424, 424*t*
inferential statistics, 116, 130–132
  analysis of variance (ANOVA), 139–141, 141*t*
  applications, 130–132
  chance (coin toss example), 131–132
  Chi-Square, 138–139, 140*t*, 141*t*
  degrees of freedom, 137
  nonparametric tests, 137, 138*t*
  other tests of significance, 144
  parametric tests, 136, 138*t*
  probability, 131
  sampling distribution, 137
  statistical symbols for, 136*t*
  t-statistic, 139, 140*t*, 141*t*
  testing for differences between groups, 137–142, 138*t*
  testing for relationships among variables, 142–144, 138*t*
informed consent, 54, 61, 62*t*, 63–64
  components, 64*t*
Institutional Review Board (IRB), 21, 54, 66–70, 377
  application, information required for, 67
  approval of research, criteria for, 68–69, 69*t*
  exempt reviews, 68
  expedited review, 68
  full board review, 68
  functions, 66–67
  members, 66, 67
  purpose of, 66
  reviews, levels of, 67–68
instrument bias, 99

instruments, 6
  qualitative research, 245
  quantitative research, 98–101
  reliability, 99–100
  sensitivity, 100–101
  specificity, 101
  validity, 100
intellectual conflicts, 59
intention-to-treat analysis, 161, 227
inter-item reliability. *See* internal consistency reliability
inter-rater reliability, 99, 373, 374*t*
  described, 268
  vs. consensus coding, 267–268
internal consistency reliability, 99–100, 373, 374*t*
internal validity, 87, 88
  defined, 90
  threats to, 88
interrupted time series design with control group, 169*t*, 170
interrupted time series designs, 169–171, 169*t*, 170*f*, 170*t*
interval measurement, 116, 117, 118*t*
intervention group, 6
intervention research, 15–16, 156
  defined, 15, 20*t*
  examples, 20*t*
  researcher interview, 178–179
interventions, 15, 156, 157
  effectiveness, 16
  RCTs, 163
interviewer errors, 378
interviews
  for data collection, 260–261
  as data collection tools, 255–256
  semistructured, 256
  structured, 255
  unstructured, 255
intraclass correlation coefficient (ICC), 99
intramural NIH research, 419
Introduction section, research article, 102–103
  evaluating, 222–224, 222*t*
  writing of, 395–396, 395*f*
Intuitive Eating Scale score, 141
IRB. *See* Institutional Review Board (IRB)
IRB review, 54, 67–69

J

jottings, 261
Journal of Nutrition Education and Behavior, 302
  qualitative reviewer guidelines, 303*f*
Journal of the Academy of Nutrition & Dietetics (JAND), 32–34, 400
  "Research" section, 33–34
Journal of the American Medical Association, 32*t*
journals, 32
  described, 33–36
  digital object identifier (DOI), 35–36
  examples, 32*t*
  Impact Factor, 35–36
  nutrition-related, 35, 36*t*
  open-access, 35–36
  peer review, 33
  research articles (*See* research article(s))
  scholarly/academic, 32, 32*t*
  scientific literature not found in, 36–37
  vs. magazine/newspapers and trade publications, 32*t*
judgment/purposive sampling, 95, 96*t*
justice, 55

K

Kaplan-Meier survival plot, 208–209, 209*f*
Karmally, Wahida, 22–24
keywords
  advantages and disadvantages, 39*t*
  databases searching using, 38–39, 38*t*, 39*t*
  PubMed search using, tips for, 41–43
Kolmogorov-Smirnov test, 142
Kurtosis, 128, 128*f*

L

letter of inquiry, 425
level of significance, 84
levels of measurement
  defined, 116–117
  identification, 117
  interval, 116, 117, 118*t*
  nominal, 116, 117, 118*t*
  ordinal, 116, 117, 118*t*
  quantitative research, 81*t*
  ratio, 116, 117, 118*t*
Likert scale, 366, 367*t*
line chart, 403, 405*f*
linear mixed models, 191
linear regression, 198–202
  multiple, 198, 200–202
  simple, 198
literature review, 102, 391
  citation tools, use of, 392
  defined, 5

for garden-based nutrition education study, 392*f*
matrix, 392–393, 393*f*
outline for, 393–394
purpose of, 102, 391
qualitative research, 246–247
evaluating, 306–307, 306*f*
quantitative research, 222, 223
writing of, 391–395
guidelines for, 394–395
transition words and phrases to connect ideas in, 394*t*
logistic regression, 198, 202–207
multiple, 203
simple, 203
longitudinal study, 6, 105, 156
longitudinal survey, 355–356, 356*t*

M

magazines, 32
examples, 32*t*
vs. newspapers, trade publications and journals, 32*t*
magnitude, 142–143
management research, researcher interview, 70–71
Mann-Whitney U test, 142
mapping, 39
masking, 161
maturation, 88
maximum variation, 254
MD. *See* mean difference (MD)
mean, 122–124
calculation, 122
defined, 122
example, 123
mean difference (MD), 144–145, 163, 326, 327
measurement, 156. *See also* levels of measurement
errors in, 99
interval, 116, 117, 118*t*
nominal, 116, 117, 118*t*
ordinal, 116, 117, 118*t*
quantitative research, 98–101
ratio, 116, 117, 118*t*
RCTs, 163
temperature, 117
measures of central tendency, 120–124
defined, 120
mean, 122–124
median, 122, 123*t*
mode, 121–122, 121*t*
measures of variability, 124–126
comparisons, 126
defined, 124
percentile, 125
range, 124, 124*t*
semiquartile range, 124–125, 125*f*
standard deviation, 125–126, 126*t*
median, 122
of age data for 20 participants, 123*t*
position of, 122
median test, 142
MEDLINE/PubMed, 37, 38
background, 39, 40
MeSH Headings, 39, 40–41, 41*f*
tips for search using keywords, 41–43
using, 39–43, 41*f*
volume of data, 39–40
member checking, 272–273
memo
defined, 268
example, 270*f*
sample, 269*f*
memoing, 268–270, 269*f*
Mendeley, 392
MeSH Headings (Medical Subject Headings), 39, 40
using, 40–41, 41*f*
meta-analysis, 34, 320, 326–332
and effect size, 326–330
and forest plot, 330–332, 332*f*, 333*f*
heterogeneity in, 330
methodological designs, 178
Methods section, research article
qualitative research (*See* data analysis; data collection)
quantitative research, 104–105
evaluating, 224–228, 226*t*
statistical tests, use of, 399*t*
writing of, 396–398, 397*f*, 399*t*
minimal risk, defined, 68
mixed methods study, 12, 250
mixed methods systematic review, 320
modality, 121
mode, 121–122, 121*t*
of age data for 20 participants, 121*t*
models. *See also specific entries*
defined, 81, 272
quantitative research, 81, 82*f*
Results section, qualitative research, 275–277, 276*f*, 277*f*
transtheoretical, 81, 82*f*
moderator, 248

multi-method research, 12
multicollinarity, 200
multimethod qualitative study, 250
multiple linear regression, 198
multiple linear regression models, 200–202, 202*t*
multiple regression analysis, 143–144
multiple time series design, 170
multisite studies, 88
multistage (multilevel) cluster sampling, 94, 95*t*
multistage sampling, 93–94, 95*t*
multivariate analysis, 116
multivariate analysis of variance (MANOVA), 141, 191

N

narrative reviews, 9, 34, 220, 320–321
National Agriculture Library (NAL), 43
National Center for Biotechnology, 40
National Collaborative on Childhood Obesity Research, 177*t*
National Commission for the Protection of Human Subjects of Biomedical and Behavioral Research, 55
National Guidelines Clearinghouse (NGC), 344
National Health and Nutrition Examination Survey (NHANES), 98, 171, 177, 352
National Institute for Food and Agriculture (NIFA), 421
National Institute of Health (NIH), 18, 39, 56, 58, 419–421
  data sources for secondary data analysis, 177*t*
National Library of Medicine (NLM) database, 39, 40
National Nutrition Monitoring and Related Research Program (NNMRRP), 352
National Research Act (1974), 55
National Science Foundations (NSF), 56, 58, 422
Nation's Restaurant News, 32*t*
negatively skewed distribution, 127–128, 127*f*
network (snowball) sampling, 96, 96*t*, 255, 360, 361, 362*t*
New York Times (newspaper), 32*t*
newspapers, 32
  examples, 32*t*
  vs. magazine, trade publications and journals, 32*t*
NHANES. *See* National Health and Nutrition Examination Survey (NHANES)
NIH. *See* National Institute of Health (NIH)
NIH RePorter, 419
nominal measurement, 116, 117, 118*t*
nondirectional hypothesis, 83
nonequivalent control group designs, 168–169, 168*t*
nonexperimental study, 220–221
nonparametric tests, 137, 138*t*
nonprobability sampling, 94–97, 360–362
  convenience sampling, 360
  with examples, 362*t*
  network/snowball sampling, 360, 361
  purposive/judgment sampling, 360
  quota sampling, 360
nonresponse bias, 91, 97, 357
nonsampling errors, 378
normal distributions, 127, 127*f*
  percentile rank based on, 129, 130*f*
  with standard deviations, 129, 129*f*
null hypothesis, 84
Nuremberg Code (1949), 55
Nurses' Health Study, 356
Nutrition Action Healthletter (magazine), 32, 32*t*
nutrition epidemiology, 186. *See also* epidemiology
Nutrition Evidence Library (NEL), 342–343, 342*t*, 343*f*
nutrition-related journals, 35, 36*t*
nutrition research
  ethics in, 53–71 (*See also* ethics)
  overview, 3–4
  purposes of, 7–9, 8*t*
  types of studies, 15–21

O

objective(s), 5, 102–103, 222, 224, 245
  examples, 103*t*
  in grant proposals, 427–428, 428*t*
observations
  for data collection, 257, 261
  data collection tool, 258–259*f*
  qualitative research, 249–250
Observed score, 87*f*
observer's comments, 261
odds ratio, 146–147, 193, 203, 329
  in case-control design, 193–196
  in logistic regression, 203–207
Office of Research Integrity (ORI), 56–57
Omni Cohort, 189
one-way ANOVA, 140
Online Survey Design Guide, 369
open-access journals, 35–36
open coding, 287
open-ended questions, 244–245, 353, 365
operational definition, 78
opinion pieces, 37
OR. *See* odds ratio (OR)
oral surveys, 353, 354*t*
ordinal measurement, 116, 117, 118*t*

ORI. *See* Office of Research Integrity (ORI)
ORI Introduction to the Responsible Conduct of Research, 57
original research article, 9, 32–33, 34, 220
outcome evaluation, 429
outcome measure, 5, 16
outcome measurements, RCTs, 163
outcome variable, 174, 227
outcomes
  categories, 16
  defined, 7, 16
  exposures, and confounder, relationship between, 200, 200*f*
outcomes research, 16–17, 17*t*
  defined, 16, 20*t*
  examples, 20*t*
  researcher interview, 107–108
overhead costs, 430

P

P-value (probability value), 84, 172
panel survey, 356
paper surveys, 353, 354*t*
parallel forms reliability, 373, 373*f*, 374*t*
parametric tests, 136, 138*t*
pass-through grant, 418
patient outcomes, 16
PBRNs. *See* practice-based research networks (PBRNs)
Pearson's *r* statistic (Pearson product–moment correlation), 142–143
peer review, 33, 421
  frequent, 273
percentage distributions, 119–120, 119*t*
  standard deviation and, 129*f*
percentile, 125
performance bias, 326
personal conflicts, 59
phenomenology, 286, 288–289, 302
  strengths and limitations, 289
phenomenon, 286
PHI (protected health information), 65
PICOS, using, 38*t*, 388
Pie chart, 403, 405*f*
pilot testing, 257, 370
piloting, 257
placebo, 160
plagiarism, 60
population
  accessible, 92, 93*f*
  target, 92, 93*f*
  sample, 92, 93*f*
population parameters, 116
position of the median, 122
positive mealtime environment (PME), 290
positively skewed distribution, 128, 128*f*
positivist paradigm, 10
poster, 408
  effective, 409
  layout for evidence-based practice poster, 410*f*
  making of, 409–410
  presenting of, 410
  quality, creation of, 411*t*
power, 363
  defined, 89, 97
power analysis, 97, 363–364
practice, theory, and research, relationships among, 82–83, 82*f*
practice-based research networks (PBRNs), 21
precaution adoption process model, 81*t*
precision, 90
predictive correlational designs, 104
  epidemiological research, 197–211
predictive validity, 100, 375
predictor variable, 174
prepositions, 42
presentations, 408–409, 408*f*
Press Ganey, 352
pretest-posttest design, RCTs, 162, 162*t*
pretesting questionnaire, 370–371, 371*t*
prevalence, defined, 186
prevalence ratio, 187
primary documents, 250
primary research, 9
primary research articles, 33
principal investigator (PI), 67, 429
PRISMA group, 233, 324
  PRISMA 2009 checklist, 461
  PRISMA 2009 flow diagram, 322, 324, 324*f*
privacy, 65–66, 65–66*t*
Privacy Rule *(Standards for Privacy of Individually Identifiable Health Information),* 65–66
Privacy Rule Authorization, 65
probability, 131
probability-based statistics, 358
probability sampling, 93–94, 359–360
  cluster random sampling, 93, 94*f*
  examples, 95*t*
  with examples, 361*t*
  simple random sampling, 93, 359
  stratified random sampling, 93, 94*f*, 359
  systematic random sampling, 93, 359
probability value (*P*-value), 84, 172

problem statement, 4, 102, 222
 examples, 103*t*
 qualitative research, 245–246
process evaluation, 429
project budget, 430–431, 430*t*
proposal, 427
prospective, 6
prospective cohort studies, 8–9, 188–192, 188*f*
 example, 9, 191–192
prospective study, 105, 225
protected health information (PHI), 65
protocol, 67
PsycINFO, 44
Public Health Service, 55
publication bias, 91, 321
publications, 32, 32*t*, 408
PubMed. *See* MEDLINE/PubMed
purposive/judgment sampling, 95, 96*t*
purposive sampling, 360, 362*t*

Q

QCC. *See* Quality Criteria Checklist (QCC)
qualitative research, 10–13, 220, 244–278. *See also* quantitative research
 coding process, 262–268, 263–264*f*
 data analysis, 262–273
 data collection, 260–262
 data collection methods, 248–251
 data collection tools, 255–257
 data organization, 262
 defined, 10
 discussion and conclusions, 278
 evaluation, 301–313
  conclusions, 312–313
  data analysis, 310
  data collection, 309–310
  design, 308
  discussion, 311–312
  literature review, 306–307, 306*f*
  overview, 301–302
  results, 311
  review criteria, 302
  statement of problem, 302–305, 305*t*
  subject selection, 309
  trustworthiness, 313
 inductive, 244
 join with quantitative research, 12–13
 literature review, 246–247
 memoing, 268–270, 269*f*
 methods, 247–262
 overview, 244–245
 piloting, 257
 problem statement, 245–246
 researcher (training), 257, 260
 researcher interview, 294–296
 results, 273–277
 subjects and sampling, 251, 253–255
 theming, 270–271
 theory development, 271–272
 trustworthiness, 272–273
 vs. quantitative research, 10, 11–12*t*
qualitative research designs, 285–296
 case studies, 286, 292–293
 characteristics, summary, 293, 294*f*
 evaluating, 308
 grounded theory, 286, 289–292
 phenomenology, 286, 288–289
 thematic analysis, 285, 286–288
qualitative reviewer guidelines, *Journal of Nutrition Education and Behavior,* 303*f*
qualitative software, 262
Quality Criteria Checklist (QCC), 232–233, 334, 335–336*t*
quality improvement (QI)
 defined, 14
 steps in, 14*f*
Quality Rating Summary, 334
quantitative research, 5, 10–13, 78–108, 220. *See also* qualitative research
 bias, 90–92, 91*t*
 categories, 104–105
 concepts, 78–80
 constructs, 78–80
 defined, 10
 error, 90–92
 evaluation, 219–235
  additional tools, 232–233
  discussion and conclusion, 230–232, 231*t*
  introduction of article, 222–224, 222*t*
  methods, 224–228, 226*t*
  overview, 219–220
  research title and authors, 220–221, 221*t*
  results, 228–230, 229*t*
 foundations, 78–86
 framework, 82
 hypothesis, 83–85
 instruments, 98–101
 join with qualitative research, 12–13
 levels of measurement, 81*t*
 measurement, 98–101

models, 81, 82*f*
overview, 78
reliability, 86, 87*f*
research article, 101–107
sampling, 92–98
statistical significance and effect size, 86
theories, 80, 81*t*
theory, research, and practice, relationships among, 82–83, 82*f*
validity, 86–90
variables, 78–80, 79*f*, 80*t*
vs. qualitative research, 10, 11–12*t*

quantitative research designs
additional types, 177–178
descriptive, 171–176 (*See also* descriptive quantitative designs)
experimental, 157–168 (*See also* experimental designs)
features, 156–157
methodological designs, 178
quasi-experimental, 168–171 (*See also* quasi-experimental designs)
secondary data analysis, 177–178, 177*t*
secondary research, 178

quasi-experimental designs, 104, 157, 168–171, 220
interrupted time series designs, 169–171, 169*t*, 170*f*, 170*t*
nonequivalent control group designs, 168–169, 168*t*

questionnaire, 352. *See also* questions
laying out, 369
pretesting of, 370–371

questions, 365
closed-ended, 353, 365
open-ended, 353, 365–366
sequence of, 369
writing of, considerations in, 366

quota sampling, 95, 96*t*, 360, 362*t*

R

R-squared, 199

random error, 90
example of, 91

random sampling, 80*t*, 93, 95*t*

random sequence generation, 325

randomization, 80*t*, 88
experimental designs, 157, 159
RCTs, 163 (*See also* randomized controlled trials (RCTs))
simple, 159, 159*f*

randomized block design, 159, 159*f*

randomized controlled trials (RCTs), 6, 160–165, 220, 225. *See also* controlled clinical trials (CCT)
attrition, 161
blinding, 161, 163
defined, 15, 160
efficacy demonstration in, 15–16
in experimental designs, 160–165
intervention, 163
measurements, 163
outcome measurements, 163
participants, 163
pretest-posttest design, 162, 162*t*
randomization, 163
results, 163–165, 164*t*
statistical analysis, 163

range, 124, 124*t*

rank order scale, 367*t*

ratio measurement, 116, 117, 118*t*

RCR. *See* Responsible Conduct of Research (RCR)

RCTs. *See* randomized controlled trials (RCTs)

recall bias, 99

referred journal, 33

Registered Dietitian Nutritionists (RDNs), 7, 423
evidence-based practice, 31–32
translational research for, 18–19, 19*t*

regression, 104–105

regression analysis, 186, 197–200
using least squares method, 198–199, 199*f*

regression coefficient, 144, 199

regression models, 198
linear regression, 198–202
logistic regression, 198, 202–207

regression to the mean, 88, 169

relative risk (RR), 145–146, 189, 328

reliability, 272, 372–373, 374*t*
defined, 86
equivalence, 373, 374*t*
instruments, 99–100
internal consistency, 373, 374*t*
of measures, 89
quantitative research, 86
test-retest, 372–373, 372*f*, 374*t*
of treatment implementation, 89

repeated cross-sectional study, 171–172, 173*t*

repeated cross-sectional survey, 355

repeated measures, 165
ANOVA, 191

reporting bias, 326

research. *See also* nutrition research
analytic, 8

research (*cont.*)
- applied, 13–14
- basic, 13–14
- classifying, 9–14
- criteria for IRB approval, 68–69, 69*t*
- defined, 4–7, 14
- descriptive, 8
- ethics standards/norms, 54 (*See also* ethics)
- examples, 8*t*
- facts about, 4
- human subjects (*See* human subjects research)
- hypothesis, 5–6
- literature review, 5
- methods, 6
- mixed methods, 12
- objective (*See* objective)
- primary, 9
- purposes, 7–9, 8*t*
- qualitative, 10–13, 11–12*t* (*See also* qualitative research)
- quantitative, 10–13, 11–12*t* (*See also* quantitative research)
- research question, 4
- scientific method, 4–7, 5*f*
- secondary, 9
- statement of the problem, 4
- tertiary, 9
- theory, practice and, relationships among, 82–83, 82*f*
- variables, 5–6

research article(s). *See also* scientific writing; *scientific writing*
- abstract, 102
- checklist for selection, 44–45
- commentary articles, 34
- Conclusion section, 105–106, 107*t*, 230–232, 231*t*
- databases, using, 37–44 (*See also* databases)
- Discussion section, 105–106, 230–232, 231*t*
- format, 101–102, 101*t*, 102*f*
- Introduction section, 102–103, 222–224, 222*t*
- literature review, 102
- Methods section, 104–105, 224–228, 226*t*
- original, 32–33, 34, 220
- publications, 32
- Results section, 105–106, 228–230, 229*t*
- types of, 33–35

"Research Brief," 33

research design, 6, 156, 225. *See also specific designs*

research editorial, 34

research framework, 82

Research Grants (R Series), NIH, 419, 420*t*

research hypothesis, 83

research methods, 6

research misconduct, 60

research objective. *See* objective

research paper, 4

research problem, 102, 224, 244
- problem statement, 103*t*

research proposal and paper, writing of, 387–407
- conclusion, 406
- Discussion section, 404–406
- Introduction, 395–396
- Literature Review, 391–395
- Methods section, 396–398
- Results section, 402–404, 403*t*
- style manual to format paper, use of, 398, 400
  - AMA style, 400–401, 402*t*
  - APA style, 401, 402*t*
- table of contents for thesis, 389*t*
- title and abstract, 406–407, 407*f*
- topic identification and research question, 388–390, 389*t*

research question, 4, 156

research title, 220–221, 221*t*

researcher, qualitative (training), 257, 260

researcher bias, 256. *See also* bias(es)

researcher interview
- bioactive compounds in fruits and vegetables, 46–47
- epidemiology, 211–212
- food science/sensory evaluation, 233–235
- intervention research, 178–179
- management research, 70–71
- outcomes research, 107–108
- qualitative research, 294–296
- translational research, 22–24

respect for persons, 55

respect for subjects, in human research, 61, 62*t*

response bias, 99
- examples, 99

response errors, 378

response formats, 366–369
- for close-ended questions, 367*t*–368*t*
- scales in, use of, 366

response rate, 378

Responsible Conduct of Research (RCR), 56–60
- conflict of interest, 57–59
- research misconduct, 60

Results section, research article
- qualitative research
  - evaluating, 311
  - themes, 273–275, 274*f*
  - theories and models, 275–277, 276*f*, 277*f*
- quantitative research, 105–106
  - evaluating, 228–230, 229*t*

retrospective, 6
retrospective cohort studies, 188, 188*f*
retrospective study, 105
retrospective survey, 355, 356*t*
review(s)
  evidence analysis library, 34
  exempt, 68
  expedited, 68
  full board, 68
  levels, conducted by IRB, 67–68
  narrative, 34, 220
  systematic, 34, 220
rigor, 10, 92
Risica, Patricia Markham, 211–212
risk-benefit ratio, favorable, 61, 62*t*
risk ratio (relative risk), 145–146, 189–190, 328
risks-benefits, 67
RR (relative risk), 145–146
Rule of 68–95–99.7, 128–130, 129–130*f*

S

sample bias, 97
sample size, 97–98
  in qualitative research, 254
  in surveys, 363–364
sample statistics, 116
sample variance. *See* sampling error
sample(s), 225, 358, 358*f*
  bias, 357–358
  defined, 92, 93*f*
  described, using frequencies, 118–120, 118*t*, 119*t*
  picking of, 357, 362
    nonprobability sampling methods, 360–361, 362*t*
    random probability methods for, 359–360, 361*t*
  size, 97–98, 363–364
    calculators, 364
    and power analysis, 363–364
sampling
  key concepts, 92
  multistage, 93–94, 95*t*
  nonprobability, 94–97, 96*t*
  probability, 93–94, 95*t*
  qualitative research, 251, 253–255
  quantitative research, 92–98
  random, 93, 95*t*
  sample size, 97–98, 363–364
  techniques and strategies, 254–255
  theoretical, 290
  variance(error), 96–97
sampling distribution, 137
sampling error, 131–132, 357
sampling frame, 358, 358*f*
  defined, 92
sampling variance (error), 96–97
scales, 366
scatterplot, 174, 174*f*
  correlations (positive and negative), 175–176, 175*f*
scholarly journals, 32, 32*t*. *See also* journals
Science Direct, 37, 38
scientific journals. *See* journals
scientific literature, not found in journals, 36–37
scientific method, 4–7, 5*f*
  example, 4–7, 5*f*
scientific validity, human subjects research and, 60–61, 62*t*
scientific writing. *See also* research article(s)
  principles, 45–46
Scopus, 37, 38
secondary data analysis, 6, 177–178, 177*t*
  data sources for, 177*t*
secondary documents, 250
secondary research, 9, 178, 220, 320
selection bias, 97, 325–326, 357
self-care, 87
semantic differential scale, 367*t*
seminal articles, 247
semiquartile range, 124–125, 125*f*
semistructured interviews, 256
sensitivity, instrument, 100–101
Shanklin, Carol W., 70–71
Shape (magazine), 32, 32*t*
sign test, 142
signed rank test, 142
significance
  defined, 84
  level of, 134–136, 135*f*
  tests of, 132
significant financial interest, 58, 58*f*
simple hypothesis, 83
simple interrupted time series design, 169–171, 169*t*, 170*t*
simple linear regression, 198
simple logistic regression, 203
simple random sampling, 93, 95*t*, 359, 361*t*
simple randomization, 159, 159*f*
single-blind study, 161
skewed (asymmetric) distributions, 127–128, 127–128*f*
  negatively skewed, 127–128, 127*f*
  positively skewed, 128, 128*f*
SMD. *See* standardized mean difference (SMD)
snowball (network) sampling, 96, 96*t*, 255

social cognitive theory (as example), 80
social desirability bias, 99
social value, human subjects research and, 60, 62*t*
software, qualitative, 262
Solomon four-group design, 167–168, 167*t*
source population, 358, 358*f*
  defined, 92, 93*f*
specificity, instrument, 101
stability reliability, 99. *See* also test-retest reliability
Stage, Virginia C., 294–296
stages of change model (transtheoretical model), 81, 81*t*, 82*f*
standard deviation(s), 125–126, 126*t*
  of age data, 130*f*
  normal distributions with, 129, 129*f*
  and percentage distribution, 129*f*
standard intervention (SI), 223
Standard Intervention group, 227
standardized mean difference (SMD), 145, 328
Standards for Privacy of Individually Identifiable Health Information (Privacy Rule), 65–66
Standards of Professional Performance, Academy of Nutrition and Dietetics, 31–32
statement of the problem, 4, 102, 222
  evaluation, qualitative research, 302–305, 305*t*
statistical analysis, RCTs, 163
statistical conclusion validity, 87, 89, 89*t*
  defined, 90
  threats to, 89, 89*t*
statistical hypothesis, 84
statistical significance, 84–86, 145
statistical tables, tips for reading, 148*t*
statistical tests/testing
  analysis of variance (ANOVA), 139–141, 141*t*
  Chi-Square tests, 139–139, 140*t*, 141*t*
  for differences between groups, 137–142
  inferential statistics, 136–144
  nonparametric, 137, 138*t*
  other tests of significance, 144
  parametric, 136, 138*t*
  for relationships among variables, 142–144
  t-tests, 139, 140*t*, 141*t*
  violation of assumptions of, 89, 227
statistically nonsignificant values, 132
statistically significant values, 132
statistics
  background, 116
  defined, 116
  descriptive, 116, 130 (*See also* descriptive statistics)
  inferential, 116, 130–132 (*See also* inferential statistics)
  risk, 145–147
  symbols, 117*t*, 136*t*
  that look at associations, 158*t*
  that look at differences, 158*t*
stratified random sampling, 93, 94*f*, 95*t*, 359, 360*f*, 361*t*
STROBE Statement, 233, 457
structured interviews, 255
study objective. *See* objective
study protocol, 160
study variables, 5. *See also* variables
subject headings, databases searching using, 38–39
  advantages and disadvantages, 39*t*
subjects, qualitative research, 251, 253–255
  selection, evaluating, 308
survey, 351–381. *See also* sample(s)
  in agricultural research, 352–353
  in clinical nutrition research, 352
  closed-ended questions in, 353
  cross-sectional, 355, 356*t*
  data collection and analysis, 377–381
  definition of, 352
  electronic, 353, 354*t*
  face-to-face, 355*t*
  longitudinal, 355–356, 356*t*
  methods, 353
    advantages and disadvantages of, 354–355*t*
    selection of, factors in, 355
  in nutrition epidemiology research, 352
  in nutrition program evaluation, 352
  in nutrition research, 352
  open-ended questions in, 353
  oral, 353, 354*t*
  paper, 353, 354*t*
  pretesting, 370–371
  questionnaire in, use of, 352 (*See also* Questionnaire)
  reliability of, 372–373, 374*t*
  retrospective, 355, 356*t*
  steps in process, 357, 357*t*
  types of, on frequency of administration, 355–356, 356*t*
  usefulness of, 353
  validity of, 373–377, 375*t*
SurveyMonkey, 352
survival analysis, 207–211
survival time, 207
symbols, statistical
  for descriptive statistics, 117*t*
  for inferential statistics, 136*t*
systematic error. *See* bias(es)
systematic random sampling, 93, 95*t*, 359, 361*t*
systematic review, 9, 34, 220, 319–332
  assessing quality of, guidelines for, 325*t*

definition of, 320
for Evidence Analysis Library, 332–338
interpreting forest plots, 330–332
meta-analysis, 323–332
mixed methods, 320
and narrative review, 320–321
PRISMA 2009 flow diagram, 322, 324, 324*f*
steps in, 321–324, 322*t*–323*t*

T

T1, 19–20, 19*t*, 20*t*
T2, 19, 19*t*, 20, 20*t*
T3, 19, 19*t*
t-statistic, 139, 140*t*, 141*t*
tables, use of, 403
tailedness, distribution patterns, 128–130, 129–130*f*
target population, 358
defined, 92, 93*f*
technical reports, 37
telephone survey, 354*t*
temperature measurement, 117
tertiary research, 9, 320
test-retest reliability, 99, 372–373, 374*t*
thematic analysis, 285, 286–288, 302
strengths and limitations, 287–288
theme(s), 270–271
Results section, qualitative research, 273–275, 274*f*
"Too Big" (example), 274–275, 274*f*
theming, in qualitative research, 270–271
theoretical definition, 78
theoretical sampling, 290
theory of planned behavior, 81*t*
theory(ies)
defined, 80
development, in qualitative research, 271–272, 290
examples, 81*t*
quantitative research, 80, 81*t*
research, practice and, relationships among, 82–83, 82*f*
Results section, qualitative research, 275–277, 276*f*, 277*f*
theses, 36
time-to-event, 207–211
Today's Dietitian, 32
"Too Big," theme, 274–275, 274*f*
tools. *See also* data collection tools
defined, 255
trade magazines, 32
trade publications
examples, 32*t*
vs. magazine, newspapers and journals, 32*t*
traditional ordinal rating scale, 367*t*
training, qualitative researcher, 257, 260
transcript, 261
transcription, 262
translational research, 18–20, 19*t*
defined, 18, 20*t*
examples, 20*t*
phases, 19*t*
for RDNs, 18–19, 19*t*
researcher interview, 22–24
transtheoretical model (stages of change model), 81, 81*t*, 82*f*
treatment fidelity, 80*t*
triangulated design, 12
triangulation, 273
True Score, 87*f*
truncation, 41–42
trustworthiness. *See also* reliability; validity
in qualitative research, 272–273
evaluating, 313
Tuskegee study, 55
two-way ANOVA, 140
type I error (α error), 85, 85*t*, 97, 133–134, 134*t*
level of significance, 134–136, 135*f*
type II error (β error), 85, 85*t*, 97, 133–134, 134*t*
level of significance, 134–136, 135*f*

U

ungrouped format, 118–119
categorical data in, 118*t*
unimodal data, 121
univariate analysis, 116
unstructured interviews, 255
U.S. Department of Agriculture (USDA), 43, 56, 353
data sources for secondary data analysis, 177*t*

V

validity, 86–90, 272, 374–377, 375*t*
construct, 87, 90, 377
content, 375
criterion, 375, 377
defined, 86
definitions, 90
external, 87, 88–89
face, 374
instruments, 100
internal, 87, 88
quantitative research, 86–90
statistical conclusion, 87, 89, 89*t*
types of, 87

variability, measures of. *See* measures of variability
variables, 5
  associative relationship, 79, 79*f*
  categorical, 5, 80
  confounding, 79
  continuous, 5, 80
  defined, 156
  dependent, 5–6, 78–79, 198*t*, 221
  dichotomous, 78, 117
  extraneous, 6, 79, 80*t*, 156
  independent, 5, 6, 78–79, 198*t*, 221
  outcome, 174
  predictor, 174
  quantitative research, 78–80, 79*f*, 80*t*
  testing for relationships among, 142–144
variance, sampling, 96–97
vegetables, bioactive compounds in (researcher interview), 46–47
verbal frequency scale, 367*t*
verbatim (word-for-word) transcripts, 262
visual analog scales (VAS), 368*t*
visual model of coding process, qualitative research, 263, 263*f*
vulnerable populations, 63*t*

W

Washington Post (newspaper), 32*t*
washout period, 165
Web of Knowledge, 40
Web of Science, 35, 37, 38
weight management program (12-month period)
  outcomes research, 17*t*
Wilcoxin matched pairs test, 142
within-groups design, 165
World Medical Association, 55
World War II, 54, 55
writing research proposal/paper, 387–407

Z

Zotero, 392